Practical Haematology

For Churchill Livingstone

Commissioning Editor: Lowri Daniels
Project Editor: Dilys Jones
Copy Editor: Julie Gorman
Design Direction: Erik Bigland
Production: Kay Hunston
Sales Promotion Executive: Douglas McNaughton

Practical Haematology

Sir John V. Dacie MD (Lond) FRCPath FRS
Emeritus Professor of Haematology, University of London,
Royal Postgraduate Medical School, London

S. M. Lewis BSc MD (Cape Town) DCP (Lond) FRCPath
Emeritus Reader in Haematology, University of London;
Senior Research Fellow, Royal Postgraduate Medical School;
Consultant Haematologist, Hammersmith Hospital, London

EIGHTH EDITION

CHURCHILL LIVINGSTONE
EDINBURGH   HONG KONG   LONDON   MADRID   MELBOURNE   NEW YORK   AND
TOKYO 1995

CHURCHILL LIVINGSTONE
Medical Division of Longman Group Limited

Distributed in the United States of America by Churchill
Livingstone Inc., 650 Avenue of the Americas, New York,
N.Y. 10011, and by associated companies, branches and
representatives throughout the world.

First edition 1950
Second edition 1956
Third edition 1963
Fourth edition 1968
Fifth edition 1975
Sixth edition 1984
Seventh edition 1991
Eighth edition 1995

ISBN 0 443 04931 9

British Library Cataloguing in Publication Data
A catalogue record for this book is available from the British
Library.

Library of Congress Cataloging in Publication Data
A catalog record for this book is available from the Library of
Congress.

The
publisher's
policy is to use
**paper manufactured
from sustainable forests**

Printed in Hong Kong
NPC/01

Contents

Contributors   vii
Preface   ix
Units of measurement   x

1. Collection and handling of blood   1

2. Reference ranges and normal values   9

3. Laboratory organization and
   management   21
   (Written in collaboration with J. Stuart)

4. Quality assurance   35

5. Basic haematological techniques   49
   (Revised by B. Bain)

6. Preparation and staining methods for blood
   and bone-marrow films   83

7. Blood-cell morphology in health and
   disease   97
   (Written in collaboration with D. M. Swirsky)

8. Red cell cytochemistry   131

9. Leucocyte cytochemical and immunological
   techniques   143
   (By D. Catovsky)

10. Bone-marrow biopsy   175

11. Diagnosis of blood cell disorders   191
    (Revised by J. Parker-Williams)

12. Laboratory methods used in the investigation
    of the haemolytic anaemias   197

13. Investigation of the hereditary haemolytic
    anaemias: membrane and enzyme
    abnormalities   215
    (Revised by L. Luzzatto and D. Roper)

14. Investigation of abnormal haemoglobins and
    thalassaemia   249
    (Revised by Milica Brozović and Joan Henthorn)

15. Laboratory methods used in the investigation
    of paroxysmal nocturnal haemoglobinuria
    (PNH)   287
    (Revised by L. Luzzatto and P. Hillmen)

16. Investigation of haemostasis   297
    (Revised by M. A. Laffan and A. Bradshaw)

17. Investigation of a bleeding tendency   317
    (Revised by M. A. Laffan and A. Bradshaw)

18. Investigation of a thrombotic tendency   351
    (Revised by M. A. Laffan and A. Bradshaw)

19. Laboratory control of anticoagulant,
    thrombolytic and anti-platelet therapy   367
    (Revised by M. A. Laffan and A. Bradshaw)

20. Use of radionuclides in haematology   381
    (Revised by M. J. Myers)

21. Blood volume, erythrokinetics and platelet
    kinetics   391

22. Investigation of megaloblastic anaemia   417
    (By B.F.A. Jackson and A.V. Hoffbrand)

23. Iron deficiency anaemia   437
    (By M. Worwood)

24. Red cell blood-group antigens and antibodies
    445
    (Revised by A. H. Waters)

25. Platelet and neutrophil antigens and
    antibodies   465
    (By A. H. Waters)

26. Laboratory aspects of blood transfusion   479
   (Revised by A. H. Waters)

27. Serological investigation of the auto-immune
   and drug-induced immune haemolytic
   anaemias   499
   (Revised by A. H. Waters)

28. DNA techniques in haematology   529
   (By T. Vulliamy and J. Kaeda)

29. Miscellaneous tests   559

30. Appendices   575

Index   593

Contributors

Barbara J. Bain MB BS MRCPath FRACP
Senior Lecturer in Haematology, St Mary's
Hospital Medical School, Imperial College of
Science, Technology and Medicine, London, UK

A. E. Bradshaw BSc FIBMS DMLM
Principal Biomedical Scientist, Department of
Haematology, Royal Postgraduate Medical
School, London, UK

Milica Brozović MD FRCPath
Retired Consultant Haematologist, Central
Middlesex Hospital, London, UK

D. Catovsky DSc (Med) FRCP FRCPath
Professor and Head, Academic Department of
Haematology, Royal Marsden Hospital and
Institute of Cancer Research, London, UK

Sir John V. Dacie MD FRCP FRCPath FRS
Emeritus Professor of Haematology, University
of London, Royal Postgraduate Medical School,
London, UK

J. S. Henthorn FIBMS
Head of Laboratory, Department of Haematology,
Central Middlesex Hospital, London, UK

Dr P. Hillmen MB ChB MRCP
Research Fellow, Department of Haematology,
Royal Postgraduate Medical School; Honorary
Senior Registrar, Hammersmith Hospital,
London, UK

A. Victor Hoffbrand MA DM FRCP FRCPath
FRCP (Edin) DSc
Professor of Haematology, Royal Free Hospital
School of Medicine, London, UK

B. F. A. Jackson FAIMS
Chief Medical Laboratory Scientific Officer,

Department of Haematology, Royal Free
Hospital, London, UK

Jaspal Singh Kaeda FIBMS MIBiol
Senior Medical Laboratory Scientific Officer,
Department of Haematology, Royal Postgraduate
Medical School, London, UK

M. A. Laffan DM MRCP MRCPath
Senior Lecturer, Department of Haematology,
Royal Postgraduate Medical School,
Hammersmith Hospital, London, UK

S. M. Lewis BSc MD (Cape Town) DCP (Lond)
FRCPath
Emeritus Reader in Haematology, University of
London; Senior Research Fellow, Royal
Postgraduate Medical School; Consultant
Haematologist, Hammersmith Hospital, London,
UK

L. Luzzatto MD FRCP FRCPath
Professor of Haematology, Royal Postgraduate
Medical School; Consultant Haematologist,
Hammersmith Hospital, London, UK

M. J. Myers PhD FInstPSM
Principal Physicist, Department of Medical
Physics, Hammersmith Hospital, London, UK

E. J. Parker-Williams MB BS FRCPath
Senior Lecturer and Honorary Consultant
Haematologist, St George's Hospital and
Medical School, London, UK

D. R. Roper MSc FIBMS
Chief Biomedical Scientist, Department of
Haematology, Royal Postgraduate Medical
School, Hammersmith Hospital, London, UK

John Stuart MD FRCP (Edin) FRCPath
Professor of Haematology, The Medical School,
University of Birmingham, Birmingham, UK

David M. Swirsky FRCP MRCPath
Senior Lecturer in Haematology, Royal
Postgraduate Medical School; Honorary
Consultant, Hammersmith Hospital, London,
UK

Tom Vulliamy PhD
Clinical Scientist, Department of Haematology,
Royal Postgraduate Medical School,
Hammersmith Hospital, London, UK

A. H. Waters PhD FRCPath FRCP
Professor of Haematology, St Bartholomew's
Hospital Medical College; Honorary Consultant
Haematologist, The Royal Hospitals NHS Trust,
London, UK

Mark Worwood BSc PhD FRCPath
Reader in Haematology, University of Wales
College of Medicine, Cardiff, UK

Preface

With the continuing expansion of the practice of haematology, the biggest challenge in the preparation of a new edition of *Practical Haematology* has been to provide a volume which is up to date and which reflects the advancing technology of the 1990s without excessively increasing its size. This has meant that some obsolescent techniques have perforce been omitted or set in small print.

While automated procedures are by now widely employed, we recognize that basic manual methods continue to be used in many laboratories. Past editions of this book have been found to be useful at all levels of laboratory practice — from primary health centres, where only a few diagnostic tests can be carried out, to reference centres which use sophisticated technology. We hope that this will be true also of this new edition. Every chapter and topic has been closely scrutinized and revised where necessary and amongst new material added has been a chapter on DNA technology as applied to haematological problems, including the antenatal diagnosis of blood disorders. Particular attention has been paid to laboratory management and organization. Additional colour slides have been included where these illustrate specific features of blood cells better than black-and-white photographs could.

Throughout the book, we stress the value of standards and reference reagents and quality control applied to all tests, and the tests which we describe conform to the recommendations of the International Council for Standardization in Haematology where these are available.

London, 1995

J.V.D.
S.M.L.

Units of measurement

In keeping with recommendations of the World Health Organization, the International Council for Standardization in Haematology and other international authorities we have used the Système International (SI) for expressing quantities and units (p. 581). In this system the basic unit of volume is the litre; and in keeping with the recommended convention haemoglobin is expressed in g/l.

1. Collection and handling of blood

Venous blood   1
Serum   2
Anticoagulants   3
Effects of storage on morphology   4

Effects of storage on quantitative estimations   6
Peripheral blood   6
Differences between peripheral and venous blood   7

Venous blood is preferred for most haematological examinations. Peripheral samples can be almost as satisfactory for some purposes if a free flow of blood is obtained (see p. 6), but this procedure should be avoided, if possible, in any patient considered to be a possible carrier of transmissible disease.

Biohazard precautions

When collecting a blood sample the operator should, wherever possible, wear disposable plastic thin rubber gloves, especially if the patient is uncooperative or when collecting peripheral blood. The operator is also strongly advised to wear gloves if he or she has any cuts, abrasions or skin breaks on the hands. Care must be taken to prevent injuries when handling syringes and needles. After being used they should be placed, without separating the needles, in a puncture-resistant container for disposal or subsequent decontamination (see p. 31). The specimens must be sent to the laboratory in individual closed plastic bags, separated from the request forms to prevent their contamination should there be any leakage from the specimens.

VENOUS BLOOD

This is best withdrawn from an antecubital vein by means of a dry glass syringe. If available, a disposable plastic syringe should be used. The needles should not be too fine or too long; those of 19 or 20 SWG* are suitable, and short needles with shafts about 15 mm long are particularly valuable for use in children. The skin should be cleaned with 70% alcohol (e.g. isopropanol) and allowed to dry before being punctured.

When a series of samples is required or when the blood sampling is to be followed by a transfusion, it is convenient to collect the blood by means of a butterfly needle connected to a length of plastic tubing attached to the patient's arm by adhesive tape. If a large volume of blood is required, and a large syringe is not available, a needle of larger bore, e.g. 16 SWG, provided with a short length of plastic tubing should be used; with this equipment 100 ml of blood or more can be easily withdrawn.

Except in the case of very young children it should be possible with practice to obtain venous blood even from patients with difficult veins. Successful venepuncture may be facilitated by keeping the subject's arm warm, applying to the upper arm a sphygmomanometer cuff kept at approximately diastolic pressure and smacking the skin over the site of the vein. In obese patients it

---

*The nearest equivalent American gauges and diameters are as follows: 16 SWG = 14 (1.625 mm); 19 SWG = 18 (1.016 mm); 20 SWG = 19 (0.914 mm); 23 SWG = 22 (0.610 mm).

1

may be easier to use a vein on the dorsum of the hand, after warming it by immersion in warm water. When the hand is dried and the fist clenched, veins suitable for puncture will usually become apparent. If the veins are very small, a 23 SWG needle should be used and this should enable at least 2 ml of blood to be obtained satisfactorily. Vein punctures in the dorsum of the hand tend to bleed more readily than at other sites. The arm should be elevated after withdrawal of the needle and pressure should be applied for several minutes before an adhesive dressing is placed over the puncture site.

If possible, congestion should be completely avoided so as to prevent haemoconcentration. In practice, it is usually necessary to use a tourniquet. This should be loosened once the needle has been inserted into the vein. The piston of the syringe should be withdrawn slowly and no attempt made to withdraw blood faster than the vein is filling. After detaching the needle, the blood should be delivered carefully from the syringe into a container, and if it is desired to prevent coagulation it should be promptly and thoroughly but gently mixed with the anticoagulant.

Ideally, blood films should be made immediately the blood has been withdrawn. For this it is convenient to deliver a small drop of blood directly on to a glass slide but this may not be good practice when handling biohazardous specimens, unless special precautions are observed (p. 31). In practice, blood samples are often collected by the clinical staff and sent to the laboratory after a variable delay. Films should be made in the laboratory from such blood as soon as is practicable. After carefully and thoroughly mixing it, a glass capillary can be used to sample the blood and to deliver a drop of the right size on to a slide so that films can be made.

The differences between films made of fresh blood (no anticoagulant) and anticoagulated blood are dealt with on p. 4. It is convenient to use as containers for blood samples disposable glass or plastic flat-bottomed tubes fitted with caps; except for coagulation studies, the choice between glass and plastic is a matter of availability or personal preference. Because of the possibility of infection of personnel when blood has leaked from the container or when removing the cap causes an aerosol discharge of the contents, it is essential to use containers designed to minimize these risks. Design requirements for this and other specifications have been described in a number of national and international standards, e.g. that of the International Organization for Standardization (ISO 6710: 1993).

The most common disposable containers available from commercial sources contain dipotassium or tripotassium or disodium EDTA as anticoagulant and are marked at the 2.5 or 5 ml level to indicate the correct amount of blood to be added (see p. 4). Containers are also available containing trisodium citrate, heparin or acid citrate dextrose.

Haemolysis can be avoided or minimized by using clean apparatus, withdrawing the blood slowly, not using too fine a needle, delivering the blood gently into the receiver and avoiding frothing during the withdrawal of the blood and subsequent mixing with the anticoagulant.

Evacuated containers have been designed to be used in conjunction with a double-ended needle for collecting blood without the need for a syringe. The vacuum should ensure that the container will fill to within ±10% of the prescribed volume to ensure that the correct blood/anticoagulant ratio is obtained. As the containers must maintain their vacuum during storage before use, they are made of glass and have an expiry date. Design requirements have been specified by the International Organization for Standardization (ISO 6710: 1993), by the European Committee for Clinical Laboratory Standards[6] and by the US National Committee for Clinical Laboratory Standards.[14] With a special adaptor it is possible to fill several tubes in succession from one venepuncture.

SERUM

Blood collected in order to obtain serum should be delivered into sterile tubes or screw-capped bottles and allowed to clot undisturbed for 1–2 h at 37°C. When the blood has firmly clotted and the clot has started to retract, the sample may be left in a refrigerator overnight at 4°C, so that clot retraction may become complete under conditions unfavourable for the growth of bacteria. If the clot fails to retract, it may be gently detached from the wall of the container by means of a platinum wire or thin glass rod. If it is roughly treated, lysis is certain to follow. However, exactly how serum should be obtained depends also on what it is required for. For instance, if complement is to be estimated, the serum should be separated and then frozen at –20°C or below with the minimum of delay.

When serum is required urgently or when both serum and cells are required, as in the investigation of certain types of haemolytic anaemia, the sample can be defibrinated. This can be simply performed by placing the blood in a receiver such as a conical flask containing a central glass rod on to which small pieces of glass capillary have been fused (Fig. 1.1). The blood is whisked around the central rod by moderately rapid rotation of the flask. Coagulation is usually complete within 5 min, most of the fibrin collecting upon the central rod. When fibrin formation seems complete, the defibrinated blood may be centrifuged and serum obtained quickly and in relatively large volumes. Blood defibrinated in this way should not undergo any visible degree of lysis. The morphology of the red cells and the leucocytes is well preserved.

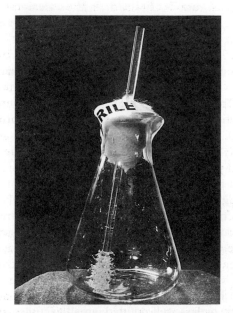

Fig. 1.1   Flask for defibrinating 10–50 ml of blood. The glass rod has had some small pieces of drawn-out glass capillary fused to its lower end.

If cold agglutinins are to be titrated, the blood must be kept at 37°C until the serum has separated, and if cold agglutinins are known to be present in high concentration it is best to bring the patient to the laboratory and to collect blood into a previously warmed syringe and then to deliver the blood into containers which have been kept warm at 37°C. When filled the containers should be promptly replaced in the 37°C water-bath. In this way it is possible to obtain serum free from haemolysis even when cold antibodies are present capable of causing agglutination at temperatures as high as 30°C. A practical way of warming the syringe is to place it in its container for 10 min in an oven at approximately 50°C or for 30 min or so in a 37°C incubator. When the clot has retracted in the sample and clear serum has been expressed, the serum is removed by a Pasteur pipette and transferred to a tube which has been warmed by being allowed to stand in a water-bath. It is then rapidly centrifuged so as to rid it of any suspended red cells.

Standardized procedure

As described below, and in Chapter 2, the method used for blood collection may affect the sample. The constituents of the blood may be altered after the blood has been collected by the anti-coagulant used and by storage of the specimen. In-vivo variation occurs in specimens collected at different times of the day ('diurnal'), after meals or exercise, whether the person is standing, sitting or lying. It is thus important to have a standard procedure for collecting and handling of blood specimens.

Recommendations for organizing a phlebotomy service and for standardizing the procedure have been published.[8,15]

ANTICOAGULANTS

For various purposes a number of different anti-coagulants are available.

Ethylenediamine tetra-acetic acid (EDTA)

The sodium and potassium salts of EDTA are powerful anticoagulants and they are especially suitable for routine haematological work. EDTA acts by its chelating effect on the calcium molecules in blood. To achieve this requires a concentration of 1.2 mg of the anhydrous salt per ml of blood (c 4 μmol). The anticoagulant recommended by the International Council for Standardization in Haematology[12]* is the dipotassium salt at a concentration of 1.50 ± 0.25 mg/ml of blood. At this concentration the tripotassium salt produces some shrinkage of red cells which results in a 2–3% decrease in packed cell volume (PCV) and followed by a gradual mean cell volume (MCV), increase on standing,[12,18] whereas there are negligible changes when the dipotassium salt is used.

Excess of EDTA, irrespective of which of its salts, affects both red cells and leucocytes, causing shrinkage and degenerative changes. EDTA in excess of 2 mg/ml of blood may result in a significant decrease in PCV by centrifugation and increase in mean cell haemoglobin concentration (MCHC).[10,16] The platelets are also affected; excess of EDTA causes them to swell and then disintegrate, causing an artificially high platelet count, as the fragments are large enough to be counted as normal platelets. Care must therefore be taken to ensure that the correct amount of blood is added, and that by repeated inversions of the container the anticoagulant is thoroughly mixed in the blood added to it. The dipotassium salt is very soluble (1650 g/l) and is to be preferred on this account to the disodium salt which is considerably less soluble (108 g/l).[11] Rapid solution of the EDTA can be ensured by coating the container with a thin film of the salt.

The dilithium salt of EDTA is equally effective as an anticoagulant,[17] and its use has the advantage that the same sample of blood can be used for chemical investigation. However, it is less soluble than the dipotassium salt (160 g/l).

EDTA is not suitable for use in the investigation of coagulation problems and should not be used in the estimation of prothrombin time.

Trisodium citrate

100–120 mmol/l   trisodium   citrate   (32 g/l

Na$_3$C$_6$H$_5$O$_7$.2H$_2$O) is the anticoagulant of choice in coagulation studies. Nine volumes of blood are added to 1 volume of the sodium citrate solution and immediately well mixed with it. Sodium citrate is also the anticoagulant most widely used in the estimation of the sedimentation rate (ESR); for this 4 volumes of venous blood are diluted with 1 volume of the sodium citrate solution.

Heparin

This may be used at a concentration of 10–20 IU per ml of blood. Heparin is an effective anticoagulant and does not alter the size of the red cells; it is a good dry anticoagulant when it is important to reduce to a minimum the chance of lysis occurring after blood has been withdrawn. However, heparinized blood should not be used for making blood films as it gives a faint blue colouration to the background when the films are stained by Romanowsky dyes. This is especially marked in the presence of abnormal proteins. Heparin is the best anticoagulant to use for osmotic fragility tests; otherwise it is inferior to EDTA for general use and should not be used for leucocyte counts as it tends to cause the leucocytes to clump.

EFFECTS OF STORAGE ON BLOOD-CELL MORPHOLOGY

If blood is allowed to stand in the laboratory before films are made, degenerative changes occur. The changes are not solely due to the presence of an anticoagulant for they also occur in defibrinated blood.

Irrespective of anticoagulant, films made from blood which has been standing for not more than 1 h at room temperature (18–25°C) are not easily distinguished from films made immediately after collection of the blood. By 3 h changes may be discernible and by 12–18 h these become striking. Some but not all neutrophils are affected; their nuclei may stain more homogeneously than in fresh blood, the nuclear lobes may become separated and the cytoplasmic margin may appear ragged or less well defined; small vacuoles appear in the cytoplasm (Fig. 1.2). Some or many of the large mononuclears develop marked changes; small

*Or International Committee for Standardization in Haematology, ICSH.

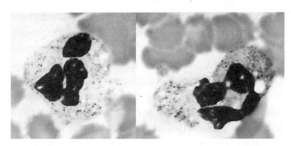

Fig. 1.2 Effect of storage on leucocyte morphology.
Photomicrographs of polymorphonuclear neutrophils in a film made from EDTA–blood after 18 h at 20°C.

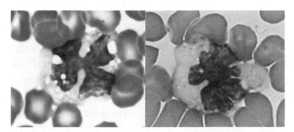

Fig. 1.3 Effect of storage on leucocyte morphology.
Photomicrographs of monocytes in a film made from EDTA–blood after 18 h at 20°C.

vacuoles appear in the cytoplasm and the nucleus undergoes irregular lobulation which may almost amount to disintegration (Fig. 1.3). Some of the lymphocytes, too, undergo a similar type of change; a few vacuoles may be seen in the cytoplasm and the nucleus may undergo major budding so as to give rise to nuclei with two or three lobes (Fig. 1.4). Other lymphocyte nuclei may stain more homogeneously than usual.

The red cells (of normal blood at least) are little affected by standing for up to 6 h at room temperature (18–25°C). Longer periods lead to progressive crenation and sphering (Fig. 1.5).

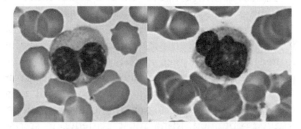

Fig. 1.4 Effect of storage on leucocyte morphology.
Photomicrographs of lymphocytes in a film made from EDTA–blood after 18 h at 20°C.

The cells in defibrinated blood undergo degenerative changes at about the same rate as those in EDTA blood, but with an excess of EDTA (p. 4) a marked degree of crenation occurs within a few hours.

All the above changes are retarded but not abolished in blood kept at 4°C. Their occurrence underlines the importance of making films as soon as possible after withdrawal. But delay of up to 1–3 h or so is certainly permissible.

The practice of making films of blood before it is added to the anticoagulant is to be commended, especially when screening for lead toxicity, as the granules of punctate basophilia may stain less obviously in anticoagulated blood. In fresh blood films, however, the platelets usually clump and it is less easy to estimate the platelet count from

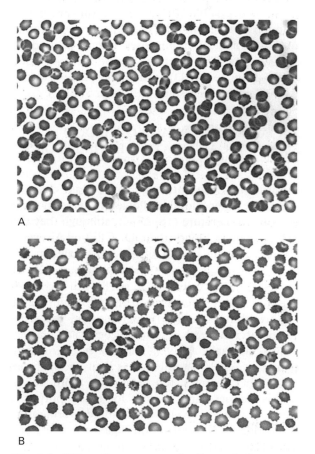

Fig. 1.5 Effect of storage on red cell morphology.
Photomicrographs of red cells in films made from blood after storage at 20°C in different concentrations of dipotassium EDTA. (A) 24 h at 1.3 mg/ml; (B) 12 h at 3.5 mg/ml.

inspection of the films. Such films are nevertheless of particular value in investigating patients suspected of suffering from purpura, as in certain rare conditions the absence of platelet clumping is a useful pointer to the diagnosis (see p. 127).

MODE OF ACTION OF ANTICOAGULANTS

EDTA and sodium citrate remove calcium which is essential for coagulation. Calcium is either precipitated as insoluble oxalate (crystals of which may be seen in oxalated blood) or bound in a non-ionized form. Heparin works in a different way; it neutralizes thrombin by inhibiting the interaction of several clotting factors in the presence of a plasma co-factor, antithrombin III. Sodium citrate or heparin can be used to render blood incoagulable before transfusion. For better long-term preservation of red cells for certain tests and for transfusion purposes citrate is used in combination with dextrose in the form of acid-citrate-dextrose (ACD), citrate-phosphate-dextrose (CPD) or Alsever's solution (see p. 575).

EFFECTS OF STORAGE OF BLOOD BEFORE QUANTITATIVE ESTIMATIONS ARE PERFORMED

Regardless of the anticoagulant, certain changes take place when blood is allowed to stand in vitro at room temperature (18–25°C), although they are less marked in blood in ACD, CPD or Alsever's solution than in EDTA blood and greater in the tripotassium salt than in the dipotassium salt of EDTA. The red cells start to swell, with the result that the MCV increases, osmotic fragility and prothrombin time slowly increase and the sedimentation rate decreases; the leucocyte and platelet counts gradually fall.[2,18] There is no significant change in MCV if the blood is kept overnight at 4°C. Other changes, too, take place more slowly at this temperature, so that for many purposes blood may safely be allowed to stand overnight in the refrigerator if precautions against freezing are taken. Nevertheless, it is best to count leucocytes and especially platelets within 2 h. The fall in leucocyte count, however, may become marked within 1–2 h if there is an excessive amount of

EDTA (>4.5 mg/ml).[10] Degenerative changes in leucocyte morphology (p. 4) will affect automated differential counts (see p. 75). Reticulocyte counts are unchanged when the blood is kept in either EDTA or ACD anticoagulant for 24 h at 4°C, but at room temperature the count begins to fall within 6 h. Nucleated red cells disappear from the blood specimen within 1–2 days at room temperature.[1] The advisability of making films as soon as possible has already been stressed.

Haemoglobin remains unchanged for days, provided that the blood does not become infected, as shown by lysis with turbidity or discolouration of the specimen.

The importance of effectively mixing blood after collection, particularly if it has been stored and is cold and viscid, cannot be over-emphasized. If cold, the blood should first be allowed to warm up to room temperature, then mixed, preferably by rotation, for at least 2 min. The difficulty of mixing stored blood adequately is a strong point in favour of performing blood counts without delay.

PERIPHERAL ('CAPILLARY') BLOOD

Peripheral blood is liable to give erroneous results, and should be used only when it is not possible to obtain venous blood. Furthermore, there is greater likelihood of contamination and risk of transmission of disease than with venesection. The blood can be obtained from an ear-lobe or finger of an adult or from the heel of an infant. A free flow of blood is essential, and only the very gentlest squeezing is permissible; ideally, large drops of blood should exude slowly but spontaneously. If it is necessary to squeeze firmly in order to obtain blood, the results are unreliable. If the poor flow is due to the part being cold and cyanosed, too high figures for red cell count, Hb content and leucocyte count are usually obtained.

The discrepancies between peripheral and venous samples are more marked if the ear-lobe rather than the finger is chosen as the site for puncture.[3,13] However, if the ear is rubbed well (with a piece of lint or cotton wool) until it is pink and warm, a good spontaneous flow of blood can be obtained from most patients if sterile lancets are used as prickers. Under these circumstances the figures for red cell count, Hb content and leucocyte count approximate closely to those of venous blood.

Ear-lobe puncture is carried out as follows. Rub the ear with lint until warm. Then prick the ear-lobe to a depth of 2–3 mm with a sterile lancet by a single stabbing action. Wipe away the first few drops and collect the sample when the blood is flowing spontaneously, usually in about 30 s. A separate lancet must be used for each patient.

When a finger is used this should be the distal digit of the 3rd or 4th finger on its palmer surface, about 3–5 mm lateral from the nail bed, or on its dorsal surface proximal to the nail bed.

Heel blood

Satisfactory samples can be obtained in infants by a deep puncture using a steel lancet, but only if the heel is really warm—it may be necessary to bathe it in hot water. Appropriate sites are the lateral or medial parts of the plantar surface of the heel. The central plantar area and the posterior curvature should not be punctured in small infants to avoid the risk of injury to the underlying tarsal bones.

COLLECTION OF PERIPHERAL BLOOD FOR QUANTITATIVE STUDIES

The usual procedure is to use a micropipette to draw up the correct amount of blood (usually 20 µl). An alternative method is to use disposable capillary tubes cut to size so as to contain the exact volume of blood when completely filled. The capillary tube is filled by capillarity and then dropped into a tube containing the appropriate amount of diluent solution. Apart from the potential biohazard, another disadvantage is the presence of contaminating blood on the outside of the capillary where it has been in contact with the source. Such blood is difficult to wipe off without causing the loss of a portion of the blood contained within the capillary. In another system (Unopette) the calibrated capillary, which is to be completely filled with blood, is attached by a special holder directly to a reservoir containing the premeasured volume of diluent*.[7]

As an alternative method the capillary can be connected to a rubber teat and its contents can then be discharged into the diluent by squeezing the teat**. These methods are particularly suitable for use by the bedside or in the 'field', as less technical skill is required to draw up the correct amount of blood than in the micropipette method.

DIFFERENCES BETWEEN PERIPHERAL AND VENOUS BLOOD

Venous blood and peripheral blood are not quite the same, even if the latter is freely flowing, and it is likely that free flowing blood obtained by skin puncture is more nearly arteriolar in origin.[9] The PCV, red-cell count and Hb content of peripheral blood are slightly greater than in venous blood. The total leucocyte and neutrophil counts are higher by about 8%, the monocyte count by about 12%, and in some cases by as much as 100%, especially in children;[4,5] this occurs in both finger and ear-lobe, but neutrophils and monocytes especially tend to accumulate in the ear-lobe if the blood is not free flowing.[13]

Conversely, the platelet count appears to be higher in venous than in peripheral blood; this is on average by about 9% and in some cases by as much as 32%.[4,5] This may be due to adhesion of platelets to the site of the skin puncture.

---

*Becton Dickinson Ltd.
**e.g. Drummond Microcaps or 'Volupettes', Scientific Supplies Co. Ltd.

REFERENCES

[1] BAER, D. M. and KRAUSE, R. B. (1968). Spurious laboratory values resulting from simulated mailing conditions. *American Journal of Clinical Pathology*, **50**, 111.

[2] BRITTIN, G. M., BRECHER, G., JOHNSON, C. A. and ELASHOFF, R. M. (1969). Stability of blood in commonly used anticoagulants. *American Journal of Clinical Pathology*, **52**, 690.

[3] BRÜCKMANN, G. (1942). Blood from the ear lobe: preliminary report. *Journal of Laboratory and Clinical Medicine*, **27**, 487.

[4] DAAE, L. N. W., HALLERUD, M. and HALVORSEN, S. (1988). A comparison between haematological parameters in "capillary" and venous blood samples from hospitalized children aged 3 months to 14 years. *Scandinavian Journal of Clinical and Laboratory Investigation*, **51**, 651.

[5] DAAE, L. N. W., HALVORSEN, S., MATHISON, P. M. and

MIRONSKA, K. (1988). A comparison between haematological parameters in 'capillary' and venous blood from healthy adults. *Scandinavian Journal of Clinical and Laboratory Investigation*, **48,** 723.

6   EUROPEAN COMMITTEE FOR CLINICAL LABORATORY STANDARDS (1984). *Standard for Specimen Collection Part 1: Blood Containers*. ECCLS Document Vol 1, No. 1, 1–6. Beuth-Verlag, Berlin.

7   FREUNDLICH, M. H. and GERARDE, H. W. (1963). A new, automatic, disposable system for blood counts and hemoglobin. *Blood*, **21,** 648.

8   GARZA, D., BECAN-MCBRIDE, K. (1989). *Phlebotomy Handbook*, 2nd edn. Appleton & Lange, Norwalk, CN.

9   GIBSON, J. G. 2nd, SELIGMAN, A. M., PEACOCK, W. C., AUB, J. C., FINE, J. and EVANS, R. D. (1964). The distribution of red cells and plasma in large and minute vessels of the normal dog, determined by radioactive isotopes of iron and iodine. *Journal of Clinical Investigation*, **25,** 848.

10   GOOSSENS, W., VAN DUPPEN, V. and VERWILGHEN, R. H. (1991). K_2- or K_3-EDTA: the anticoagulant of choice in routine haematology? *Clinical and Laboratory Haematology*, **13,** 291.

11   HADLEY, G. G. and WEISS, S. P. (1955). Further notes on use of salts of ethylenediamine tetraacetic acid (EDTA) as anticoagulants. *American Journal of Clinical Pathology*, **25,** 1090.

12   INTERNATIONAL COUNCIL FOR STANDARDIZATION IN HAEMATOLOGY (1993). Recommendations for EDTA-anticoagulation of blood for hematology testing. *American Journal of Clinical Pathology*, **100,** 371.

13   LUCEY, H. C. (1950). Fortuitous factors affecting the leucocyte count in blood from the ear. *Journal of Clinical Pathology*, **3,** 146.

14   NATIONAL COMMITTEE FOR CLINICAL LABORATORY STANDARDS (1976). *Standard for Evacuated Tubes for Blood Specimen Collection*, 2nd edn. NCCLS, Villanova, PA.

15   NATIONAL COMMITTEE FOR CLINICAL LABORATORY STANDARDS (1991). *Procedures for the Collection of Diagnostic Blood Specimens by Venipuncture*, 3rd edn. Document H3-A3, Vol 11, No 10. NCCLS, Villanova, PA.

16   PENNOCK, C. A. and JONES, K. W. (1966). Effect of ethylene-diamine-tetraacetic acid (dipotassium salt) and heparin on the estimation of packed cell volume. *Journal of Clinical Pathology*, **19,** 196.

17   SACKER, L. S., SAUNDERS, K. E., PAGE, B. and GOODFELLOW, M. (1959). Dilithium sequestrene as an anticoagulant. *Journal of Clinical Pathology*, **12,** 254.

18   VAN ASSENDELFT, O. W. and PARVIN, R. M. (1988). Specimen collection, handling and storage. In *Quality Assurance in Haematology*. Eds. S. M. Lewis and R. L. Verwilghen, p. 5. Baillière Tindall, London.

2. Reference ranges and normal values

Reference ranges   9
  Statistical procedure   10

Physiological variation   11
  Hb, PCV and RBC   11
  Leucocyte count   15
  Platelet count   16

A number of factors affect haematological values in apparent health. These include:

1. The sex, age, occupation, body build, ethnic background and environment, especially altitude.
2. The physiological conditions under which the specimens are obtained, including the subject's diet, his posture when the sample was taken, whether ambulant or confined to bed.
3. The technique and timing of specimen collection, transport and storage.
4. Variation in the analytical methods used.

Furthermore, it is difficult to be certain in any survey of a population for the purposes of obtaining data from which normal ranges may be constructed that the 'normal' subjects are completely healthy and do not have mild chronic infections, parasitic infestations or nutritional deficiencies.

The borderline between health and ill-health is indefinite; so it is with haematological values, for the normal and abnormal undoubtedly overlap. For instance, a value well within the recognized normal range may be definitely pathological in a particular subject, e.g. a total leucocyte count of $10.0 \times 10^9/1$ is abnormal for a man whose count usually ranges between 4.0 and $6.0 \times 10^9/1$. For these reasons the concept of 'normal values' and 'normal ranges' is being replaced by 'reference values' and 'reference limits' in which the variables are defined when establishing the values for the reference population in a particular test.[27,30] A desirable goal is to have a data bank of reference values which take account of the physiological variables mentioned above, so that an individual's result can be expressed and interpreted relative to a comparable normal. Such data are at present available for only a limited number of haematological tests, mainly for red cell indices in different age groups.[32,43]

REFERENCE RANGES

A reference range for a population can be established from measurements on a relatively small number of subjects (see below) if they are assumed to be representative of the population as a whole.[21,27,57] The conditions for obtaining samples from the individuals must be standardized and data should be analysed separately for different variables such as individuals in bed or ambulant, smokers or non-smokers. The samples should be collected at about the same time of day, preferably in the morning before breakfast; the last meal should have been eaten not later than 9 p.m. on the previous evening and at that time alcohol should have been restricted to one bottle of beer or an equivalent amount of other alcoholic drink.[28]

STATISTICAL PROCEDURE[29]

It is usually assumed that the data will fit a specified type of pattern, either symmetric (Gaussian) or asymmetric with a skewed distribution (non-Gaussian) (p. 584). If the data (x_1, x_2 etc.) fit a Gaussian distribution the arithmetic mean ($\bar{x}$) and SD may be calculated as described on p. 584.

Alternatively, a frequency histogram is plotted (Fig. 2.1). Taking the modal value (mode) and the calculated standard deviation (SD) as reference points, a Gaussian curve is superimposed. From this curve practical reference limits can be determined even if the original histogram included outlying results from some subjects not belonging to the normal population. Limits representing the 95% range (reference interval) are calculated from arithmetic mean ± 2 SD (or more accurately ± 1.96 SD). When there is a log normal (skew) distribution of measurements, the range to –2 SD may extend below zero (Fig. 2.2). To avoid this

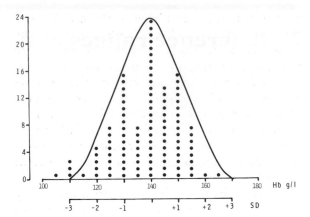

Fig. 2.1   Example of establishing a reference range. Histogram of data of haemoglobin measurements in a population, with Gaussian curve superimposed. The ordinate shows the number at each reference point.

anomaly the data should be converted to their logarithms by means of log-tables or a calculator with the appropriate facility. The mean and SD are calculated in the usual way (p. 584); the figures are then converted to their antilogs in order to express the data in the original scale.

When it is not possible to make an assumption about the type of distribution a non-parametric

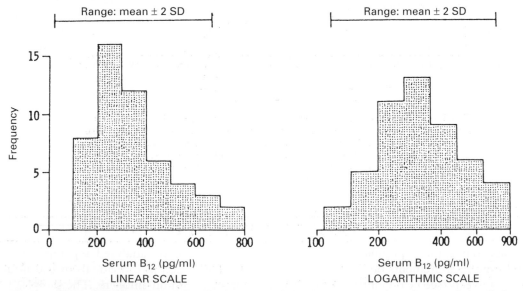

Fig. 2.2   Example of log normal distribution. Data of vitamin B_{12} measurements in a population. Left: arithmetic scale; Right: geometric scale. Arithmetic mean 343 pg/ml and SD 161 pg/ml; 2 SD range would thus be 21–665 pg/ml. When the data are converted to their logarithms as described on p. 584, the geometric mean is 308 pg/ml, and a 2 SD range is 121–783 pg/ml. Reproduced with permission from J. M. England (1975) *Medical Research: A Statistical and Epidemiological Approach*, p. 20, Churchill Livingstone, Edinburgh.

procedure may be used instead. For this the data are sorted out and ranked according to increasing numerical values. The total number of results = n; subsequent calculations are based on n + 1. The lower reference limit will correspond to the rank number at which 2.5% of n + 1 results occur; the upper reference limit is similarly taken as the rank number at which 97.5% of n + 1 results have accumulated. If these numbers are not integers it may be necessary to interpolate between two adjacent rank values.

In any of the methods of analysis a reasonably reliable estimate can be obtained with 40 values, although a larger number (120 or more) is preferable (Fig 2.3).[29,45] When a large set of reference values is unattainable and precise estimation impossible, a smaller number of values may still serve as a useful clinical guide.

The data given in Table 2.1 provide a rough guide to normal reference values which are applicable to most healthy individuals. The data have been derived from various sources; some are based on observations from the authors' own laboratory. The range of ±2 SD from the mean indicates the limits which should cover 95% of normal subjects; 99% of normal subjects will be included in a range of ±3 SD. Age and sex differences have been taken into account for some values. Even so, the wide ranges which are shown for some tests reflect the influence of various factors as described on p. 9. Narrower ranges would be expected under standardized conditions.

A 'normal range' for 95% of normal subjects has been given without SD when the distribution does not show a recognizable pattern or when the data are too scanty for full analysis.

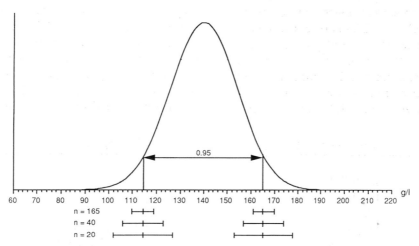

Fig. 2.3 Effect of sample size on reference values. A smoothed distribution graph was obtained for haemoglobin measurement from a group of normal women: the ordinate shows the density probability. The 0.95 reference interval was calculated; this was 115–165 g/l, as shown by the perpendicular lines on the graph. The confidence levels for lower and upper reference limits are shown for three sample sizes of 20, 40 and 165 values, respectively.

PHYSIOLOGICAL VARIATION

PHYSIOLOGICAL VARIATION IN Hb CONTENT, PCV AND RED CELL COUNTS

It is well known that there is considerable variation in the red cell count and Hb content at different periods of life. At birth the Hb is higher than at

any period subsequently (Table 2.1). The red cell count is high immediately after birth[7,14,35] and values for Hb greater than 200 g/l, red cell count higher than 6.0×10^{12}/l and a packed cell volume (PCV) of 0.65 are encountered frequently when the cord is tied late after delivery. Probably it is the

Table 2.1 Haematological values for normal adults expressed as a mean ±2 SD (95% range)

Red blood cell count	
Men	$5.0 \pm 0.5 \times 10^{12}/l$
Women	$4.3 \pm 0.5 \times 10^{12}/l$
Haemoglobin	
Men	150 ± 20 g/l
Women	135 ± 15 g/l
Packed cell volume (PCV) or haematocrit (Hct) value	
Men	0.45 ± 0.05 (l/l)
Women	0.41 ± 0.05 (l/l)
Mean cell volume (MCV)	
Men and women	92 ± 9 fl
Mean cell haemoglobin (MCH)	
Men and women	29.5 ± 2.5 pg
Mean cell haemoglobin concentration (MCHC)	
Men and women	330 ± 15 g/l
Red cell distribution width (RDW)	
As coefficient of variation (CV)	12.8 ± 1.2 %
As standard deviation (SD)	42.5 ± 3.5 fl
Red cell diameter (mean values)	
Dry films	6.7–7.7 μm
Red cell density	1092–1100 g/l
Reticulocyte count	0.5–2.5% ($50–100 \times 10^9/l$)
Blood volume	
Red cell volume: men	30 ± 5 ml/kg
women	25 ± 5 ml/kg
Plasma volume	45 ± 5 ml/kg
Total blood volume	70 ± 10 ml/kg
Red cell life-span	120 ± 30 days
White blood cell count	$7.0 \pm 3.0 \times 10^9/l$
Differential white cell count	
Neutrophils	$2.0–7.0 \times 10^9/l$ (40–80%)
Lymphocytes	$1.0–3.0 \times 10^9/l$ (20–40%)
Monocytes	$0.2–1.0 \times 10^9/l$ (2–10%)
Eosinophils	$0.02–0.5 \times 10^9/l$ (1–6%)
Basophils	$0.02–0.1 \times 10^9/l$ (<1–2%)
Platelet count	$150–400 \times 10^9/l$
Bleeding time (Ivy's method)	2–7 min
(Template method)	2.5–9.5 min
Prothrombin time	11–16 s
Partial thromboplastin time (APTT)	30–40 s
Thrombin time	15–19 s
Plasma fibrinogen	2.0–4.0 g/l

Table 2.1   *(Continued)*

Fibrinogen titre	≥ 128
Plasminogen	
Function	0.75–1.35 u/ml
Antigen	0.76–1.36 u/ml
Euglobulin lysis time	90–240 min
Antithrombin III	
Function	0.86–13.2 u/ml
Antigen	0.79–1.11 u/ml
β-*Thromboglobulin*	< 50 ng/ml
Platelet factor 4	< 10 ng/ml
Protein C	
Function	0.70–1.40 u/ml
Antigen	0.61–1.32 u/ml
Protein S	
Total	0.78–1.37 u/ml
Free	0.68–1.52 u/ml
Heparin co-factor II	55–145%

Osmotic fragility (at 20° and pH 7.4)

NaCl (g/l)	Before incubation (% lysis)	After incubation for 24 h at 37°C (% lysis)
2.0	100	95–100
3.0	97–100	85–100
3.5	90–99	75–100
4.0	50–95	65–100
4.5	5–45	55–95
5.0	0–6	40–85
5.5	0	15–70
6.0	0	0–40
6.5	0	0–10
7.0	0	0–5
7.5	0	0
8.0	0	0
8.5	0	0

Median corpuscular fragility (MCF) (g/l NaCl)

4.0–4.45	4.65–5.9

Autohaemolysis (37°C)	
48 h without added glucose	0.2–2.0
48 h with added glucose	0–0.9%
Cold agglutinin titre (4°C)	< 64
Serum iron	13–32 μmol/l (0.7–1.8 mg/l)
Total iron-binding capacity	45–70 μmol/l (2.5–4.0 mg/l)
Transferrin	1.2–2.0 g/l

Table 2.1   *(Continued)*

Ferritin	
Men	20–300, median 100 µg/l
Women	15–150, median 30 µg/l
Serum vitamin B₁₂	160–760 ng/l
Serum folate	3–20 µg/l
Red cell folate	160–640 µg/l
Plasma haemoglobin	10–40 mg/l
Serum haptoglobin	
By radial immunodiffusion	0.8–2.7 g/l
By haemoglobin binding capacity	0.3–2.0 g/l
Hb A₂	2.2–3.5%
Hb F	< 1.0%
Methaemoglobin	< 2.0%
Sedimentation rate (1 h at 20 ± 3°C) (upper limits)	
Men 17–50 yr	10 mm
51–60 yr	12 mm
61–70 yr	14 mm
> 70 yr	30 mm
Women 17–50 yr	19 mm
51–60 yr	19 mm
61–70 yr	20 mm
> 70 yr	35 mm
Plasma viscosity	
25°C	1.50–1.72 mPa/s
37°C	1.16–1.33 mPa/s
Heterophile (anti-sheep red cell) agglutinin titre	< 80
After absorption with guinea-pig kidney	< 10

cessation of pulsation of the umbilical artery in the cord as well as the uterine contractions which result in much of the blood contained in the placenta re-entering the infant's circulation. After the immediate post-natal period the Hb falls fairly steeply to a minimum of about 100 g/l at about the 3rd month.[7,14,35] The red cell count and PCV also fall, though less steeply and the cells may become microcytic with the development of 'physiological' iron-deficiency anaemia.

In the neonate the average mean cell haemoglobin concentration (MCHC) is 300 g/l with a SD of 27 g/l; it does not alter significantly during the first 3 yr but the SD diminishes. The mean MCV is 120 fl in the neonate, 100 at 2 months, 95 at 3 months and within the adult range by 3 yr.

The Hb content and red cell count normally rise gradually to almost adult levels by the time of puberty; thereafter the levels in women tend to be significantly lower than those of men.[24,32] Factors influencing the difference between men and women include a hormonal influence on haemopoiesis and menstrual blood loss; the extent to which the latter is a significant factor is not clear, as a loss of up to 100 ml of blood with each period does not appear to cause a fall in Hb although it results in lower levels of serum iron.[13,23] Moreover, arrest of menstruation by oral contraceptives causes an increase in serum iron without affecting the haemoglobin level.[8]

In normal pregnancy there is an increase in erythropoietic activity. However, at the same time an increase in plasma volume occurs and this results in a fall in Hb and red cell count.[10,33] The level returns to normal about a week after delivery. Serum ferritin falls in early pregnancy and usually remains low throughout pregnancy, even when supplementary iron is given.[25]

In old age Hb is reported to fall progressively; in one study this was found to be, in men, to a mean level of 134 g/l at 65, 129 g/l at 75 and 122 g/l at over the age of 85.[51] Lesser differences have been recorded by others.[24,32,43] By contrast, in older women the level tends to rise, so that a sex difference of 20 g/1 in younger age groups is reduced to 10 g/l or less in old age, although in women there is also a progressive fall with time, on average 0.35 g/l per year.[13,36,40] There is a concomitant increase in serum iron although serum ferritin levels remain higher in men than in women. In healthy men and women Hb, red cell count, PCV and related parameters remain remarkably constant until the 6th decade.[47]

In addition to the permanent effects of age and sex, there seem to be transient fluctuations, the significance of which is often difficult to assess. Muscular activity, if at all strenuous, raises the red cell count and Hb, largely due to reduction in plasma volume and to a lesser extent to the re-entry into the circulation of cells previously sequestered in the spleen;[1,2] increases in red cells amounting to 0.5×10^{12}/l and in Hb to 15 g/l may be observed. Posture, too, appears to cause transient alterations in the plasma volume, and thus in Hb and PCV. There is a small but significant increase as the posture changes from lying to sitting especially in women[19] and, conversely, change from walking about to lying down results in a 5–10% fall in the Hb and PCV. This occurs within 20 min, after which time, the PCV is stabilized at the lower level.[16,37] Consistently similar findings have also been reported by Eisenberg in a study of 25 subjects.[15] He also showed that the position of the arm during venous sampling affected the magnitude of the increase in PCV; it was 2–4% lower when the arm was held at the atrial level instead of being dependent.

It is not clear whether emotion or light exercise raises the red cell count or Hb significantly above the baseline observed with the subject at rest; the effects may be small enough to be submerged in the technical errors of estimation.[53] Athletes tend to have slightly lower Hb levels than non-athletes, with significantly higher total red cell volume which is partly obscured by a concomitant increase in plasma volume.[6] Diurnal variation is usually slight[17] but fluctuations as much as 15% have been reported;[54] in most cases Hb was highest in the morning and lowest in the evening, the mean difference being about 8%. Pronounced diurnal variations are seen in serum iron and ferritin in healthy as well as in anaemic subjects.[44,46,52]

It has been suggested that seasonal variations also occur, but the evidence for this is conflicting.[42,49] There may be an ethnic difference in red cell indices; lower levels of Hb and MCV have been reported in healthy Africans and West Indians living in Britain, not related to nutritional status.[22]

The effect of altitude is to raise the Hb and increase the number of circulating red cells; the magnitude of the polycythaemia depends on the degree of anoxaemia.[26] At an altitude of 2 km (c 6500 ft) the Hb is c 10 g/l higher than at sea level; at 3 km (c 10 000 ft) it is c 20 g/l higher. Corresponding increases occur at intermediate altitudes. These increases appear to be due both to increased erythropoiesis as a result of the anoxic stimulus and to the decrease in plasma volume which occurs at high altitudes.[34,41] Smokers have slightly higher Hb values and PCV.[31,56] This is probably in consequence of the accumulation of carboxyhaemoglobin in the blood. After a single cigarette the carboxyhaemoglobin level increases by about 1%,[48] and in heavy smokers the carboxyhaemoglobin may constitute c 4–5% of the total haemoglobin.[30] There may be polycythaemia.[50]

PHYSIOLOGICAL VARIATIONS IN THE TOTAL LEUCOCYTE COUNT[24,53]

The effect of age is indicated in Table 2.1; at birth the neutrophil polymorphonuclears predominate, reaching a peak of $c\ 13.0 \times 10^9$/l at 12 h and then falling to a mean of $c\ 4.0 \times 10^9$/l over the next

2–3 days, at which level the count remains steady. The lymphocytes fall during the first 3 days of life to a low level of c 2.0–2.5 $\times$ 10^9/l and then rise up to the 10th day;[50] after this time they are the predominant cell (up to about 60%) until the 5th–7th yr when they give way to the neutrophils. There are slight sex differences; the total leucocyte count and the neutrophil count may be slightly higher in women than men.[18] After the menopause the counts fall in women so that they tend to become lower than in men of similar age.[12,13,18]

People differ considerably in their leucocyte counts. Some tend to maintain a relatively constant level over long periods of time;[5] others have counts which may vary by as much as 100% at different times. In some subjects there appears to be a rhythm, occurring in cycles of 14–23 days, and in women this may be related to some extent to the menstrual cycle.[39] Some forms of oral contraception have been reported to raise the leucocyte count.[18] There is also diurnal variation which differs on an hour-to-hour basis as well as from day to day;[53] it affects the total leucocyte count as well as all the individual cell types. The minimum count is found in the morning with the subject at rest; the maximum in the afternoon. Random activity may raise the count slightly; strenuous exercise causes rises of up to 30 $\times$ 10^9/l, chiefly due to decreased splenic blood flow resulting in reduced pooling of neutrophils in the spleen, and to some extent to liberation into the blood stream of neutrophils formerly sequestered in shut-down capillaries and in the spleen.[2] Large numbers of lymphocytes and monocytes also enter the blood stream during strenuous exercise.

Adrenaline injection causes an increase in the leucocyte count; here, too, increases in the numbers of all major types of leucocytes (and platelets) occur.[9] The rise has been thought to be a reflection of the extent of the reservoir of mature blood cells present not only in the bone marrow and spleen but also in other tissues and organs of the body. Emotion may possibly cause an increase in the leucocyte count in a similar way. The effect of ingestion of food is uncertain. Cigarette smoking causes a significant increase in the leucocyte count.[11,24,56] A moderate leucocytosis of up to 15 $\times$ 10^9/l is common during pregnancy, with the peak about 8 weeks before parturition. The count returns to normal levels a week or so after delivery.[12] The rise in leucocytes is due to neutrophilia.

Diurnal variation of the eosinophil count is especially marked.[53] The height of the count is controlled at least in part by the adrenal cortex, increased adrenocortical activity leading to a fall in the number of circulating eosinophils; diurnal fluctuations parallel diurnal glucocorticoid fluctuation.

The environment may influence the leucocyte count. Thus in tropical Africa there is a tendency for a reversal of the neutrophil:lymphocyte ratio in individuals with a low total leucocyte count.[58] This may be partly due to endemic parasitic and protozoal disease; however, genetics are also likely to play a part as significantly lower leucocyte counts, especially neutrophil counts, have been observed in Africans living in Britain.[4] In some tropical areas reactive eosinophilia or monocytosis is sufficiently common to be regarded as a reference value for that population.

PHYSIOLOGICAL VARIATION IN THE PLATELET COUNT

There may be a sex difference; thus, in women the count has been reported to be about 20% higher than in men.[55] A fall in the platelet count may occur in women at about the time of menstruation and there is some evidence of a cycle with a 21–35 day rhythm.[38] There is no evidence that oral contraceptives affect the platelet count. There is a variation during the course of a day as well as from day to day.[53] Within the wide normal reference range there are no significant ethnic differences, but in healthy West Indians and Africans platelet counts may on average be 10–20% lower than those in Europeans living in the same environment.[3] There are no obvious age differences; at birth and in the first few weeks of infancy, however, the platelet count tends to be at the lower level of the adult normal reference range, rising to adult values at about 6 months. Strenuous exercise causes a 30–40% increase in platelet count;[2] the mechanism is similar to that which occurs with leucocytes.

Modern blood counting systems provide a high

level of precision, so that even small differences in successive measurements may be significant. It is thus most important to establish and understand the limits of physiological variation etc. for the various tests. With this proviso, present-day blood count data can now provide sensitive indications of minor abnormalities which may be important in clinical interpretation and health screening.

Table 2.2 Haematological values for normal infants and children

	At birth (full term)	Day 3	1 month	2–6 months	2–6 years	6–12 years
Red blood cell count ($\times 10^{12}$/l)	6.0 ± 1.0	5.3 ± 1.3	4.2 ± 1.2	3.8 ± 0.8	4.6 ± 0.7	4.6 ± 0.6
Haemoglobin (g/l)	165 ± 30	185 ± 40	140 ± 30	115 ± 20	125 ± 15	135 ± 20
Packed cell volume/haematocrit	0.54 ± 0.10	0.56 ± 0.11	0.43 ± 0.12	0.35 ± 0.07	0.37 ± 0.03	0.40 ± 0.05
Mean cell volume (MCV) (fl)	110 ± 10	108 ± 13	104 ± 19	91 ± 17	81 ± 6	86 ± 8
Mean cell haemoglobin (MCH) (pg)	34 ± 3	34 ± 3	34 ± 6	30 ± 5	27 ± 3	29 ± 4
Mean cell haemoglobin concentration (MCHC) (g/l)	330 ± 30	330 ± 40	330 ± 40	330 ± 30	340 ± 30	340 ± 30
Reticulocytes (%)	2–5	1–4.5	0.3–1	0.4–1	0.2–2	0.2–2
White blood cell count ($\times 10^9$/l)	18 ± 8	15 ± 8	12 ± 7	12 ± 6	10 ± 5	9 ± 4
Neutrophils ($\times 10^9$/l)	5–13	3–5	3–9	1.5–9	1.5–8	2–8
Lymphocytes ($\times 10^9$/l)	3–10	2–8	3–16	4–10	6–9	1–5
Monocytes ($\times 10^9$/l)	0.7–1.5	0.5–1	0.3–1	0.1–1	0.1–1	0.1–1
Eosinophils ($\times 10^9$/l)	0.2–1	0.1–2.5	0.2–1	0.2–1	0.2–1	0.1–1

Expressed as mean ±2 SD or 95% range.

REFERENCES

[1] ALLSOP, P., PETERS, A. M., ARNOT, R. N., STUTTLE, A. W. J., DEENMAMODE, M., GWILLIAM, H., MYERS, M. J. and HALL, G. M (1992). Intrasplenic blood cell kinetics in man before and after brief maximal exercise. *Clinical Science*, **83**, 47.

[2] ALLSOP, P., ARNOT, R., GWILLIAM, M., HALL, G. M. and LEWIS, S. M. (1988). Does splenic autotransfusion occur during high intensity cycle exercise in man? *Journal of Physiology (London)*, **407**, 24P.

[3] BAIN, B. J. and SEED. M. (1986). Platelet count and platelet size in healthy Africans and West Indians. *Clinical and Laboratory Haematology*, **8**, 43.

[4] BAIN, B. J., SEED, M. and GODSLAND, I. (1984). Normal values for peripheral blood white cell counts in women of four different ethnic origins. *Journal of Clinical Pathology*, **37**, 188.

[5] BOOTH, K. and HANCOCK, R. E. T. (1961). A study of the total and differential leucocyte counts and haemoglobin levels in a group of normal adults over a period of two years. *British Journal of Haematology*, **7**, 9.

[6] BROTHERHOOD, J., BROZOVIC, B. and PUGH, L. G. C. (1975). Haematological status of middle and long distance runners. *Clinical Science and Molecular Medicine*, **48**, 139

[7] BURMAN, D. (1972). Haemoglobin levels in normal infants aged 3 to 24 months and the effect of iron. *Archives of Diseases in Childhood*, **47**, 261.

[8] BURTON, J. L. (1967). Effect of oral contraceptives on haemoglobin, packed cell volume, serum-iron and total iron-binding capacity in healthy women. *Lancet*, **i**, 978.

[9] CHATTERJEA, J. B., DAMESHEK, W. and STEFANINI, M. (1953). The adrenalin (epinephrin) test as applied to hematologic disorders. *Blood*, **8**, 211.

[10] CHESLEY, L. C. (1972). Plasma and red cell volumes during pregnancy. *America Journal of Obstetrics and Gynecology*, **112**, 440

[11] CORRE, F., LELLOUCH, J. and SCHWARTZ, D. (1971). Smoking and leucocyte counts; results of an epidemiological survey. *Lancet*, **ii**, 632.

[12] CRUICKSHANK, J. M. (1970). The effects of parity on the leucocyte count in pregnant and non-pregnant women. *British Journal of Haematology*, **18**, 531.

[13] CRUICKSHANK, J. M. and ALEXANDER, M. K. (1970). The effect of age, parity, haemoglobin level and oral contraceptive preparations on the normal leucocyte count. *British Journal of Haematology*, **18**, 541.

[14] DEMARSH, Q. B., ALT, H. L., WINDLE, W. F. and HILLIS, D. S. (1941). The effect of depriving the infant of its placental blood. *Journal of American Medical Association*, **116**, 2568.

[15] EISENBERG, S. (1963). The effect of posture and position of the venous sampling site on the hematocrit and serum protein concentration. *Journal of Laboratory and Clinical Medicine*, **51**, 755.

16 EKELUND, L. G., EKLUND, B. and KAIJSER, L. (1971). Time course for the change in hemoglobin concentration with change in posture. *Acta Medica Scandinavica*, **190**, 335.

17 ELWOOD, P. C. (1962). Diurnal haemoglobin variation in normal male subjects. *Clinical Science*, **23**, 379.

18 ENGLAND, J. M. and BAIN, B. J. (1976). Total and differential leucocyte count. *British Journal of Haematology*, **33**, 1.

19 FELDING, P., TRYDING, N., HYLTOFT PETERSEN, P. and HORDER, M. (1980). Effects of posture on concentration of blood constituents in healthy adults: practical application of blood specimen collection procedures recommended by the Scandinavian Committee on Reference Values. *Scandinavian Journal of Clinical and Laboratory Investigation*, **40**, 615.

20 GALEA, G. and DAVIDSON, R. J. L. (1985). Haematological and haemorheological changes associated with cigarette smoking. *Journal of Clinical Pathology*, **38**, 978.

21 GARBY, L. (1970). The normal haemoglobin level (Annotation). *British Journal of Haematology*, **19**, 429.

22 GODSLAND, I. F., SEED, M., SIMPSON, R., BROOM, G. and WYNN, V. (1983). Comparison of haematological indices between women of four ethnic groups and the effect of oral contraceptives. *Journal of Clinical Pathology*, **36**, 184.

23 HALLBERG, L., HOGDAHL, A. M., NILSSON, L. and RYBO, G. (1966). Menstrual blood loss and iron deficiency. *Acta Medica Scandinavica*, **180**, 639.

24 HELMAN, N. and RUBENSTEIN, L. S. (1975). The effects of age, sex and smoking on erythrocytes and leukocytes. *American Journal of Clinical Pathology*, **63**, 35.

25 HOWELLS, M. R., JONES, S. E., NAPIER, J. A. F., SAUNDERS, K. and CAVILL, I. (1986). Erythropoiesis in pregnancy. *British Journal of Haematology*, **64**, 595.

26 HURTADO, A., MERINO, C. and DELGADO, E. (1945). Influence of anoxemia on the hemopoietic activity. *Archives of Internal Medicine*, **75**, 284.

27 INTERNATIONAL COMMITTEE FOR STANDARDIZATION IN HAEMATOLOGY (1981). The theory of reference values. *Clinical and Laboratory Haematology*, **3**, 369.

28 INTERNATIONAL COMMITTEE FOR STANDARDIZATION IN HAEMATOLOGY (1982). Standardization of blood specimen collection procedures for reference values. *Clinical and Laboratory Haematology*, **4**, 83.

29 INTERNATIONAL FEDERATION OF CLINICAL CHEMISTRY AND INTERNATIONAL COMMITTEE FOR STANDARDIZATION IN HAEMATOLOGY (1987). The theory of reference values. Part 5. Statistical treatment of collected reference values. Determination of reference limits. *Journal of Clinical Chemistry and Clinical Biochemistry*, **25**, 645.

30 INTERNATIONAL FEDERATION OF CLINICAL CHEMISTRY AND INTERNATIONAL COUNCIL FOR STANDARDIZATION IN HAEMATOLOGY (1987). The Theory of Reference Values Part 6: Presentation of observed values related to reference values. *Journal of Clinical Biochemistry*, **25**, 657.

31 ISAGER, H. and HAGERUP, L. (1971). Relationship between cigarette smoking and high packed cell volume and haemoglobin levels. *Scandinavian Journal of Haematology*, **8**, 241.

32 KELLY, A. and MUNAN, L. (1977). Haematologic profile of natural populations: red cell parameters. *British Journal of Haematology*, **35**, 153.

33 LARGE R. D. and DYNESIUS, R. (1973). Blood volume changes during normal pregnancy. *Clinics in Haematology*, **2**, 433.

34 LEVIN, N. W., METZ, J., HART, D., VAN HEERDEN, D. R., BOARDMAN, R. G. and FARBER, S. A. (1960). The blood volume of healthy adult males resident in Johannesburg (altitude 5740 feet). *South African Journal of Medical Sciences*, **28**, 132.

35 MATOTH, Y., ZAIZON, R. and VARSANO, I. (1971). Post-natal changes in some red cell parameters. *Acta Paediatrica Scandinavica*, **60**, 317.

36 MATTILA, K. S., KUUSELA, V., PELLINIEMI, T. T., RAJAMAKI, A., KAIHOLA, H. L. and JUVA, K. (1986). Haematological laboratory findings in the elderly; influence of age and sex. *Scandinavian Journal of Clinical and Laboratory Investigation*, **46**, 411.

37 MOLLISON, P. L. (1983). *Blood Transfusion in Clinical Medicine*, 7th edn., p. 77. Blackwell Scientific Publications, Oxford.

38 MORLEY, A. (1969). A platelet cycle in normal individuals. *Australasian Annals of Medicine*, **18**, 127.

39 MORLEY, A. (1973). Correspondence. *Blood*, **41**, 329.

40 MYERS, A. M. SAUNDERS, C. R. G. and CHALMERS, D. G. (1968). The haemoglobin level of fit elderly people. *Lancet*, **ii**, 261.

41 MYHRE L. D., DILL, D. B., HALL, F. G. and BROWN, D. K. (1970). Blood volume changes during three-week residence at high altitude. *Clinical Chemistry*, **16**, 7.

42 NATVIG, H., BJERKEDAL, T. and JONASSEN, O. (1963). Studies on hemoglobin values in Norway. III. Seasonal variations. *Acta Medica Scandinavica*, **174**, 351.

43 NILLSON-EHLE, H., JAGENBURG, R., LANDAHI, S., SVANBORG, A. and WESTIN, J. (1989). Decline of blood haemoglobin in the aged: a longitudinal study of an urban Swedish population from age 70 to 81. *British Journal of Haematology*, **71**, 437.

44 PITON, V. A., HOWANITZ, P. J., HOWANITZ, J. H. and DOMRES, N. (1981). Day-to-day variation in serum ferritin concentration in healthy subjects. *Clinical Chemistry*, **27**, 78.

45 REED, A. H., HENRY, R. J. and MASON, W. B. (1971). Influence of statistical method used on the resulting estimate of normal range. *Clinical Chemistry*, **17**, 275.

46 ROMSLO, I. and TALSTAD, I. (1988). Day-to-day variations in serum iron, serum iron binding capacity, serum ferritin and erythrocyte protoporphyrin concentration in anaemic subjects. *European Journal of Haematology*, **40**, 79.

47 ROSS, D. M., AYSCUE, L. H., WATSON, J. and BENTLEY, S. A. (1988). Stability of hematologic parameters in healthy subjects: intra-individual versus inter-individual variation. *American Journal of Clinical Pathology*, **90**, 262.

48 RUSSEL, M. A. H., WILSON, C., COLE, P. V., IDLE, M. and FEYERABEND, C. (1973). Comparison of increases in carboxyhaemoglobin after smoking 'extramild' and 'non mild' cigarettes. *Lancet*, **ii**, 687.

49 SAUNDERS, C. (1965). Some erythrocyte parameters on a cross section of U. K. A. E. A. employees. *Laboratory Practice*, **14**, 1390.

50 SMITH, J. R. and LANDOW, S. A. (1978). Smoker's polycythemia. *New England Journal of Medicine*, **298**, 6.

51 SMITH, J. S. and WHITELAW, D. M. (1971). Hemoglobin values in aged men. *Canadian Medical Association Journal*, **105**, 816.

52 STATLAND, E. E. and WINKEL, P. (1976). Variation in serum iron concentration in young healthy men: within-day and day-to-day changes. *Clinical Biochemistry*, **9**, 26.

53 STATLAND, B. E., WINKEL P., HARRIS, S. C., BURDSALL, M. J. and SAUNDERS, A. M. (1978). Evaluation of biologic

sources of variation of leukocyte counts and other hematologic quantities using very precise automated analyzers. *American Journal of Clinical Pathology*, **69**, 48.

[54] STENGLE, J. M. and SCHADE, A. L. (1957). Diurnal-nocturnal variations of certain blood constituents in normal human subjects: plasma iron, siderophilin, bilirubin, copper, total serum protein and albumin, haemoglobin and haematocrit. *British Journal of Haematology*, **3**, 117.

[55] STEVENS, R. F. and ALEXANDER, M. K. (1977). A sex difference in the platelet count. *British Journal of Haematology*, **37**, 295.

[56] TIBBLIN, E., BENGTSSON, C., HALLBERG, L. and LENNARTSSON, J. (1979). Haemoglobin concentration and peripheral blood cell counts in women. The population study of women in Goteborg, 1968–1969. *Scandinavian Journal of Haematology*, **22**, 5.

[57] VITERI, F. E., DE TUNA, V. and GUZMAN, M. A. (1972). Normal haematological values in the Central American population. *British Journal of Haematology*, **23**, 189.

[58] WOODLIFF, H. J., KATAAHA, P. K., TIBALEKA, A. K. and NZARO, E. (1972). Total leucocyte count in Africans. *Lancet*, **ii**, 875

[59] XANTHOU, M. (1970). Leucocyte blood picture in healthy full-term and premature babies during neonatal period. *Archives of Disease in Childhood*, **45**, 242.

3. Laboratory organization and management

Written in collaboration with J. Stuart

Human resource management   21
Strategic and business planning   22
Workload   23
Instrumentation   24
Laboratory computers   27
Pre-analytical and post-analytical stages of testing   28

Customized services   29
Healthy and safety   31
   Handling biohazardous specimens   31
   Toxic or carcinogenic reagents   32
Laboratory audit and accreditation   33
Future trends   33

The essential function of a haematology laboratory is to provide accurate and timely data to assist in the diagnosis of disease and in monitoring its response to treatment. Advancing technology and increasing health care legislation have both added to the complexity of modern laboratory practice whose area of responsibility now extends to include both the pre-analytical stage (test ordering, blood collection, specimen transport) and the post-analytical stage (transmission of results) of the test cycle. As a consequence, laboratory organization and management have become increasingly important determinants of good laboratory practice.[31] The principles outlined in this chapter can be generalized to small as well as to large departments despite the more complex management issues that arise in the latter.

HUMAN RESOURCE MANAGEMENT

Management structure

The management structure of a haematology laboratory should indicate a clear line of accountability of each member of staff to the head of department. In turn, the head of department may be managerially accountable to a clinical director (of laboratories) and thence to a hospital or health authority executive. This structure is best displayed as a management tree, with explanatory text, to be issued to all staff. The head of department is responsible for departmental leadership, for ensuring that the laboratory has effective political representation within the hospital, and for ensuring that managerial and administrative tasks are performed efficiently. Where the head of department delegates managerial tasks to others, this should be stated so that responsibilities are clear.

Staff development and appraisal

Laboratory staff are the most valuable and costly asset of the department and their personal development should be allocated the highest priority via a programme of managerial as well as scientific development. All staff should receive some training in laboratory management, relevant aspects of which can be selected from Table 3.1 according to grade.

A staff development scheme includes the setting and achievement of goals for each individual and an element of appraisal is usually included. Most individuals who work in health care are highly dedicated; the main value of appraisal is to ensure that such dedication is channelled in the same direction as the strategic aim of the department. Not all individuals are natural team players

21

Table 3.1   Suggested components of a management training programme for laboratory staff

Strategic and business planning
Implementing change
Communication skills
Workload assessment and costing of tests
Budget management
Working as a team
Delegation
Health and safety
Quality assurance
Audit and accreditation

and some may follow personal interests that are not in the mainstream of the departmental strategic plan; they need to be reminded to work on the right things.[11]

The appraisal process should cascade down from the head of department, and appropriate training must be given at successive levels to each appraiser. It is useful for the appraiser, before the appraisal interview, to send the appraisee a short list of topics to be discussed. The appraisee can then add to and return the list so that each understands the topics to be covered. An appraisal interview usually requires 1–2 hours and should be a constructive dialogue of the appraisee's need for development and the progress made to date. The working relationship between appraiser and appraisee, and how to make this relationship maximally effective, should also be discussed. Ideally, appraisees should leave the interview with the knowledge that their personal development and future progress is of importance to the department, that priorities have been identified, that an action plan with milestones and a time-scale has been agreed, and that progress will be monitored. Formal appraisal interviews (annually for senior staff and more often for others) should be complemented by less formal follow-up discussions to monitor progress. Documentation of formal interviews can be limited to a short list of agreed objectives.

Performance appraisal can have lasting value in the personal development of individuals,[31] but the process can easily be mishandled[17] and should not be started without training in how to hold an appraisal interview.

STRATEGIC AND BUSINESS PLANNING

The head of department is responsible for determining the long-term (usually up to 5 years) strategic direction of the department. Strategic planning requires awareness of any national and local legislation that may affect the laboratory and of changes in local clinical practice that may alter workload. It is conventional to perform an analysis of the internal *strengths* and *weaknesses* of the laboratory and its ability to respond to external *opportunities* and *threats* (SWOT analysis). Expansion of a major clinical service, such as organ transplantation, may pose both an external opportunity and threat to the laboratory depending on its ability to respond to the consequential increase in workload. Internal strengths may include technical or scientific expertise, whereas a heavy workload that precludes any additional developmental work would be a weakness. The stages involved in developing a strategic plan are listed in Table 3.2 and the concept of strategic management is discussed further by Greenley.[15]

A business plan is primarily concerned with determining short-term objectives that will allow the strategy to be implemented over the next financial year or so. Planning of these objectives should involve all staff as this will heighten awareness of the issues and will develop 'ownership' of the strategy. In all but the smallest laboratory, a business manager is required to coordinate such planning and to liaise with the equivalent business managers in other clinical and laboratory areas. Business planning also requires a sophisticated laboratory accounting process with an up-to-date record of workload and costs so that the price of tests can be established.

Table 3.2   Stages of strategic and business planning

1. Perform a SWOT* analysis
2. Define the present role and future direction of the laboratory
3. Formulate, and then select from, strategic options
4. Determine specific objectives (within a business plan) to achieve the strategy
5. Implement the plan according to a timetable with agreed milestones
6. Monitor progress

*Strength, weaknesses, opportunities and threats (see text).

Workload assessment and costing of tests

Health care legislation in different countries determines the extent to which a laboratory requires to monitor workload and to cost its tests for clinical users. Even when this is not a legislative requirement, all laboratories should maintain accurate records of workload and costs in order to apportion resources to each section. Computerization of laboratories has greatly facilitated this process.

Methods for determining the workload of individual laboratory sections, adjusted for test complexity, include those of the College of American Pathologists,[8] the Canadian Workload Measurement System,[30] and the Welcan system as used in the United Kingdom.[5] In the Welcan system, one unit of workload corresponds to one minute of productive (excluding waiting) time of technical, clerical and aide staff. Examples are given in Table 3.3. Welcan units encompass the total time taken from receipt of a specimen to issue of the report and are based on timing studies from a range of laboratories. Welcan units exclude, however, training time and the absence of staff for annual leave or sickness. Continuous refinement has increased the value of Welcan units for assessing workload, particularly for tests that are performed in high volume.

When the total number of workload units is known, this can be divided into total laboratory cost to determine the cost per Welcan unit, for example (I. Cavill, personal communication):

Table 3.3 Examples of Welcan units for haematological tests

Test	Welcan unit value
Automated blood count	3
Prothrombin time (manual method)	5
ABO and Rh(D) blood group (manual method)	5
Blood film morphology including differential white cell count	8
Venepuncture	8
Reticulocyte count (manual method)	9
Vitamin B_{12} (isotope method)	10
Haemoglobin electrophoresis (agar gel)	25
Coagulation factor (one-stage, manual, clotting assay)	60
Red cell survival	180

$$\frac{\text{Total laboratory cost}}{\text{No. of operators} \times \text{Welcan units} \times \text{Efficiency}}$$
$$\text{(hours per annum)} \qquad \text{index}\star$$

$\star$effective bench time (e.g. 0.55 for 55% efficiency)

The limitations of using Welcan units for determining costs have been described.[9,32] The approach can, however, facilitate comparison of the relative labour costs between different sections of a department which share common overhead costs. Limitations of the approach become apparent when non-labour costs are apportioned to Welcan units and when different departments are compared as there is no standardized method of determining and apportioning overhead costs. Full absorption costing includes all overheads (e.g. building maintenance, portering services, transport, laboratory cleaning, personnel management), but the apportionment of such indirect costs remains highly variable.

Costing of tests is greatly facilitated by computer software programmes that offer spreadsheets. The latter comprise a matrix of columns and rows of financial numerical data that allow costs to be calculated for different levels of workload, staffing or automation. Individual cells of the matrix may contain not only numerical data but also a mathematical instruction; a library of such mathematical formulae allows complex data analysis to be performed. Various software packages are available for calculating laboratory costs and for the modelling exercises necessary to determine prices (Audit Commission Pathology Costing System, Audit Commission, Bristol; Data Tree, Data Tree Software Ltd., Bodelwyddan;[14] Pathology Manager, Lynx Management Systems Ltd., London). Such software packages are invaluable for determining laboratory test prices, particularly in countries with a health care system that encourages competition between hospital laboratories with consequential pressure on test prices.

Cost-effective working

Most laboratories are now expected by management to have an annual programme of continuous improvement (based on the Japanese concept 'kaizen'),[29] including increased cost-effectiveness. Each laboratory section should therefore aim for incremental improvements in productivity; these can often achieve revenue savings of up to 5% per annum. Larger savings are usually beyond the ability of a continuous improvement programme and require more fundamental restructuring of departments.

Most organizations tend to specialize and become more segmented with time. This can occur within haematology laboratories so that a previously fluid network of integrated sections can become rigidly segmented into work areas that operate as independent kingdoms. In some countries, the pathology disciplines may be separate and located in different buildings; in other countries, national legislation determines that laboratories in adjacent hospitals must provide an independent and comprehensive service. A first step to cost-effective working is to remove these segmental barriers in order to achieve economies of scale and cross-fertilization between laboratories.

The overnight and week-end emergency service is an important cost factor in many large departments, some laboratories retaining a disproportionately large day-time establishment to provide cover for the emergency service. Approaches to lowering costs include the employment of part-time staff for emergency work, extending the routine working day until the workload peak has passed (e.g. 8 p.m.), moving to a 24-hour service, or sharing a common emergency service between hospitals. Turnaround time, safety of blood transfusion practice, and other quality measures of the emergency service must be maintained, however.

Automation is another means of lowering revenue costs, if the number of staff is thereby reduced, but automated equipment must be used to high capacity and ideally throughout a 24-hour service. Computer spreadsheets are useful for determining the optimal mix of staff and automation for different levels of workload. If the equipment is purchased, and thereby added to the capital assets of the laboratory, then the consequential cost of any capital asset charge and of eventually replacing the equipment (e.g. 10% per annum of total value) must be taken into account. Leasing equipment can be a better alternative and, in some countries, most equipment is obtained in this way. Careful calculation of the lease cost is required, as this can be up to 20% higher than outright purchase. Advantages of leasing include flexibility to upgrade equipment should workload increase or technology change. Inclusion of consumables and maintenance costs in the lease agreement allows outgoings to be known for the duration of the lease.

When automation is coupled with centralization of the service to another site, care must be taken to maintain service quality. Loss of contact between clinical users and laboratory staff will compromise, in particular, the pre-analytical phase of the test process and may lead to inappropriate requests, excessive requests, and test samples that are of inadequate volume or are poorly identified. When services are centralized, attention must be paid to all phases (pre-analytical, analytical and post-analytical) of the test process. Failure to do so will encourage clinicians to establish independent satellite laboratories.

INSTRUMENTATION

Equipment evaluation

Evaluation of equipment to match the nature and volume of laboratory workload is a critically important exercise. Protocols for evaluating blood cell counters and other haematology instruments have been published by the International Committee (now Council) for Standardization in Haematology.[19–21] The following are usually included in such evaluations:

1. Verification of instrument requirements for space and services.
2. Extent of technical training required to operate the instrument.
3. Clarity and usefulness of instruction manual.

4. Assessment of safety (mechanical, electrical, microbiological and chemical).
5. Determination of:
   (a) linearity;
   (b) precision;
   (c) carry-over;
   (d) accuracy by comparison with measurement by definitive or reference methods;
   (e) comparability with an established method used in the laboratory;
   (f) sensitivity (i.e. determination of the smallest change in analyte concentration which gives a measured result);
   (g) specificity (i.e. extent of errors caused by interfering substances).
6. Throughput time and number of specimens that can be processed within a normal working day.
7. Cost per test.
8. Reliability of the instrument when in routine use and adequacy of service and maintenance provided.
9. Staff acceptability, impact on laboratory organization and level of technical expertise required to operate the instrument.

As a rule, this type of evaluation is carried out by a reference laboratory on behalf of a national consumer organization or government health agency such as the Medical Devices Agency of the Department of Health, London. After an instrument has been purchased and installed, however, a less extensive check of performance with regard to precision, linearity, carry-over and comparability is often useful and details are given below.

Precision

Carry out appropriate measurements 10–20 times consecutively on three or more specimens selected in the pathological range so as to include a low, a high and a normal concentration of the analyte. Calculate standard deviation (SD) and coefficient of variation (CV) as derived on p. 584.

Linearity

This demonstrates the effects of dilution. Prepare a specimen with a high concentration of the analyte to be tested and, as accurately as possible, make a series of dilutions in plasma so as to obtain 10 samples with evenly spaced concentration levels between 10% and 100%. Measure each sample and calculate the means. Plot results on arithmetic graph paper. All points should fall on a straight line which should pass through the zero of the horizontal and vertical axes. Inspection of the graph will show whether there is linearity throughout the range or whether it is limited to part of the range. The actual results should lie within the limits of the CVs obtained from the analysis of precision (see above) at low, intermediate and high levels of the analyte.

Carry-over

This indicates the extent to which measurement of an analyte in a specimen is likely to be affected by the preceding specimen. Measure a specimen with a high concentration in triplicate, immediately followed by a specimen with a low concentration of the analyte.

$$\text{Carry-over (\%)} = \frac{l_1 - l_3}{h_3 - l_3} \times 100$$

where l_1 and l_3 are the results of the first and third measurements of the samples with a low concentration and h_3 is the third measurement of the sample with a high concentration.

Comparability

This tests whether the new instrument (or method) gives results which agree satisfactorily with those obtained with an established procedure. Test specimens should be measured alternately, or in batches, by the two procedures. If results by the two methods are analysed by correlation coefficient (r), a high correlation does not mean that the two methods agree. Correlation coefficient is a measure of relation and not agreement. It is better to use the limits of agreement method.[6] Plot the differences between paired results on the vertical axis of linear graph paper against the means of the pairs on the horizontal axis (Fig. 3.1); differences between the methods are then readily

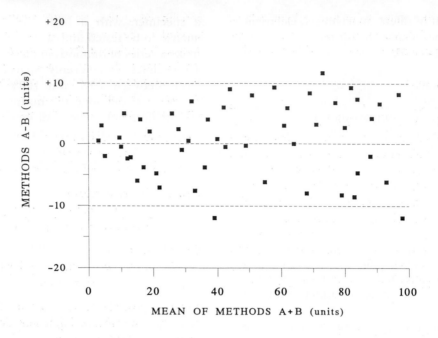

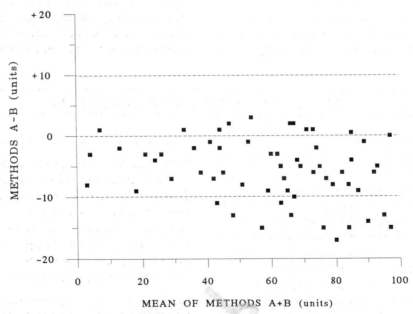

Fig. 3.1   Limits of agreement method. Shows mean values for paired results by two methods A plus B (horizontal axis) plotted against the differences (A minus B) between the paired results (vertical axis). Horizontal lines represent equality with range of ±10 units (mean ±SD). Upper figure shows no bias between methods A and B, whereas lower figure shows false high results (negative values) for method B.

apparent over the range from low to high values. If the scatter of differences increases at high values, logarithmic transformed data should be plotted.

Maintenance logs

All laboratory equipment should be inspected regularly and specific maintenance procedures carried out. Each item of laboratory equipment should have a maintenance log to document what maintenance is required, the desired frequency and when it was last carried out. The log includes servicing and repairs by the manufacturer. Equipment used to test biological specimens must be cleaned thoroughly before a maintenance procedure is carried out to reduce the biohazard. The procedure for such cleaning must be documented (as a standard operating procedure) together with the name of the cleaner and the date.

Efficiency of laboratory tests

To evaluate the diagnostic efficiency of an individual laboratory test, it is necessary to calculate test sensitivity and specificity.[13] Sensitivity is the percentage of true positive results when a test is applied to patients known to have the relevant disease. Specificity is the percentage of true negative results when the test is applied to healthy subjects. Test efficiency is the percentage of results that are true results, whether positive or negative. These parameters are calculated as follows:

$$\text{Test sensitivity in disease} = \frac{\text{True positive results}}{\text{True positive + False negative results}} \times 100$$

$$\text{Test specificity in health} = \frac{\text{True negative results}}{\text{True negative + False positive results}} \times 100$$

$$\text{Test efficiency} = \frac{\text{True positive + True negative results}}{\text{All results}} \times 100$$

It is not possible to have both 100% sensitivity and 100% specificity. High sensitivity is necessary when a disease is serious and should not be missed; high specificity is desirable when a false positive result may have a significant psychological or other adverse effect on the patient.

LABORATORY DATA PROCESSING

It is essential that accurate records of laboratory results are kept for whatever period is stipulated by national legislation. Computer assisted data handling is essential for all but the smallest laboratory. For long-term storage of data, possibilities include a printed (hard) copy, a microfiche, and the newer compact disc read-only memory (CD-ROM) or write once, read-many (WORM) systems that are read using a modified personal computer.

Laboratory results are usually issued as numerical data with, whenever possible, abnormal results highlighted for the clinician. Report forms should be reader friendly. Serial data are particularly useful to illustrate any trend with time and may be in the form of a cumulative numerical display or a graph. The latter is widely used to facilitate adjustment of dosage of drugs that suppress bone marrow activity. An arithmetical scale should be used to display haemoglobin, red cell count and reticulocytes, while platelet and leucocyte counts are best displayed on a logarithmic scale.

LABORATORY COMPUTERS

Developments in computer technology have made available powerful microcomputers and sophisticated computer software at moderate prices. Such computers may be an integral part of an analytical instrument or interfaced to it by cable. Stand-alone personal computers, requiring data to be keyed in manually, also have wide application in haematology laboratories (Table 3.4).

Table 3.4 Some uses of laboratory personal computers

Statistics
Graphics
Word processing
Desktop publishing
Database files
Spreadsheets
Workload recording
Test costing and invoicing
Managing budgets
Audit systems
Expert systems – clinical decision support
– teaching/training
Stock control

When purchasing a laboratory personal computer, a random access memory (RAM) capacity of 4 megabytes, with potential for further expansion, is now desirable to run sophisticated programs. There is considerable attraction in interconnecting such computers within a local area network to allow flexibility and data interchange. Printers and plotters can then be shared and multiple users can use a common database.

Larger computer systems catering for all the pathology disciplines require a larger RAM (e.g. 30–60 megabytes) and the purchase or lease of such systems requires considerable planning as to the necessary specification. Much time and effort are involved in the procurement process and expert advice is needed.

PRE-ANALYTICAL AND POST-ANALYTICAL STAGES OF TESTING

The area of influence of a haematology laboratory should nowadays extend to the pre-analytical stage (test requesting, blood sample collection and transport to the laboratory) and to the post-analytical stage (return of results to the clinician) of the test cycle.

Test requesting

There is considerable variation between clinicians in their test ordering patterns and pathologists have historically exerted little influence on test request patterns; sustained educational programmes have sometimes achieved more selective testing.[2] Innovations in modifying requesting patterns have included use of problem-orientated request forms[12,36] and computer-assisted ordering of tests according to protocols written by specialist clinical teams.[25] Computerized laboratories have the advantage that test requests can be stratified according to clinician, or clinical directorate, of origin but non-computerized laboratories can achieve similar information by manual sampling of request forms.

Sample collection and delivery

Blood sample collection by phlebotomists and manual delivery of specimen tubes to the laboratory by porters are traditionally performed by different work teams whose activities are not co-ordinated. Blood samples may therefore remain in clinical areas awaiting collection by porters who then follow a fixed circuit of other hospital areas before eventually reaching the laboratory. Once responsibility for blood collection and transport is held by the laboratory, however, these separate activities can be co-ordinated. Alternative and faster means of specimen delivery to laboratories include rail track (Telelift (UK) Ltd., Emsworth) or pneumatic tube (Air Tube Conveyors Ltd., Warley) conveyor systems.[22]

Return of results

Computer-assisted reporting of results to linked printers located in clinical areas is an ideal, but most hospitals rely on manual transport of result sheets and this can significantly prolong request completion times. Pneumatic tube and rail track conveyor systems used for the pre-analytical stage can also be used for rapid return of results to wards and clinics. Return of results is, of course, no guarantee that ward or clinic staff will react in a timely way to change a patient's treatment or file report forms in the patient's medical record. Audit trials of selected test results (e.g. action taken on a haemoglobin electrophoresis result that recommends further study of the family or issue of a medical card) are helpful in determining whether the sequence from requesting a test to taking clinical action has been completed.

Test turnaround time

Test turnaround time is most easily measured as the time lapse between arrival of a blood specimen in the laboratory and issue of the validated result. It is possible, but tedious, to use a date/time stamp to record manually the arrival and issue times for each request/report form. In a computerized laboratory, however, it is relatively easy to record these times and then to analyze the data to calculate the median time for completing each test (the distribution is usually not Gaussian) and the 95th percentile; the percentage of tests completed within a pre-selected time is also of value.[34,35] Computer-assisted graphical presentation of the frequency distribution of completed tests is a useful way of displaying turnaround times for individual tests (Fig. 3.2).

Test turnaround time, as defined above, refers to the analytical stage of testing and excludes the time delay of the pre-analytical and post-analytical stages of testing. Laboratories should hold the budget and have responsibility for all three stages. If then becomes possible to extend the measurement of analytical turnaround time to the more meaningful parameter of request completion time (total time from initiation of the request to delivery of the result to a clinician). Request completion time is becoming an increasingly important criterion of laboratory quality.[16]

CUSTOMIZED SERVICES

Near-patient testing

Specialist clinical areas within hospitals have an increasing need for a customized laboratory service to meet their particular requirements for patient care. When a fast results service is the particular requirement, laboratory testing within the clinical area is an option. Intensive care units have a long established need for near-patient monitoring of blood gases, but other clinicians use laboratory tests for monitoring ill patients and for making rapid decisions on treatment (such as the early diagnosis of myocardial infarction prior to thrombolytic therapy[10]), and this has increased demand for a rapid results service. Haematology, oncology, and diabetes out-patient clinics also require a rapid service. Instrument manufacturers are now developing haematology analysers for this market so that demand for haematology testing nearer the patient will increase.

Hospital architects have often located diagnostic laboratories in areas of the hospital that are remote from critical care and out-patient areas. Rapid transit systems, including pneumatic tubes (see above), are often the preferred alternative to multiple satellite testing areas, particularly when the main laboratory already offers a 24-hour rapid results service. Knowledge of test turnaround time (Fig. 3.2) is required to make an informed decision on the need for near-patient testing in satellite areas. When near-patient testing equipment is the preferred option, the satellite laboratory and its equipment must be the responsibility of the appropriate pathology discipline. This is essential for purposes of quality control, safety and accreditation whether the satellite is staffed by laboratory staff, as in busy locations, or used

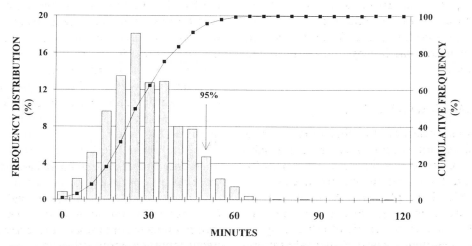

Fig. 3.2   Frequency histogram, cumulative percentage (■-■-■), and 95th percentile (arrow) showing analytical completion time for non-urgent prothrombin times.

by medical staff or nurses as a marginal activity. A designated member of laboratory staff should supervise this service, visiting each test location daily and ensuring that all results and quality control data are integrated into the main laboratory computer system. Some instruments designed for near-patient testing will store quality control data on a computer floppy disk which can be removed and taken to the main laboratory. Essential criteria for satisfactory near-patient working are described by Marks.[24]

The concept of near-patient testing is further developed in patient-centred care, or patient-focused, hospitals. This involves the restructuring of a hospital into a series of mini-hospitals, each of which comprises a specialist care area for patients requiring similar clinical resources (e.g. orthopaedic surgery). Ancillary services, such as basic radiology and simple laboratory testing, are then provided at ward level. Hospital staff are retrained to form multi-skilled, multi-disciplinary care teams that cross traditional professional boundaries to combine, for example, nursing and pathology testing. Pilot studies of the cost-effectiveness of this approach are in progress in North America and the United Kingdom.[23]

Laboratory services for general practitioners

The customers of a haematology laboratory include not only hospital clinicians but also general practitioners working in primary health care; they can provide up to 30%, but more usually 10%, of a laboratory's workload. A hospital laboratory that wishes to attract work from primary health care must provide a customized service which should be planned in close co-operation with general practitioners as they have different priorities from hospital practitioners. Failure to provide a customized service will favour the independent development of pathology services within large polyclinics in primary care as another variant of near-patient testing. The main components of a customized service include the following.

Quality assurance

General practitioners are not specialists in laboratory medicine and require evidence that a haema-

tology laboratory provides a service of high quality. Such evidence may include accreditation of the laboratory, participation in external quality control schemes, a good local reputation amongst other laboratory users, and a willingness to collaborate with general practitioners in a mutually beneficial audit programme.

Pre-analytical service

Education of the general practitioner is important. This may include a users' handbook or wallchart (to show the correct specimen container and volume of blood required), reference ranges, requirements for patient preparation (e.g. fasting), the timing of any medication that may affect the test result, and the turnaround time for each test. The latter is important so that patients can be given a follow-up appointment to be told the result. Handbooks should be of loose-leaf format to facilitate updating. An occasional laboratory newsheet may also be of value, particularly when a new test or service is introduced. Education should also cover safety aspects, such as how to deal with blood spillage or a needlestick injury.

Specimen collection and transport are also of high priority. A general practitioner may require health centre staff to be trained and accredited for collecting blood samples. A specimen transport system at an agreed time of day (so that patients can be given a suitable appointment for blood collection) is particularly important. Request forms should be standardized, with the ideal being one request form for all pathology requests.

Post-analytical service

The general practitioner needs a fast report service for abnormal test results to a direct telephone number at the health centre. To facilitate contact with the laboratory there should be a direct dial help-line to the haematologist of the day. Transmission of results by telefax becomes too time-consuming for laboratories when many results are involved and there is also the problem of confidentiality unless a computer-assisted call-back system is used to identify the correct recipient number before the data are transmitted. Direct transfer of encoded data via telephone from the laboratory computer to that of the practice may be justified for major users.

Close attention to the general practitioner's needs is an important mark of laboratory quality and is important to the hospital's practice as referral of patients from primary care often follows the initial use of laboratory services.

HEALTH AND SAFETY

Good safety practice must be extended to all aspects of the laboratory's work, including satellite near-patient test areas and satellite storage refrigerators for blood and blood products. Each haematology laboratory should designate a safety officer who has sufficient seniority, and is given the authority, to implement departmental safety policy in all sections of the laboratory. The safety officer should be responsible for day-to-day management of safety issues and should be directly accountable to the head of department. Departmental safety policy should be documented in booklet form which is readily accessible in each section of the laboratory and issued to each member of staff. A loose-leaf format facilitates updating. This booklet will refer to relevant local and national safety legislation but must provide a comprehensive account of departmental safety policy. This will include known and potential hazards in relation to infection, fire, radiation, and other injury. Where a hazard cannot be eliminated, the risk should be reduced so far as is reasonably practicable by, for example, reducing the frequency or period of exposure, as risk is a function of hazard and probability. Other aspects of safety policy relevant to a haematology laboratory are listed in Table 3.5. Useful references to laboratory safety legislation within the United Kingdom are given by Telfor Brunton.[33]

It is particularly important to have a clear policy in the event of needlestick injury to a member of staff, with immediate referral to the appropriate hospital department of occupational health which should provide a 24-hour advisory service.

The safety officer must have the training and time to do the job well and provide training for other staff. The officer should represent the laboratory on relevant safety committees and work closely with hospital occupational health, control of infection, and radiation protection officers.

Within the department, a statutory safety committee should be established as a useful forum for safety audit.

HANDLING BIOHAZARDOUS SPECIMENS

All material of human origin should be regarded as capable of transmitting infection. Material from patients suffering from, or at risk of, hepatitis or human immunodeficiency virus (HIV) infection requires particular care. The laboratory safety policy must define the special precautions required when blood is collected from such patients and when specimens are handled in the laboratory. Laboratories that receive specimens from high-risk clinical groups (e.g. haemophilia unit, liver unit) may need to adopt such safety

Table 3.5 Some aspects of safety policy within the remit of a haematology department safety officer

---

Blood collection from high-risk patients
Labelling, transport and reception of specimens
Handling and containment of high-risk specimens
Location of protective equipment
Needlestick injury
Sharps disposal
Blood spillage
Hazard risk assessment for all substances in the laboratory
Near-patient testing
Protective clothing
Health records of staff, including immunization
Equipment maintenance and log books
Visitors to the department
Waste disposal including access to an autoclave
Electrical equipment testing
Recording of accidents
Safety cabinet monitoring
Laboratory cleaning policies
Laboratory security, including out-of-hours working
Policy for postal specimens
Radiation protection
Fire precautions
Training in safety
Safety inspections
Advisory service to general practitioners

---

precautions for all specimens received irrespective of whether or not the specimens are labelled as biohazardous.

Universal precautions for good safety practice include:

1. Experienced staff to perform procedures.

2. Venepucture to be performed wearing disposable plastic or thin rubber gloves. A fresh pair of gloves must be used for each patient. Institutions that consider that routine gloving for all phlebotomies is not necessary should periodically re-evaluate their policy. Care must be taken to prevent injuries when handling syringes and disposing of the needles. Do not recap used needles by hand; do not detach the needle from the syringe or break, bend, or otherwise manipulate used needles by hand. Used disposable syringes and needles (and other sharp items such as glass slides) must be placed in a puncture-resistant container for disposal.

3. Specimens to be handled in a microbiological safety cabinet (if the procedure involves generation of an aerosol) or in a clearly segregated and designated area of the laboratory.

4. Specimens to be handled using protective clothing (close-fitting disposable plastic or thin rubber gloves, disposable plastic apron, glasses or goggles).

5. Centrifugation to be performed in sealed centrifuge buckets.

6. Disposable plastic should be used instead of glassware and sharp-pointed instruments (e.g. scissors) should not be used.

7. On completion of the work, the laboratory bench must be disinfected immediately using freshly prepared 1% w/v sodium hypochlorite solution (10 000 p.p.m. available chlorine). Disposable pipettes should be used but, if reusable pipettes are essential, they must be soaked in this solution for 30 min or longer. Absorbent granules containing sodium dichloro*iso*cyanurate, which releases chlorine when wet, or organic chlorine-releasing compounds (e.g. chloramine), are useful for containment of liquid spillages.

8. Some automated equipment can be disinfected by flushing several times with 10% w/v sodium hypochlorite, or with 2% w/v glutaraldehyde, followed by several flushes with water. Only glutaraldehyde should be used in instruments with a metal surface as hypochlorite causes corrosion. Other instruments have special requirements for decontamination; always refer to the manufacturer's instructions.

9. Used material to be placed in designated biohazard plastic sacs and transported with care to an autoclave.

Laboratory centrifuges require particular attention, as they develop high energies, and should be checked frequently for corrosion and hair-line cracks. Any spillage of blood should be dealt with immediately and the bowl, head and buckets (including rubber pads) should be disinfected regularly with 2% w/v glutaraldehyde solution. Centrifuges should never be cleaned using hypochlorite solution or other metal corrosives. Special care is required when a glass or plastic tube breaks in a centrifuge (Table 3.6).

Toxic or carcinogenic reagents

All potentially hazardous substances in a laboratory must be documented in a risk assessment which also contains instructions on safe handling. Such reagents must be stored in a secure place with restricted access, they should be handled only by experienced staff wearing protective clothing, and weighing should be carried out in a fume cupboard whose air flow is regularly monitored (face velocity of around 0.8 m/s).

Laboratories contain many and varied hazards but the actual risk to staff is small. Good safety practice is essential, however, to minimize the risk of illness arising from occupational exposure and safety should therefore be accorded the highest priority.

Table 3.6 Recommended procedure when a specimen tube breaks during centrifugation

1. Switch off centrifuge motor and do not open lid for 30 min. Inform the safety officer.
2. When breakage involves a known high risk specimen in a sealed bucket, gloves, goggles and a protective apron must be worn and the bucket opened in a safety cabinet.
3. Strong gloves must be worn and forceps used when removing solid debris. All broken tubes, fragments of glass or plastic, buckets, trunnions and rotor should be placed in 2% w/v glutaraldehyde solution for 24 hours.
4. The centrifuge bowl should be washed with 2% w/v glutaraldehyde solution, left to dry, and washed again.
5. All contaminated disposable material must be placed in appropriate bags for autoclaving.

LABORATORY AUDIT AND ACCREDITATION

Laboratory audit can be defined as the systematic and critical analysis of the quality of the laboratory service. The essence of audit is that it should be continuous and designed to achieve incremental improvement in quality of the day-to-day service. Audit should encompass the pre-analytical, analytical, and post-analytical stages of laboratory practice; some examples are given in Table 3.7.

The first stage of audit is to define the standard to be achieved and this may be in the form of a protocol for test ordering, a surgical maximum blood order schedule, a standard operating procedure for an analytical procedure,[26] or a laboratory policy that states a target turnaround time. These standards will have been agreed within the laboratory and, whenever possible, in conjunction with relevant users of the laboratory. To monitor performance against agreed standards, each laboratory section should form its own audit group or, if there is an audit group for the whole department, it should be open to all grades of staff to allow peer review and to take advantage of the educational value of audit. Laboratory staff should feel that they own and lead the audit process rather than having it imposed upon them. It is good practice to make a short report of each audit meeting, recording attendance, the items identified for improvement, and an action list.

The audit process improves quality simply by examining and questioning established standards; even the process of agreeing standards will itself improve quality. For more sophisticated aspects of audit involving quantitative data, computer-assisted audit can be invaluable.[28] External quality assessment schemes and national accreditation programmes are important aspects of external audit; the more specialist areas of laboratory practice will also require external audit at regional or national level.

The purpose of laboratory accreditation schemes is to allow external audit of a laboratory's organization, management, quality assurance programme, and level of user satisfaction. The advantage to the accredited laboratory is that it can declare to clinical users a defined standard of practice that has been independently confirmed by external peer review. Such review should include access by clinical users, structure (laboratory facilities such as staff and equipment), process (test analyses), outcome (quality of test results including timeliness and interpretation), and use of resources.[4,27] Published descriptions of national accreditation programmes are available for the United States of America,[3] Australia,[18] and the United Kingdom.[1] An overview of the evolution of these and other laboratory accreditation schemes has been prepared by Burnett.[7]

FUTURE TRENDS

The laboratory service of the future is likely to be managed as a network of different test sites with the area of responsibility extending from the main central laboratory to near-patient testing in hospital out-patient and critical care areas and to testing of patients in general practitioner surgeries. The pre-analytical, analytical, and post-analytical areas of this service will be closely integrated to ensure timeliness of test reporting as this will become an increasingly important quality criterion for the pathology service. The ever increasing need for cost effectiveness is likely to forge closer working relationships between the different pathology disciplines, as well as between laboratories within the same discipline. This changing laboratory environment will highlight the need for continuous training of haematology staff in good laboratory management.

Table 3.7   Examples of laboratory audit

Education of laboratory users
Appropriateness of test requests
Appropriateness of blood samples (e.g. adequate volume)
Interpretation of abnormal results
Timeliness of reports
Quality control performance
Cost effectiveness of specialist tests
Telephone reporting of abnormal results
Compliance with safety policies
Use of blood and blood products
Frequency and cause of transfusion reactions
Turnaround time for emergency requests
Satisfaction of out-patients undergoing venepuncture
Satisfaction of laboratory users

REFERENCES

[1]ADVISORY TASK FORCE ON STANDARDS TO THE AUDIT STEERING COMMITTEE OF THE ROYAL COLLEGE OF PATHOLOGISTS (1991). Pathology department accreditation in the United Kingdom: a synopsis. *Journal of Clinical Pathology*, **44**, 798.

[2]BAREFORD, D. and HAYLING, A. (1990). Inappropriate use of laboratory services: long term combined approach to modify request patterns. *British Medical Journal*, **301**, 1305.

[3]BATJER, J. D. (1990). The College of American Pathologists Laboratory Accreditation Programme. *Clinical and Laboratory Haematology*, **12** (Suppl. 1), 135.

[4]BATSTONE, G. F. (1992). Medical audit in clinical pathology. *Journal of Clinical Pathology*, **45**, 284.

[5]BENNETT, C. H. N. (1991). Welcan UK: its development and future. *Journal of Clinical Pathology*, **44**, 617.

[6]BLAND, J. M. and ALTMAN, D. G. (1986). Statistical methods for assessing agreement between two methods of clinical measurement. *Lancet*, **i**, 307.

[7]BURNETT, D. (1993). Laboratory accreditation – an overview. *Journal of the International Federation of Clinical Chemistry*, **5**, 146.

[8]COLLEGE OF AMERICAN PATHOLOGISTS WORKLOAD AND PERSONNEL MANAGEMENT COMMITTEE (1992). *Workload Recording Method and Personnel Management Manual*, College of American Pathologists, Northfield, Ill.

[9]DICK, H. M. (1991). Costing of pathology services in the United Kingdom National Health Service. *Journal of Clinical Pathology*, **44**, 705.

[10]DOWNIE, A. C., FROST, P. G., FIELDEN, P., JOSHI, D. and DANCY, C. M. (1993). Bedside measurement of creatine kinase to guide thrombolysis on the coronary care unit. *Lancet*, **341**, 452.

[11]DRUCKER, P. F. (1990). *Managing the Non-Profit Organization*, p. 155. Butterworth-Heinemann, Oxford.

[12]FRASER, C. G. and WOODFORD, F. P. (1987). Strategies to modify the test-requesting patterns of clinicians. *Annals of Clinical Biochemistry*, **24**, 223.

[13]GALEN, R. S. and GAMBINO, S. (1975). *Beyond Normality: The Predictive Value and Efficiency of Medical Diagnoses*, Wiley, New York.

[14]GOZZARD, D. I., MACAULAY, M. E., NUTTALL, D. S. and JONES, E. R. M. (1992). A pragmatist's approach to pathology costing: the Welsh Datatree project. *Journal of Clinical Pathology*, **45**, 650.

[15]GREENLEY, G. E. (1989). *Strategic Management*, Prentice Hall, London.

[16]HILBORNE, L. H., OYE, R. K., MCARDLE, J. E., REPINSKI, J. A. and RODGERSON, D. O. (1989). Use of specimen turnaround time as a component of laboratory quality. A comparison of clinician expectations with laboratory performance. *American Journal of Clinical Pathology*, **92**, 613.

[17]HUGHES, J. M. (1989). The pathology of performance appraisal. *Institute of Medical Laboratory Sciences Gazette*, **33**, 303.

[18]HYNES, A. F., LEA, A. R. and HAILEY, D. M. (1989). Pathology laboratory accreditation in Australia. *Australian Journal of Medical Laboratory Science*, **10**, 12.

[19]INTERNATIONAL COMMITTEE FOR STANDARDIZATION IN HAEMATOLOGY (1978). Protocol for type testing equipment and apparatus used for haematological analysis. *Journal of Clinical Pathology*, **31**, 275.

[20]INTERNATIONAL COUNCIL FOR STANDARDIZATION IN HAEMATOLOGY (1994). Guidelines for the evaluation of blood cell analysers including those used for differential leucocyte and reticulocyte counting and cell marker applications. *Clinical and Laboratory Haematology*, **16**, 157.

[21]INTERNATIONAL COUNCIL FOR STANDARDIZATION IN HAEMATOLOGY (EXPERT PANEL ON BLOOD RHEOLOGY). (1993). ICSH recommendations for measurement of erythrocyte sedimentation rate. *Journal of Clinical Pathology*, **46**, 198.

[22]KESHGEGIAN, A. A. and BULL, G. E. (1992). Evaluation of a soft-handling computerized pneumatic tube specimen delivery system. Effects on analytical results and turnaround time. *American Journal of Clinical Pathology*, **97**, 535.

[23]LEE, J. G., CLARKE, R. W. and GLASSFORD, G. H. (1993). Physicians can benefit from a patient-focused hospital. *Physician Executive*, **19**, 36.

[24]MARKS, V. (1988). Essential considerations in the provision of near-patient testing facilities. *Annals of Clinical Biochemistry*, **25**, 220.

[25]MUTIMER, D., MCCAULEY, B., NIGHTINGALE, P., RYAN, M., PETERS, M. and NEUBERGER, J. (1992). Computerised protocols for laboratory investigation and their effect on use of medical time and resources. *Journal of Clinical Pathology*, **45**, 572.

[26]NATIONAL COMMITTEE FOR CLINICAL LABORATORY STANDARDS (1984). Clinical laboratory procedure manuals. Approved guideline. *NCCLS Publication GP2-A*, **4**(2), 27. NCCLS, Villanova, PA.

[27]PEDDECORD, K. M. (1989). A regulatory model for clinical laboratories: an empirical evaluation. *Clinical Chemistry*, **35**, 691.

[28]PETERS, M., BROUGHTON, P. M. G. and NIGHTINGALE, P. G. (1991). Use of information technology for auditing effective use of laboratory services. *Journal of Clinical Pathology*, **44**, 539.

[29]SMITH, R. (1990). Medicine's need for kaizen. Putting quality first. *British Medical Journal*, **301**, 679.

[30]STATISTICS CANADA (1989). *Canadian Workload Measurement System. A Schedule of Unit Values for Clinical Laboratory Procedures*, 1989–90 edn. Canadian Government Publishing Centre, Ottawa.

[31]STUART, J. and HICKS, J. M. (1991). Good laboratory management: an Anglo-American perspective. *Journal of Clinical Pathology*, **44**, 793.

[32]TARBIT, I. F. (1990). Laboratory costing system based on number and type of test: its association with the Welcan measurement system. *Journal of Clinical Pathology*, **43**, 92.

[33]TELFER BRUNTON, W. A. (1992). Safety in the laboratory. *Journal of Clinical Pathology*, **45**, 949.

[34]VALENSTEIN, P. N. and EMANCIPATOR, K. (1989). Sensitivity, specificity, and reproducibility of four measures of laboratory turnaround time. *American Journal of Clinical Pathology*, **91**, 452.

[35]WESTGARD, J. O., BURNETT, R. W. and BOWERS, G. N. (1990). Quality management science in clinical chemistry: a dynamic framework for continuous improvement of quality. *Clinical Chemistry*, **36**, 1712.

[36]WONG, E. T. and LINCOLN, T. L. (1983). Ready! Fire! . . . Aim! An inquiry into laboratory test ordering. *Journal of the American Medical Association*, **250**, 2510.

4. Quality assurance

Reference preparations: haemoglobin and
  blood cells 36
Quality control materials for blood counts 37
  Preparation of stabilized whole blood control 38
  Quality control for blood count analysers 39
Analysis of data 40
  Standard deviation of control specimens 40

Control charts 40
Cumulative sum method (CUSUM) 40
Duplicate tests on patients' specimens 42
Use of normal haematological data for quality control 42
Use of patient data for quality control 42
External Quality Assessment (EQA) 44
Routine quality assurance programme 46

Quality assurance in the haematology laboratory is intended to ensure the reliability of the laboratory tests. The objective is to achieve precision and accuracy. *Accuracy* refers to the closeness of the estimated value to that considered to be true. *Precision* refers to the reproducibility of a result, whether accurate or inaccurate. Inaccuracy and/or imprecision occurs as a result of improper standards or reagents, incorrect instrument calibration, or poor technique, e.g. consistently faulty dilution or the use of a method that gives a reaction that is incomplete or not specific for the test.

Precision can be controlled by replicate tests, check tests on previously measured specimens and statistical evaluation of results. Accuracy can, as a rule, be checked only by the use of reference materials which have been assayed by independent methods of known precision. In general, reference materials are either assayed samples that can be measured alongside each batch of routine specimens without being identifiable during the test, or standard preparations handled in a special way.

A quality assurance programme has four separate aspects, namely, internal quality control, external quality assessment, proficiency surveillance and standardization.

Internal quality control is based on monitoring the haematology test procedures that are performed in the laboratory. It includes measurements on specially prepared materials, and repeated measurements on routine specimens, as well as statistical analysis, day by day, of data obtained from the tests which have been routinely carried out. Internal quality control is intended to ensure that there is continual evaluation of the reliability of the work of the laboratory and that control is exercised over the release of test results. However, it is primarily a check of precision (i.e. reproducibility) but not necessarily accuracy.

External quality assessment is the objective evaluation by an outside agency of the performance by a number of laboratories on material which is supplied specially for the purpose; this is usually organized on a national or regional basis. Analysis of performance is retrospective. The objective is to achieve comparability, but again not necessarily accuracy unless the specimens have been assayed by a reference laboratory, using methods of known precision, alongside a reference preparation of known value.

Proficiency surveillance implies critical supervision of all aspects of laboratory tests, whereas internal quality control and external quality assessment relate only to the actual analysis. Thus, account must be taken of collection, labelling, delivery and storage of specimens before the tests are performed (see Chapter 1) and of reading and reporting of results. Proficiency includes maintenance and

35

control of equipment and apparatus. It is also necessary, for correct interpretation of test results, for the laboratory to establish normal reference values that are valid for their test methods and their local population (see Chapter 2).

Standardization refers to both materials and methods. A material standard or reference preparation is used to calibrate analytic instruments and to assign a quantitative value to calibrators. Where possible it must be traceable to a defined physical or chemical measurement based on the metrological units of length (metre), mass (kilogram), amount of substance (mole) and time (seconds). A reference method is an exactly defined technique which provides sufficiently accurate and precise data for it to be used to assess the validity of other methods. The main international authorities concerned with primary standards in haematology are the World Health Organization (WHO)[32] and the International Council for Standardization in Haematology (ICSH)*.[19] The method and/or material standards which are available for various tests are referred to in the sections where tests are described. International reference preparations are not freely available for routine use but are intended to act as standards for assigning values to commercial (or laboratory produced) 'secondary standards' or calibrators. In some countries national standards have been established, while in Europe the Bureau of Reference of the European Community (BCR)** has produced a number of certified reference materials for haematology and clinical chemistry.[16]

REFERENCE PREPARATIONS: HAEMOGLOBIN AND BLOOD CELLS

The availability of an international reference preparation[10] has contributed to improved accuracy of Hb measurement. In several countries working standards are prepared which conform to the international standard and the appropriate national authority certifies that this is so. A limited quantity of the international standard can be obtained from WHO* or ICSH* and a comparable certified reference material which conforms to it is available in Europe**. A method for preparing a lysate is described on p. 38.

As whole blood can be kept only for a short time, it cannot be used as an alternative to a haemiglobincyanide (HiCN) standard for calibration purposes. However, both whole blood and lysates are of use in quality assurance as differences in results obtained with these preparations help to distinguish errors due to incorrect dilution from those due to inadequate mixing or failure of a reagent to bring about complete lysis. Whole-blood reference samples should be introduced into a batch of blood samples and all the samples assayed together.

Red blood cells

Reference preparations for the red cell count are essential for the calibration of electronic particle counters, especially automated systems which can be adjusted arbitrarily. This means that to obtain a true result the machine has to be calibrated using a reference preparation with assigned values of known accuracy (see above).

Natural blood, collected into EDTA, is of no value as a reference preparation because of its short life in the laboratory. Blood will, however, keep for a few weeks at 4°C if acid citrate dextrose (ACD) or citrate phosphate dextrose (CPD) has been added to it. Even so, the mean cell volume (MCV) slowly increases and some of the red cells lyse, with the result that the blood cannot be regarded as a reference material, although it can be used as a control to check the precision and reliable functioning of a cell counting system over relatively short periods of time.[15]

Attempts have been made to provide suitably sized particles in stable suspension as substitutes

---

*WHO: World Health Organization, Biological Standards Division, 1211 Geneva 27, Switzerland.
*ICSH: International Council for Standardization in Haematology, Executive Secretary, Department of Haematology, Western Infirmary, Glasgow, G11 6NT, UK.
**BCR: Community Bureau of Reference of the Commission of the European Union; (now called *Measurement and Testing Programme*), Rue de la Loi 200, B-1049, Brussels, Belgium.

for normal blood cells. These include fixed red cells and spherical latex particles.[16] The cells can be permanently stabilized by fixation, especially in glutaraldehyde solution. The glutaraldehyde causes red cells to shrink in size immediately, and the shrinking process continues for 3–4 days. Thereafter, the cells remain constant in size and shape, and the results of cell counts and cell size distribution remain the same for months or even years. Unfortunately there are disadvantages in using these as a cell reference preparation: in most counting systems, natural (fresh) red blood cells become spherical when diluted, whereas the fixed red cells remain biconcave discs; they are too inflexible and have different flow properties so that they cannot be used to calibrate an instrument for subsequent measurement of natural blood.[24,27] Latex spheres are now available in a series of defined sizes between 2 and 12 μm in diameter; these preparations may be used as primary reference materials for sizing red cells provided that a reliable 'shape factor' can be established.[20]

Platelets

Glutaraldehyde or formaldehyde fixed platelets can provide a useful reference preparation for platelet counting, as they retain their natural shape in dilute suspension. They are derived from platelet-rich plasma. The procedure was described in the 7th edition; it is somewhat laborious and it is important to ensure that aggregation and irreversible clumping of the platelets does not occur. A simpler reliable method using whole blood is described on p. 38.

Leucocytes

Three types of material are suitable as reference materials for leucocyte counts:

1. Leucocytes concentrated from human blood and fixed in the following solution:[28]
   Glacial acetic acid 42 mg
   Sodium sulphate 7 g
   Sodium chloride 7 g
   Water to 1 litre.
2. Glutaraldehyde-fixed turkey or chicken erythrocytes resuspended in leucocyte-free mammalian whole blood.[15]
3. Latex particles 5–6 μm in diameter.[20]

Leucocytes undergo changes when a fresh blood sample is diluted for measurement in an automated counting system. These size changes and other physical properties of the different types of leucocyte are not paralleled in the reference materials. They are thus unsuitable as direct standards for leucocyte sizing and for automated differential counts based on the identification of cells by their physical properties.

QUALITY CONTROL MATERIALS FOR BLOOD COUNTS

Either preserved or stabilized blood provides suitable material for internal quality control procedures for haemoglobin, red cell and leucocyte counts. Human, horse or donkey blood is collected into ACD or CPD (see p. 575) and passed through a blood-infusion set to remove any clots. For lysates, blood in EDTA or heparin is also suitable. One unit of blood (500 ml) will be sufficient to provide about 75 ml of lysate or 200 ml of resuspended stabilized cells. In the procedures described below, care should be taken at all stages to avoid contamination. Where possible sterile glassware and reagents should be used and aseptic handling procedures adopted. To help maintain sterility broad spectrum antibiotics should be added to the product, e.g. 25–50 mg of penicillin together with 25–50 mg of gentamycin per 500 ml.

When human blood is used it should, if possible, first be checked to ensure that it is hepatitis antigen and HIV-antibody negative. If this information is not available it should be handled in the same way as a patient's sample (see p. 31).

Preparation of preserved blood

Collect a unit of blood into a blood transfusion

donor bag containing ACD or CPD. Run the blood through a transfusion-giving set into a sterile 2-litre round-bottomed flask. The contents of the flask must be mixed continuously*.

Adjust the red cell count and leucocyte count as required:

1. To increase the red cell count let the cells settle over exit vents of the pack and then run them into the flask with a minimum of plasma.

2. To lower the red cell count, add compatible plasma or a solution containing 1.5 volumes of ACD and 10 volumes of 9 g/l NaCl.

3. To raise the leucocyte count add fixed avian cells (p. 39).

4. To lower the leucocyte count, pass blood through a leucocyte filter.** Add antibiotic (see above). With continuous mixing, dispense into sterile containers*** and cap tightly. Store at 4°C. Assign values for Hb, red cell and leucocyte counts and packed cell volume (PCV) by 5–10 replicate measurements on each of three vials, using the counter on which the subsequent tests will be performed. The coefficient of variation (CV) should not exceed 2%. Check homogeneity of dispensing by repeated counts on five randomly selected vials. Before analysis, mix a sample on a roller mixer or continuously by hand for 5 min before opening. Unopened vials of human blood should keep in good condition for about 3 weeks at 4°C, equine blood for up to 2 months.[15]

Preparation of lysate

Collect blood as described above into a blood transfusion donor bag. Centrifuge at c 2000*g* for 20 min and remove the plasma aseptically. Add an equal volume of 9 g/l NaC1, mix well, transfer to a sterile centrifuge bottle and re-centrifuge; discard the supernatant and the buffy coat. Repeat the saline wash three times to ensure complete removal of the plasma, leucocytes and platelets. Add to the washed cells half their volume of carbon tetrachloride, cap and then shake vigorously on a mechanical shaker or vibrator for 1 h. Then keep overnight at 4°C to allow the lipid/cell debris to form a semi-solid surface between the carbon tetrachloride and lysate. On the following day, centrifuge at c 2500*g* for 20 min, remove the upper lysate layers and pool them in a clean bottle.

Using gentle vacuum suction, e.g. by water-pump, filter the lysate through Whatman No. 1 filter paper in a Buchner funnel. Repeat filtration using Whatman No. 42 filter paper, changing the paper whenever the filtration slows down. It is important not to overload the funnel with lysate. To each 70 ml of lysate add 30 ml of glycerol. Mix well; if it is necessary to lower the Hb concentration, add 30% glycerol in saline. Add antibiotic (see p. 37). Mix well and dispense aseptically into sterile containers*** and cap tightly.

Assign a value for Hb concentration by the spectrophotometric method (p. 50); carry out 10 replicate tests, taking samples at random from several vials of the batch. The CV should be less than 2%. Stored at 4°C, the product should retain its assigned value for at least several months.

Fixed cell preparations are suitable for use only in some types of counter. With fully automated systems they must be pre-diluted before being introduced into the instrument.

PREPARATION OF STABILIZED WHOLE BLOOD CONTROL[23]

Reagent

Formaldehyde 37–40%	6.75 ml
Glutaraldehyde 50%	0.75 ml
Trisodium citrate	26 g
Distilled water to	100 ml.

Method

Obtain whole blood in CPD or ACD. This should be as fresh as possible and not more than 48 h old. Filter through a 40 μm blood filter and measure the volume. Add 1 volume of reagent to 50 volumes of the blood. If required, raise or lower the red cell or leucocyte count as described above. Add antibiotic (p. 37).

Mix well and then with continuous mixing dispense into sterile containers; cap tightly and seal

---

*A mixing unit which is particularly suitable has been designed specifically for this.[5,29]
** e.g. Sepacell R-500 (Asahi Medical Co., Tokyo).
***γ-Irradiated containers are available from most laboratory suppliers. Autoclaving and dry heat sterilization distort some containers and caps, subsequently causing leakage when filled.

with plastic tape. Refrigerate at 4°C until needed. Unopened vials should keep in good condition for several weeks at 4°C.

For analysis, the sample should be gently mixed on a roller mixer or by hand before opening. Assign values for Hb and cell counts by 5–10 replicate tests on each of three vials from the batch under standardized conditions. The CV should not exceed 2%. Note, however, that the PCV by centrifugation will be c 10% lower than the haematocrit obtained by automated counters.

QUALITY CONTROL FOR BLOOD COUNT ANALYSERS

The method described below provides a suitable preparation for control of total red cell, leucocyte and platelet counting by an electronic instrument as well as haemoglobin. It should be stable for c 3 weeks if kept at 4°C.

Method

Collect a unit of human blood into CPD anti-coagulant (p. 575). Carry out the subsequent procedure no later than 1 day after collection.

Filter the blood through a blood transfusion recipient set into a 500 ml glass bottle.

Add 1 ml of fresh 40% formaldehyde. Mix well by inverting and then leave on a roller mixer for 1 h.

Leave at 4°C for 7 days, mixing by inverting a few times each day. At the end of this period of storage mix well on a roller mixer for 20 min and then with constant mixing by hand dispense in 2-ml volumes into sterile containers.

Preparation of stabilized cell suspension (pseudo-leucocytes)[30]

Chicken and turkey red blood cells are nucleated, and when fixed their size as recognized on electronic cell counters is within the leucocyte range. They are thus suitable to serve as pseudo-leucocytes.

For use as a white blood cell (WBC) control, 25 ml of blood collected into any anticoagulant will suffice; after processing, an appropriate amount is added to preserved whole blood. Sterility must be maintained throughout the procedure. Centrifuge blood at c 2000g for 20 min and remove the plasma aseptically. Add an equal volume of 0.15 mol/l phosphate buffer, pH 7.4 (p. 578); mix and transfer to a sterile centrifuge bottle; recentrifuge and discard the supernatant and buffy coat. Repeat the wash and centrifugation twice. To the washed cells add 10 times their volume of glutaraldehyde fixative (0.25% in 0.15 mol/l phosphate buffer, pH 7.4). Leave overnight at 4°C. On the next day shake vigorously to ensure complete resuspension. Mix on a mechanical mixer for 1 h. To check that fixation has been complete, centrifuge 2–3 ml of the suspension, discard the supernatant and add water to the deposit. If lysis occurs, the stock glutaraldehyde requires replacement.

When fixation is complete (i.e. after 18 h exposure), centrifuge the suspension at c 2000g for 10 min and discard the supernatant. Add an equal volume of water to the fixed cell deposit, resuspend and mix by stirring and shaking; recentrifuge at c 2000g for 10 min and discard the supernatant; repeat twice. Resuspend the fixed cells to c 30% concentration in 9 g/l NaCl. Mix well with vigorous shaking. If it is intended to keep this preparation as a stock, autoclave at 121°C for 15 min, add antibiotic (see p. 37), cap tightly, seal with plastic tape and store at 4°C.

When required, resuspend by vigorous hand shaking or on a vortex mixer until no clumps remain at the base of the container, and then mix on a rotary mixer for at least 20 min before opening the vial. The cells in unopened vials should be stable for several years.

For use as a WBC surrogate, after resuspension as described above, transfer an appropriate amount to a volume of preserved blood (p. 37) from which the leucocytes have been depleted by filtration (p. 38). Establish the count by 5–10 replicate measurements from each of three vials from the batch. The CV should be 5%.

If it is intended to simulate other cellular components, dilute appropriately in a solution of 60 vol glycerol and 40 vol 9 g/l NaCl. Mix well for at least 20 min and then with continuous mixing in a mixing unit (p. 38) or constant shaking by hand dispense into sterile containers with two or three 3 mm glass beads. Cap tightly and seal with a plastic seal. For use, resuspend by vigorous shaking by hand for least 10 min before opening the tube.

Cap tightly and seal with plastic tape. Store at 4°C. Before use mix the vials on a roller mixer for 10–20 min at room temperature. Establish the count for each parameter by 10 replicate measurements on each instrument for which it is intended as a control.

An occasional batch may be found to be unsatisfactory and should be discarded.

ANALYSIS OF DATA

STANDARD DEVIATION OF CONTROL SPECIMENS

If a value is assigned to a specimen a number of times, dispersion of results around the mean will indicate the error of reproducibility. This can be expressed as the standard deviation (SD). Subsequently, 95% of results on the same specimen should be within ±2 SD and 99.7% within ±3 SD. Thus, by chance alone 1 in 20 of the measurements might be expected to fall outside ±2 SD but only 1 in 333 outside ±3 SD. If the measurements are more widely dispersed, this indicates an error in the test.

To determine the SD, 10–20 identical tests are carried out on samples of the specimen. The standard deviation is then calculated as shown on p. 584.

Calculating the coefficient of variation (CV) provides an alternative way of expressing the dispersion of results. The advantage of the CV is that it relates the SD to the level of the measurements. It is calculated as shown on p. 584.

CONTROL CHARTS

The use of control charts, originally described by Shewhart,[26] were first applied in clinical chemistry by Levey and Jennings.[13] They are now widely used in haematology.[7,9]

Samples of the control specimen are included in every batch of patients' specimens and the results checked on a control chart. To check precision it is not necessary to know the exact value of the control specimen. If, however, its value has been determined reliably by a reference method, the same material can also be used to check accuracy or to calibrate an instrument. If possible, controls with high, low and normal values should be used. It is advisable to use at least one control sample per batch even if the batch is very small. As the controls are intended to simulate random sampling, they must be treated exactly like the patients' specimens. The results obtained with the control samples can be plotted on a chart as described below.

The mean value and SD of the control specimen should first be established, as described above, in the laboratory where the tests on specimens are performed. It is not appropriate to use control limits provided by manufacturers of materials. Using arithmetical graph paper a horizontal line is drawn to represent the mean (as a base) and on an appropriate scale of quantity and unit, lines representing +2 SD and –2 SD are drawn above and below the mean (Fig. 4.1). The results of successive control sample measurements are plotted. If the test is satisfactory, sequential results will oscillate about the mean value and less than 5% of the results will fall outside 2 SD. The following indicate a fault in technique or in the instrument or reagent used:

Two or more results on or outside the + 2 SD and – 2 SD limits.
Consecutive values rising.
Consecutive values falling.
Consecutive values on one side of the mean.

It is, however, important to check that the material itself has not become infected or has deteriorated in any other way.

CUMULATIVE SUM METHOD (CUSUM)[3,9,25]

The CUSUM is the running total of the difference

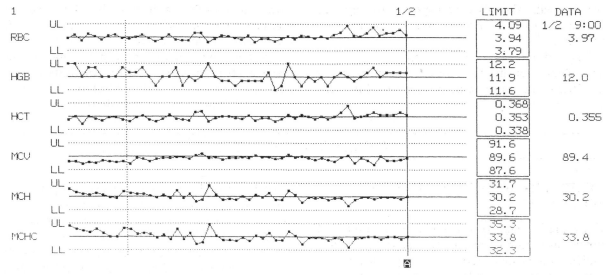

Fig. 4.1 **Control chart.** The upper and lower limits for satisfactory performance have been set at +2 SD and –2 SD, respectively.

between each measurement and the established mean of the control tests. Taking the plus and minus signs into account, it provides another way to display the data obtained in the precision test. It can indicate more sensitively than a control chart a faulty technique or instrument, and it is especially useful for detecting a change in performance due to drift, a consistent error in one direction (bias) or a *slight* progressive drift away from the original mean.

The size of the change that the test is designed to detect (i.e. sensitivity of analysis) can be varied for the individual test, taking account of the clinical significance of changes in the result.

Graphical presentation of CUSUM

Establish the mean value and SD of the control specimen as for the control chart (p. 40). Subtract this mean value from each subsequent observed value for the control specimen and plot the difference on arithmetical graph paper (Fig. 4.2).

Random changes tend to cancel each other out, so that, if the observed values are close to the established mean value, with only random differences, some of the differences will be positive and some negative: the CUSUM will then oscillate around zero, and the charted data will form an

approximately horizontal line. Consistent differences in values will result in all the values being either above or below the zero line, or in a change of the slope of the plotted line; the differences become significant if they reach 2 SD of the mean. The scale used for plotting the results should be such that each unit on the horizontal axis (e.g. 1 day) corresponds in scale to 1 SD on the vertical axis.

Numerical analysis of CUSUM[3,9]

1. Establish the mean and SD of the control preparation; decide on the minimum consistent change which should be detected. This 'decision interval' (DI) might be 2–3 SD or a percentage (e.g. 3%) of the mean.

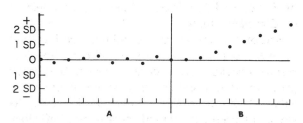

Fig. 4.2 **CUSUM chart.** A illustrates satisfactory performance; B indicates a small consistent error.

2. Calculate the following values for the control:

Upper reference value (URV) = m + DI
Lower reference value (LVM) = m – DI

where m = mean

3. Analyse a sample of the control after every 10–20 patient samples. Start with the CUSUM as zero, and begin to record results only if the measured value of the control falls outside the URV or LRV. If so, record the difference between the result (x) and the appropriate reference value (i.e. x–URV or LRV–x).

4. With each subsequent test add the difference between the result and the *same* reference value to the previous CUSUM score (observing the sign) to give the new CUSUM.

If the CUSUM changes direction but its value does not exceed the opposite reference value, stop recording it. Restart the calculation only if the value again falls outside one of the reference values.

If, on the other hand, the CUSUM changes sign and this causes the result to lie outside the opposite reference value, there has been an abrupt calibration shift or a sporadic 'blunder'. A repeat test on further samples of the control specimen may help to elucidate the cause.

If the CUSUM exceeds the decision interval a significant change in accuracy has probably occurred. Check and correct calibration and then start a new CUSUM as described above.

DUPLICATE TESTS ON PATIENTS' SPECIMENS

This provides another way of checking the precision of routine work.[2] Test ten consecutive specimens in duplicate under careful conditions. Calculate the differences between the pairs of results and derive the SD (p. 584). Subsequent duplicate tests should not differ from each other by more than 2 SD. This method will detect random errors but it is not sensitive to gradual drift nor will it detect incorrect calibration. If the test is always badly done or has an inherent fault the SD will be wide. This procedure is impractical for routine blood counts in a busy laboratory. In this case a few consecutive specimens in a batch should be tested in duplicate from time to time as a rough check.

Another method is to repeat measurement on a few specimens which have been measured originally in an earlier batch. The two tests should agree with each other within 2 SD in the majority of cases.[4] This procedure will detect any deterioration of apparatus and reagents which may have developed between tests, if it is certain that the earlier specimen has not altered on standing.

USE OF NORMAL HAEMATOLOGICAL DATA FOR QUALITY CONTROL

In healthy individuals the blood count remains virtually constant day by day, subject only to the physiological changes already discussed (p. 11). It is possible to use observations on healthy individuals for quality control in routine laboratory work by analysing the results of blood counts from 5–10 healthy subjects at intervals and calculating means and SD for MCV, MCH and MCHC (p. 584). On each occasion the mean should not vary by more than 2 SD and the SDs themselves should remain constant. A significant difference in mean indicates a constant error, e.g. incorrect calibration; random errors will result in an increase in SD although the mean may be unaffected.

USE OF PATIENT DATA FOR QUALITY CONTROL

In hospitals with at least 100 patients investigated each day, there should be no significant day-to-day variability in the means of their red cell indices obtained by an automated blood counter provided that the population of patients remains stable and that samples from a particular clinical source are not processed all in the same set, thus disproportionately influencing the mean. Assuming that the sample population is stable, any significant change in the means of the red cell indices will indicate a change in instrument calibration or a drift due to a fault in its function.

To start this programme it is first necessary to assay samples from at least 300–500 patients in an automated blood counter and to establish the means of MCV, MCH and MCHC. Then, using an algorithm proposed by Bull,[12] and a computer, it is possible to analyse the results in successive batches of 20 specimens. By plotting these results (x_B) on a graph any drift from the three indices can be readily recognized and used to identify instrument faults (Fig. 4.3).[1] The algorithm is now incorporated in some automated blood counters. This method appears to be as accurate and precise as the use of preserved blood controls[14] and is especially sensitive to changes in RBC.[22]

In laboratories using manual methods a simple adaptation of the same principle can be applied, confined to MCHC. From the daily means for all measurements on 11 consecutive working days

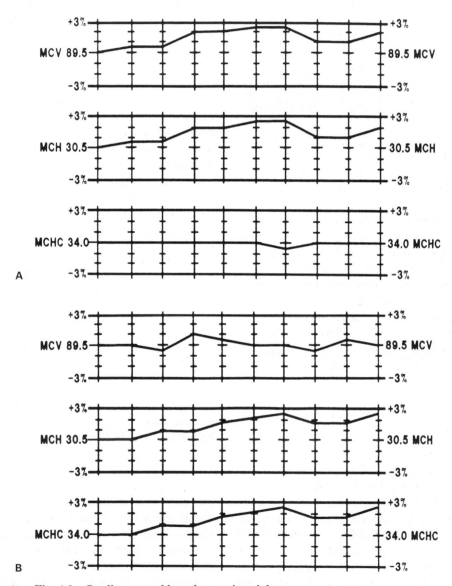

Fig. 4.3   Quality control based on patients' data.
(A) Synchronous elevation of MCV and MCH, due to partial blockage of red-cell aperture, commonly caused by protein build-up. (B) Synchronous elevation of MCH and MCHC indicates a fall in red-cell count or an increase in Hb; this might be caused by deterioration in the diluent giving rise to excessive turbidity or lysis of some of the red cells. Reproduced, with permission, from Bull and Hay[1]

an overall daily mean and SD are established. The mean MCHC is then calculated at the end of each day. If the test does not vary by more than 2 SD it is considered to be satisfactory provided that there is not a simultaneous error in the same direction in both Hb and PCV. The results may be displayed graphically as illustrated in Fig. 4.4. It is useful in validating successive batches of calibrators.

Correlation check

This implies that any unexpected result of a test must be checked to see whether it can be explained on clinical grounds or whether it correlates

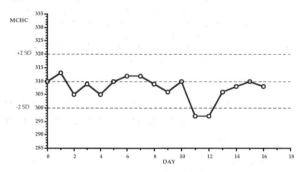

Fig. 4.4   Quality control of manual counts by MCHC. The limits for satisfactory performance have been set at ±2 SD. The values which occurred outside the lower limit were due to either a decrease in Hb or an elevation of PCV.

with other tests. Thus, for example, an unexpectedly higher or lower haemoglobin might be explained by a blood transfusion or a haemorrhage, respectively. A low MCHC should be confirmed by demonstrating hypochromic red cells on a Romanowsky-stained blood film; a high MCV must correlate with macrocytosis; similarly the blood films should be examined to confirm a leucocytosis or leucopenia, a thrombocytosis or thrombocytopenia – but be careful as the blood film itself may be misleading if not correctly made and stained.

Recording blood count data on cumulative report forms is good clinical practice as well as providing an inbuilt quality control system by making it easy to detect an aberrant result when compared with a previously determined baseline. This is especially useful in detecting the occasional wild errors caused by incorrect labelling, inadequate mixing, partial clotting of a blood sample or deterioration on storage.

A formal way of testing for aberrant results is known as the 'delta check'. The blood count parameters should not differ in subsequent tests by more than a certain amount which takes into account both test CV and physiological variation. With automated counters, the differences should generally be not more than 10% for Hb and RBC and 20–25% for WBC and platelets, assuming that the patient's clinical condition has not altered significantly.

EXTERNAL QUALITY ASSESSMENT[8,11,17,18]

External quality assessment (EQA) is an important supplement to the internal control system used by an individual laboratory. Even when all possible precautions are taken to achieve accuracy and precision in the laboratory, errors arise which are only detectable by objective external assessment. The principle is that the same material is sent from a national or regional centre to a large number of laboratories. All the laboratories send results back to the centre where they are analysed and interpreted by one of several procedures.

Deviation index

From the results returned from the participants the median or mean and SD are calculated.

An individual laboratory can then compare its performance in the survey with that of other laboratories and with its own previous performance from the 'deviation index'. This is calculated as the difference between the individual laboratory's result and the median or mean (calculated from the results of all laboratories) related to the SD.

Thus,
Deviation index =

$$\frac{\text{Actual results} - \text{Weighted median or mean for test*}}{\text{Weighted SD*}}$$

A deviation index (score) of less than 0.5 denotes excellent performance; a score between 0.5 and 1.0 is satisfactory, and a score between 1.0 and 2.0 is still acceptable. A score above 2.0 indicates that there is a defect requiring attention.

Assigned values

Values are assigned to the test materials by expert laboratories who also establish the SD of the method under optimal conditions. This will usually be lower than the SD derived from the participants' results.

Performance by participants is judged by the extent of deviation from the assigned value: less than 1 SD denotes excellent performance; 1–2 SD is satisfactory; 2–3 SD warns that there is a possibility of a problem which might require checking whilst >3 SD indicates a defect needing immediate attention.

Youden (xy) plot

This is a useful method for relating measurements on two samples in a survey to provide a graphic display and, when a participant's results are unsatisfactory, to distinguish between a consistent bias and random error. Results for the two samples are plotted on the horizontal (x) and the vertical (y) axis, respectively, and the standard deviations (2 SD or 3 SD) for the two sets are drawn, as shown in outline in Fig. 4.5.

Results which fall in block A are satisfactory; those in blocks B indicate a consistent bias which may be positive (to right) or negative (to left), while results in other areas indicate random errors (inconsistency) in the two samples.

Clinical significance

In assessing performance, using limits based on the SD will, in some cases, be too rigid, and in others be too lenient. To ensure that results are clinically reliable, they should be within a certain percentage of the assigned value. This must take account of unavoidable imprecision of the method

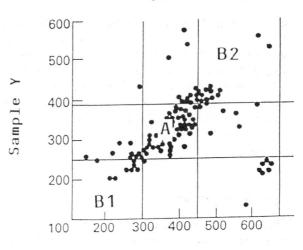

Fig. 4.5 Youden (xy) graph. The SDs of the results with the two samples are drawn on the x and y axis, respectively, and individual paired results are plotted. Results in block A are satisfactory; those in B demonstrate a consistent bias with measurements that are too low (B1) or too high (B2), while results in other areas indicate random errors.

as well as normal diurnal variations. The following limits are adequate to meet these requirements in practice:

Hb and RBC (by counter)	3–4%
PCV, MCV, MCH, MCHC	4–5%
Leucocyte count	8–10%
Platelet count	10–15%
Vitamin B_{12}, folate, iron, ferritin	20%
HbA_2 and HbF quantitation	20%

In addition to providing guidance on the laboratory's general level of performance, a major purpose of EQA is to achieve harmonization or concordance between laboratories. Specimens used for surveys must remain stable during transit. In general, material used for internal quality control (p. 38) is suitable for EQA surveys. However, some blood cell counters handle preserved blood differently from routine specimens and, even if correctly calibrated, different types of counter

---

*Weighted results are obtained by recalculation of the mean after excluding results outside ±3 SD. When distribution is non-Gaussian, the median should be used rather than the mean, without excluding outliers. The SD is calculated as: Central 50% spread ÷ 1.349.

may differ in their responses to EQA samples;[21,31] it may thus be necessary to analyse results separately for different groups of instruments. When there are unexplained differences in counts on EQA samples with different instruments in a laboratory, counts should be made on fresh EDTA blood samples with the different instruments in order to check their comparative performance.

In assessing qualitative or interpretative tests (e.g. blood film morphology), results are compared with the consensus obtained from a panel of referees or from 75–80% of the participants.

ROUTINE QUALITY ASSURANCE PROGRAMME: A SUMMARY

The procedures which should be included in a comprehensive programme will vary with the tests undertaken, the instruments used and (especially if these include a fully-automatic counting system) the size of the laboratory and the numbers of specimens handled, the computer facilities available and the amount of time which can be devoted to the programme. Some at least of the following must be carried out:

1. **Calibration of instruments** (at intervals; some daily, others weekly, always after maintenance service): by means of reference preparations and standards; e.g. HiCN reference preparations, preserved blood (in ACD or CPD), stabilized blood cell standards, calibrators with certified values.

2. **Calibration of pipettes and diluting systems** (initially and at intervals when indicated).

3. **Tests on control specimens** (daily): control sample with each batch of specimens; control chart; CUSUM; duplicate measurements on patients' specimens (five or more).

4. **Statistical analysis of patient data** (daily): mean of MCV, MCH and MCHC.

5. **Interlaboratory (EQA) surveys** (at intervals; usually monthly or 3-monthly).

6. **Correlation assessment** (at all times): by means of cumulative report forms; blood film appearances and numerical data; clinical state.

REFERENCES

[1] BULL, B. S. and HAY, K. L. (1990). Interlaboratory quality control using patients' data. *Methods in Haematology*, **22**, 185.

[2] CARSTAIRS, K. C., PETERS, E. and KUZIN, E. J. (1977). Development and description of the 'random duplicates' method of quality control for a hematology laboratory. *American Journal of Clinical Pathology*, **67**, 379.

[3] CAVILL, I. (1990). Intralaboratory quality confirmation using control samples. *Methods in Hematology*, **22**, 154.

[4] CEMBROWSKI, G. S., LUNETZKY, E. S., PATRICK, C. C. and WILSON, M. K. (1988). An optimized quality control procedure for hematology analyzers with the use of retained patient specimens. *American Journal of Clinical Pathology*, **89**, 203.

[5] CHAPPELL, D. A. and WARD, P. G. (1978). Safe and sterile mixer for biological fluids. *Laboratory Equipment Digest*, **16**, 75.

[6] COMMUNITY BUREAU OF REFERENCE (1992). *BCR Reference Materials*. Commission of the European Communities, Brussels.

[7] ENGLAND, J. M. (1984). Internal quality control and calibration. In *Automation and Quality Assurance in Haematology*. Eds. J. M. England and R. M. Rowan, p. 8–17. Blackwell Scientific Publications, Oxford.

[8] EUROPEAN COMMITTEE FOR CLINICAL LABORATORY STANDARDS (1986). *Standard for Quality Assurance, Part 5: External Quality Assessment in Haematology*. ECCLS Document, Vol. 3, No. 1. Beuth Verlag, Berlin.

[9] EUROPEAN COMMITTEE FOR CLINICAL LABORATORY STANDARDS (1987). *Standard for Quality Assurance, Part 4: Internal Quality Control in Haematology*. ECCLS Document, Vol. 4, No. 2. Beuth Verlag, Berlin.

[10] INTERNATIONAL COMMITTEE FOR STANDARDIZATION IN HAEMATOLOGY (1987). Recommendations for reference methods of haemiglobinometry in human blood (ICSH Standard 1986) and specifications for international haemiglobincyanide reference preparation, 5th edn. *Clinical and Laboratory Haematology*, **9**, 73.

[11] KOEPKE, J. A. (1986). The College of American Pathologists Survey Programme. In *Automation and Quality Assurance in Haematology*. Eds. J. M. England and R. M. Rowan, p. 62–83. Blackwell Scientific Publications, Oxford.

[12] KORPMAN, R. A. and BULL, B. S. (1976). The

implementation of a robust estimator of the mean for quality control on a programmable calculator or a laboratory computer. *American Journal of Clinical Pathology*, **65**, 252.

[13] LEVEY, S. and JENNINGS, E. R. (1950). The use of control charts in the clinical laboratory. *American Journal of Clinical Pathology*, **20**, 1059.

[14] LEVY, W. C., HAY, K. L. and BULL, B. S. (1986). Preserved blood versus patient data for quality control – Bull's algorithm revisited. *American Journal of Clinical Pathology*, **85**, 719.

[15] LEWIS, S. M. (1975). Standards and reference preparations. In *Quality Control in Haematology*. Eds. S. M. Lewis and J. F. Coster, p. 79. Academic Press, London.

[16] LEWIS, S. M. (1981). The philosophy of value assignment. In *Advances in Hematological Methods: The Blood Count*. Eds. O. W. van Assendelft and J. M. England, p. 231. CRC Press, Boca Raton, FL.

[17] LEWIS, S. M. (1986). External quality assessment in Europe. In *Automation and Quality Assurance in Haematology*. Eds. J. M. England and R. M. Rowan, p. 18. Blackwell Scientific Publications, Oxford.

[18] LEWIS, S. M. (1990). Quality assessment schemes. *Methods in Hematology*, **22**, 14.

[19] LEWIS, S. M. (1990). Standardization and harmonization of the blood count: the role of International Committee for Standardization in Haematology (ICSH). *European Journal of Haematology*, **45** (Suppl 53), 9.

[20] LEWIS, S. M., ENGLAND, J. M. and ROWAN, R. M. (1991). Current concerns in haematology 3: Blood count calibration. *Journal of Clinical Pathology*, **44**, 881.

[21] LEYSSEN, M. H. J., DE BRUYERE, M. J. G., VAN DRUPPEN, V. J. M. and VERWILGHEN, R. L. (1985). Problems related to CPD preserved blood used for NEQAS trials in haematology. *Clinical and Laboratory Haematology*, 7, 239.

[22] LUNETZKY, E. S. and CEMBROWSKI, G. S. (1987). Performance characteristics of Bull's algorithm for the quality control of multichannel hematology analyzers. *American Journal of Clinical Pathology*, **88**, 634.

[23] REARDON, D. M., MACK, D., WARNER, B. and HUTCHINSON, D. (1991). A whole blood control for blood count analysers, and source material for an external quality assessment scheme. *Medical Laboratory Sciences*, **48**, 19.

[24] RICHARDSON JONES, A. (1982). Counting and sizing of blood cells using aperture-impedance systems. In *Advances in Hematological Methods: The Blood Count*. Eds. O. W. van Assendelft and J. M. England, p. 50. CRC Press, Boca Raton, FL.

[25] RICKETTS, C. (1982). Intralaboratory quality control using control samples. *Methods in Hematology*, **4**, 151.

[26] SHEWHART, W. A. (1931). *Economic Control of Quality of Manufactured Products*. Van Nostrand, New York.

[27] THOM, R. (1972). Hemocytometry: method and results by improved electronic blood-cell sizing. In *Modern Concepts in Hematology*. Eds. G. Izak and S. M. Lewis, p. 91. Academic Press, New York.

[28] TORLONTANO, G. and TATA, A. (1972). Stable standard suspension of white blood cells suitable for calibration and control of electronic counters. In *Modern Concepts in Hematology*. Eds. G. Izak and S. M. Lewis, p. 230. Academic Press, New York.

[29] WARD, P. G., CHAPPELL, D. A., FOX, J. G. C. and ALLEN, B. V. (1975). Mixing and bottling unit for preparing biological fluids used in quality control. *Laboratory Practice*, **24**, 577.

[30] WARD, P. G., WARDLE, J. and LEWIS, S. M. (1982). Standardization for routine blood counting – the role of interlaboratory trials. *Methods in Hematology*, **4**, 102.

[31] WARDLE, J., WARD, P. G. and LEWIS, S. M. (1985). Response of various blood counting systems to CPD-A1 preserved whole blood. *Clinical and Laboratory Haematology*, 7, 245.

[32] WORLD HEALTH ORGANIZATION (1984). *Biological Substances: International Standards Reference Preparations and Reference Reagents*. WHO, Geneva.

5. Basic haematological techniques

Revised by B. J. Bain

Manual techniques   50
  Estimation of haemoglobin concentration   50
    Haemiglobincyanide method   50
    Oxyhaemoglobin method   52
    Alkaline haematin method   53
    Other methods   53
  Red blood cell count   54
  Determination of packed cell volume   57
  Determination of red cell indices   58
    Estimation of mean cell volume   58
    Estimation of mean cell haemoglobin content   58
    Estimation of mean cell haemoglobin concentration   59
  White blood cell counts   59
    Estimation of total white blood cell count   59
    Differential count and estimation of absolute white blood cell counts   60
    Absolute eosinophil count   62
    Absolute basophil count   63
  Platelet count   63
  Reticulocyte count   65

Automated techniques   68
  Haemoglobin concentration and red cell parameters   69
    Estimation of haemoglobin concentration   69
    Red blood cell count   69
    Estimation of haematocrit   72
    Estimation of mean cell volume   72
    Estimation of mean cell haemoglobin   74
    Estimation of mean cell haemoglobin concentration   74
    Determination of red cell size distribution   75
    Determination of red cell haemoglobin distribution   75
  White cell parameters   75
    Total white blood cell count   75
    Differential count   75
    New white cell parameters   77
  Platelet parameters   77
    Platelet count   77
    Mean platelet volume   78
    Other platelet parameters   78
  Reticulocyte count   78
  Calibration of automated counters   79

It is possible to use manual, semi-automated or automated techniques to determine the various elements of the full blood count (FBC). Manual techniques are generally low cost with regard to equipment and reagents but are labour intensive; automated techniques entail high capital costs but permit rapid performance of a large number of blood counts by a small number of laboratory workers. Automated techniques are more precise and, if instruments are correctly calibrated, can be as accurate as manual techniques. Many laboratories now use automated techniques almost exclusively, but manual techniques remain the basis of haematological practice and accordingly they will be described first.

All the tests discussed in this chapter can be performed on venous or free-flowing capillary blood which has been anticoagulated with K_2EDTA. Thorough mixing of the blood specimen before sampling is essential for accurate test results. Ideally, tests should be performed within 6 h of obtaining the blood specimen, since some test results are altered by longer periods of storage. However, results of acceptable accuracy are obtained on blood stored for up to 24 h at 4°C.

MANUAL TECHNIQUES

ESTIMATION OF HAEMOGLOBIN CONCENTRATION (Hb)

The haemoglobin concentration (Hb) of a solution may be estimated by several methods: by measurement of its colour, by its power of combining with oxygen or carbon monoxide or by its iron content. The clinical methods to be described are all colour or light-intensity matching techniques, which measure at the same time with different degrees of efficiency any proportion of inert pigments, i.e. methaemoglobin (Hi) or sulphaemoglobin (SHb), that may be present. The oxygen-combining capacity of blood is 1.34 ml O_2 per g haemoglobin. Ideally, as a functional estimation of Hb, measurement of oxygen capacity should be carried out, but this is hardly practicable in clinical work. It gives results at least 2% lower than the other methods because a small proportion of inert pigment is probably always present. The iron content of haemoglobin can be estimated accurately,[87] but again the method is impracticable for routine purposes. Estimations based on iron content are generally taken as authentic, but iron bound to inactive pigment is included. Iron content is converted into Hb content by assuming the following relationship: 0.347 g iron = 100 g haemoglobin.[37]

MEASUREMENT OF HAEMOGLOBIN CONCENTRATION (Hb) USING A SPECTROMETER* OR PHOTOELECTRIC COLORIMETER

In the following section three procedures will be described and their merits and disadvantages discussed:

1. The cyanmethaemoglobin (haemiglobincyanide (HiCN) method.
2. The oxyhaemoglobin (HbO_2) method.
3. The alkaline-haematin method.

There is little to choose in accuracy between the methods, although the alkaline-haematin procedure is probably less accurate than the others. A major advantage of the HiCN method is the availability of a stable and reliable reference preparation. Sahli's acid-haematin method is less accurate than any of the methods mentioned above as the colour develops slowly, is unstable and begins to fade almost immediately after it reaches its peak.

HAEMIGLOBINCYANIDE (CYANMETHAEMOGLOBIN) METHOD

The basis of the method is dilution of blood in a solution containing potassium cyanide and potassium ferricyanide.[23] Haemoglobin, Hi and HbCO (but not SHb) are converted to HiCN. The absorbance of the solution is then measured in a spectrometer* at a wavelength of 540 nm or a photoelectric colorimeter with a yellow-green filter (e.g. Ilford 625).

Diluent

This is based on Drabkin's cyanide-ferricyanide solution.[23] The original Drabkin reagent had a pH of 8.6. The following modified solution, which has a pH of 9.6, is less likely to cause turbidity from precipitation of plasma proteins; it consists of potassium ferricyanide 200 mg, potassium cyanide 50 mg, water to 1 litre.

The above solution reacts relatively slowly, and the diluted blood must stand for at least 15 min to ensure complete conversion of Hb. The following further modification, as recommended by the International Committee for Standardization in Haematology,[37] results in a shorter conversion time (3–5 min), although it has the disadvantage that the presence of a detergent causes some degree of frothing:

Potassium ferricyanide 200 mg
Potassium cyanide 50 mg
Potassium dihydrogen phosphate 140 mg
Non-ionic detergent 1 ml
Water to 1 litre.

---

*Elsewhere in this book this is alternatively referred to as a "spectrophotometer".

The pH should be 7.0–7.4. Suitable non-ionic detergents include Nonidet P40 (Sigma), Saponic 218 (Alcoac Inc.) and Triton X-100 (Rohm and Haas).

The diluent should be clear and pale yellow in colour. When measured against water as blank in a photoelectric colorimeter at a wavelength of 540 nm, absorbance must be zero. If stored at room temperature in a brown borosilicate glass bottle, the solution keeps for several months. It must not be allowed to freeze, as this can result in its decomposition.[88] The reagent must be discarded if it becomes turbid, or if the pH is found to be outside the 7.0–7.4 range or if it has an absorbance other than zero at 540 nm against a water blank.

Haemiglobincyanide (HiCN) reference preparation

With the advent of HiCN as a stable solution other standards have become outmoded. The International Committee for Standardization in Haematology has defined specifications on the basis of a molecular weight* of 64 458 and a millimolar coefficient extinction of 44.0*.[37] These specifications have been widely adopted; in Britain they have been incorporated into a British Standard (BS 3985: 1966) for a HiCN solution for photometric haemoglobinometry, a WHO International Standard has been established, and a comparable European standard is also available from the Community Bureau of Reference (BCR) (see p. 36).

Solutions of HiCN are stable for at least several years. Reference solutions that conform to the international specifications are available commercially. They contain 550–850 mg of haemoglobin per litre and the exact concentration is indicated on the label. The solution is dispensed in 10 ml sealed ampoules, and, to ensure that contamination is avoided, any unused solution should be discarded at the end of the day on which the ampoule is opened. In use, the reference solution is regarded as a dilution of whole blood, and the original Hb that it represents is obtained by multiplying the figure stated on the label by the dilution to be applied to the blood sample. Thus, if the standard solution contains 600 mg of

haemoglobin per litre, it will have the same optical density as that of a blood sample containing 120 g haemoglobin per litre diluted 1 in 200, or as one containing 150 g haemoglobin per litre diluted 1 in 250.**

The HiCN reference preparation is intended primarily for direct comparison with blood which is also converted to HiCN. It can also be used for the standardization of a whole-blood standard in the HbO_2 method and for the calibration of Gibson and Harrison's standard used in the alkaline-haematin method (see p. 53).

Method

Add 20 μl of blood to 4 ml of diluent. Stopper the tube containing the solution and invert it several times. After being allowed to stand at room temperature for a sufficient period of time to ensure the completion of the reaction (3–5 min, see above), the solution of HiCN is ready to be compared with the standard and a reagent blank in a spectrophotometer at 540 nm or in a photoelectric colorimeter with a suitable filter.*** Open an ampoule of HiCN standard (brought to room temperature if previously stored in a refrigerator) and measure the absorbance of the solution in the same spectrophotometer or photoelectric colorimeter against the blank. The standard should be discarded at the end of the day and during the day must be kept in the dark. The absorbance of the test sample must be measured within 6 h of its being diluted.

Calculation

$$Hb \text{ (g/l)} = \frac{^\dagger A^{540} \text{ of test sample}}{A^{540} \text{ of standard}} \times \text{Conc. of standard}$$

$$\times \frac{\text{Dilution factor (e.g. 201)}}{1000}$$

---

*i.e. the absorbance of a solution containing 4×55.8 mg of haemoglobin iron per litre at 540 nm.
**Within the SI system many measurements are now expressed in terms of substance concentration, using the mole as unit. For clinical purposes, there are practical advantages in continuing to express Hb in mass concentration, i.e. as g/l; if substance concentration is used, the monomer should be the elementary entity used in calculation.[86]
***e.g. Ilford 625, Wratten 74 or Chance 0 Gr 1.
†i.e. absorbance; formerly called optical density. In some instruments, measurements are read as percentage transmittance.

*relative molecular mass

Preparation of standard curve and standard table

When many blood samples are to be tested it is convenient to read the results from a standard curve or table relating absorbance readings to Hb in g/l for the individual instrument. These can be prepared as follows.

Open an ampoule of HiCN reference solution (brought to room temperature) and measure in the same photometer as is to be used for the subsequent haemoglobinometry the absorbance or transmittance of the solution against a blank of cyanide-ferricyanide reagent. Make readings with the same standard solution diluted with the reagent 1 in 2, 1 in 3, 1 in 4, etc. Translate the Hb value of the solutions into terms of g/l, as described above. If the readings record absorbance, plot them on linear graph paper using arithmetical scales, with absorbance as ordinates (vertical scale). If the readings are in percentage transmittance, use semilogarithmic paper with the transmittance recorded on the vertical (log) scale. As Lambert-Beer's law is valid for HiCN, the points should fit a straight line that passes through the origin. This provides a check that the calibration of the photometer is linear (assuming that the standard has been correctly diluted). From the standard curve it is possible to construct a table of readings and corresponding Hb values. The table may be more convenient than the graph when large numbers of measurements are made. Prepare a calibration curve whenever a new photometer is put into use.

It is important that the performance of the instrument should not vary and that its calibration remains constant in relation to Hb measurements. To ensure this, the reference preparations should be measured at frequent intervals, preferably with each batch of blood samples.

The main advantages of the HiCN method for Hb determination are that it allows direct comparison with the HiCN standard and that the readings need not be made immediately after dilution; it also has the advantage that all forms of haemoglobin, except SHb, are readily converted to HiCN. The use of KCN in the preparation of Drabkin's solution is a potential hazard. To avoid using cyanide, lauryl sulphate has been proposed as a non-hazardous substitute, as lauryl sulphate has similar properties to HiCN.[45] However, as Drabkin's solution contains only 50 mg of KCN per litre, it is relatively innocuous; 600–1000 ml would have to be swallowed to produce serious effects. As already referred to, a possible disadvantage is that the diluted blood has to stand for a period of time to ensure complete conversion of the haemoglobin. Also, the rate of conversion of blood containing HbCO is markedly slowed. This difficulty can be overcome by prolonging the reaction time to 30 min.[83]

Abnormal plasma proteins or a high leucocyte count may result in turbidity when the blood is diluted in the cyanide-ferricyanide reagent. The turbidity can be avoided by centrifuging the diluted sample or by increasing the concentration of potassium dihydrogen phosphate to 33 mmol/l (4.0 g/l).[51]

OXYHAEMOGLOBIN METHOD

This is the simplest and quickest method for general use with a photoelectric colorimeter. Its disadvantage is that it is not possible to prepare a stable HbO_2 standard. The reliability of the method is not affected by a moderate rise in plasma bilirubin but it is not satisfactory in the presence of HbCO, Hi or SHb.

Method

Wash 20 µl of blood into 4 ml of 0.4 ml/l ammonia (sp gr 0.88) contained in a tube provided with a tightly fitting stopper. Mix by inverting the tube several times. The solution of HbO_2 is then ready for matching in the colorimeter at 540 nm or with a yellow-green filter (e.g. Ilford 625). If the absorbance of the haemoglobin solution exceeds 0.7, dilute the blood further with an equal volume of water.

Standard

At a dilution of 1 in 200, blood containing 146 g/l, haemoglobin placed in a 1 cm cell, gives an extinction coefficient of 0.475, using a yellow-green filter (Ilford 625, Wratten 74 or Chance 0 Gr 1) or at 540 nm. A neutral grey filter of 0.475 density (Ilford or Chance) can, therefore, be used as a 146 g/l standard.

Colorimeters and light filters unfortunately differ sufficiently one from the other to make it essential to check the chosen standard at frequent intervals against a HiCN reference preparation in the colorimeter in which it is going to be used. It is probably preferable to use a new fresh whole-blood sample each day as a secondary standard after measuring its Hb by the HiCN method. Preserved blood (p. 37) or lysate (p. 38) can be used instead.

As originally used, a disadvantage of the HbO_2 method was the tendency for the solution of HbO_2 to fade.[75] This has been found to be due to the high dilution of the solution and the unnecessary high pH, resulting from the use of 1 g/l sodium carbonate solution or relatively strong ammonia solution as diluent. However, using 0.4 ml/l ammonia, the solution appears to be stable for a day or more at room temperature.

ALKALINE-HAEMATIN METHOD

The alkaline-haematin method is a useful ancillary method under special circumstances as it gives a true estimate of total Hb even if HbCO, Hi or SHb is present. A true solution is obtained and plasma proteins and lipids have little effect on the development of colour, although they cause turbidity unless the blood and alkali are quickly and thoroughly mixed.

A disadvantage of the method is that certain forms of haemoglobin are resistant to alkali denaturation, in particular Hb F and Hb Bart's, but this can be overcome by heating the solution in a boiling water-bath for 4 min. In normal circumstances the method is more cumbersome and less accurate than the HiCN or HbO_2 methods, and is thus unsuitable for use as a routine method.

Two methods will be described:

1. The standard method[17] using Gibson and Harrison's standard.[30]
2. The acid-alkali method.

Standard method

Add 50 μl of blood to 4.95 ml of 0.1 mol/l NaOH and heat in a boiling water-bath for exactly 4 min. Cool the sample rapidly in cold water and when cool match against the standard in a photoelectric colorimeter at 540 nm or using a yellow-green filter (e.g. Ilford 625).

Standard

This is a mixture of chromium potassium sulphate, cobaltous sulphate and potassium dichromate in aqueous solution. The solution is equal in colour to a 1 in 100 dilution of blood containing 160 g haemoglobin per litre.

It is essential to heat the standard along with the test sample. Only after heating, which alters the ionization of the salts it contains, does the ability of the standard to absorb green light approximate closely to that of alkaline haematin. A fresh sample of standard should be heated on each occasion and then discarded.

Acid-alkali method

A disadvantage of the alkaline-haematin method, as previously described, is that the solution of haemoglobin in alkali has to be heated to ensure complete denaturation. This procedure can be omitted if the blood is collected first into acid and, after standing for 20–30 min, sufficient alkali is added to neutralize the acid and convert the acid haematin into alkaline haematin.

Wash 50 μl of blood into 4.0 ml of 0.1 mol/l HCl and mix immediately. After the tube has stood for 20–30 min, add 0.95 ml of 1 mol/l NaOH and invert the tube several times. After a further 2 min, measure the test sample in a photoelectric colorimeter at 540 nm or with a yellow-green filter (e.g. Ilford 625) employing as a standard heated Gibson and Harrison's standard (see above) or a grey filter or solution[79] previously calibrated against blood of known Hb treated by acid and then alkali as described above.

OTHER METHODS OF HAEMOGLOBINOMETRY

Direct-reading haemoglobinometers

These instruments have a built-in filter and a scale calibrated for direct reading of Hb in g/dl or g/l. They are generally based on the oxyhaemoglobin method but a number of instruments are now available which are standardized to give the same results as with the cyanmethaemoglobin method, with a light-emitting diode of appropriate wavelength.* The calibration of this type of instrument should be checked regularly to ensure maintenance of accuracy and precision, using HiCN reference solutions or a secondary standard of preserved blood (p. 37) or lysate (p. 38).

---

*e.g. HemoCue (HemoCue AB, Helsingborg).

Spectrophotometry

The Hb of blood can be determined accurately by spectrophotometry. The blood is diluted suitably (1 to 200 or 1 to 250) with cyanide-ferricyanide reagent (see p. 50) and the absorbance is measured at 540 nm. The Hb is calculated as follows:

$$Hb\ (g/l) = \frac{A^{540}HiCN \times 64\ 500 \times Dilution\ factor}{44.0 \times d \times 1000}$$

where $A^{540}HiCN$ = absorbance of the solution at 540 nm, 64 500 = molecular weight of haemoglobin (derived from 64 458), dilution = 201 when 20 μl of blood are diluted in 4 ml of reagent, 44.0 = millimolar extinction coefficient, d = layer thickness in cm, and 1000 = conversion factor for mg to g.

The spectrophotometric method gives a direct measurement of the Hb of the diluted blood. Calibration of the spectrophotometer should be checked from time to time by verifying that it gives an accurate value for the HiCN standard. Slight deviations from the expected $A^{540}HiCN$ value for the standard may be used to correct the results of test samples for a bias in measurement.[37]

Range of Hb in health

(See pp. 12 and 17.)

THE TOTAL RED BLOOD CELL COUNT (RBC)

The red blood cell count (RBC) is itself of use in diagnostic haematology, but it is also of importance because it permits the mean cell volume (MCV) and mean cell haemoglobin (MCH) to be calculated. However, a manual red cell count in which cells are counted visually is so time consuming and has such poor precision that both it and the red cell indices derived from it are of limited use in routine practice. The reference method for the RBC is an automated rather than a manual count.

MANUAL RED BLOOD CELL COUNT

Make a 1:200 dilution of blood in formal-citrate solution. This is most conveniently done by washing 20 μl of blood taken into a micropipette into 4 ml of diluting fluid contained in a glass or plastic 75 × 12 mm tube. After sealing the tube with a tightly fitting rubber or plastic bung, mix the diluted blood in a mechanical mixer or by hand for at least 2 min by tilting the tube through an angle of about 120° combined with rotation, thus allowing the air bubble to mix the suspension.

Fill a clean dry counting chamber, with its cover-glass already in position, without delay. This is simply accomplished with the aid of a Pasteur pipette or a length of stout capillary glass tubing which has been allowed to take up the suspension by capillarity. Care should be taken that the counting chamber is filled in one action and that no fluid flows into the surrounding moat. Leave the chamber undisturbed on a bench for at least 2 min for the cells to settle, but not much longer, for drying at the edges of the preparation initiates currents which cause movement of the cells after they have settled. The bench must be free of vibrations and the chamber not exposed to draughts or to direct sunlight or other sources of heat. It is important that the cover-glass should be of a special thick glass and perfectly flat, so that when laid on the counting chamber, diffraction rings are seen. The cover-glass should be of such a size that when placed correctly on the counting chamber the central ruled areas lie in the centre of the rectangle to be filled with the cell suspension. The preparation must be discarded and the filling procedure repeated using another clean dry chamber if any of the following filling defects occur:

1. Overflow into moat.
2. Chamber area incompletely filled.
3. Air bubbles anywhere in chamber area.
4. Any debris in chamber area.

The type of counting chamber used and the arrangement of the rulings are matters of personal preference and availability. The Neubauer and improved Neubauer chambers have been the commonest types in general use. The visibility of the rulings is as important as the accuracy of calibration.

Count the cells using a ×40 dry objective and ×6 or ×10 eyepieces. It is important to count as many cells as possible, for the accuracy of the count is increased thereby (see below); 500 cells should be considered the absolute minimum. With a Neubauer chamber (Figs 5.1 and 5.2), count the cells in 4 or 8 horizontal rectangles of 1 mm × 0.05 mm (80 or 160 small squares) or in 5 or 10 groups of 16 small squares, including the cells which touch the bottom and left-hand margins of the small squares.

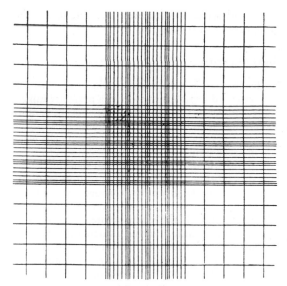

Fig. 5.1 Neubauer counting chamber. The total ruled area is 3 mm × 3 mm; the central ruled area is 1 mm × 1 mm. In the central area 16 groups of 16 small squares are separated by triple rulings.

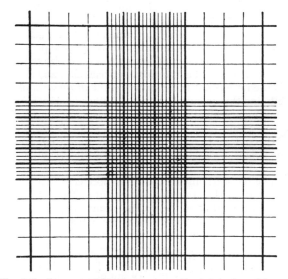

Fig. 5.2 Improved Neubauer counting chamber. The central area consists of 25 groups of 16 small squares separated by closely ruled triple lines (which appear as thick black lines in the photograph).

Calculation

Red cell count (per litre) =

$$\frac{\text{No. of cells counted}}{\text{Volume counted (μl)}} \times \text{Dilution} \times 10^6$$

Thus, when the cells in 80 small squares of an improved Neubauer chamber are counted (total

volume = 0.02 μl) and the blood is diluted 1:200, the red cell count will be:

$$\frac{\text{N}}{0.02} \times 200 \times 10^6 \text{ per litre}$$

Red cell diluting fluid

A solution of 10 ml of 40% formalin, made up to 1 litre with 32 g/l trisodium citrate is recommended. The solution is simple to prepare; it keeps well and does not need to be sterilized. The red cells maintain their normal disc-like form and are not agglutinated. The cells are well preserved and counts may be performed several hours after the blood has been diluted.

Occasionally, when the patient's blood is auto-agglutinated, as in some cases of auto-immune haemolytic anaemia, it is advantageous to use as a diluting fluid 32 g/l trisodium citrate solution without the addition of formalin. Agglutinates may disperse and enable a count to be carried out in the absence of formalin which appears to prevent, possibly by its fixing action, the clumps of agglutinated cells from breaking up.

Range of red cell counts in health

(See pp. 12 and 17.)

ERRORS IN RED CELL COUNTING

The errors associated with the manual red cell count are of two main kinds: those due to inaccurate apparatus, indifferent technique or unrepresentative nature of the blood counted ('technical' errors); and that due to the distribution of the suspension of red cells in the counting chamber—the 'inherent' or 'field' error. The former errors can be minimized by careful technique; the latter error can be diminished by counting a large number of cells.

Technical errors

These include bad technique in obtaining the blood specimen; insufficient mixing of the blood specimen; inaccurate pipetting and the use of badly calibrated pipettes or counting chambers; inadequate mixing of the red cell suspension; faulty filling of the counting chamber, and careless counting of cells within the chamber.

It is essential that the accuracy of the apparatus be known so that, if necessary, appropriate correction factors can be applied.[66] The British Standard for Haemocytometer and Particle Counting Chambers (BS 748: 1982) specified a tolerance of dimensions which provides reasonable accuracy. But even so, the chance summation of all the tolerances for different parts of the apparatus in a single counting chamber would result in an error as large as ±7%. The exact chamber depth depends also on the cover-glass, which should be free from bowing and sufficiently thick so as not to bend when pressed on the chamber. It must be free from scratches, and even the smallest particle of dust may cause unevenness in its lie on the chamber.

Bulb diluting pipettes are not recommended; they are difficult to calibrate and easily broken. The volumes of blood used are unnecessarily small and the pipettes are difficult to label and handle. In particular, filling the counting chamber so that the exact amount of fluid is delivered from the pipette is an art difficult to master. 20 μl pipettes are relatively inexpensive and easy to calibrate. By the use of 4 ml of diluting fluid in a glass or plastic tube provided with a tightly fitting rubber or plastic bung, a suspension easy to label and handle is obtained, and with a little practice a perfect filling of the counting chamber can regularly be accomplished with the aid of a fine Pasteur pipette or stout glass capillary.

The accuracy of 20 μl pipettes may be checked, after careful cleaning, by filling them to the mark with clean mercury, expelling the mercury and weighing it.[74] 20 μl of mercury weigh 272 mg; 50 μl weigh 680 mg. It is convenient to draw up the mercury to the mark in the pipette by attaching to the pipette a small length of pressure tubing, one end of which has been closed. The measured column of mercury is then expelled on to a previously weighed watch-glass and weighed in a balance sensitive to a difference of 1 mg.*

Automatic diluter units are useful. These consist of a dual metering system which enables a volume of diluent and the appropriate volume of blood to be dispensed consecutively into a tube. A variety of automatic diluting systems are now available which have good accuracy and precision. Hand-held semi-automatic microsamplers with a detachable tip (e.g. Eppendorf, Oxford, Labora) are designed to operate as 'to deliver' pipettes.

Pipetting errors apply to all tests which involve dilution of the blood sample and they also occur with autodiluters which are liable to error with viscid fluids and when the delivery volume of the unit is not correctly adjusted. The inherent error, discussed below, is unique to counting.

Inherent error

The distribution of cells in a counting chamber is of an irregular (random) pattern even in a perfectly mixed sample. However, the pattern of distribution conforms to a definite type. Theoretical considerations indicate that variation between the numbers of red cells which settle in areas similar in size should conform to a Poisson distribution (see p. 584) and that the deviation of the distribution of the number of cells in areas of equal size should be given by $\sqrt{\lambda}$ where λ is the total number of cells in each area. However, the movement of the cells in the chamber during the filling process causes them to collide and this influences their distribution which thus differs from the theoretical expectation of the variance.[48] This is given instead by $\sigma = 0.92 \sqrt{\lambda}$. This means that if a counting chamber is filled with a red cell suspension so that the number of cells in an area (say 80 small squares) in 100, σ would be 9.2. Then, if it were possible to count the number of cells in each of 100 similar areas, in 95 areas the number of cells encountered would range between 82 and 118, i.e. $100 \pm 2\sigma$; in the remaining five areas the counts would be outside this range.

Clearly, this random distribution has a very important bearing on the accuracy of visual blood counts, for no amount of mixing will minimize the inherent variation in numbers between area and area.

The ratio σ/λ is the variation of the *distribution* of cells and this calculated as a percentage gives a convenient way of expressing the inherent error of blood counts.

By contrast to σ, the standard deviation (SD) and coefficient of variation (CV) are measures of variance between each result (see p. 584). The inherent error can be reduced only by counting more cells in a preparation. The calculations set out in Table 5.1 demonstrate that, in theory, the count varies in proportion to the square root of the number of cells counted, i.e. if four times the number of cells are counted, the variation is halved. For example, if the imaginary (ideal) figures given in Table 5.1 are studied, it will be seen that 19 out of 20 counts based on the number of cells in 80 small squares will lie within the wide range of 5.16 to 6.04×10^{12}/l. If the

---

*When water is used instead of mercury, a balance of this sensitivity is adequate for weighing volumes > 0.1–0.2 ml. For 20 μl volumes a much more sensitive balance is necessary.

Table 5.1 Error of the visual red-cell count

No. of small squares counted	No. of cells counted (λ)	$(0.92 \times \sqrt{\lambda}) = \sigma$	Range (95%) $\lambda \pm 2\sigma$	Calculated red cell count ($\times 10^{-12}$/l)*	Count variation (%)
80	560	22	516–604	5.16–6.04	3.9
160	1120	31	1058–1182	5.29–5.91	2.8
320	2240	44	2152–2328	5.38–5.82	2.0
640	4480	62	4356–4604	5.44–5.75	1.4

Shows how the inherent error of red-cell counting may be reduced by counting large numbers of red cells.
*If the red cell count (RBC) is 5×10^{12}/l then 5 is the RBC/l $\times 10^{-12}$.

cells in 320 small squares are counted, the range will be considerably narrower—5.38 to 5.82 × 10^{12}/l. Causes of error of red cell counts include personal bias from foreknowledge of what the result should be, selection of counting areas and uneven distribution of cells within the counting chamber due to the momentum given to the cells as the chamber is filled.[66]

The method of making serial counts and taking the mean has been widely (perhaps unconsciously) used as a means of reducing the error of the red cell count. If a sufficient number of counts are done, the truth is likely to reveal itself; and there is also a chance that errors in technique will cancel each other out.

Clearly, the errors of blood counting by visual means are very considerable. That due to the random distribution of the cells in the counting chamber can be reduced by counting the cells in a larger area, as already mentioned (see Table 5.1), but in ordinary laboratory practice there is rarely time to count carefully the cells in more than 160 small squares—about 1000 cells in a normal count. The practice of making counts in duplicate is a good one, but does not necessarily increase accuracy: it is always possible that the second count will be further from the truth than the first, due to the random distribution of cells. It is better to repeat a count using a second chamber and pipette than to count double the number of cells in a single filling of the counting chamber.

DETERMINATION OF PACKED CELL VOLUME (PCV) OR HAEMATOCRIT (Hct) VALUE

Haematocrit (literally 'blood separation') tubes are in daily use in many haematological laboratories where automated blood-count systems are not available, as the measurement of the PCV can be used as a simple screening test for anaemia. In addition, in conjunction with estimations of Hb and red cell count, knowledge of the PCV enables the calculation of red cell indices (see p. 58). Furthermore, it can be used as a reference method for calibrating automated blood count systems.[39] The macro-method of Wintrobe is no longer in routine use, having been replaced by the micro-haematocrit.

MICRO-HAEMATOCRIT

The use of capillary tubes is very convenient for routine determination of the PCV. The centrifuge used provides a centrifugal force of c 12 000g and 3–5 min centrifugation results in a constant PCV. When the PCV is greater than 0.5, it may be necessary to centrifuge for a further 5 min. When packing is as complete as possible the column of cells will appear translucent. The amount of trapped plasma is less than with the Wintrobe method. Garby and Vuille reported a mean of 1.3% (range 1.1–1.5%).[29] Pearson and Guthrie reported a slightly higher amount with normal blood (mean 1.53%, SD 0.166)[58] and other authors have reported values of 2–3%.[25] Plasma trapping is increased in macrocytic anaemias,[25]

spherocytosis, thalassaemia, hypochromic anaemias and sickle-cell anaemia;[58] it may be as high as 20% in sickle-cell anaemia if all the cells are sickled.[25]

Method

Capillary tubes 75 mm in length and having an internal diameter of about 1 mm are required. They can be obtained plain or coated inside with 2 IU of heparin. The latter type are suitable for the direct collection of capillary blood. Plain tubes are used for anticoagulated venous blood.

Allow the blood to enter the tube by capillarity, leaving at least 15 mm unfilled. Then seal the tube by a plastic seal, e.g. Cristaseal (Hawksley, Lancing, Sussex) or by heating the dry end of the tube rapidly in a fine flame, e.g. the pilot light of a Bunsen burner, combined with rotation. After centrifugation for 5 min, measure the PCV using a reading device.

Accuracy of micro-haematocrit

Failure to mix the blood sample adequately will produce an inaccurate result. EDTA anticoagulant in excess of 1.5 mg/ml may cause a falsely low PCV as a consequence of cell shrinkage. The degree of oxygenation of the blood also affects the result, as the PCV of venous blood is c 2% higher than that of fully aerated blood (which has lost CO_2 and taken up O_2). Variation of the bore of the tubes may, too, cause serious errors if they are not manufactured within the narrow limits of precision that conform to defined standards, e.g. British Standard for Apparatus for Measurement of Packed Red Cell Volume (BS 4316: 1968).

Other errors are caused by difficulty in heat-sealing the lower end of the tube so as to obtain a flat base and difficulties in reading. To avoid errors in reading with the special reading device, a magnifying glass should be used. Alternatively, the ratio of red cell column to whole column (i.e. red cells plus plasma) can be calculated from measurements obtained by placing the tube against arithmetic graph paper or against a ruler. In routine practice it is not customary to correct for trapped plasma. But when the PCV is required for calculating blood volume, the observed

PCV should be reduced by a 2% correction factor when the PCV is less than 0.5. When it is more than 0.5, centrifugation should be continued for a further 5 min and 3% should be deducted from the observed reading.[38] When accuracy is especially important the amount of trapped plasma can be determined using radioactive human serum albumin as an indicator.[58]

There is no advantage in applying an arbitrary correction when using a micro-haematocrit to calibrate an automated counter; this practice has a disadvantage in that the micro-haematocrit and the automated haematocrit will then differ.

Range of packed cell volume in health

(See pp. 12 and 17.)

CALCULATION OF THE VOLUME, HAEMOGLOBIN CONTENT AND HAEMOGLOBIN CONCENTRATION OF RED CELLS (RED CELL INDICES)

From the measured Hb, PCV and RBC it is possible to derive other values which indicate the red cell volume and haemoglobin content and concentration; these values are commonly referred to as the red cell indices. They are the mean cell volume (MCV), the mean cell haemoglobin (MCH) and the mean cell haemoglobin concentration (MCHC). The red cell indices are of considerable clinical importance and are widely used in the classification of anaemia.

The precision and accuracy of these derived values is inferior to that of the primary measurements from which they are derived, since the errors in the primary measurements are additive. If a manual red cell count is used to determine red cell indices the precision is generally poor. The ready availability of precise automated values (see p. 72) has increased the clinical usefulness of the red cell indices.

Calculation of mean cell volume (MCV)

If the PCV and the number of red cells per litre are known, the MCV can be calculated:

e.g. if the PCV is 0.45, 1 litre of blood contains 0.45 litre of red cells. Therefore, if there are 5×10^{12} red cells per litre, they occupy a volume of 0.45 litre. Therefore,

$$\text{Volume of 1 cell} = \frac{0.45}{5 \times 10^{12}}$$

$$= 90 \text{ femtolitres (fl)}$$

In practice, the PCV (0.45) is divided by the red cell count per litre $\times 10^{-12}(5.0)$ and multiplied by 1000 to give the MCV in femtolitres (90).

Calculation of mean cell haemoglobin (MCH)

This can be calculated if the Hb and red cell count are known:

e.g. if there are 150 g of Hb per litre of blood, and if there are 5×10^{12} red cells per litre, the mean cell Hb is

$$\frac{150}{5 \times 10^{12}} = \frac{3}{10^{11}} \text{ g} = 30 \text{ picograms (pg)}$$

In practice, the Hb in g/l (150) is divided by the RBC per litre $\times 10^{-12}$/l (5) to give the MCH in picograms (30).

Calculation of mean cell haemoglobin concentration (MCHC)

This can be calculated if the Hb per litre of blood and the PCV are known:

e.g. if there are 150 g of Hb per litre of blood, of PCV 0.45, the MCHC is

$$150 \div 0.45 = 333 \text{ g/l.}$$

Range of MCV, MCH and MCHC in health

(See pp. 12 and 17.)

WHITE BLOOD CELL COUNT

TOTAL WHITE BLOOD CELL COUNT (WBC) OR LEUCOCYTE COUNT

Make a 1 in 20 dilution of blood by adding 20 µl of blood to 0.38 ml of diluting fluid in a 75 × 10 mm glass or plastic tube. Bulb pipettes are not recommended (see p. 56). After tightly corking the tube, mix the suspension by rotating in a cell-suspension mixer for at least 1 min. Fill the Neubauer counting chamber by means of a Pasteur pipette or stout glass capillary, as for red cell counts (p. 56).

The red cells are lysed by the diluting fluid (see below) but the leucocytes remain intact, their nuclei staining deep violet-black. View the preparation using a × 40 objective and × 6 eyepieces or a × 10 objective and × 6 or × 10 eyepieces. Count at least 100 cells in as many 1 mm² areas (0.1 µl in volume) as may be necessary—the ruled area in an improved Neubauer chamber consists of nine of these areas.

Calculation

Count (per litre) =
$$\frac{\text{No. of cells counted}}{\text{Volume counted (µl)}} \times \text{Dilution} \times 10^6$$

Thus, if N cells are counted in 0.1 µl, then the leucocyte count per litre is:

$$\frac{N}{0.1} \times 20 \times 10^6 = N \times 200 \times 10^6$$

e.g. if 115 cells are counted, the WBC is
$$115 \times 200 \times 10^6/l = 23 \times 10^9/l$$

Diluting fluid

2% (20 ml/l) acetic acid coloured pale violet with gentian violet.

Error of the total white cell count

The factors causing errors in counting leucocytes by the visual method are the same as in counting red cells. As many leucocytes as possible should be counted; 100 cells is a reasonable and practical figure for visual counts. The inherent distribution error (σ) of a 100-cell count is approximately $\sqrt{100} = 10$, and the count variation is thus 10% (see p. 56); 95% of counts of mean value 100 would thus lie within the range $100 \pm 2\sigma = 80$ to 120. Translated into actual results, this means that 95% of observed counts on a blood of true value 5.0×10^9 cells per litre would lie within the range 4.0–6.0.

Fortunately, error in the leucocyte count is not as critical as error in red cell counts; even an error as high as 20% does not matter much—the difference between 5.0 and 6.0×10^9 cells per litre is of little practical significance. The error can be reduced by counting more cells, and with high counts this can be accomplished without the expenditure of much extra time. If 400 cells are counted, the error is reduced to 5%.

Other potential causes of error include mistaking dirt or clumped red cell debris for leucocytes and the clumping of leucocytes. The latter—usually several leucocytes stuck to debris—seems to occur particularly in heparinized blood, especially when the concentration of heparin exceeds 25 IU per ml of blood. The clumps are most frequently seen in blood which has been allowed to stand for several hours before undertaking the count.

Range of WBC in health

(See pp. 12 and 17.)

DIFFERENTIAL WHITE CELL COUNT

Differential white cell counts are usually performed by visual examination of blood films which are prepared on slides by the spread or 'wedge' technique. Unfortunately, even in well-spread films the distribution of the various cell types is not totally random (see below).

For a reliable differential count on films spread on slides the film must not be too thin and the tail of the film should be smooth. To achieve this the film should be made with a rapid movement using a smooth glass spreader (see p. 83). This should result in a film in which there is some overlap of the red cells, diminishing to separation near the tail, and in which the white cells in the body of the film are not too badly shrunken. If the film is made too thinly, or if a rough-edged spreader is used, many of the white cells, perhaps even 50% of them, accumulate at the edges and in the tail (Fig. 5.3). Moreover, a gross qualitative irregularity in distribution is the rule: polymorphonuclear neutrophils and monocytes predominate at the margins and the tail, and lymphocytes in the middle of the film (Fig. 5.4). This separation probably depends upon differences in stickiness, size and specific gravity among the different classes of cells.

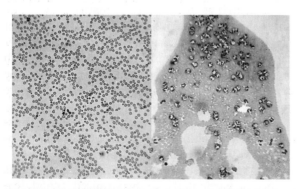

Fig. 5.3 Centre (left) and tail (right) of a badly made blood film. The centre of the film is almost devoid of white cells; in the tail neutrophils, particularly, are present in large numbers. ×100.

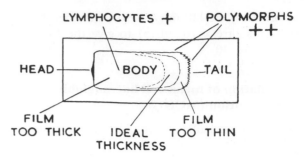

Fig. 5.4 Schematic drawing of a blood film made on a slide. The film has been spread from left to right. An indication is given of the way the white blood cells are distributed (see text).

Various systems of performing the differential count have been advocated. The problem is to overcome the differences in distribution of the various classes of cells, which are probably always present to a small extent even in well made films. No system of counting will compensate for the gross irregularities in distribution in a badly made film. It is a waste of time to attempt a differential count on such a film and, if this is attempted, futile to count only the cells in the centre of the film, where lymphocytes probably predominate, and to neglect altogether the tail, where most of the neutrophils lie. If the film had been well made, and many leucocytes are present in the body of the film and there is no great accumulation at the tail, the following technique of counting is recommended.

MANUAL DIFFERENTIAL WHITE CELL COUNT

Count the cells using a × 40 dry or × 100 oil-immersion lens, in a strip running the whole length of the film. Avoid the lateral edges of the film. Inspect the film from the head to the tail, and if less than 100 cells are encountered in a single narrow strip, examine one or more additional strips until at least 100 cells have been counted. Each longitudinal strip represents the blood drawn out from a small part of the original drop of blood when it has spread out between the slide and spreader (Fig. 5.5). If all the cells are counted in such a strip, the differential totals will approximate closely to the true differential count. This technique is liable to error if cells in the thick part of the film cannot be identified; also it

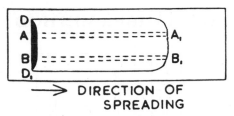

→ DIRECTION OF SPREADING

Fig. 5.5 Schematic drawing illustrating the longitudinal method of performing differential leucocyte counts. The original drop of blood spreads out between spreader and slide (D–D$_1$). The film is made in such a way that representative strips of films, such as A–A$_1$ and B–B$_1$ are formed from blood originally at A and B, respectively. In order to perform an accurate differential count, all the leucocytes in one or more strips, such as A–A$_1$ and B–B$_1$, should be inspected and classified.

does not allow for any excess of neutrophils and monocytes at the edges of the film, but this preponderance is slight in a well-made film and in practice makes little difference to the result.

The above technique is easy to carry out; with high counts $(10–30 \times 10^9$ cells per litre) a short, 2–3 cm, film is desirable. In patients with very high counts (as in leukaemia) the method has to be abandoned and the cells should be counted in any well spread area where the cell types are easy to identify. Other systems of counting, such as the 'battlement' count,[47] are more elaborate but may minimize error due to variation of distribution of cells between the centre and the edge of the film.

Most workers find it possible to remember accurately the differential counts of small groups of 20 to 25 cells, writing the results on paper when each small group has been surveyed. However, a multiple manual register is a help in recording the results of a count. With some sophisticated electronic registers, the differential count is entered directly into a computerized data processor alongside the results of the automated blood count.

The observed differential count depends not only on artefactual differences in distribution due to the process of spreading, but also on 'random' distribution; together they are by far the most important cause of unreliable differential counts.[26] Distribution of the counts of a major cell population is Gaussian; that of a minor population is a Poisson distribution (see p. 584). In practical terms the random distribution means that, if a total of 100 cells are counted, with a true neutrophil proportion of 50%, the range (± 2 SD) within which 95% of the counts will fall, is of the order of ± 14%, i.e. 36–64% neutrophils.

A 200-cell count can provide a more accurate estimate; in the above example, the ± 2 SD range will be about 40–60%. In a 500-cell count the range would be reduced to 44–56% neutrophils. In the case of a minor population, if the true count is 3% in a 100-cell differential count, in 95 out of 100 counts, the count would range between 0% and 6%, whilst a true count of 10% is likely to be counted as anything between 5% and 15%. Even 500-cell counts are little better for accurate counting of cells present in low percentages, but if abnormal cells are present in small numbers they are more likely to be detected when 200–500 cell counts are performed than with a 100-cell count.[61] In practice a 100- or 200-cell count is recommended as a routine procedure.

Reporting the differential white cell count

The differential count, expressed as the percentage of each type of cell, should be related to the total leucocyte count and the results reported in absolute numbers $(\times 10^9/l)$. Nucleated red blood cells (NRBC) may be either included or excluded in the differential count. If excluded, they are expressed as NRBC/100 WBC and the total nucleated cell count is corrected to a true WBC so that absolute leucocyte counts are correct. If they are included, they are expressed as a percentage of the total nucleated cell count. Since most automated blood counters include some or all of any NRBC in the 'WBC' it is more convenient, if relating a manual differential count to an automated 'WBC', to *include* the NRBC in the differential count and to redesignate the 'WBC' the 'total nucleated cell count' (TNCC). Myelocytes and metamyelocytes, if present, are recorded separately from neutrophils. Band (stab) cells are generally counted as neutrophils but it may be useful to record them separately. They normally constitute less than 6% of the neutrophils; an increase may point to an inflammatory process even in the absence of an absolute leucocytosis.[50]

Range of differential white cell counts in health

(See pp. 12 and 17.)

EOSINOPHIL COUNT BY A COUNTING-CHAMBER METHOD

Although total eosinophil counts can be roughly calculated from the total and differential leucocyte counts, the staining properties of eosinophils make it possible to count them directly and more accurately in a counting chamber.

The principles underlying the counting-chamber or 'wet' eosinophil count were reviewed by Spiers.[73] Ideally, the diluent should stain the eosinophil granules brightly and distinctly and at the same time lyse the red cells and all other types of leucocyte.

Diluting fluids for eosinophil counts

The acetone group of diluents, introduced by Dunger,[24] contain:

1. An acid dye, such as eosin or phloxine
2. Water to lyse the red cells and rupture the leucocyte membranes (the eosinophils seem more resistant than other leucocytes in this respect)
3. Acetone to inhibit the lytic action of water on the leucocytes according to the proportion used—about 5–10% seems to be the most useful concentration.

In later modifications of Dunger's diluent small amounts of a detergent[24] or alkali[73] were added to accelerate the staining of the eosinophil granules.

Method

Add 20 µl of EDTA blood to 0.38 ml of diluting fluid to give a 1 in 20 dilution. Mix the suspension for not longer than 30 s, and then fill the counting chamber using a stout glass capillary or Pasteur pipette. The eosinophils may be counted as soon as they have settled or the count may be postponed for up to 30 min or so if the counting chamber is placed in a moist chamber (a Petri dish with cover containing a pledget of damp cotton wool).

Counting chamber

A chamber with the Fuchs–Rosenthal ruling is suitable. The ruled area in a Fuchs–Rosenthal chamber is a 4 mm square (Fig. 5.6) and the chamber is 0.2 mm in depth (area 16 mm^2 and volume 3.2 µl)*. With counts at the upper limit of the normal range the whole ruled area should be surveyed and the total number of eosinophils recorded. With lower counts several fillings of the counting chamber should be surveyed. It is convenient to use a × 10 objective and × 10 eyepieces. In a good clean preparation the eosinophils should be easily identified; their granules stain deep red and the cells containing them should be intact.

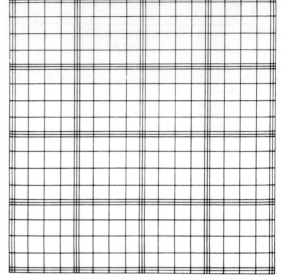

Fig. 5.6   Fuchs–Rosenthal counting chamber. The total ruled area is 4 mm × 4 mm, divided into 16 large squares (1 mm × 1 mm), each containing 16 small squares.

As in ordinary leucocyte counts the accuracy of the count is largely determined by the number of cells counted. In a serious investigation 100 cells should be looked upon as the minimum, the counting chamber being filled several times, if necessary. The CV due to the random distribution of the cells is c 10% in a 100-cell count.

Calculation

$$\text{Count (per litre)} = \frac{\text{No. of cells counted}}{\text{Volume counted (µl)}} \times \text{Dilution} \times 10^6$$

Thus, if N eosinophils are counted in 3.2 µl, then the total eosinophil count per litre is:

$$\frac{N \times 20 \text{ (dilution)}}{3.2} \times 10^6 = N \times 6.25 \times 10^6$$

Diluting fluid

Aqueous eosin (200 g/l) 10 ml
Acetone 10 ml
Water 80 ml.

---

*A modified version is also available in which the ruled area is a 3 mm square, total area 9 mm^2.

The fluid will keep for 2–3 weeks at 4°C. It must be filtered before use.

Eosinophils slowly disintegrate in the diluting fluid and the count should not be delayed for more than 30 min. It is probably best to fill the counting chamber as soon as the blood is diluted and to avoid prolonged mixing, for in this way, clumping of eosinophils may be prevented.[8]

Range of eosinophil count in health

(See pp. 12 and 17.)

There is normally considerable diurnal variation in the eosinophil count and differences amounting to as much as 100% have been recorded. The lowest counts are found in the morning (10 a.m. to noon) and the highest at night (midnight to 4 a.m.)[12,64,81] Muehrcke et al.[56] found that the counts of 42 healthy but fasting young males conformed to a log-normal distribution.

BASOPHIL COUNTS BY A COUNTING-CHAMBER METHOD

Alcian blue stains basophil granules specifically and at a low pH the contrast between the stained basophils and other (unstained) leucocytes is excellent.[31]

Diluting fluid

Solution A: EDTA 1 g/l in 9 g/l NaCl.
Solution B: Cetyl pyridinium chloride
monohydrate 0.76 g
Lanthanum chloride $6H_2O$ 7 g
NaCl 9 g
Tween 20 2.1 ml
Alcian blue 8 GX (CI 74240) 1.43 g
Water to 1 litre.
Solution C: HCl 1 mol/l.

Method[31]

Dilute 0.1 ml of EDTA blood with 0.4 ml of Solution A. Add 0.45 ml of Solution B; mix gently for 1 min. Add 0.05 ml of Solution C; mix gently for a few seconds and then fill a Fuchs-Rosenthal counting chamber, using a stout glass capillary or Pasteur pipette.

Leave for 5–10 min in a moist chamber (a Petri dish with cover containing a pledget of damp cotton wool). Count the stained cells in the whole ruled area.

Calculation

$$\text{Count (per litre)} = \frac{\text{No. of cells counted}}{\text{Volume counted (}\mu l)} \times \text{Dilution} \times 10^6$$

Thus, if N cells are counted in the entire chamber, (i.e. 3.2 μl),

$$\text{Count/l} = \frac{N \times 10}{3.2} \times 10^6$$
$$= N \times 3.13 \times 10^6$$

Range of basophils in health[70]

(See pp. 12 and 17.)

Gilbert and Ornstein[31] reported a 95% distribution in normal subjects of $0.01–0.08 \times 10^9$/l. There are no age or sex differences although serial counts have shown lower levels during ovulation.[53]

PLATELET COUNT

The platelet count is an important component of the blood count. Automated full blood counters produce platelet counts with a precision which is much superior to that of manual platelet counts. Manual counts are still necessary if there is a significant proportion of giant platelets.

Platelet counts are best performed on EDTA-anticoagulated blood which has been obtained by clean venepuncture. They can also be carried out on peripheral blood but the results are less satisfactory than those on venous blood. Peripheral blood counts are significantly lower than counts on venous blood and less constant;[14] a variable number of platelets are probably lost at the site of the skin puncture.

Manual platelet counts are performed by visual examination of diluted whole blood.

MANUAL PLATELET COUNT OF WHOLE BLOOD[13,44]

The diluent consists of 1% aqueous ammonium oxalate in which the red cells are lysed. There is a possibility that red cell debris may be mistaken for platelets but with some experience this should not cause any difficulties. The method is recommended in preference to that using formal-citrate as diluent, which leaves the red cells intact and is more likely to give incorrect results, when the platelet count is low.

Reagent

10 g/l ammonium oxalate. Not more than 500 ml should be made at a time, using scrupulously clean glassware and fresh glass-distilled or deionized water. The solution should be filtered through a micropore filter (0.22 μm) and kept at 4°C. For use, a small part of the stock is refiltered and dispensed in 1.9 ml volumes in 75 × 12 mm tubes.

Method

It is convenient to make a 1 in 20 dilution of the blood in the diluent by adding 0.1 ml of blood to 1.9 ml of the diluent. Mix the suspension on a mechanical mixer for 10–15 min.

Fill a Neubauer counting chamber with the suspension, using a stout glass capillary or Pasteur pipette. Place the counting chamber in a moist Petri dish and leave untouched for at least 20 min to give time for the platelets to settle.

Examine the preparation with the × 40 objective and × 6 or × 10 eyepieces. The platelets appear under ordinary illumination as small (but not minute) highly refractile particles, if viewed with the condenser racked down; they are usually well separated and clumps are rare if the blood sample has been skilfully collected. They are more easily seen with the phase-contrast microscope. A special thin-bottomed (1 mm) counting chamber is best for optimal phase-contrast effect.

The number of platelets in one or more areas of 1 mm^2 should be counted. The total number of platelets counted should always exceed 200.

Calculation

$$\text{Count (per litre)} = \frac{\text{No. of cells counted}}{\text{Volume counted (μl)}} \times \text{Dilution} \times 10^6$$

Thus if N is the number of platelets counted in an area of 1 mm^2 (0.1 μl in volume), the number of platelets per litre of blood is:

$$N \times 10 \times 20 \text{ (dilution)} \times 10^6 = N \times 200 \times 10^6$$

Accuracy and precision

Accuracy in visual platelet counting can be achieved only by the most careful regard to detail, particularly with respect to the cleanliness of the preparation, and by experience, which alone can help in deciding what is and what is not a platelet. As mentioned, the use of phase-contrast microscopy helps considerably in recognizing and counting platelets.

With manual platelet counts the coefficient of variation (CV) is 8–10%.

Range of platelet counts in health

In health there are approximately 150–400 × 10^9 platelets per litre of blood. The counts in individual subjects have been reported as being relatively constant,[13,72] although there is some evidence of a diurnal variation. There may also be a sex difference (see p. 16); in women there is cycling with a slightly lower count at about the time of menstruation.[55]

THE RETICULOCYTE COUNT

Reticulocytes are juvenile red cells; they contain remnants of the ribosomal ribonucleic acid which was present in larger amounts in the cytoplasm of the nucleated precursors from which they were derived. Ribosomes have the property of reacting with certain basic dyes such as azure B, brilliant cresyl blue or New methylene blue to form a blue precipitate of granules or filaments. This reaction takes place only in vitally stained unfixed preparations. The most immature reticulocytes are those with the largest amount of precipitable material; in the least immature only a few dots or short strands are seen. Stages of maturation can be identified by their morphological features.[4,32] Reticulocytes can be classified into four groups ranging from the most immature reticulocytes, with a large clump of reticulin (group I), to the most mature, with a few granules of reticulin (group IV) (Fig. 5.7).

If a blood film is allowed to dry and is afterwards fixed with methanol, reticulocytes appear as red cells staining diffusely basophilic if the film

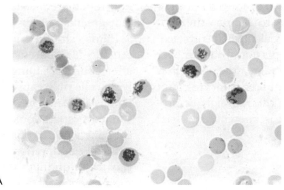

A

Fig. 5.7   (A) Photomicrograph of reticulocytes in haemolytic anaemia. Stained supravitally by New methylene blue.

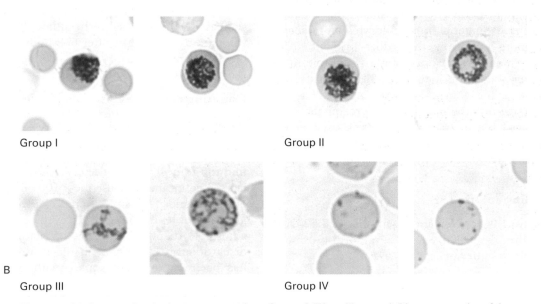

Group I   Group II

B

Group III   Group IV

Fig. 5.7   (B) Stages of reticulocyte maturation. Groups I–IV are illustrated. I is representative of the most immature group; II and III are intermediate stages and IV is representative of the most mature group.

is stained with basic dyes. Complete loss of basophilic material probably occurs as a rule in the blood stream and, particularly, in the spleen[7] after the cells have left the bone marrow.[67] The ripening process is thought to take 2–3 days, of which about 24 h are spent in the circulation.

The number of reticulocytes in the peripheral blood is a fairly accurate reflection of erythropoietic activity, assuming that the reticulocytes are released normally from the bone marrow, and that they remain in circulation for the normal period of time. These assumptions are not always valid as an increased erythropoietic stimulus leads to premature release into the circulation. The maturation time of these so-called 'stress' or stimulated reticulocytes may be as long as 3 days. In such cases, it is possible to deduce the reticulocyte maturation time and calculate a 'corrected' reticulocyte count by using plasma-iron turnover data.[33,34] Nevertheless, adequate information is usually obtained from a simple reticulocyte count recorded as a percentage of the red cells or preferably, if the red cell count is known, expressed as absolute numbers.

MANUAL COUNT

Better and more reliable results are obtained with New methylene blue than with brilliant cresyl blue. New methylene blue stains the reticulo-filamentous material in reticulocytes more deeply and more uniformly than does brilliant cresyl blue, which varies from sample to sample in its staining ability. Purified azure B is a satisfactory substitute for New methylene blue; it has the advantage that the dye does not precipitate[52] and it is available in pure form.[85] It is used in the same concentration and the staining procedure is the same as with New methylene blue.

Staining solution

Dissolve 1.0 g of New methylene blue (CI 52030)* or azure B (p. 86) in 100 ml of iso-osmotic phosphate buffer pH 7.4 (p. 578).

Method

Deliver 2 or 3 drops of the dye solution into a 75 × 10 mm glass or plastic tube by means of a Pasteur pipette. Add 2–4 volumes of the patient's EDTA-anticoagulated blood to the dye solution and mix. Keep the mixture at 37°C for 15–20 min. Resuspend the red cells by gentle mixing and make films on glass slides in the usual way. When dry, examine the films without fixing or counterstaining.

The exact volume of blood to be added to the dye solution for optimal staining depends upon the red cell count. A larger proportion of anaemic blood, and a smaller proportion of polycythaemic blood, should be added than of normal blood. In a successful preparation the reticulo-filamentous material should be stained deep blue and the non-reticulated cells stained diffusely shades of pale greenish blue.

Films should not be counterstained. The reticulo-filamentous material is not better defined after counterstaining and precipitated stain overlying cells may cause confusion. Moreover, Heinz bodies will not be visible in fixed and counterstained preparations. If the stained preparation is examined under phase contrast, both the mature red cells and reticulocytes are well defined. By this technique late reticulocytes characterized by the presence of remnants of filaments or threads are readily distinguished from cells containing inclusion bodies. Satisfactory counts may be made on blood that has been allowed to stand (unstained) for as long as 24 h, although the count will tend to fall slightly after 6–8 hours unless the blood is kept at 4°C.

Counting reticulocytes

An area of film should be chosen for the count where the cells are undistorted and where the staining is good. A common fault is to make the film too thin; however, the cells should not overlap. To count the cells, use the × 100 oil-immersion objective and if possible eyepieces provided with an adjustable diaphragm. If eyepieces with an adjustable diaphragm are not available, a paper or cardboard diaphragm, in the centre of which has been cut a small square with sides about

---

*New methylene blue is chemically different from methylene blue which is a poor reticulocyte stain.

4 mm in length, can be inserted into an eyepiece and used as a less convenient substitute.

The counting procedure should be appropriate to the number of reticulocytes present. Very large numbers of cells have to be surveyed if a reasonably accurate count is to be obtained when only small numbers of reticulocytes are present.[67] When the count is less than 10% a convenient method is to survey successive fields until at least 100 reticulocytes have been counted and to count the total cells in at least ten fields in order to determine the average number of cells per field.

Calculation

Number of reticulocytes in n fields = x
Average number of cells per field = y
Total number of cells in n fields = $n \times y$

$$\text{Reticulocyte percentage} = \frac{x}{n \times y} \times 100\%$$

Absolute reticulocyte count = $\% \times RBC$

Thus when the reticulocyte percentage is 3.3 and the RBC is $5 \times 10^{12}/l$ the absolute reticulocyte count per litre is:

$$\frac{3.3}{100} \times 5 \times 10^{12} = 165 \times 10^9$$

It is essential that the reticulocyte preparation be well spread to ensure an even distribution of cells in successive fields.

When the reticulocyte count exceeds 10% only a relatively small number of cells will have to be surveyed to obtain a standard error of 10%.*

An alternative method is based on the principle of 'balanced sampling', using a Miller ocular.** This is an eyepiece giving a square field, in the corner of which is a second ruled square, one-ninth the area of the total square. Reticulocytes are counted in the large square and the total number of cells in the small square. The number of fields which should be surveyed to obtain a desired degree of accuracy depends on the proportion of reticulocytes (Table 5.2).

It is essential that the reticulocyte preparation be well spread and well stained. Other important factors which affect the accuracy of the count are the visual acuity and patience of the observer and the quality and resolving power of the microscope.

Table 5.2 Accuracy of reticulocyte counts with Miller ocular

Reticulocytes		Standard error (σ)		
%	Proportion (p)	2%	5%	10%
1	0.01	27500	4400	1100
2	0.02	13600	2180	550
5	0.05	5280	845	210
10	0.10	2500	400	100
25	0.25	835	135	35

Columns 3–5 indicate the total number of red cells to be counted *in the small squares* so as to give the required standard error at different reticulocyte levels. It is derived from:

$$\sigma = \sqrt{\frac{p(1-p)}{\lambda}}$$

where p = $\dfrac{\text{Number of reticulocytes in n large squares}}{\text{Number of red cells in n small squares} \times f}$
 f = ratio of large to small squares (i.e. 9), and
 λ = approximate total number of cells in n large squares.

The most accurate counts are carried out by a conscientious observer who has no knowledge of the supposed reticulocyte level, thus eliminating the effect of conscious or unconscious bias.

The decision as to what is and what is not a reticulocyte may be difficult, as the most mature reticulocytes contain only a few dots or threads of reticulo-filamentous material. Fortunately, in well-stained preparations, viewed under the light microscope, the Pappenheimer (iron-containing) type of granular material—usually present as a single small dot, less commonly as multiple dots—stains a darker shade of blue than does the reticulo-filamentous material of the reticulocyte. As described above, phase contrast will help to distinguish them. If there is any doubt, Pappenheimer's bodies can be identified by overstaining the film for iron by Perls's reaction (see p. 132).

HbH undergoes denaturation in the presence of brilliant cresyl blue or New methylene blue, resulting in round inclusion bodies which stain greenish-blue (Fig. 8.7, p. 136). These can be easily differentiated from reticulo-filamentous material (Fig. 5.7).

---

*Standard error (σ) = $\sqrt{\dfrac{p(1-p)}{\lambda}}$ where p is the proportion of reticulocytes and λ is the total number of cells surveyed.
**e.g. Graticules Ltd, Morley Road, Tonbridge, Kent.

Heinz bodies are also stained by New methylene blue, but they stain a lighter shade of blue than the reticulo-filamentous material of reticulocytes (Figs. 8.5 and 8.6, p. 135).

Reticulocytes can be counted by fluorescence microscopy.[43,82] Add 1 volume of acridine orange solution (50 mg/100 ml of 9 g/l NaCl) to 1 volume of blood. Mix gently for 2 min; make films on glass slides, dry rapidly and examine in a fluorescent microscope.

RNA gives an orange-red fluorescence whilst nuclear material (DNA) fluoresces yellow. However, the method is not suitable for routine use for reticulocyte counting. Although the amount of fluorescence is proportional to the amount of RNA, the brightness and colour of the fluorescence fluctuates and the preparation quickly fades when exposed to light; also, it requires a special fluorescence microscope.

Fluorescent staining combined with flow cytometry has been developed as a method for automated reticulocyte counting (see p. 78).[65,76,84]

Range of reticulocyte count in health

(See pp. 12 and 17.)
    Adults and children 0.5–2.5%
    Infants (full term, cord blood) 2–5%.

In absolute numbers the normal reticulocyte count in health is about $50–100 \times 10^9/l$.

AUTOMATED TECHNIQUES

A variety of automated instruments for performing blood counts have been developed and are now in widespread use. Semi-automated instruments require some steps, for example dilution of a blood sample, to be carried out by the operator. Fully automated instruments require only that an appropriate blood sample is presented to the instrument. Semi-automated instruments often measure only a small number of variables, for example WBC and Hb. Fully automated multi-channel instruments usually measure from 8 to 20 variables including some new parameters which do not have any equivalent in manual techniques. Automated instruments usually have a high level of precision which, for cell counting and cell sizing techniques, is greatly superior to that which can be achieved with manual techniques. If instruments are carefully calibrated and their correct operation is assured by quality control procedures they produce test results that are generally accurate. When blood has abnormal characteristics the results for one or more parameters may be inaccurate; instruments are designed so that such aberrant results consequent on unusual characteristics of the blood are 'flagged' for subsequent review. The abnormal characteristics which lead to inaccurate counts vary between instruments, so that it is important for instrument operators to be familiar with the types of factitious results to which their instrument is prone. The most recently developed blood cell counters have automated systems of sample recognition (for example by bar-coding), ensure that adequate sample mixing occurs, sample the blood automatically and have a system for detection of clots and samples of inadequate size. Ideally, blood sampling is by piercing the cap of a closed tube so that samples which carry an infection hazard can be handled with maximum safety.

Laboratories performing large numbers of blood counts each day require fully automated blood counters capable of the rapid production of accurate and precise blood counts. Such instruments should perform a platelet count and may perform an automated differential count, either three-part or five-part. The sample throughput required varies with the workload and the timing of arrival of blood specimens in the laboratory, but for most large laboratories a throughput of 80–100 samples per hour is required. Sample size and the availability of a 'pre-dilute' mode are particularly relevant if the laboratory receives many paediatric specimens. Choice of an instrument for an individual laboratory should also consider: the necessary capital expenditure and running costs, including maintenance and reagents; size of instrument; likelihood of generation of heat, vibration and noise; requirement for environmental temperature and humidity control and for services such as water, compressed air, drainage and an electricity supply with stable voltage; the need for storage for the often bulky reagents; ease of operation; and the likely level of support which can be expected from the manufacturer. Guidelines have been published to help in the choice of an instrument suitable for the needs of an individual laboratory and also to assess its performance, as compared with the claims of the manufacturer, when it has been installed and is being used in routine practice.[40,42,68] Choice of instrument may be aided by reference to published reports of instrument evaluations and to reports available in the United Kingdom from the National Health Service Medical Devices Directorate. A number of monographs are available which aid in the interpretation of the numerical and graphical output of automated instruments.[4,9,63,69]

Some semi-automated instruments aspirate a sample of accurately determined volume and so can perform absolute cell counts and accurate estimations of Hb. Most automated instruments, however, count for a specified period of time rather than on an exact volume of blood; they therefore require calibration by means of the direct counts derived from instruments counting cells in a defined volume of diluted blood. For some parameters instruments are calibrated by the manufacturer, but others require calibration in the laboratory (see p. 79). Performance characteristics of an instrument vary over time so that periodic recalibration is needed, both when quality control procedures indicate the necessity and when certain components are replaced.

The principles underlying the performance of specific measurements by automated counters will now be discussed.

HAEMOGLOBIN CONCENTRATION (Hb)

Most automated counters measure Hb by a modification of the manual haemiglobincyanide (HiCN) method. Modifications include alterations in the concentration of reagents and in the temperature and pH of the reaction. A non-ionic detergent is included to ensure rapid cell lysis and to reduce turbidity due to cell membranes and plasma lipids. Measurements of absorbance are made at a set time interval after mixing of blood and the active reagents but before the reaction is completed.

In some Sysmex (Toa) instruments, HiCN has been replaced with a method using a non-toxic chemical, sodium lauryl sulphate, in order to reduce possible environmental hazards from disposal of large volumes of cyanide-containing waste. This has been found to be a reliable routine method with estimations of Hb being generally equivalent to those produced by the HiCN method.[45]

RED BLOOD CELL COUNT (RBC)

Red cells and other blood cells may be counted electronically in systems based on aperture impedance or light-scattering technology. Cells are counted as they pass in a stream through an aperture. Large numbers of cells can be counted so that the precision of an electronic red cell count is much better than that of a manual count and the count is available in a fraction of the time. As a consequence, electronic counts have rendered the RBC and the red cell indices derived from it (the MCV and the MCH) of much more clinical relevance than when only a slow and imprecise manual RBC was available.

Impedance counting

Impedance counting, first described by Wallace Coulter in 1956,[19] depends on the fact that red cells are poor conductors of electricity whereas certain diluents are good conductors; this difference forms the basis of the Coulter Counting System and is also used in the Sysmex (Toa) counters and in several other more recently developed counters.

For a cell count, blood is highly diluted in a buffered electrolyte solution. An external vacuum initiates movement of a mercury siphon which causes a measured volume of the sample to flow through an aperture tube of specific dimensions, e.g. 100 μm in diameter and 70 μm in length. By means of a constant source of electricity a direct current is maintained between two electrodes, one in the sample beaker or the chamber surrounding the aperture tube and another inside the aperture tube. As a blood cell is carried through the aperture it displaces some of the conducting fluid and increases the electrical resistance. This produces a corresponding change in potential between the electrodes which lasts as long as the red cell takes to pass though the aperture; the height of the pulses produced indicates the volume of the cells passing through. The pulses can be displayed on an oscillograph screen. The pulses are led to a threshold circuit provided with an amplitude discriminator for selecting the minimal pulse height which will be counted (Fig. 5.8). The height of the pulses is used to determine the volume of the red cells (see p. 73).

Light scattering

Red cells and other blood cells may be counted by means of electro-optical detectors.[80] A diluted cell suspension flows through an aperture so that the cells pass, in single file, in front of a light source; light is scattered by the cells passing through the light beam. Scattered light is detected by a photomultiplier or photodiode which converts it into electrical impulses which are

accumulated and counted. The amount of light scattered is proportional to the surface area and therefore the volume of the cell so that the height of the electrical pulses can be used to estimate the cell volume (see p. 73). The high intensity coherent laser beams used in current instruments have superior optical qualities to the noncoherent tungsten light of earlier instruments. Sheathed flow allows cells to flow in an axial stream with a diameter not much greater than that of a red cell; light can be very precisely focused on this stream of cells. Electro-optical detectors are employed for red cell sizing and counting in Ortho and Technicon counters (and for white cell differential counting in a number of other instruments).

RELIABILITY OF ELECTRONIC COUNTERS

Electronic counts are precise but care needs to be taken so that they are also accurate. The recorded count on the same sample may vary from instrument to instrument and even between different models of the same instrument. Inaccuracy may be introduced by coincidence (that is, by two cells passing through an orifice simultaneously and being counted as one cell, or

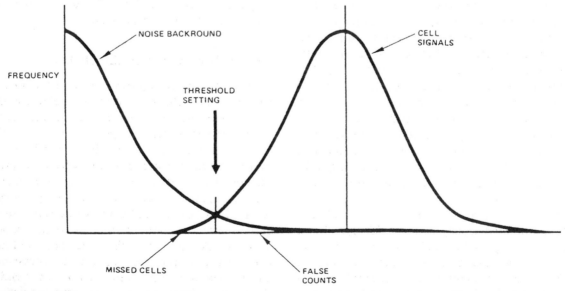

Fig. 5.8   Effect of threshold discrimination (horizontal axis) in separating cell signals from background noise.

by a pulse being generated during the electronic dead time of the circuit), by recirculation of cells which have already been counted, by red cell agglutination (which causes a clump of cells to be counted as one cell) and by the counting of bubbles or extraneous particles as cells. Faulty maintenance may lead to variation in the volume aspirated or the flow rate. Single channel instruments may have their thresholds set incorrectly and multi-channel instruments may be incorrectly calibrated.

A statistical correction may be applied for coincidence (coincidence correction); in some instruments this is done automatically by electronic editing. Errors of coincidence can be detected by carrying out a series of measurements at various dilutions of the same specimen, plotting the data on graph paper and then extrapolating the graph to the baseline for the true value. Alternatively, the need for coincidence correction can be avoided by having the dimensions and flow characteristics of the aperture through which the cells pass such that cells can only pass in single file; this may be achieved by sheath flow or hydrodynamic focusing in which diluted blood is injected into a sheath of fluid as it flows into the sensing zone. This induces the cells to pass through the centre of the sensing zone in single file and free of distortion. Coincidence can be more effectively reduced with sheathed flow and precisely focused light in an electro-optical detector than in an impedance counter so that less dilution of the blood sample is needed.[80] Electrical impulses generated by recirculation of cells can be eliminated by electronic editing or, alternatively, recirculation of cells in the region of the aperture can be prevented by 'sweep flow' in which a directed stream of diluent sweeps cells and debris away from the aperture, thus preventing cells from being recounted and debris from being counted as cells.

Inaccurate counts consequent on red cell agglutination are usually due to cold agglutinins. They are recognized as erroneous because of an associated marked factitious elevation of the MCV. A correct count can be achieved by pre-warming the blood sample and, if necessary, also pre-warming the diluent.

A correct red cell count and, particularly, a correct measurement of the MCV is dependent on the use of an appropriate diluent. For impedance counters pH, temperature and rate of ionization have to be standardized and remain constant, since changes alter the electrical field and may lead to artefactual alterations in the size, shape and stability of the blood cells in the diluent. Diluents must be free of particles and give a background count of less than 50 particles in the measured volume. The correct diluent for each individual instrument must be used; other diluents, even those made by the same manufacturer, may not be interchangeable. Any laboratories using diluents other than those recommended by the manufacturer of the instrument must satisfy themselves that no error is being introduced.

For red cell counting in simple single channel counters a suitable diluent requires a pH of 7.0–7.5 and osmolality of 340 ± 10 mmol. Physiological saline (9 g/l NaCl) or phosphate buffered saline (p. 579) which have the advantages of simplicity and ready availability, can be used as a red cell diluent, provided that the counts are performed immediately after dilution in order to avoid errors due to sphering. Commercial solutions of saline (for intravenous use) are usually particle-free. Other solutions may require filtration through a 0.22 or 0.45 μm micropore filter to remove dust.

Setting discrimination thresholds

An accurate RBC requires that thresholds be set so that all red cells, but a minimum of other cells, are included in the count. Some counters have a lower threshold but no upper threshold so that white cells are included in the 'red cell count'. Since the white cell count is usually very low in relation to the red cell count this is not usually of practical importance; however, an appreciable error can be introduced if the white cell count is greatly elevated, particularly if the patient is also anaemic. The setting of the lower threshold is of considerable importance since it is necessary to ensure that microcytic red cells are included in the count without also counting large platelets.

Current multi-channel instruments, both impedance counters and counters employing light-scattering technology, have thresholds which are either pre-calibrated by the manufacturer or are automatically adjusted, depending on the characteristics of individual blood samples. Single channel impedance instruments capable of performing a direct red cell count require setting of thresholds so as to separate pulses generated by red cells from background noise and from pulses generated by platelets. This is done by adjusting the aperture current and the pulse amplification. A simple method is to dilute a fresh blood sample and carry out successive counts on the suspension, whilst the lower threshold control is moved incrementally from its maximum to its minimum position. At the maximum position the count should be zero or close to zero, and the counts will rise as the amplitude is reduced. The counts at each setting are plotted on arithmetic graph paper (Fig. 5.9). The correct threshold setting is at the left of the horizontal part of the graph before the line begins to slope. It is important to

check that the setting selected is valid for microcytic cells. The threshold can be defined more precisely for an individual sample by means of a pulse height analyser linked to the counting system. The lower threshold is correctly set if beyond this point there are fewer than 0.5% of the counts at the peak (mode) of the pulse size distribution curve (Fig. 5.8).

PACKED CELL VOLUME (PCV) AND MEAN CELL VOLUME (MCV)

Modern automated blood cell counters estimate packed cell volume (PCV) by technology which has little connection with packing red cells by centrifugation. It is sometimes convenient to use different terms to distinguish the manual and automated tests, and for this reason the International Council for Standardization in Haematology (ICSH) has suggested that the term 'haematocrit' (Hct) rather than packed cell volume (PCV) should be used for the automated

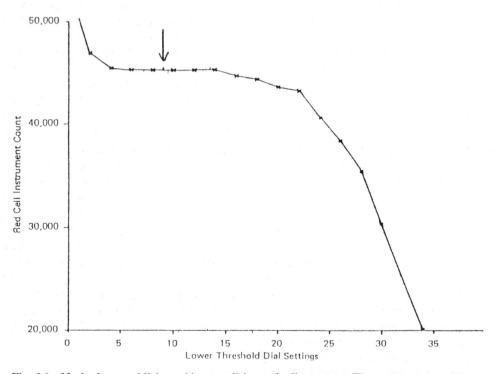

Fig. 5.9   Method to establish working conditions of cell counters. The correct setting of the threshold (at arrow) is intended to exclude noise pulses without loss of the signal pulses produced by the blood cells.

measurement. However, it should be noted that in the past the terms 'packed cell volume' and 'haematocrit' have been used interchangeably for the manual procedure.

With automated instruments the derivation of the RBC, PCV and MCV are closely interrelated. The passage of a cell through the aperture of an impedance counter or through the beam of light of a light-scattering instrument leads to the generation of an electrical pulse the height of which is proportional to cell volume. The number of pulses generated allows the RBC to be determined, as discussed above. Pulse height analysis allows either the MCV or the PCV to be determined. If the average pulse height is computed this is indicative of the MCV and the PCV can be derived by multiplying the estimated MCV by the RBC. Similarly, if the pulse heights are summed this figure is indicative of the PCV and the MCV can, in turn, be derived by dividing the PCV by the RBC.

Automated instruments require calibration before the PCV or MCV can be determined. Calibration of the PCV can be based on manual PCV determinations. Alternatively, the MCV can be calibrated by means of the pulse heights generated by latex beads,* stabilized cells or some other calibrant containing particles of known size; however, unfixed human red cells which are biconcave and flexible will not necessarily show the same characteristics in a cell counter as latex particles or some other artificial calibrant. Aperture-impedance systems measure an apparent volume which is greater than the true volume, being influenced by a 'shape factor';[27] this factor is less than 1.1 for young, flexible red cells, is between 1.1 and 1.2 for fixed biconcave cells, and is about 1.5 for fixed spheres, whether they be fixed cells or latex spheres.[27,80]

The MCV and therefore the PCV as determined by an automated counter will vary with certain cell characteristics other than volume. As indicated above, such characteristics include shape which in turn is partly determined by flexibility. With impedance counters the normal disc-shaped red cell becomes elongated into a cigar shape as it passes through the aperture; this is caused by deformation in response to shear force which occurs in cells of normal flexibility. Cells with a reduced haemoglobin concentration undergo more elongation than normal cells; this leads to a reduced 'shape factor', a reduced pulse height in relation to the true size of the cell and underestimation of the MCV. Conversely, cells with abnormally rigid membranes and cells such as spherocytes with a high haemoglobin concentration will undergo less deformation than normal and the MCV will be overestimated. Earlier light-scattering instruments also underestimated the volume of red cells with a reduced haemoglobin concentration since light scattering was affected by the haemoglobin concentration.[54] These artefacts are seen even with normal red cells of varying haemoglobin concentration but are more apparent with red cells from patients with defects in haemoglobin synthesis such as those from patients with iron deficiency. Several recent light-scattering instruments (Technicon H1 and H2) have sought to avoid artefacts of this type. Cells are isovolumetrically sphered so that their light-scattering characteristics are uniform and should follow the laws of physics. Light scattering by each individual cell is measured at two angles, which permits computation of both its volume and its haemoglobin concentration;[54,62] the latter measurement is designated the cellular haemoglobin concentration mean (CHCM) to distinguish it from the traditional MCHC derived from the Hb and the PCV. If all measurements are accurate the CHCM and the MCHC should give the same results, thus providing an internal quality control mechanism.

The automated MCV and PCV are prone to certain errors which do not occur or are less of a problem with manual methods. Alterations in plasma osmolarity occurring, for example, in severe hyperglycaemia cause factitious elevation of the MCV and PCV.[28,35] Cold agglutinins are a relatively common cause of factitious elevation of the MCV since clumps of cells are sized as if they were single cells. Since the RBC is underestimated the PCV is less affected, although it is also inaccurate. It is rare for warm agglutinins to cause a similar problem.

---

*Available as certified reference materials from the Commission of the European Union (see p. 36).

MEAN CELLULAR HAEMOGLOBIN (MCH) AND MEAN CELLULAR HAEMOGLOBIN CONCENTRATION (MCHC)

As is the case for manual blood counts, the MCH and the MCHC are derived parameters. The MCH is derived from the Hb and the RBC. With instruments that measure the PCV and calculate the MCV, the MCHC is derived in the traditional manner from the Hb and the PCV. With instruments that measure the MCV and calculate the PCV, the MCHC is derived from the Hb, MCV and RBC according to the formula:

$$\text{MCHC (g/l)} = \frac{\text{Hb (g/l)} \times 1000}{\text{MCV (fl)} \times \text{RBC/l} \times 10^{-12}}$$

e.g. if Hb is 150 g/l, MCV is 90 fl and RBC is $5 \times 10^{12}/l$,

$$\text{MCH} = \frac{150 \times 1000}{90 \times 5}$$
$$= 333 \text{ g/l}$$

As mentioned above, the CHCM of the H1 and H2 counters is a more directly measured equivalent of the MCHC.

As automated counters were developed and introduced it was noted that the lowered MCHC which, with manual methods, had been a useful indicator of hypochromia in early iron deficiency was a less sensitive indicator of developing iron deficiency. The explanation of this is complex. In iron deficiency there is not only true hypochromia but also increased plasma trapping within the column of red cells in a microhaematocrit tube which increases the PCV and exaggerates the fall in the MCHC. The lowered MCHC is thus partly a true reflection of hypochromia and partly an artefact. When the MCHC is derived by automated counters the artefact of increased plasma trapping is no longer present but the instruments are also less sensitive to a true reduction of the MCHC because of the underestimation of the size of hypochromic red cells described above. Since the MCHC is calculated from the formula given above the underestimation of the MCV leads to an overestimation of the MCHC. The MCHC thus shows little alteration as cells become hypochromic. The MCHC as derived using the H1 and H2

counters has regained some of the sensitivity to iron deficiency of the manual methods since, although the artefact of increased plasma trapping is not reproduced by the automated instrument, the MCHC and the CHCM fall as hypochromia develops.[62]

THE DISTRIBUTION OF RED CELL VOLUMES—RED CELL DISTRIBUTION (RDW)

Automated instruments produce volume distribution histograms which allow the presence of more than one population of cells to be appreciated. Instruments may also assess the percentage of cells falling above and below given MCV thresholds and 'flag' the presence of an increased number of microcytes or macrocytes. Such measurements may indicate the presence of a small but significant increase in the percentage of either microcytes or macrocytes before there has been any change in the MCV.

Most instruments also produce a quantitative measurement of the variation in cell volume, an equivalent of the microscopic assessment of the degree of anisocytosis. This new parameter has been named the 'red cell distribution width' (RDW). The RDW is derived from pulse height analysis and can be expressed either as the standard deviation (in fl) or as the coefficient of variation (%) of the measurements of the red cell volume. Current Coulter and Technicon instruments express the RDW as the SD, and Sysmex(Toa) instruments express it as either the SD or the CV. Widely different reference ranges have been reported for the RDW with the CV varying between 7.4 and 13.4%[9,10,59,63] It is therefore important for laboratories to determine their own reference ranges. The RDW expressed as the CV has been found of some value in distinguishing between iron deficiency (RDW usually increased) and thalassaemia trait (RDW usually normal) and between megaloblastic anaemia (RDW often increased) and other causes of macrocytosis (RDW more often normal).

Range of RDW values in health

(See p. 12.)

THE DISTRIBUTION OF RED CELL HAEMOGLOBINIZATION—HAEMOGLOBIN DISTRIBUTION WIDTH (HDW)

Instruments which determine the haemoglobin concentration of individual red cells (Technicon H1 and H2) provide distribution curves of the haemoglobin concentration and are able to 'flag' the presence of increased numbers of hypochromic cells and hyperchromic cells. Since the volume of individual red cells is also determined it is possible to distinguish between hypochromic microcytes, which are indicative of a defect in haemoglobin synthesis, and hypochromic macrocytes, which often represent reticulocytes.[5] The identification of an increased percentage of hyperchromic cells may be caused by the presence of spherocytes, 'irregularly contracted cells' or sickled cells. The degree of variation in red cell haemoglobinization is quantified as the haemoglobin distribution width or HDW; this is the CV of the measurements of haemoglobin concentration of individual cells. The normal 95% range is 1.82–2.64.

TOTAL WHITE BLOOD CELL COUNT (WBC)

The total white cell count is determined in whole blood in which red cells have been lysed. The lytic agent is required to destroy the red cells and reduce the red cell stroma to a residue which causes no detectable response in the counting system without affecting leucocytes in such a manner that the ability of the system to count them is altered. Various manufacturers recommend specific reagents and for multi-channel instruments which also perform an automated differential count use of the recommended reagent is essential. For a simple single-channel impedance counter the following fluid is satisfactory:

Cetrimide 20 g
10% formaldhyde (in 9 g/l NaCl) 2 ml
Glacial acetic acid 16 ml
NaCl 6 g
Water to 1 litre.

Relatively simple instruments are also available which determine the Hb and the WBC by consecutive measurements on the one blood sample. The diluent contains a reagent to lyse the red cells and another to convert haemoglobin to haemiglobin cyanide. Hb is measured by a modified HiCN method and white cells are counted by impedance technology. Apart from the reagents specified by the manufacturers a diluent containing potassium cyanide and potassium ferricyanide together with ethylhexadecyldimethylammonium bromide can be used.[6,71]

Fully automated multi-channel instruments perform white cell counts by either impedance or light-scattering technology or both. Residual particles in a diluted blood sample are counted after red cell lysis or, in the case of some light-scattering instruments, after the red cells have been rendered transparent. Thresholds are set to exclude normal platelets from the count, although giant platelets are included. Some or all of any nucleated red cells present are usually included, so that when nucleated red cells are present the count approximates more to the total nucleated cell count (TNCC) than to the white cell count.

Factitiously low automated white cell counts occasionally occur as a consequence of white cell agglutination. Factitiously high counts are more common and usually result from failure of lysis of red cells; with certain instruments this may occur with the cells of neonates or be consequent on uraemia or on the presence of an abnormal haemoglobin such as haemoglobin S or haemoglobin C.

AUTOMATED DIFFERENTIAL COUNT

Automated differential counters which are now available generally use flow cytometry incorporated into a full blood counter rather than being stand-alone differential counters. Differential counters based on pattern recognition in stained blood films were initially preferred by many haematologists but they were relatively slow, and since they could count only a small number of cells in a reasonable time the precision of the automated count was no better than that of a manual count.

Increasingly, automated blood cell counters have a differential counting capacity, providing either a three-part or a five- to seven-part differential count. Counts are performed on diluted whole blood in which red cells are either lysed or are rendered transparent. A three-part differential count assigns cells to categories usually designated: (i) 'granulocytes' or 'large cells'; (ii) 'lymphocytes' or small cells; or (iii) 'monocytes', 'mononuclear cells' or 'middle cells'. In theory, the granulocyte category includes eosinophils and basophils, but in practice it is common for an appreciable proportion of cells of these types to be excluded from the granulocyte category and to be counted instead in the monocyte category.[2,16] Five-part or six- to seven-part differential counts classify cells, at a minimum, as neutrophils, eosinophils, basophils, lymphocytes and monocytes.[16,18,49,62,69] The automated differential count of the H1 and H2 counters have a sixth category, designated 'large unstained cells'.[62] These are cells which are larger than normal lymphocytes and lack peroxidase activity; this category includes atypical lymphocytes and various other abnormal cells. The Cobas Argos 5000 counter identifies seven categories of white cell including large immature cells (composed of blasts and immature granulocytes) and atypical lymphocytes (including small blasts). Automated instruments performing three-part or five- to seven-part differential counts are able to 'flag' or reject counts from the majority of samples with nucleated red cells, myelocytes, promyelocytes,

blasts and atypical lymphocytes.[18,60,62,69] To a lesser extent instruments incorporating a three-part differential count, although not capable of enumerating eosinophils or basophils, are able to flag a significant proportion of samples which have an increased number of one of these cell types.[21]

Both impedance counters and light-scattering instruments are capable of producing three-part differential counts from a single channel; the categorization is based on the different volume of various types of cell following partial lysis and cytoplasmic shrinkage. Most five- to seven-part differential counts require two or more channels in which cell volume and other characteristics are analysed by various modalities (Table 5.3). Analysis may be dependent only on volume and other physical characteristics of the cell or also on activity of cellular enzymes such as peroxidase. Technologies employed to study cell characteristics include light scattering and absorbance, and impedance measurements with low- and high-frequency electromagnetic current or radiofrequency current. Cells may have been exposed to lytic agents or a cytochemical reaction may have occurred before cell characteristics are studied. Two-parameter analysis or more complex discriminant functions divide cells into clusters which can be matched with the position of the various white cell clusters in normal blood. Thresholds, some fixed and some variable, divide

Table 5.3   Automated full blood counters with a five-, six- or seven-part differential counting capacity

Instrument and manufacturer	Technology employed in automated differential count
Coulter STKS (Coulter Electronics Ltd)	Impedance with low-frequency electromagnetic current. Impedance with high-frequency electromagnetic current. Laser light scattering
Sysmex NE-8000 (Toa Medical Electronic Co)	Impedance with low-frequency direct current. Impedance with radiofrequency current
H1, H2 and H3 (Technicon Division of Bayer)	Light scattering and absorbance following peroxidase reaction. Two-angle light scattering following differential cytoplasmic stripping
Cell-Dyn 3500 (Abbott Diagnostics Division)	Four light-scattering parameters: forward light scatter, orthogonal light scatter, narrow-angle light scatter, depolarized orthogonal light scatter
Cobas Argos 5 Diff (Roche Diagnostics Systems)	Electrical impedance with intact cells and following differential cytoplasmic stripping. Light absorbance

clusters from one another, permitting cells in each cluster to be counted.

Automated differential counters employing flow cytometry classify far more cells than is possible with a manual differential count. Automated counts are consequently much more precise than manual counts; however, with certain cell categories—specifically monocytes and basophils—the degree of precision is sometimes less than would be expected for the number of cells counted, indicating that such cells are not always classified in a consistent manner. The accuracy of automated counters is less impressive than their precision. With all types of counter, unusual cell characteristics or ageing of a blood specimen can lead to misclassification of cells. Although the majority of samples containing abnormal cells are 'flagged' this is not invariably so; the presence of nucleated red cells, immature granulocytes, atypical lymphocytes and blasts (even occasionally quite large numbers of blasts) may not give rise to a 'flag'. However, human observers performing a 100-cell manual differential count also miss significant abnormalities. In general, automated counts have compared reasonably favourably with routine manual counts if the instruments are assigned only two functions—performing differential counts on normal samples, and 'flagging' abnormal samples. If a differential count shows other than distributional abnormalities there is, as yet, no substitute for the human observer for the recognition and enumeration of abnormal cells.

The instrument–reagent systems which have been developed to permit automated differential counts often include some but not all nucleated red cells in the total 'white cell count'. Thus, in the presence of a significant number of nucleated red cells the total count is neither a true 'white cell count' nor a true 'total nucleated cell count' and the absolute white cell counts calculated from the total will necessarily be somewhat erroneous. This differs from the situation with earlier instruments which included any nucleated red cells in the 'white cell count'. It may be possible to make some assessment of the proportion of the nucleated red cells included in the total count by studying the graphical output of the instrument, but if accurate absolute counts of different leucocyte types are needed it is necessary to revert to earlier instruments to provide the total nucleated cell count.

New white cell parameters

Automated white cell counters analyse cell characteristics by novel technologies and identify cell types by features which differ greatly from those used when a blood film is examined visually. It is possible, for example, to identify eosinophils by the ability of their granules to polarize light[18] or to detect a left shift or the presence of blasts by the reduced light-scattering of the nuclei of more immature granulocytes. There is also the potential to produce information which is not directly analogous with that available from a manual differential count. Instruments, such as the H1 and H2, that incorporate a cytochemical reaction, yield information on enzyme activity expressed as the mean peroxidase activity index (MPXI). An increased MPXI has been observed in infections, in some myelodysplasias and leukaemias, in the acquired immune deficiency syndrome (AIDS) and in megaloblastic anaemia, whereas a reduced MPXI occurs in inherited and acquired neutrophil peroxidase deficiency.[22,62,69,78] Such measurements may prove to be clinically useful.

PLATELET COUNT

Platelets can be counted in whole blood using the same techniques of electrical or electro-optical detection as are employed for counting red cells. An upper threshold is needed to separate platelets from red cells and a lower threshold to separate platelets from debris and electronic noise. Recirculation of red cells near the aperture should be prevented or pulses produced may simulate those generated by platelets. Three techniques for setting thresholds have been used: (i) platelets can be counted between two fixed thresholds, for example between 2 and 20 fl; (ii) pulses between fixed thresholds can be counted with subsequent fitting of a curve and extrapolation so that platelets falling outside the fixed thresholds are included in the computed count; and (iii) thresholds can vary automatically, depending of the characteristics of individual blood samples, to make allowance for microcytic or fragmented red cells or for giant platelets.

Platelet count in health

(See pp. 12 and 17.)

Platelet counts are somewhat higher in women than in men.[1] Lower platelet counts have been observed in apparently healthy West Indians and Africans than in Caucasians.[3] (See p. 16).

Mean platelet volume (MPV) and other platelet parameters

The same techniques which are used to size red cells can be applied to platelets. The calculated mean platelet volume (MPV) is very dependent on the technique of measurement and on length and conditions of storage prior to testing the blood. When MPV is measured by impedance technology it has been found to vary inversely with the platelet count in normal subjects. If this curve is extrapolated it has been found that data fit the extrapolated curve when thrombocytopenia is caused by peripheral platelet destruction; however, the MPV is lower than predicted when thrombocytopenia is caused by megaloblastic anaemia or bone marrow failure.[11] The MPV is generally greater than predicted in myeloproliferative disorders, but differentiating essential thrombocythaemia from reactive thrombocytosis on this basis has not been very successful.

Other platelet parameters which can be computed by automated counters include the platelet distribution width (PDW) which is a measure of platelet anisocytosis and the 'plateletcrit' which is the product of the MPV and platelet count and, by analogy with the haematocrit, may be seen as indicative of the volume of circulating platelets in a unit volume of blood. The PDW has been found to be of some use in distinguishing essential thrombocythaemia (PDW increased) from reactive thrombocytosis (PDW normal). The plateletcrit does not appear to provide any information of clinical value.

RETICULOCYTE COUNT

An automated reticulocyte count can be performed utilizing the fact that various fluorochromes combine with the RNA of reticulocytes. Fluorescent cells can then be enumerated by using a flow cytometer, either a general purpose flow cytometer (such as the Becton Dickinson FACScan or the Coulter Electronics EPIC Profile) or a committed automated reticulocyte counter (such as the Toa-Sysmex R-1000 or R-3000 Automated Reticulocyte Analyzer). Some automated full blood counters also now incorporate a reticulocyte counting capacity.

A variety of fluorochromes have been employed; some produce a high level of background fluorescence and some require a long period of incubation with counts being dependent on temperature as well as time. Ethidium bromide and auramine 0, both of which are rapidly taken up by reticulocytes, and thiazole orange, which requires 30 min incubation, are generally suitable.

Automated reticulocyte counts correlate well with manual reticulocyte counts, although absolute counts may differ since automated counts are dependent on the conditions of incubation and the method of calibrating the instrument. Precision is much superior to that of the manual count since many more cells are counted and the subjective element inherent in recognizing late reticulocytes is eliminated. Potential sources of inaccuracy are the inclusion of some leucocytes and platelets and, less often, Howell-Jolly bodies or malarial parasites, in the 'reticulocyte' count.

An automated reticulocyte counter also permits assessment of reticulocyte maturity since the most immature reticulocytes, produced when erythropoietin levels are high, have more RNA and fluoresce more strongly than the mature reticulocytes normally present in the peripheral blood. Parameters indicating reticulocyte immaturity have potential clinical relevance. For example, an increase in mean fluorescence intensity has been noted as an early sign of engraftment following bone marrow transplantation.[15]

Automated reticulocyte counts are stable in blood which has been stored for 1–2 days at room temperature or up to 3–5 days at 4°C.

Reticulocyte counts in health

Reference ranges reported for automated reticulocyte counts have varied considerably between methods. Ranges of $19–59 \times 10^9/l$ $(0.2–1.6\%)$[57] and $40–140 \times 10^9/l$ $(1–3\%)$[15] have been reported for thiazole orange with a Coulter Epic Flow Cytometer. With the Sysmex R-1000, absolute ranges have been reported as $19–98$,[36] $20–70$,[20] and $10–90 \times 10^9/l$,[77] and percentage ranges as $0.4–2.1$[36] and $0.27–2.11$.[77]

CALIBRATION OF AUTOMATED BLOOD CELL COUNTERS

There are three satisfactory methods for calibrating an automated blood cell counter:[41,44,46]

1. Using fresh normal blood specimens to which values have been assigned for Hb, PCV, RBC, WBC and platelet count.
2. Using a stable calibrant (either preserved blood or a substitute) to which values appropriate for the instrument in question have been assigned by comparison with fresh normal blood.
3. By use of a commercial calibrant with assigned values suitable for the instrument in question.

For reasons of convenience and economy, control materials are commonly used as calibrants; this practice is not recommended. Such materials are not sufficiently stable to serve as calibrants. They are designed to give test results within a stated range over a stated period of time rather than a specific result.

The procedure for assigning values to fresh blood samples and indirectly to a stable calibrant is as follows.

1. 4 ml blood specimens are obtained from three haematologically normal volunteers and are anticoagulated with K_2EDTA.
2. The Hb value is assigned by using the haemiglobincyanide method (see p. 50) and the mean of two measurements.
3. The PCV is assigned by the microhaematocrit method (see p. 57), taking the mean of measurements in four microhaematocrit tubes.
4. The RBC is assigned by performing counts on a single channel aperture-impedance counter capable of performing a direct cell count; the mean of two dilutions, each counted twice, is used.
5. The MCV is assigned by calculation from the RBC and PCV.
6. The WBC is assigned by performing counts on a single channel aperture-impedance instrument capable of performing direct cell counts; the mean of two dilutions, each counted twice, is used.
7. The platelet count is assigned by using a counter capable of measuring the ratio of platelets to red cells, the platelet count being calculated from the ratio and an independently measured RBC.

To calibrate the automated counter directly from the fresh blood samples, perform two counts with each sample and take the mean. If the measured counts differ from those assigned, recalibrate the counter appropriately.

To calibrate a stable calibrant, perform two counts on the calibrant and on each fresh sample using the automated instrument, A, and take the mean. From the ratio of the test results on fresh blood to those on the calibrator, assign corrected values to the calibrator by using the following calculations.

Corrected calibrator value =

$$A_C \times \sqrt[3]{\frac{D_{F1}}{A_{F1}} \times \frac{D_{F2}}{A_{F2}} \times \frac{D_{F3}}{A_{F3}}}$$

where: A_C = measurement of calibrator by automated counter

A_F = measurement of the fresh bloods (1, 2 and 3) by automated counter

D_F = direct measurement of the fresh bloods (1, 2 and 3).

Considerable care is required to ensure that the initial measurements on the fresh blood are as accurate as possible. Dilutions should be made with individually calibrated pipettes and grade A volumetric flasks. The cell counter should be calibrated as described on p. 71, with a signal to noise ratio of greater than 100:1, and the count corrected for coincidence. Details of procedures to be used are described by the International Committee for Standardization in Haematology.[41]

REFERENCES

[1] BAIN, B. J. (1985). Platelet count and platelet size in males and females. *Scandinavian Journal of Haematology*, **35**, 77.

[2] BAIN, B. J. (1986). An assessment of the three population differential count on the Coulter Model S Plus IV. *Clinical and Laboratory Haematology*, **8**, 347.

[3] BAIN, B. J. and SEED, M. (1986). Platelet count and platelet size in Africans and West Indians. *Clinical and Laboratory Haematology*, **8**, 43.

[4] BAIN, B. J. (1989). *Blood Cells: a Practical Guide*. Gower Medical Publishing, London.

[5] BAIN, B. J. and CAVILL, I. (1993). Hypochromic macrocytes—are they reticulocytes? *Journal of Clinical Pathology*, **46**, 963.

[6] BALLARD, B. C. D. (1972). Lysing agent for the Coulter S. *Journal of Clinical Pathology*, **25**, 460.

[7] BERENDES, M. (1973). The proportion of reticulocytes in the erythrocytes of the spleen as compared with those of circulating blood, with special reference to hemolytic states. *Blood*, **14**, 558.

[8] BERGSTRAND, C. G. HELLSTROM, B. and JOHNSSON, B (1950). Remarks on the technique of eosinophil counting. *Scandinavian Journal of Clinical and Laboratory Investigation*, **2**, 341.

[9] BESSMAN, J. D. (1986). *Automated Blood Counts and Differentials: A Practical Guide*. John Hopkins University Press, Baltimore.

[10] BESSMAN, J. D., GILMER, P. R. and GARDNER, F. H. (1983). Improved classification of anemias by MCV and RDW. *American Journal of Clinical Pathology*, **80**, 322.

[11] BESSMAN, J. D., WILLIAMS, L. J. and GILMER, P. R. (1982). Platelet size in health and hematologic disease. *American Journal of Clinical Pathology*, **78**, 150.

[12] BEST, W. R. and SAMSTER, M. (1951). Variation and error in eosinophil counts of blood and bone marrow. *Blood*, **6**, 61.

[13] BRECHER, G. and CRONKITE, E. P. (1950). Morphology and enumeration of human blood platelets. *Journal of Applied Physiology*, **3**, 365.

[14] BRECHER, G., SCHNEIDERMAN, M. and CRONKITE, E. P. (1953). The reproducibility and constancy of the platelet count. *American Journal of Clinical Pathology*, **23**, 15.

[15] CHIN-YEE, I., KEENEY, M. and LOHMANN, C. (1991). Flow cytometric reticulocyte analysis using thiazole orange; clinical experience and technical limitations. *Clinical and Laboratory Haematology*, **13**, 177.

[16] CLARK, P. T., HENTHORN, J. S. and ENGLAND, J. M. (1985). Differential white cell counting on the Coulter Counter Model S Plus IV (Three population) and the Technicon H6000: a comparison by simple and multiple regression. *Clinical and Laboratory Haematology*, **7**, 335.

[17] CLEGG, J. W. and KING, E. J. (1942). Estimation of haemoglobin by the alkaline haematin method. *British Medical Journal*, **ii**, 329.

[18] CORNBLEET, P. J., MYRICK, D., JUDKINS, S. and LEVY, R. (1992). Evaluation of the CELL-DYN 3000 differential. *American Journal of Clinical Pathology*, **98**, 603.

[19] COULTER, W. H. (1956). High speed automatic blood cell counter and cell size analyser. *Proceedings of National Electronics Conference*, **12**, 1034.

[20] DAVIES, S. V., CAVILL, I., BENTLEY, N., FEGAN, C. D., POYNTON, C. H. and WHITTAKER, J. A. (1992). Evaluation of erythropoiesis after bone marrow transplantation: quantitative reticulocyte counting. *British Journal of Haematology*, **81**, 12.

[21] D'ONOFRIO, G., SALVATI, A. M., BERTI, P., CAPPABIANCA, M. P., MARSILI, G., QUARANTELLI, M., ZINI, G., CASINI, C., DE PHILIPPIS, C., MANGO, G. and FERRINI, P. R. (1991). Analysis of leucocyte populations with the Coulter S-Plus STKR as a screening tool for haematological abnormalities. *Clinical and Laboratory Haematology*, **13**, 51.

[22] D'ONOFRIO, G., ZINI, G., TOMMASI, M., VALENTINI, S., MAIURO, G., TAMBURRINI, E. and ORTONA, L. (1992). *Anomalie Ultramorpholigiche dei Granulociti Neutrofili Nelle Infezioni da Virus HIV*. Atti del V Incontro del Club Utilizzatori Sistemi Ematologici Bayer-Technicon, Montecatini Terme, 1991.

[23] DRABKIN, D. L. and AUSTIN, J. H. (1932). Spectrophotometric studies: spectrometric constants for common haemoglobin derivatives in human, dog and rabbit blood. *Journal of Biological Chemistry*, **98**, 719.

[24] DUNGER, R. (1910). Eine einfache Methode der Zählung der eosinophilen Leukozyten und der praktische Wert dieser Untersuchung. *Münchener medizinische Wochenschrift*, **57**, 1942.

[25] ENGLAND, J. M., WALFORD, D. M. and WATERS, D. A. W. (1972). Reassessment of the reliability of the haematocrit. *British Journal of Haematology*, **23**, 247.

[26] ENGLAND, J. M. (1979). Prospect for automated differential leucocyte counting in the routine laboratory. *Clinical and Laboratory Haematology*, **1**, 263.

[27] ENGLAND, J. M. and VAN ASSENDELFT, O. W. (1986). Automated blood counters and their evaluation. In *Automation and Quality Assurance in Haematology*. Eds. R. M. Rowan and J. M. England. Blackwell Scientific Publications, Oxford.

[28] EVAN-WONG, L. and DAVIDSON, R. J. (1983). Raised Coulter mean corpuscular volume in diabetic ketoacidosis, and its underlying association with marked plasma hyperosmolarity. *Journal of Clinical Pathology*, **36**, 334.

[29] GARBY, L. and VUILLE, J. C. (1961). The amount of trapped plasma in a high speed micro-capillary haematocrit centrifuge. *Scandinavian Journal of Clinical and Laboratory Investigation*, **13**, 642.

[30] GIBSON, Q. H. and HARRISON, D. C. (1945). An artificial standard for use in the estimation of haemoglobin. *Biochemical Journal*, **39**, 490.

[31] GILBERT, H. S. and ORNSTEIN, L. (1975). Basophil counting with a new staining method using Alcian blue. *Blood*, **46**, 279.

[32] GILMER, P. R. and KOEPKE, J. A. (1976). The reticulocyte: an approach to definition. *American Journal of Clinical Pathology*, **66**, 262.

[33] HILLMAN, R. S. (1969). Characteristics of marrow production and reticulocyte maturation in normal man in response to anemia. *Journal of Clinical Investigation*, **48**, 443.

[34] HILLMAN, R. S. and FINCH, C. A. (1969). The misused reticulocyte. *British Journal of Haematology*, **17**, 313.

[35] HOLT, J. T., DEWANDLER, M. J. and ARVAN, D. A. (1982). Spurious elevation of the electronically determined mean corpuscular volume and hematocrit caused by hyperglycemia. *American Journal of Clinical Pathology*, **77**, 561.

[36] HOY, T. G. (1990). Flow cytometry: clinical applications in haematology. *Baillière's Clinical Haematology*, **3**, 977.

37 INTERNATIONAL COMMITTEE FOR STANDARDIZATION IN HAEMATOLOGY (1978). Recommendations for reference method for haemoglobinometry in human blood and specifications for international haemiglobincyanide reference preparation. *Journal of Clinical Pathology*, **31**, 139.

38 INTERNATIONAL COMMITTEE FOR STANDARDIZATION IN HAEMATOLOGY (1980). Recommended methods for measurement of red-cell and plasma volume. *Journal of Nuclear Medicine*, **21**, 793.

39 INTERNATIONAL COMMITTEE FOR STANDARDIZATION IN HAEMATOLOGY (1980). Recommendations for reference method for determination by centrifugation of packed cell volume of blood. *Journal of Clinical Pathology*, **33**, 1.

40 INTERNATIONAL COMMITTEE FOR STANDARDIZATION IN HAEMATOLOGY (1983). Protocol for evaluation of automated blood cell counters. *Clinical and Laboratory Haematology*, **6**, 69.

41 INTERNATIONAL COMMITTEE FOR STANDARDIZATION IN HAEMATOLOGY; EXPERT PANEL ON CYTOMETRY (1988). The assignment of values to fresh blood used for calibrating automated blood cell counters. *Clinical and Laboratory Haematology*, **10**, 203.

42 INTERNATIONAL COUNCIL FOR STANDARDIZATION IN HAEMATOLOGY (1994). Guidelines for the evaluation of blood cell analysers including those used for differential leucocyte and reticulocyte counting and cell marker applications. *Clinical and Laboratory Haematology*, **16**, 157.

43 JAHANMEHR, S. A. H., HYDE, K., GEARY, C. G., CINKOTAI, K. I. and MACIVER, J. E. (1987). Simple technique for fluorescence staining of blood cells with acridine orange. *Journal of Clinical Pathology*, **40**, 926.

44 LEWIS, S. M., WARDLE, J., COUSINS, S. and SKELLY, J. V. (1979). Platelet counting—development of a reference method and a reference preparation. *Clinical and Laboratory Haematology*, **1**, 227.

45 LEWIS, S. M., GARVEY, B., MANNING, R., SHARP, S. A. and WARDLE, J. (1991). Lauryl sulphate haemoglobin: a non-hazardous substitute for HiCN in haemoglobinometry. *Clinical and Laboratory Haematology*, **13**, 279.

46 LEWIS, S. M. ENGLAND, J. M. and ROWAN, R. M. (1991). Current concerns in haematology 3: Blood count calibration. *Journal of Clinical Pathology*, **44**, 881.

47 MACGREGOR, R. G., SCOTT RICHARDS, W. and LOH, G. L. (1940). The differential leucocyte count. *Journal of Pathology and Bacteriology*, **51**, 337.

48 MAGATH, T. B., BERKSON, J. and HURN, M. (1936). The error of determination of the erythrocyte count. *American Journal of Clinical Pathology*, **6**, 568.

49 MANSBERG, H. P., SAUNDERS, A. M. and GRONER, W. (1974). The Hemalog D white cell differential system. *Journal of Histochemistry and Cytochemistry*, **22**, 711.

50 MATHY, K. A. and KOEPKE, J. A. (1974). The clinical usefulness of segmented vs. stab neutrophil criteria for differential leucocyte counts. *American Journal of Clinical Pathology*, **61**, 947.

51 MATSUBARA, T., OKUZONO, H. and SENBA, U. (1979). Modification of Van Kampen-Zijlstra's reagent for the hemiglobincyanide method. *Clinica Chimica Acta*, **93**, 163.

52 MARSHALL, P. N., BENTLEY, S. A. and LEWIS, S. M. (1976). Purified azure B as a reticulocyte stain. *Journal of Clinical Pathology*, **29**, 1060.

53 METTLER, L. and SHIRWANI, D. (1974). Direct basophil count for timing ovulation. *Fertility and Sterility*, **25**, 718.

54 MOHANDAS, N., KIM, Y. R., TYCKO, D. H., ORLIK, J., WYATT, J. and GRONER, W. (1986). Accurate and independent measurement of volume and hemoglobin concentration of individual red cells by laser light scattering. *Blood*, **68**, 506.

55 MORLEY, A. (1969). A platelet cycle in normal individuals. *Australasian Annals of Medicine*, **18**, 127.

56 MUEHRCKE, R. C., ECKERT, E. L. and KARK, R. M. (1952). A statistical study of absolute eosinophil cell counts in healthy young adults using logarithmic analysis. *Journal of Laboratory and Clinical Medicine*, **40**, 161.

57 NOBES, P. R. and CARTER, A. B. (1990). Reticulocyte counting using flow cytometry. *Journal of Clinical Pathology*, **43**, 675.

58 PEARSON, T. C. and GUTHRIE, D. L. (1982). Trapped plasma in microhematocrit. *American Journal of Clinical Pathology*, **78**, 770.

59 ROBERTS, G. T. and EL BADAWI, S. B. (1985). Red blood cell distribution width index in some hematologic diseases. *American Journal of Clinical Pathology*, **83**, 222.

60 ROBERTSON, E. P., LAI, H. W. and WEI, D. C. C. (1992). An evaluation of leucocyte analysis on the Coulter STKS. *Clinical and Laboratory Haematology*, **14**, 53.

61 ROCK, W. A., MIALE, J. B. and JOHNSON, W. D. (1984). Detection of abnormal cells in white cell differentials: comparison of the HEMATRAK automated system with manual methods. *American Journal of Clinical Pathology*, **81**, 233.

62 ROSS, D. W. and BENTLEY, S. A. (1986). Evaluation of an automated hematology system (Technicon H-1). *Archives of Pathology and Laboratory Medicine*, **110**, 803.

63 ROWAN, R. M. (1983). *Blood Cell Volume Analysis—A New Screening Technology for the Haematologist*. Albert Clark, London.

64 RUD, F. (1947). The eosinophil count in health and mental disease. *Acta Psychiatrica et Neurologica (København)*, **40** (Suppl.).

65 SAGE, B. H., O'CONNELL, J. P. and MERCOLINO, T. J. (1983). A rapid, vital staining procedure for flow cytometric analysis of human reticulocytes. *Cytometry*, **4**, 222.

66 SANDERS, C. and SKERRY, D. W. (1961). The distribution of blood cells on haemocytometer counting chambers with special reference to the amended British Standards Specification 748 (1958). *Journal of Clinical Pathology*, **48**, 298.

67 SEIP, M, (1953). Reticulocyte studies: the liberation of red blood corpuscles from the bone marrow into the peripheral blood and the production of erythrocytes elucidated by reticulocyte investigations. *Acta Medica Scandinavica*, (Suppl. 282).

68 SHINTON, N. K., ENGLAND, J. M. E. and KENNEDY, D. A. (1982). Guidelines for the evaluation of instruments used in haematological laboratories. *Journal of Clinical Pathology*, **35**, 1095.

69 SIMSON, E., ROSS, D. W. and KOCHER, W. D. (1988). *Atlas of Automated Cytochemical Hematology*. Technicon, Tarrytown, NY.

70 SHELLEY, W. B. and PARNES, H. M. (1965). The absolute basophil count. Technique and significance. *Journal of American Medical Association*, **192**, 368.

71 SKINNIDER, L. F. and MUSGLOW, E. (1972). A stromatolysing and cyanide reagent for use with the Coulter Counter Model S. *American Journal of Clinical Pathology*, **57**, 537.

72 SLOAN, A. W. (1951). The normal platelet count in man. *Journal of Clinical Pathology*, **4**, 37.

[73] Spiers, R. S. (1952). The principles of eosinophil diluents. *Blood*, **7**, 550.

[74] Stevenson C. F., Smetters, G. W. and Cooper, J. A. D. (1951). A gravimetric method for the calibration of hemoglobin micropipets. *American Journal of Clinical Pathology*, **21**, 489.

[75] Sunderman, F. W., MacFate, R. P., MacFadzean, D., Stevenson, G. F. and Copeland, B. E. (1953). Symposium on clinical hemoglobinometry. *American Journal of Clinical Pathology*, **23**, 519.

[76] Tanke, H. J., Rothbarth, P. H., Vossen, J. M. J. J., Koper, G. J. M. and Ploem, J. S. (1983). Flow cytometry of reticulocytes applied to clinical hematology. *Blood*, **61**, 1091.

[77] Tatsumi, N., Niri, M. and Tsuda, I. (1992). No correlation between reticulocyte count and erythrocyte count. *Clinical and Laboratory Haematology*, **14**, 92.

[78] Taylor, C. and Bain, B. J. (1991). Technicon H1 automated white cell parameters in the diagnosis of megaloblastic erythropoiesis. *European Journal of Haematology*, **46**, 248.

[79] Thompson, L. C. (1946). An inorganic grey solution. *Transactions of the Faraday Society*, **42**, 663.

[80] Thom, R. (1990). Automated red cell analysis. *Baillière's Clinical Haematology*, **3**, 837.

[81] Uhrbrand, H. (1958). The number of circulating eosinophils: normal figures and spontaneous variations. *Acta Medica Scandinavica*, **160**, 99.

[82] Vander, J. B., Harris, C. A. and Ellis, S. R. (1963). Reticulocyte counts by means of fluorescence miscroscopy. *Journal of Laboratory and Clinical Medicine*, **62**, 132.

[83] Van Kampen, E. J. and Zijlstra, W. G. (1983). Spectrophotometry of hemoglobin and hemoglobin derivatives. *Advances in Clinical Chemistry*, **23**, 199.

[84] Vaughan, W. P., Hall, J., Johnson, K., Dougherty, C. and Pebbles, D. (1985). Simultaneous reticulocyte and platelet counting on a clinical flow cytometer. *American Journal of Hematology*, **18**, 385.

[85] Wittekind, D. and Schulte, E. (1987). Standardized Azure B as a reticulocyte stain. *Clinical and Laboratory Haematology*, **9**, 395.

[86] World Health Organization (1977). *The SI for the Health Professions*, WHO, Geneva.

[87] Zijlstra, W. G. and Van Kampen, E. J. (1960). Standardization of hemoglobinometry. I. The extinction coefficient of hemiglobincyanide at $\lambda = 540$ mμ: ε^{540}HiCN. *Clinica Chimica Acta*, **91**, 339.

[88] Zweens, J., Frankena, H. and Zijlstra, W. G. (1979). Decomposition on freezing of reagents used in the ICSH recommended method for the determination of total haemoglobin in blood; its nature, cause and prevention. *Clinica Chimica Acta*, **91**, 339.

6. Preparation and staining methods for blood and bone-marrow films

Preparation of blood films on slides   83
Staining blood and bone-marrow films   84
   May-Grünwald-Giemsa's stain   86
   Standardized Romanowsky stain   87
   Jenner-Giemsa's stain   87
   Leishman's stain   88
   Rapid staining method   88
Thick blood films for parasites   89
Examination of blood cells in plasma   90
   Red cells   90

Rouleaux and auto-agglutination   90
   Parasites   91
   Leucocytes   91
Separation and concentration of blood cells   91
   Buffy coat   91
Specific cell populations   92
   Isolation of tumour cells from blood   92
Blood parasites   93
   Malaria   93
   Other parasites   93

PREPARATION OF BLOOD FILMS ON SLIDES

Blood films can be made on glass slides or cover-glasses. The latter have the single possible advantage of a more even distribution of the leucocytes, but in every other respect slides are to be preferred. Unlike cover-glasses, slides are not easily broken; they are simple to label and when large numbers of films are to be dealt with, slides will be found much easier to handle.

Good films may be made in the following manner, using clean slides (p. 580) wiped free from dust immediately before use.

Place a small drop of blood in the centre line of a slide about 1 or 2 cm from one end. Then, without delay, place a glass slide with a smooth edge, which is trimmed to a width of *c* 2 cm, at an angle of 45° to the slide and move it back to make contact with the drop. The drop should spread out quickly along the line of contact of the spreader with slide. The moment this occurs, spread the film by a rapid, smooth, forward movement of the spreader.

The drop should be such a size that the film is 3 or 4 cm in length (Fig. 6.1). The ideal thickness is such that there is some overlap of red cells throughout much of the film's length, but separ-

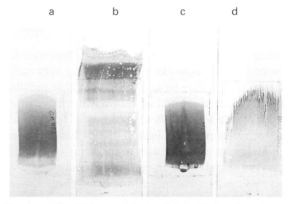

a   b   c   d

Fig. 6.1   Blood films made on slides. (a) A well-made film. (b) A film which is too long, too wide, grossly irregular in thickness and which has been made on a greasy slide. (c) A film which is too thick. (d) A film which has been spread with an irregularly- edged spreader and which shows long tails. (Slightly reduced.)

ation and lack of distortion towards the tail of the film (see p. 60). The leucocytes should be easily recognizable throughout the length of the film, although possibly with some difficulty in the thicker part at the head of the film.

Spin method

This is an automated method by which 1 or 2

drops of blood, placed in the centre of a glass slide are briefly spun at high speed in a special centrifuge (e.g. Cytospin*); the blood spreads on the slide in a monolayer. By this method leucocytes and platelets are distributed uniformly and free of distortion.[24,32] The red cells show a tendency to become distorted, but this can be overcome by diluting 2 volumes of blood with 1 volume of 9 g/l NaCl immediately prior to putting the blood on the slide.[24] With this procedure it is essential to take precautions against biohazard (p. 31).

Labelling blood films

A recommended method is to write the name of the patient and the date or a reference number in pencil (graphite) on the film itself. It will not be removed by staining. A paper label should be affixed to the slide later.

Bar-coded specimen identification labels are convenient, when available, in a computerized laboratory.

Bone-marrow films

The method for preparation of films from aspirated bone marrow is described on p. 178. They should be made without delay. Some films should be fixed in the appropriate fixatives for special staining (Chapters 8 and 9); others should be fixed and stained with a Romanowsky stain as described below.

STAINING BLOOD AND BONE-MARROW FILMS

Romanowsky stains are universally employed for staining blood films as a routine, and very satisfactory results may be obtained. As far as possible films should be stained as soon as they have dried in the air; they certainly should not be left unfixed for more than a few hours. If the films are left unfixed at room temperature for a day or more, it may be found that, in addition to distortion of morphology, the background of dried plasma stains a pale blue which is impossible to remove without spoiling the staining of the blood cells. Sometimes staining has to be postponed for up to several days, as when films are sent to the laboratory by post. It is advisable to fix such films before despatch if possible; even so, the results are likely to be less satisfactory than with freshly made films.

The remarkable property of the Romanowsky dyes of making subtle distinctions in shades of staining, and of staining granules differentially, depends on two components, namely, azure B (trimethylthionin) and eosin Y (tetrabromofluorescein).[20,33]

The original Romanowsky combination was polychrome methylene blue and eosin. Several of the stains now used routinely which are based on azure B also include methylene blue, but the need for this is debatable. Its presence in the stain is thought by some to enhance the staining of nucleoli and polychromatic red cells; in its absence normal neutrophil granules tend to stain heavily and may resemble 'toxic granules' in conventionally stained films.[19]

There are a number of causes for variation in staining. One of the main factors is the presence of contaminants in the commercial dyes and a simple combination of pure azure B and eosin Y is preferable to the more complex stains;[33,35] this was advocated by the International Council for Standardization in Haematology (ICSH).[15] It has the advantage of being standardized; it thus ensures consistent results from batch to batch. In practice absolutely pure dyes are expensive, and it is sufficient to ensure that the stains contain at least 80% of the appropriate dye.[28] Amongst the Romanowsky stains now in use, Jenner's is the simplest and Giemsa's the most complex. Leishman's stain, which occupies an intermediate position, is still widely used in the routine stain-

---

*Shandon Scientific Ltd.

ing of blood films, although the results are inferior to those obtained by the combined May-Grünwald-Giemsa, Jenner-Giemsa and azure B-eosin Y methods. Wright's stain, which is widely used in North America, gives results which are similar to those obtained with Leishman's stain. A slightly modified version of the ICSH method is described on p. 87.

A pH to the alkaline side of neutrality accentuates the azure component at the expense of the eosin and vice versa. A pH of 6.8 is usually recommended for general use, but to some extent this depends on personal preference. (When looking for malaria parasites a pH of 7.2 is recommended in order to see Schüffner's dots.) To achieve a uniform pH, 50 ml of 66 mmol/l Sörensen's phosphate buffer (p. 579) may be added to each 1 litre of the water used in diluting the stains and washing the films.

The mechanism by which certain components of a cell's structure stain with particular dyes and other components fail to do so, although staining with other dyes, depends on complex differences in binding of the dyes to chemical structures and interactions between the dye molecules.[34] Azure B in dimer form is bound to anionic molecules, e.g. phosphate groups of DNA, and eosin Y is bound as a monomer to cationic sites on proteins.

As soon as the dyes are bound, either electron interaction occurs with dye–dye aggregation[33] or the eosin Y molecule is intercalated between the azure B molecules and the complex is held together by charge effect.[21] Thus, the acidic groupings of the nucleic acids and proteins of the cell nuclei and primitive cytoplasm determine their uptake of the basic dye azure B and, conversely, the presence of basic groupings on the Hb molecule results in its affinity for acidic dyes and its staining by eosin. The granules in the cytoplasm of neutrophil leucocytes are weakly stained by the azure complexes. Eosinophilic granules contain a spermine derivative with an alkaline grouping which stains strongly with the acidic component of the dye, whereas basophilic granules contain heparin which has an affinity for the basic component of the dye.

The colour reactions of the Romanowsky effect are shown in Table 6.1; causes of variation in staining are given in Table 6.2.

Table 6.1   Colour responses of blood cells to Romanowsky staining

Cellular component	Colour
Nuclei	
Chromatin	Purple
Nucleoli	Light blue
Cytoplasm	
Erythroblast	Dark blue
Erythrocyte	Pink
Reticulocyte	Grey-blue
Lymphocyte	Blue
Metamyelocyte	Pink
Monocyte	Grey-blue
Myelocyte	Pink
Neutrophil	Pink
Promyelocyte	Blue
Basophil	Blue
Granules	
Promyelocyte (primary granules)	Red or purple
Basophil	Purple black
Eosinophil	Red-orange
Neutrophil	Purple
Toxic granules	Blue-black
Platelet	Purple
Other inclusions	
Auer body	Purple
Cabot ring	Purple
Howell-Jolly body	Purple
Döhle body	Bright blue

STAINING METHODS

Preparation of solutions of Romanowsky dyes

May–Grünwald's stain. Weigh out 0.3 g of the powdered dye and transfer to a conical flask of 200–250 ml capacity. Add 100 ml of methanol and warm the mixture to 50°C. Allow the flask to cool to *c* 20°C and shake several times during the day. After standing for 24 h, filter the solution. It is then ready for use, no ripening being required.

Jenner's stain. Prepare a 5 g/l solution in methanol in exactly the same way as described above for May–Grünwald's stain.

Giemsa's stain. Weigh 1 g of the powdered dye and transfer to a conical flask of 200–250 ml capacity. Add 100 ml of methanol and warm the mixture to 50°C; keep at this temperature for 15 min with occasional shaking, then filter the solution. It is then ready for use, but will improve on standing.

Table 6.2 Factors giving rise to faulty staining

Appearances	Causes
Too blue, nuclei blue to black	Eosin concentration too low. Incorrect preparation of stock. Stock stain exposed to light. Batch of stain solution overused
	Excess methylene blue in stain. Staining time too short. Staining solution too acid. Thick smear. Inadequate washing in buffer solution
Too pink	Incorrect proportion of azure B–eosin Y. Buffer pH too low. Excessive washing in buffer solution
Grey cytoplasm	Stain contains azure A and/or azure C
Neutrophil granules not stained	Insufficient azure B
Neutrophil granules dark blue/black (pseudo-toxic)	Excess azure B
Other stain anomalies	Various contaminating dyes and metal salts
Stain deposit on film	Stain solution left in uncovered jar. Stain solution not filtered
Blue background	Inadequate fixation or prolonged storage before fixation. Blood collected into heparin as anticoagulant

Azure B–eosin Y stock solution. Azure B, tetrafluoroborate or thiocyanate (CI 52010), >80% pure. Eosin Y (CI 45380), >80% pure.

Dissolve 0.6 g of azure B in 60 ml dimethyl sulphoxide (DMSO) and 0.2 g of eosin Y in 50 ml DMSO; preheat the DMSO at 37°C before adding the dyes. Stand at 37°C, shaking vigorously for 30 s at 5 min intervals until both dyes are completely dissolved. Add the eosin Y solution to the azure B solution and stir well. This stock solution should remain stable for several months if kept at room temperature in the dark. DMSO will crystallize below 18°C. If necessary allow it to redissolve before use.

Buffered water. Make up 50 ml of 66 mmol/l Sörensen's phosphate buffer of the required pH to 1 litre with water (see p. 579). An alternative buffer may be prepared from buffer tablets which are available commercially. Solutions of the required pH are obtained by dissolving the tablets in water.

May-Grünwald-Giemsa's stain

Dry the films in the air, then fix by immersing in a jar of methanol for 10–20 min. For bone marrow films leave for 20–25 min in the methanol. Transfer to a staining jar containing May-Grünwald's stain freshly diluted with an equal volume of buffered water. After the films have been allowed to stain for *c* 15 min, transfer them without washing to a jar containing Giemsa's stain freshly diluted with 9 volumes of buffered water, pH 6.8. After staining for 10–15 min, transfer the slides to a jar containing buffered water, pH 6.8, rapidly wash in three or four changes of water and finally allow to stand undisturbed in water for a short time (usually 2–5 min) for differentiation to take place. This may be controlled by inspection of the wet slide under the low power of the microscope; with experience the naked-eye colour of the film is often a good guide. The slides should be transferred from one staining solution to the other without being allowed to dry. As the intensity of the staining is affected by any variation in the thickness of a film, it is not easy to obtain uniform staining throughout a film's length.

When differentiation is complete, stand the slides upright to dry. When thoroughly dry, cover the films by a rectangular No. 1 cover-glass, using for this purpose a mountant, which is miscible with xylol.* For a temporary mount, cedar-wood oil may be used.

The cover-glass should be sufficiently large to overlie the whole film, including both the edges and the tail. If a neutral mounting medium is used the staining should be preserved for at least 5–10 yr if kept in the dark. Although it is probable that stained films keep best unmounted, there are objections to this course: it is almost impossible to keep the slides free from dust and from being scratched, and in the absence of a

---

*E.g. DPX Mountant (Merck).

cover-glass the observer is tempted to examine the film solely with the oil-immersion objective, a practice which is to be deprecated.

The May-Grünwald-Giemsa staining method described above is designed for staining a number of films at the same time. Single slides may be stained by flooding the slide with a combined fixative and staining solution (e.g. Leishman's stain).

A relatively prolonged fixation, at least 10 min, is required for good staining; particularly is this so in staining films of bone marrow. It is important to ensure that the methanol used as fixative is completely water-free. As little as 1% water may affect the appearance of the films and a higher water content causes gross changes (Figs 6.2 and 6.3).

The diluted stains usually retain their staining powers sufficiently well for several batches of slides to be stained in them. They must be made up freshly each day, and it is probably best to stain the day's films all at the same time, or if this is not possible in consecutive batches. There is no need to filter the stains before use unless a deposit is present.

Automatic staining machines are available which enable large batches of slides to be handled. As a rule, staining is of a uniform high standard, but,

to achieve this, reliable stains are required and the cycle time has to be carefully controlled.

Standardized Romanowsky stain[15]

Fixative. Mix 1 volume of stock solution of azure B-eosin Y with 14 volumes of methanol.

Staining solution. Immediately before use, dilute 1 volume of the stock solution with 14 volumes of HEPES buffer, pH 6.6 (p. 578). This solution is stable for about 8 h.[4]

Method. Dry the films in the air. Leave for 3 min in the fixative. Leave the slides in the diluted staining solution for 10 min. Rinse in phosphate buffer solution, pH 5.8, for 1 min. Then rinse with water, air dry and mount. For bone-marrow films, fix for 5 min and leave the slides to stain for 15–20 min.

When several batches of films are being stained in succession, the staining solution should be renewed at intervals (e.g. after each 50 slides). Loss of staining power is usually due to precipitation of the eosin Y and this will result in the nuclei staining blue instead of purple (Table 6.2).

Jenner-Giemsa's stain

Jenner's stain may be substituted for May-

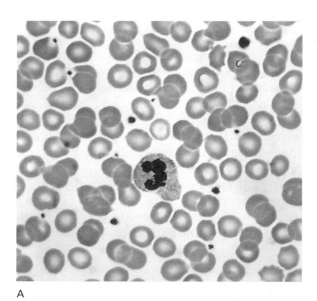

A

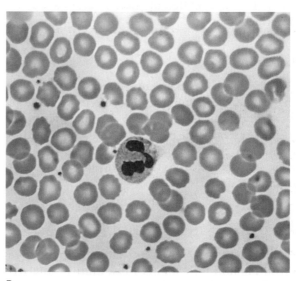

B

Fig. 6.2 Blood film appearances following methanol fixation. Photomicrographs of Romanowsky-stained blood films which have been fixed in methanol containing (A) 1% water and (B) 3% water. The red cells and leucocytes are well fixed.

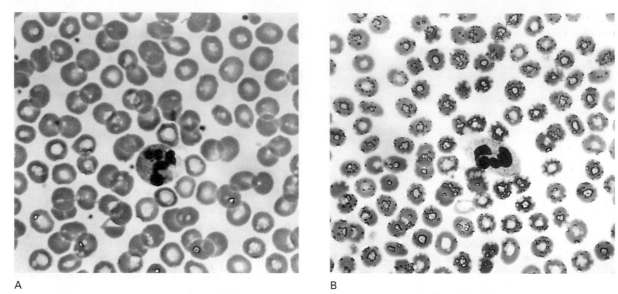

A   B

Fig. 6.3   Blood film appearances following methanol fixation. Photomicrographs of Romanowsky-stained blood films which have been fixed in methanol containing (A) 4% water and (B) 10% water. In (A) the red cells are poorly fixed; in (B) they are very badly fixed.

Grünwald's stain in the above described technique. The results are a little less satisfactory. The stain is used with 4 volumes of buffered water and the films, after being fixed in methanol, are immersed in it for approximately 4 min before being transferred to the Giemsa's stain. They should be allowed to stain in the latter solution for 7–10 min. Differentiation is carried out as described above.

Leishman's stain

Dry the film in the air and flood the slide with the stain. After 2 min add double the volume of water and stain the film for 5–7 min. Then wash it in a stream of buffered water until it has acquired a pinkish tinge (up to 2 min). After the back of the slide has been wiped clean, set it upright to dry.

RAPID STAINING METHOD

Field's method[11–13] was introduced to provide a quick method for staining thick films for malaria parasites (see below). With some modifications it can be used fairly satisfactorily for the rapid staining of thin films.

Stains

Stain A (polychromed methylene blue)

Methylene blue 1.3 g
Disodium hydrogen phosphate
   ($Na_2HPO_4.12H_2O$) 12.6 g
Potassium dihydrogen phosphate (KH_2PO_4)
   6.25 g
Water 500 ml.

Dissolve the methylene blue and the disodium hydrogen phosphate in 50 ml of water. Then boil the solution in a water-bath almost to dryness in order to 'polychrome' the dye. Add the potassium dihydrogen phosphate and 500 ml of freshly boiled water. After stirring to dissolve the stain, set aside the solution for 24 h before filtering. Filter again before use. The pH is 6.6–6.8.

Azure B may be added to the methylene blue in the proportion of 0.5 g of azure B to 0.8 g of methylene blue. In this case the dyes can be dissolved directly in the phosphate buffer solution.

Stain B (eosin)

Eosin 1.3 g
Disodium hydrogen phosphate
   ($Na_2HPO_4.12H_2O$) 12.6 g

Potassium dihydrogen phosphate (KH_2PO_4)
  6.25 g
Water 500 ml.

Dissolve the phosphates in warm freshly boiled water, and then add the dye. Filter the solution after standing for 24 h.

Method of staining

Fix the film for 10–15 s in methanol. Pour off the methanol and drop on the slide 12 drops of diluted Stain B (1 volume of stain to 4 volumes of water). Immediately, add 12 drops of Stain A. Agitate the slide to mix the stains. After 1 min rinse the slide in water, then differentiate the film for 5 s in phosphate buffer at pH 6.6, wash the slide in water and then place it on end to drain and dry.

Two-stage stains of this type are also available commercially.

Standardized azure B-eosin Y stain

The standardized stain (p. 87) can also be used for rapid staining of individual slides.
  Staining solution. Immediately before use dilute 1 volume of stock stain (p. 86) with 5 volumes of HEPES buffer pH 6.6.

Method

Cover the slide with methanol. Decant after 3 min. Without rinsing, cover the slide with staining solution for 3 min. Rinse in water, air dry and mount.

EXAMINATION OF BLOOD FILMS FOR PARASITES

In addition to standard thin films, thick films are extremely useful when parasites are scanty, but the identification of the parasites is less easy than in thin films. Mixed infections may be missed and there may be doubt as to the identification of any particular object. However, an experienced observer should be able to find and recognize with certainty parasites in badly stained thick films, whilst in a well-stained film parasites should be easily recognized even by beginners. Five minutes spent examining a thick film is equivalent to about 1 h spent in traversing a thin film. Rapid screening can also be carried out by fluorescence microscopy at low magnification, as malaria parasites fluoresce intensely with acridine orange.[17,31] Thin films should be examined for confirmation of diagnosis and identification of the species. Seldom, if ever, should there be any doubt as to whether or not an object is a malaria parasite when a film has been well stained.

Thick films, if well stained, are also useful when there is severe leucopenia. It is possible to perform differential counts (or at least estimate the proportion of polymorphonuclear to mononuclear cells) much more rapidly and more accurately than in thin films made from the same blood.

Making thick films

Make a thick film by placing a small drop of blood in the centre of a slide and spreading it out with a corner of another slide to cover an area about four times its original area. The correct thickness for a satisfactory film will have been achieved if, with the slide placed on a piece of newspaper, small print is just visible.

Allow the film to dry thoroughly for at least 30 min at 37°C before attempting to stain it. Alternatively, leave the slide on the top of a microscope lamp, where the temperature is 50–60°C, for *c* 7 min. Absolutely fresh films, although apparently dry, often wash off in the stain.

STAINING THICK BLOOD FILMS

Methods of staining have been reviewed by Field and Sandosham[13] and guidelines have been published in the USA by the National Committee for Clinical Laboratory Standards (NCCLS).[23] Field's method of staining[11,12] is quick and usually satisfactory, but the method is not practical for staining large numbers of films; for this purpose the Giemsa and azure B-eosin Y methods are more suitable.

Field's method[11-13]

The preparation of the stains is described on p. 88. Dip the slide with the dried but otherwise unfixed film on it into Stain A for 1–2 s. Rinse it in buffered water (pH 6.8–7.0) until the stain ceases to flow from the film (5–10 s). Dip into Stain B for 1 s and then rinse rapidly in buffered water for 10 s. Shake off excess water and leave the slide upright to dry. Do not blot.

Giemsa's stain

Dry the films thoroughly as above; do not fix but immerse the slides for 20–30 min in a staining jar containing Giemsa's stain freshly diluted with 20 volumes of buffered water (pH 7.2). Wash in buffered water pH 7.2 for 3 min. Stand the slides upright to dry. Do not blot.

Azure B-eosin Y

Prepare a staining solution from the stock stain, as described on p. 87, but using HEPES buffer at pH 7.2. After the films have been dried as described above, stain for 10 min in the staining solution, rinse for 1 min in buffered water, pH 7.2. Stand the slides upright to dry. Do not blot.

Sometimes the films are overlaid by a residue of stain or spoilt by the envelopes of the lysed red cells being visible. These defects can be minimized by adding 0.1% Triton X-100 to the buffer before diluting the stock stain.[22]

EXAMINATION OF BLOOD CELLS IN PLASMA

The examination of a drop of blood sealed between a slide and cover-glass is sometimes of considerable value.

The preparation may be examined in several ways; by ordinary illumination, by dark-ground or by Nomarski (interference) illumination. Chemically clean slides and cover-glasses (p. 580) must be used and the blood allowed to spread out thinly between them. If the glass surfaces are free from dust, the blood will spread out spontaneously, and pressure, which is undesirable, should not be necessary. The edges of the preparation may be sealed with a melted mixture of equal parts of petroleum jelly and paraffin wax.

Red cells

Rouleaux formation is usually seen in varying degrees in 'wet' preparations of whole blood and has to be distinguished from auto-agglutination.

Rouleaux formation versus auto-agglutination

The distinction between rouleaux formation and auto-agglutination is sometimes a matter of considerable difficulty, particularly when, as not infrequently happens, rouleaux formation is superimposed on agglutination. The rouleaux, too, may be notably irregular in haemolytic anaemias characterized by spherocytosis, while the clumping due to massive rouleaux formation of normal type may closely simulate true agglutination.

'Pseudo-agglutination' due to massive rouleaux formation may be distinguished from true agglutination in two ways:

1. By noting that the red cells, although forming parts of larger clumps, are mostly arranged side by side as in typical rouleaux.
2. By adding 3–4 volumes of 9 g/l NaCl to the preparation. Pseudo-agglutination due to massive rouleaux formation should either disperse completely or transform itself into typical rouleaux. The addition of saline to blood which has undergone true agglutination may cause the agglutination to break up somewhat, but a major degree of it is likely to persist and typical rouleaux will not be seen.

Anisocytosis and poikilocytosis can be recognized in 'wet' preparations of blood, but the tendency to crenation and the formation of rouleaux tend to make observations on shape changes rather difficult. Such changes can best be studied in a wet preparation after fixation. For this, freshly collected heparinized or EDTA blood is diluted in 10 volumes of iso-osmotic phosphate buffer, pH 7.4 (see p. 578) and immediately fixed with an equal volume of 0.3% glutaraldehyde in iso-osmotic phosphate buffer, pH 7.4. After standing for 5 min one drop of this suspension is added to 4 drops of glycerol and 1–2 drops are placed on a glass slide which is then sealed.[36]

Normally less than 2% of the circulating red cells show pitting; an increase above 4% is an indication of splenic dysfunction. The pits are readily identified by Nomarski illumination, when they have the appearance of small crater-like indentations on the cell surface.[30]

The sickling of red cells in 'wet' preparations of blood is described on p. 266.

Parasites

Wet preparations of blood are suitable for the detection of microfilariae and the spirochaetes of relapsing fever. The presence of small numbers of the latter is revealed by occasional slight agitation of groups of red cells.

Leucocytes

The motility of leucocytes can be readily studied in heparinized blood if the microscope stage can be warmed to c 37°C. Usually only the granulocytes show significant progressive movements.

Leucocytes can also be examined under darkground illumination or phase-contrast microscopy, either unstained or after supravital staining with neutral red or Janus green dyes, or with fluorescent dyes such as acridine orange or auramine.

It seems doubtful whether supravital staining or the use of the phase-contrast, interference or fluorescence microscope helps in the day-to-day problems of diagnostic haematology, and no attempt will be made to describe the appearances of cells viewed by these methods. Excellent photographs of cells viewed with the phase-contrast microscope were given by Bessis.[2] Cell shape and surface structures are particularly well demonstrated by means of Nomarski interference microscopy.[2,3] Kosenow[18] and Jackson[16] illustrated the appearances of leucocytes which had taken up fluorescent dyes.

SEPARATION AND CONCENTRATION OF BLOOD CELLS

A number of methods are available for the concentration of leucocytes or abnormal cells when they are present in only small numbers in the peripheral blood. Concentrates are most simply prepared from the buffy coat of centrifuged blood.

Making a buffy-coat preparation

Defibrinate venous blood in a flask and then centrifuge a sample for 15 min in a Wintrobe haematocrit tube at 3000 rpm ($1500g$). Remove the supernatant serum carefully with a fine pipette, and with the same pipette deposit the platelet and underlying leucocyte layers on to one or two slides. Emulsify the buffy coat in a drop of the patient's serum and then spread the films. Allow them to dry in the air and then fix and stain in the usual way.

When leucocytes are scanty or if many slides are to be made, it is worth while centrifuging the blood twice; first, c 5 ml are centrifuged and a haematocrit tube is then filled from the upper cell layers of this sample.

As an alternative to centrifugation, the blood may be allowed to sediment, with the help of sedimentation-enhancing agents such as fibrinogen, dextran, gum acacia, Ficoll (Pharmacia) or methylcellulose.[5,8] Bøyum's reagent[6,7] (methylcellulose and sodium metrizoate) is particularly suitable for obtaining leucocyte preparations with minimal red cell contamination.

Most methods of separation affect to some extent subsequent staining properties, chemical reactions and the viability of the separated cells.

The buffy coat

It is well known that atypical or primitive blood

cells circulate in small numbers in the peripheral blood in health. Thus, atypical mononuclear cells, metamyelocytes and megakaryocytes may be found. Even promyelocytes, blasts and nucleated red cells may occasionally be seen, but only in very small numbers. Efrati and Rozenszajn[9] described a method for the quantitative assessment of the numbers of atypical cells in normal blood and gave figures for the incidence of megakaryocyte fragments (e.g. mean 21.8 per 1 ml of blood) and of atypical mononuclears and metamyelocytes and myelocytes. In cord blood the incidence of all types of primitive cells is considerably greater.[10]

In disease, leaving the leukaemias and allied disorders out of consideration, abnormal cells may be seen in buffy-coat preparations in much larger numbers than in films of whole blood. For instance, megakaryocytes and immature cells of the granulocyte series are found in relatively large numbers in disseminated carcinoma.[27] Megaloblasts, if present, may help in the diagnosis of a megaloblastic anaemia. Erythrophagocytosis may be conspicuous in cases of auto-immune haemolytic anaemia (Fig. 6.4), and in systemic lupus erythematosus (SLE) a few LE cells may be found—this is, however, not the best way to demonstrate LE cells.

It is rash to attempt an accurate differential count on buffy-coat concentrates as the different leucocytes tend to sediment under the influence of gravity at different rates and form layer upon layer. However, in leucopenia there is a fairly satisfactory correlation between the buffy-coat differential count and the standard method.[26]

SEPARATION OF SPECIFIC CELL POPULATIONS

Differences in density of cells can be used to separate individual cell types, using gradient solutions of selected specific gravity.[1,7,8] These include an erythrocyte-aggregating polysaccharide (Ficoll, Pharmacia), polyvinyl pyrrolidone (PVP)-coated silica gel (Percoll, Pharmacia), and sodium metrizoate (e.g. Isopaque, Nycomed). Mixtures of Ficoll with sodium metrizoate (Lymphoprep, Nycomed), sodium metrizoate with methylcellulose and aqueous buffered solutions of sodium metrizoate (e.g. Nycodenz, Nycomed) will provide media of selected densities. In this way it is possible to separate cell populations with reasonable purity. The median values for the main haemopoietic cells are given below. There is, however, considerable overlap in the density ranges between adjacent types of cells.[7,8,25]

Erythrocytes	1100
Eosinophils	1090
Neutrophils	1085
Myelocytes	1075
Lymphocytes	1070
Monocytes	1064
Myeloblasts	1062
Platelets	1035

Isolation of tumour cells from blood

The methods used for demonstrating tumour cells in circulating blood involve elimination of the red cells and differential sedimentation or filtration of the leucocytes. Fleming and Stewart[14] assessed several methods critically and concluded that differential separation was to be preferred for routine use. They recommended a slight modification of the silicone flotation method of Seal.[29] Positive identifications are seldom made except in advanced cancer when the diagnosis is usually only too obvious.

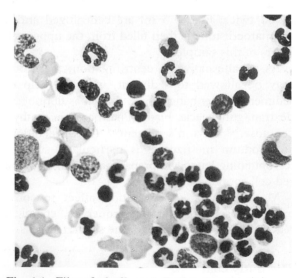

Fig. 6.4   Film of a buffy coat. Erythrophagocytosis in auto-immune haemolytic anaemia.

BLOOD PARASITES

The morphological differentiation of malaria parasites is described in Table 6.3 and illustrated in Fig. 6.5.

Apart from the Plasmodia which give rise to malaria, the most important parasites to be found in the blood are Leishmania, Trypanosoma and Microfilaria.

Leishmania causes kala-azar, oriental sore and yaws. It is identified by Leishman-Donovan bodies which are ovoid, 2–3 μm in diameter with light blue cytoplasm and red to purple chromatin. They should be looked for in splenic aspirates or in the bone marrow, where they will be found lying free or in phagocytic cells. Occasionally, they may be seen in monocytes in a blood film, especially in a buffy-coat preparation.

In trypanosomiasis the organism will be found in the lymph nodes at an early stage, and later in the blood. They are polymorphic bodies, 15–30 μm in length. The cytoplasm stains blue, the chromatin red or dark red (Fig. 6.6). In fresh blood they may be detected by their active movement which disturbs the adjacent red cells. African trypanosomiasis (*T. gambiense* and *T. rhodesiense*) causes sleeping sickness; *T. cruzi* occurs in Mexico, and in Central and South America, and causes Chagas disease.

In filariasis the microfilaria will usually be found in thick blood films stained as described on p. 89. Staining with Delafield's haematoxylin is recommended for identifying the type (e.g. *W. bancrofti*; Loa-loa). Finding and recognizing the organism is simple, as it is about 200 μm in length, coiled or with smooth curves, lying amongst the blood cells (Fig. 6.6). But species identification is more difficult and the reader should refer to a textbook on parasitology.

Table 6.3 Morphological differentiation of malaria parasites

	P. falciparum	*P. vivax*	*P. ovale*	*P. malariae*
Infected red cells	Normal size*; Maurer's clefts[†]	Enlarged; Schüffner's dots[‡]	Enlarged; oval and fimbriated; Schüffner's dots[‡]	Normal or microcytic; stippling not usually seen
Ring forms (early trophozoites)	Delicate; frequently 2 or more; accolé forms[§]; small chromatin dot	Large, thick; usually single (occasionally 2) in cell; large chromatin dot	Thick compact rings	Very small compact rings
Later trophozoites	Compact, vacuolated; sometimes 2 chromatin dots	Amoeboid; central vacuole; light blue cytoplasm	Smaller than *P. vivax*; slightly amoeboid	Band across cell; deep blue cytoplasm
Schizonts	18–24 merozoites filling 2/3 of cell (only seen in cerebral malaria)	12–24 merozoites, irregularly arranged;	8–12 merozoites filling 3/4 of cell	6–12 merozoites in daisy-head around central mass of pigment
Pigment	Dark to black clumped mass	Fine granular; yellow-brown	Coarse light brown	Dark, prominent at all stages
Gametocytes	Crescent or sausage-shaped; diffuse chromatin; single nucleus	Spherical, compact, almost fills cell; single nucleus	Oval; fills 3/4 of cell; similar to, but smaller than *P. vivax*	Round, fills 1/2 to 2/3 of cell; similar to *P. vivax*, but smaller, with no Shüffner's dots

*In *P. falciparum* it is important to report the percentage of red cells that are infected.
[†]Large, irregularly shaped, red-staining dots.
[‡]Fine stippling.
[§]i.e. marginalized to edge of cell.

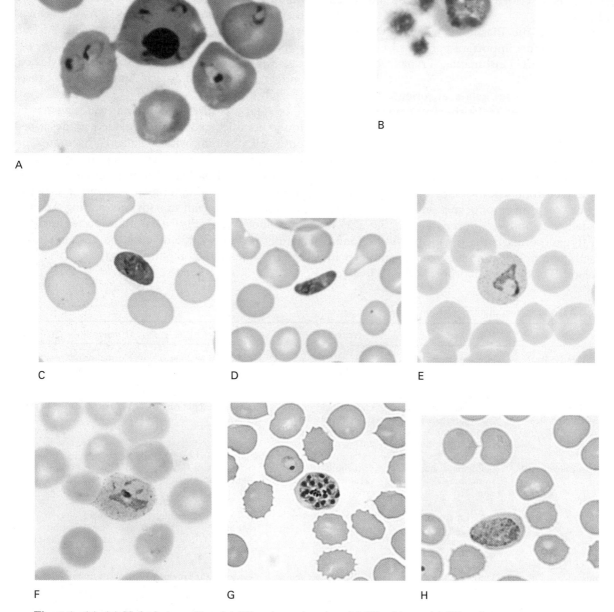

Fig. 6.5 (A)–(H) **Malaria parasites.** (A) *PF*; early trophozoites. (B) *PF*; schizont. (C) *PF*; male gametocyte. (D) *PF*; female gametocyte. (E) *PV*; trophozoite. (F) *PV*; trophozoite, Schüffner's dots are prominent. (G) *PV*; schizont and an early trophozoite. (H) *PV*; gametocyte.

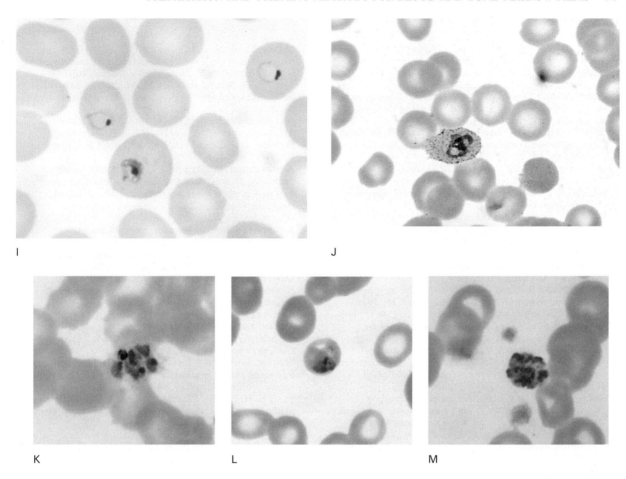

I
J

K
L
M

Fig. 6.5   (I)–(M) (I) Mixed infection *PO* and *PF*;
trophozoites. (J) *PO*; trophozoite. (K) *PO*; schizont.
(L) *PM*; trophozoite. (M) *PM*; schizont.
  *PF, Plasmodium falciparum; PV, Plasmodium vivax;
PO, Plasmodium ovale; PM, Plasmodium malariae.*

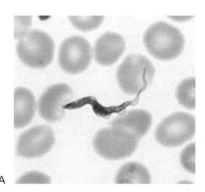

A

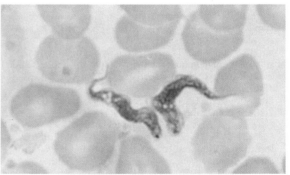

B

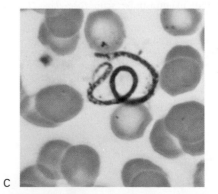

C

Fig. 6.6   Blood parasites. (A) Trypanosomiasis (*T. cruzi*).
(B) Trypanosomiasis (*T. gambiense*); higher magnification.
(C) Microfilaria.

REFERENCES

[1] ALI, F. M. K. (1986). *Separation of Human Blood and Bone Marrow Cells*. John Wright, Bristol.

[2] BESSIS, M. (1973). *Living Blood Cells and their Ultrastructure*. Springer-Verlag, Berlin.

[3] BESSIS, M. and THIÉRY, J. P. (1957). Les cellules du sang vues au microscope à interférences (Système Nomarski). *Revue d'Hématologie*, **12**, 518.

[4] BINS, M., HUIGES, W. and HALIE, M. R. (1985). Stability of azure B-eosin Y staining solutions. *British Journal of Haematology*, **59**, 73.

[5] BLOEMENDAL, H. (Ed.) (1977). *Cell Separation Methods*. Elsevier–North Holland, Amsterdam.

[6] BØYUM, A. (1964). Separation of white blood cells. *Nature (London)*, **204**, 793.

[7] BØYUM, A. (1984). Separation of lymphocytes, granulocytes and monocytes from human blood using iodinated density gradient media. *Methods in Enzymology*, **108**, 88.

[8] CUTTS, J. H. (1970). *Cell Separation: Methods in Hematology*. Academic Press, New York.

[9] EFRATI, P. and ROZENSZAJN, L. (1960). The morphology of buffy coat in normal human adults. *Blood*, **16**, 1012.

[10] EFRATI, P., ROZENSZAJN, L. and SHAPIRA, E. (1961). The morphology of buffy coat from cord blood of normal human newborns. *Blood*, **17**, 497.

[11] FIELD, J. W. (1940–41). The morphology of malarial parasites in thick blood films. Part IV. The identification of species and phase. *Transactions of the Royal Society of Tropical Medicine and Hygiene*, **34**, 405.

[12] FIELD, J. W. (1941–42). Further notes on a method of staining malarial parasites in thick films. *Transactions of the Royal Society of Tropical Medicine and Hygiene*, **35**, 35.

[13] FIELD, J. W. and SANDOSHAM, A. A. (1964). The Romanowsky stains—aqueous or methanolic? *Transactions of the Royal Society of Tropical Medicine and Hygiene*, **58**, 164.

[14] FLEMING, J. A. and STEWART, J. W. (1967). A critical and comparative study of methods of isolating tumour cells from the blood. *Journal of Clinical Pathology*, **20**, 145.

[15] INTERNATIONAL COMMITTEE FOR STANDARDIZATION IN HAEMATOLOGY (1984). ICSH reference method for staining of blood and bone marrow films by azure B and eosin Y (Romanowsky stain). *British Journal of Haematology*, **57**, 707.

[16] JACKSON, J. F. (1961). Supravital blood studies, using acridine orange fluorescence. *Blood*, **17**, 643.

[17] JAHANMEHR, S. A. H., HYDE, K., GEARY, C. G., CINKOTAI, K. I. and MacIVER, J. E. (1987). Simple technique for fluorescence staining of blood cells with acridine orange. *Journal of Clinical Pathology*, **40**, 926.

[18] KOSENOW, K. (1956). Lebende Blutzellen im Fluoreszenz und Phasenkontrastmikroscop. *Bibliotheca Haematologica (Basel)*, Fasc 4.

[19] MARSHALL, P. N. (1977). Methylene blue-azure B-eosin as a substitute for May–Grünwald–Giemsa and Jenner–Giemsa stains. *Microscopica Acta*, **79**, 153.

[20] MARSHALL, P. N. (1978). Romanowsky-type stains in haematology. *Histochemical Journal*, **10**, 1.

[21] MARSHALL, P. N. and GALBRAITH, W. (1984). On the nature of the purple coloration of leucocyte nuclei stained with azure B-eosin Y. *Histochemical Journal*, **16**, 793.

[22] MELVIN, D. M. and BROOKE, M. M. (1955). Triton X-100 in Giemsa staining of blood parasites. *Stain Technology*, **30**, 269.

[23] NATIONAL COMMITTEE FOR CLINICAL LABORATORY STANDARDS (1990). *Use of Blood Film Examination for Parasites*. Document M15, Vol. 10. NCCLS, Villanova, PA.

[24] NOURBAKHSH, M., ATWOOD, J. G., RACCIO, J. and SELIGSON, D. (1978). An evaluation of blood smears made by a new method using a spinner and diluted blood. *American Journal of Clinical Pathology*, **70**, 885.

[25] OLOFSSON, T., GÄRTNER, I. and OLSSON, I. (1980). Separation of human bone marrow cells in density gradients of polyvinyl pyrrolidone coated silica gel (Percoll). *Scandinavian Journal of Haematology*, **24**, 254.

[26] PFLIEGER, H., GAUS, W. and DIETRICH, M. (1979). Differential blood counts from cell concentrates. A comparison with routine differential blood counts. *Acta Haematologica*, **61**, 150.

[27] ROMSDAHL, M. M., McGREW, E. A., McGRATH, R. G. and VALAITIS, J. (1964). Hematopoietic nucleated cells in the peripheral venous blood of patients with carcinoma. *Cancer (Philadelphia)*, **17**, 1400.

[28] SCHENK, E. A. and WILLIS, C. T. (1989). Note from the Biological Stain Commission: certification of Wright stain solution. *Stain Technology*, **64**, 152.

[29] SEAL, S. H. (1959). Silicone flotation: a simple quantitative method for the isolation of free-floating cancer cells from the blood. *Cancer (Philadelphia)*, **12**, 590.

[30] SILLS, R. H. (1989). Hyposplenism. In *Disorders of the Spleen*. Eds. C. Pochedly, R. H. Sills and A. D. Schwartz. Marcel Dekker, New York.

[31] SODEMAN, T. M. (1970). The use of fluorochromes for the detection of malaria parasites. *American Journal of Tropical Medicine*, **19**, 40.

[32] WENK, R. E. (1976). Comparison of five methods for preparing blood smears. *American Journal of Medical Technology*, **42**, 71.

[33] WITTEKIND, D. (1979). On the nature of Romanowsky dyes and the Romanowsky Giemsa effect. *Clinical and Laboratory Haematology*, **1**, 247.

[34] WITTEKIND, D. H. (1983). On the nature of Romanowsky-Giemsa staining and its significance for cytochemistry and histochemistry: an overall view. *Histochemical Journal*, **15**, 1029.

[35] WITTEKIND, D. H., KRETSCHMER, V. and SOHMER, I. (1982). Azure B-eosin Y stain as the standard Romanowsky–Giemsa stain. *British Journal of Haematology*, **51**, 391.

[36] ZIPURSKY, A., BROWN, E., PALKO, J. and BROWN, E. J. (1983). The erythrocyte differential count in newborn infants. *American Journal of Pediatric Hematology and Oncology*, **5**, 45.

7. Blood-cell morphology in health and disease

Written in collaboration with D. M. Swirsky

Technique of examination of blood films   97
Red cell morphology   98
   Increased variation in size and shape   99
   Inadequate haemoglobin formation   101
   Damage to red cells after formation   104
   Miscellaneous changes   109
   Changes associated with compensatory erythropoiesis   115
Effects of splenectomy   116

Scanning electron microscopy   118
Leucocyte morphology   118
   Polymorphonuclear neutrophils   118
   Eosinophils   124
   Basophils   124
   Monocytes   125
   Lymphocytes   125
Platelet morphology   127

Examination of a fixed and stained blood film is an essential part of a haematological investigation, and it cannot be emphasized too strongly that for the most to be made out of the examination the films must be well spread, well stained and examined systematically. Details of the recommended technique of examination are given below.

The most important red-cell abnormalities, as seen in fixed and stained films, are described and illustrated in black and white, and some notes on their significance and importance in diagnosis are added. Leucocyte and platelet abnormalities are also described and, where appropriate, are illustrated in colour.

TECHNIQUE OF EXAMINATION OF BLOOD FILMS

The point has already been made that blood films must be well spread, well fixed and well stained and examined systematically. It is useless to place a drop of immersion oil anywhere on the film and then to examine it straightaway using the high-power ×100 objective.

First, the film should be covered with a cover-glass using a neutral medium as mountant. Next, it should be inspected under a low magnification (with a ×10 objective) in order to get an idea of the quality of the preparation, whether red-cell agglutination or excessive rouleaux is present, and the number, distribution and staining of the leucocytes, and to find an area where the red cells are evenly distributed and are not distorted.

Having selected a suitable area, a ×40 objective or ×60 oil-immersion objective should then be used. A much better appreciation of variation in red cell size, shape and staining can be obtained with these objectives than with the ×100 oil-immersion lens. The latter in combination with ×6 eyepieces should be reserved for the final examination of unusual cells and for looking at fine details such as cytoplasmic granules, punctate basophilia, etc.

As the diagnosis of the type of anaemia or abnormality present usually depends upon a comprehension of the whole picture which the film presents, the red cells, leucocytes and platelets should all be sytematically examined.

RED-CELL MORPHOLOGY

In *health*, the red blood cells vary relatively little in size and shape (Fig. 7.1). In well spread dried films the great majority of cells have round smooth contours and have diameters within the comparatively narrow range (mean ±2 SD) of 6.0 to 8.5 μm. As a rough guide, normal red cell size appears to be about the same as that of the nucleus of a small lymphocyte on the dried film. The red cells stain quite deeply with the eosin component of Romanowsky dyes, particularly at the periphery of the cell in consequence of the cell's normal biconcavity. A small but variable proportion of cells in well made films (usually less than 10%) are definitely oval rather than round and a very small percentage may be contracted and have an irregular contour or appear to be cells which have lost part of their substance as the result of fragmentation. There may be a very occasional pyknocyte or schistocyte (see p. 105 and p. 108). According to Marsh the percentage of 'pyknocytes' and schistocytes in normal blood does not exceed 0.1% and the proportion is usually considerably less than this;[14] in normal full-term infants the proportion is higher, 0.3–1.9%, and in premature infants still higher, up to 5.6%.[14]

Normal and pathological red cells are subject to considerable distortion in the spreading of a film and, as already referred to, it is imperative to scan films carefully to find an area where the red cells are least distorted before attempting to examine the cells in detail. Such an area can usually be found towards the tail of the film, although not actually at the tail. Rouleaux often form rapidly in blood after withdrawal from the body and may be conspicuous even in films made at a patient's bedside. They are particularly noticeable in the thicker parts of a film which have dried more slowly. Ideally, red cells should be examined in an area in which there are no rouleaux, but the film in the chosen area must not be so thin as to cause red cell distortion. The very different appearances of different areas of the same blood film are illustrated in Figs. 7.2–7.4. The area illustrated in Fig. 7.2 would clearly be the best for looking at red cells critically.

The advantages and disadvantages of examining red cells suspended in plasma have been referred to briefly in Chapter 6 (p. 90). By this means red cells can be seen in the absence of artefacts produced by drying, and abnormalities in size and shape can be better and more reliably appreciated than in films of blood dried on slides. However, the ease and rapidity with which dried films can be made, and their permanence, confer to the

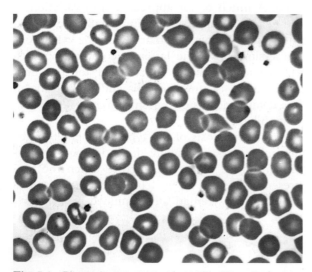

Fig. 7.1   Photomicrograph of a blood film. Film of a healthy adult.

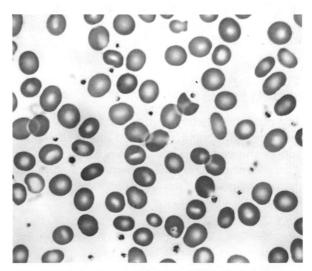

Fig. 7.2   Photomicrograph of a blood film. Ideal thickness for examination.

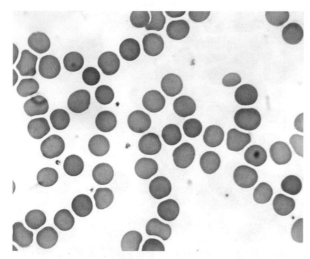

Fig. 7.3   Photomicrograph of a blood film. Film too thin. From same slide as Fig. 7.2.

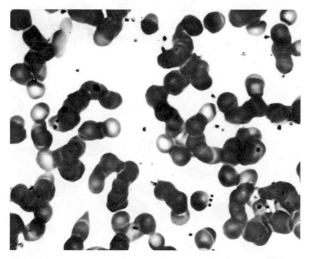

Fig. 7.4   Photomicrograph of a blood film. Film too thick. From same slide as Fig. 7.2.

conventional dried-film technique an overwhelming advantage in routine studies.

In *disease*, abnormality in the red cell picture stems from four main causes:

1. Abnormal erythropoiesis which may be effective or ineffective.
2. Inadequate haemoglobin formation.
3. Damage to, or changes affecting, the red cells after leaving the bone marrow.
4. Attempts by the bone marrow to compensate for anaemia by increased erythropoiesis.

These processes result, respectively, in the following abnormalities of the red cells:

1. Increased variation in size and shape (*anisocytosis* and *poikilocytosis*).
2. Reduced or unequal haemoglobin content (*hypochromasia* or *anisochromasia*).
3. *Spherocytosis*, irregular contraction or fragmentation (*schistocytosis*).
4. Signs of immaturity (*polychromasia*, *punctate basophilia* and *erythroblastaemia*).

INCREASED VARIATION IN SIZE AND SHAPE

Anisocytosis (ἄνισός, unequal) and poikilocytosis (πόικιλός, varied)

These are non-specific features of almost any blood disorder. The terms imply more variation in size than is normally present (Fig. 7.5). Anisocytosis may be due to the presence of cells larger than normal (*macrocytosis*) or cells smaller than normal (*microcytosis*); frequently both macrocytes and microcytes are present together (Fig. 7.6).

Macrocytes

Classically found in megaloblastic anaemias (Fig. 7.7), they are also present in aplastic anaemia (and other dyserythropoietic anaemias). In one

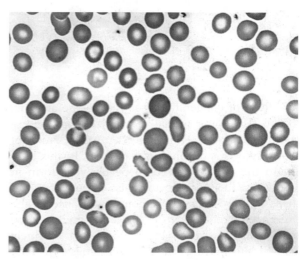

Fig. 7.5   Photomicrograph of a blood film. Shows a moderate degree of anisocytosis and anisochromasia.

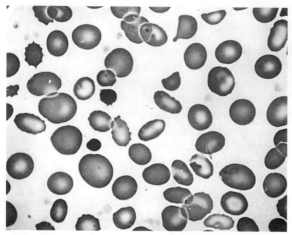

Fig. 7.6   Photomicrograph of a blood film. Shows a marked degree of anisocytosis caused by the presence of both microcytes and macrocytes.

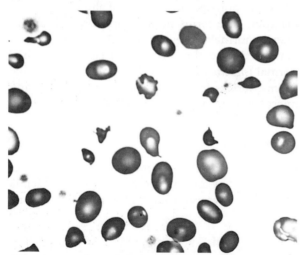

Fig. 7.7   Photomicrograph of a blood film. Shows macrocytes, poikilocytes, cell fragments (schistocytes), and extreme anisocytosis.

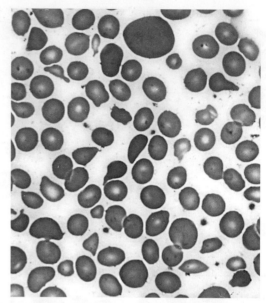

Fig. 7.8   Photomicrograph of a blood film. Congenital dyserythropoietic anaemia type III. Shows unusually large macrocytes.

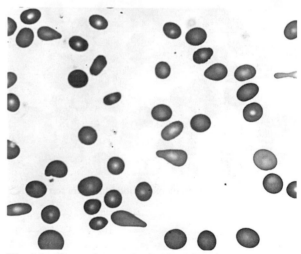

Fig. 7.9   Photomicrograph of a blood film. Myelosclerosis. Shows poikilocytosis and moderate anisocytosis.

rare form of congenital dyserythropoietic anaemia (Type III), some of the macrocytes may be exceptionally large (Fig. 7.8). Another cause of macrocytosis is chronic liver disease. In this condition the red cells tend to be fairly uniform in size and shape. Macrocytosis also occurs whenever there is increased erythropoiesis, because of the presence of reticulocytes. These are identified by their staining slightly basophilically in routinely stained films, giving rise to polychromasia (p. 115) and their presence can be easily confirmed by special stains (e.g. New methylene blue).

Microcytes

Result from fragmentation of normally sized red cells (normocytes) or macrocytes, as occurs with many types of abnormal erythropoiesis, e.g. megaloblastic anaemia (Fig. 7.7). Microcytes are formed as such, or result from fragmentation, in iron-deficiency anaemia (Fig. 7.14) and thalass-

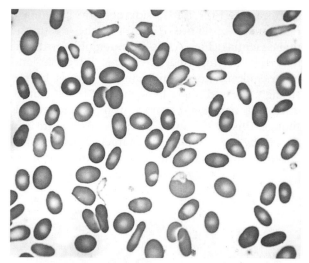

Fig. 7.10   Photomicrograph of a blood film. Myelosclerosis. Almost all the cells are elliptical or oval (cf. Fig. 7.11).

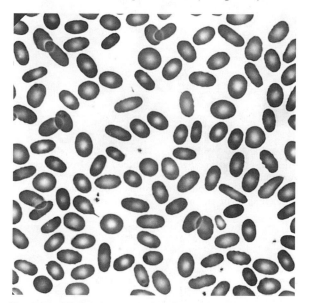

Fig. 7.11   Photomicrograph of a blood film. Hereditary elliptocytosis. Almost all the cells are elliptical.

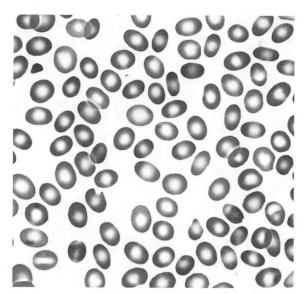

Fig. 7.12   Photomicrograph of a blood film. Hereditary ovalocytosis. The majority of the cells are oval; a few are moderately elliptical.

microangiopathic haemolytic anaemia. Poikilocytosis (and anisocytosis) are illustrated in Figs. 7.7, 7.9, 7.17 and 7.28–7.31.

Elliptocytosis

In disease many more oval or elliptical red cells may be found than in health. Elliptical or oval cells are thus frequent in megaloblastic anaemias and in hypochromic anaemias (Fig. 7.14); they may, too, be conspicuous in myelosclerosis (Fig. 7.10). The highest percentages are found in hereditary elliptocytosis (Fig. 7.11) and hereditary ovalocytosis (Fig. 7.12), in which 90% or more of the adult red cells may be markedly elliptical or oval, and in the South-East Asia variant of hereditary ovalocytosis (SEAHO) (Fig. 7.13). Remarkably, the reticulocytes in the above conditions are round in contour; that is to say, the cell assumes an abnormal shape only in the late stages of maturation.

INADEQUATE HAEMOGLOBIN FORMATION

Hypochromasia (υπόρ, under)

Present when red cells stain unusually palely. (In

aemia (Fig. 7.17). In haemolytic anaemias, microcytes result from the process of spherocytosis or from fragmentation (Figs. 7.19–7.32).

Poikilocytes

Produced in many types of abnormal erythropoiesis, e.g. megaloblastic anaemia, iron-deficiency anaemia, thalassaemia, myelosclerosis, they also result from damage to circulating red cells, as in

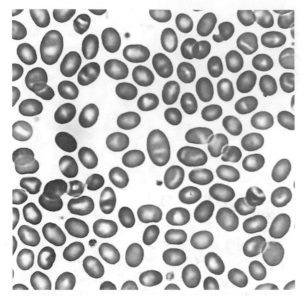

Fig. 7.13 Photomicrograph of a blood film. South-East Asian hereditary ovalocytosis. Some cells show a duplicated central pallor.

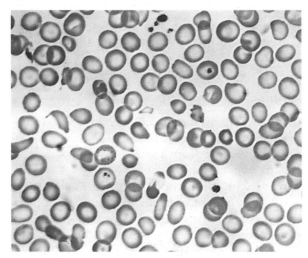

Fig. 7.14 Photomicrograph of a blood film. Iron-deficiency anaemia. Shows a marked degree of hypochromasia, microcytosis and anisocytosis, and a few poikilocytes and cell fragments.

doubtful cases it is wise to compare the staining of the suspect film with that of a normal film stained at the same time.) There are two possible causes: a lowered haemoglobin concentration and abnormal thinness of the red cells. A lowered haemoglobin concentration results from impaired haemoglobin synthesis. This may stem from failure of haem synthesis—iron deficiency is a very com-

mon cause (Fig. 7.14), sideroblastic anaemia a rare cause—or failure of globin synthesis as in the thalassaemias (Fig. 7.17). Haemoglobin synthesis may also be impaired in chronic infections and other inflammatory conditions. It cannot be too strongly stressed that a hypochromic blood picture does not necessarily mean iron deficiency, although this is the most common cause. In iron deficiency the red cells are characteristically hypochromic and microcytic, but the extent of these

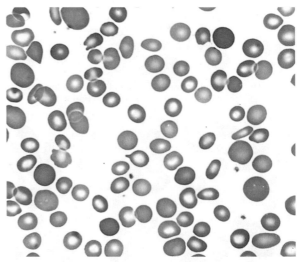

Fig. 7.15 Photomicrograph of a blood film. Iron-deficiency anaemia. Shows anisochromasia following treatment with iron. A macrocytic and orthochromic population contrasts with a microcytic and hypochromic one (dimorphic picture).

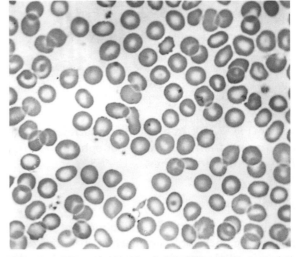

Fig. 7.16 Photomicrograph of a blood film. β-Thalassaemia trait.

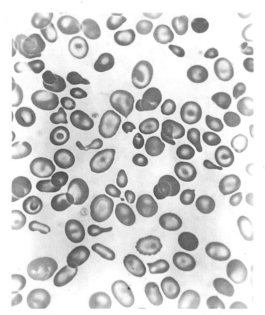

Fig. 7.17   Photomicrograph of a blood film. β-Thalassaemia major. Shows hypochromasia and anisocytosis, and numerous poikilocytes and cell fragments.

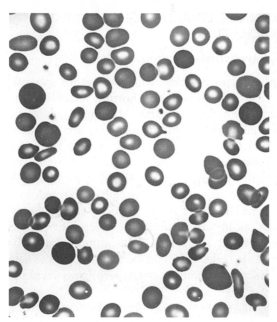

Fig. 7.18   Photomicrograph of a blood film. Acquired sideroblastic anaemia. Shows marked anisocytosis and anisochromasia (cf. Fig. 7.15).

abnormalities depends on the severity; hypochromasia may be overlooked if the Hb exceeds 100 g/l. In homozygous β-thalassaemia, the abnormalities are greater than in iron deficiency at the same level of Hb (cf. Figs. 7.14 and 7.17), but it may not be possible to distinguish heterozygous β-thalassaemia from iron deficiency by the blood film (cf. Figs. 7.14 and 7.16).

Anisochromasia

Some but not all of the red cells stain palely. It can be seen in several circumstances: in a patient with an iron-deficiency anaemia responding to iron therapy (Fig. 7.15), after the transfusion of normal blood to a patient with a hypochromic anaemia; and in sideroblastic anaemia (Fig. 7.18). Such blood pictures have been referred to as 'dimorphic'.

Hyperchromasia (υπέρ, over)

Unusually deep staining of the red cells may be seen in macrocytosis when the red cell thickness is increased and the haemoglobin concentration normal, as in neonatal blood and megaloblastic anaemias, and in spherocytosis in which the red-

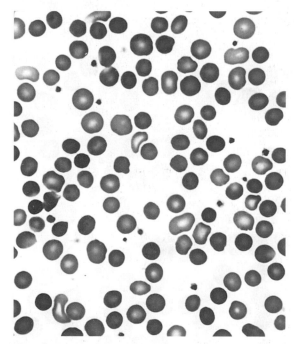

Fig. 7.19   Photomicrograph of a blood film. Hereditary spherocytosis. Shows a moderate degree of spherocytosis and anisocytosis. Note the round contour of the spherocytes.

cell thickness is greater than normal and the MCHC may be slightly increased (Figs. 7.19–7.25).

DAMAGE TO RED CELLS AFTER FORMATION

Spherocytosis (σφαιρα, a sphere)

Spherocytes are cells which are more spheroidal (i.e. less disc-like) than normal red cells. Their diameter is less and their thickness greater than normal. Only in extreme instances are they almost spherical in shape. Spherocytes may result from genetic defects of the red cell membrane as in hereditary spherocytosis (Figs. 7.19 and 7.20), from the interaction between immunoglobulin- or complement-coated red cells and phagocytic cells, as in ABO haemolytic disease of the newborn (Fig. 7.21) and auto-immune haemolytic anaemia (Figs. 7.22 and 7.23) and from the action of bacterial toxins, e.g. *Cl. perfringens* lecithinase (Fig. 7.24).

Spherocytes typically appear perfectly round in contour in stained films; they have to be carefully distinguished from 'spherical forms' or 'crenated spheres' (Fig. 7.52), the end-result of crenation or acanthocytosis (see p. 110). 'Spherical forms' can develop as artefacts especially in blood which

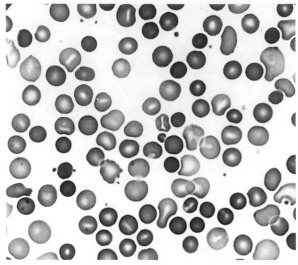

Fig. 7.21   Photomicrograph of a blood film. ABO haemolytic disease of the newborn. Spherocytosis is intense.

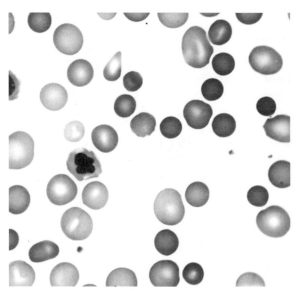

Fig. 7.22   Photomicrograph of a blood film. Auto-immune haemolytic anaemia. Shows a moderate degree of spherocytosis and anisocytosis.

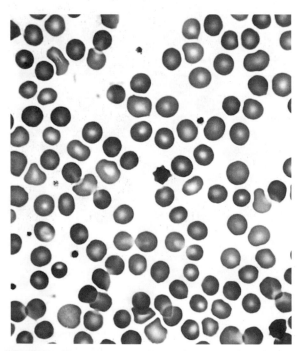

Fig. 7.20   Photomicrograph of a blood film. Hereditary spherocytosis. Clinically mild case; shows a lesser degree of spherocytosis than in Fig. 7.19.

has been allowed to stand before films are spread. In rare and atypical hereditary haemolytic anaemias spherocytes may have an irregular contour (Fig. 7.25) and in haemolytic hereditary elliptocytosis any spherocytes present tend to be oval rather than round (Fig. 7.11). The blood film of a patient who has been transfused with stored blood may show a proportion of spherocytes.

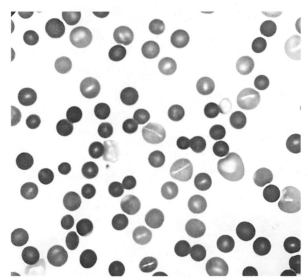

Fig. 7.23 Photomicrograph of a blood film. Auto-immune haemolytic anaemia, warm-antibody type. The majority of the cells are spherocytes.

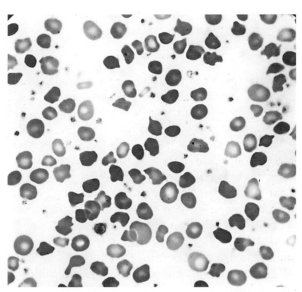

Fig. 7.25 Photomicrograph of a blood film. Atypical hereditary spherocytosis. Severe HS that did not respond fully to splenectomy. Densely-staining spherocytes with irregular contours are conspicuous in this film 23 years after splenectomy.

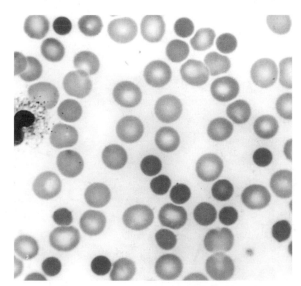

Fig. 7.24 Photomicrograph of a blood film. *Cl. perfringens* septicaemia. Shows an extreme degree of spherocytosis; note the round contour of the spherocytes. A markedly dimorphic picture.

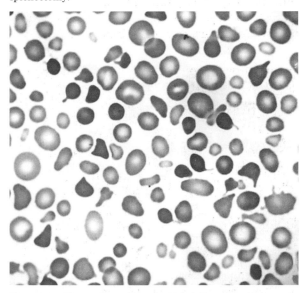

Fig. 7.26 Photomicrograph of a blood film. Hereditary haemolytic anaemia, a variant of hereditary ovalocytosis (pyropoikilocytosis). Shows spherocytes and numerous cell fragments, and a few ovalocytes.

Schistocytosis (fragmentation) (σχιστός, cleft)

Schistocytes, of varying shapes, are found in many blood diseases. Thus fragmentation occurs:

1. In certain genetically determined disorders, e.g. thalassaemias (Fig. 7.17) and hereditary elliptocytosis and allied disorders (Fig. 7.26).

2. In acquired disorders of red cell formation, e.g. megaloblastic (Fig. 7.7) and iron-deficiency anaemias (Fig. 7.14).

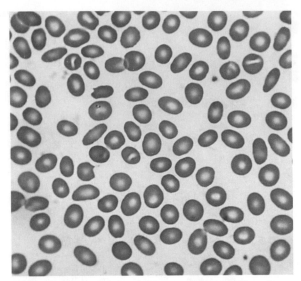

Fig. 7.27   Photomicrograph of a blood film. Mother of patient whose film is shown in Fig. 7.26. Many oval or elliptic cells are present.

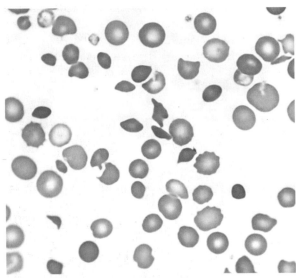

Fig. 7.28   Photomicrograph of a blood film. Microangiopathic haemolytic anaemia; renal cortical necrosis. Shows numerous small poikilocytes and cell fragments.

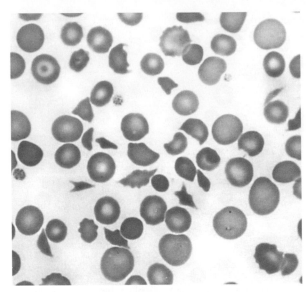

Fig. 7.29   Photomicrograph of a blood film. Microangiopathic haemolytic anaemia; haemolytic-uraemic syndrome. Shows spherocytosis and cell fragments and marked crenation.

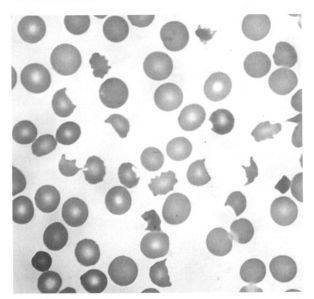

Fig. 7.30   Photomicrograph of a blood film. Microangiopathic haemolytic anaemia; disseminated carcinoma of breast. Shows many bizarre-shaped cells, crenation, cell fragments and 'burr' cells.

3. As the consequence of mechanical stresses, e.g. in the microangiopathic haemolytic anaemias (Figs. 7.28–7.30) and in cardiac haemolytic anaemias which are usually caused by peri-valvular leak accompanied by turbulence of left ventricular flow. (Fig. 7.31).

4. As the result of direct thermal injury as in severe burns (Fig. 7.32).

In all conditions in which fragmentation is occurring three types of cell can be distinguished:

1. Small fragments of cells of varying shape, sometimes with sharp angles or spines (spurs), sometimes round in contour, usually staining

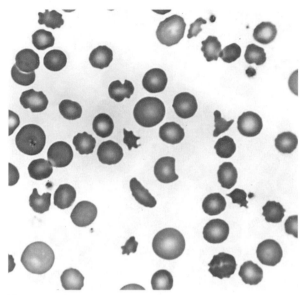

Fig. 7.31 Photomicrograph of a blood film. Post-cardiac surgery haemolytic anaemia. Shows numerous irregularly-shaped cell fragments. Note presence of platelets.

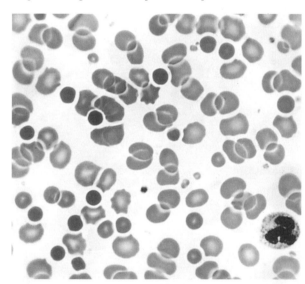

Fig. 7.32 Photomicrograph of a blood film. Severe burns. Shows many very small rounded cell fragments and a little crenation.

deeply but occasionally palely as the result of loss of haemoglobin at the time of fragmentation.

2. Larger cells, of irregular or mainly rounded contour from which fragments have been split off—these include 'helmet' cells.

3. Normal unfragmented adult red cells and reticulocytes.

Not infrequently, as for instance in the haemolytic-uraemic syndrome in children, the blood picture is made more bizarre by the superimposition of varying degrees of crenation (Fig. 7.29).

Irregularly-contracted red cells

Several types of irregularly-contracted cells can be distinguished. In drug- or chemical-induced haemolytic anaemias a proportion of the red cells are smaller than normal and unusually densely stained, i.e. they appear contracted, and their margins are slightly irregular and may be partly concave (Figs. 7.33 and 7.34). These may be cells from which Heinz bodies have been extracted by the spleen. Similar cells may be seen in films of some unstable haemoglobinopathies before splenectomy, e.g. that due to the presence of Hb Köln (Fig. 7.35). Heinz bodies are not normally visible in Romanowsky-stained blood films but they may be seen in such films as pale purple-staining bodies in severe unstable haemoglobin haemolytic anaemias after splenectomy (Fig. 7.36). An extreme degree of irregular contraction is characteristic of severe favism, and it is typical to see that in some

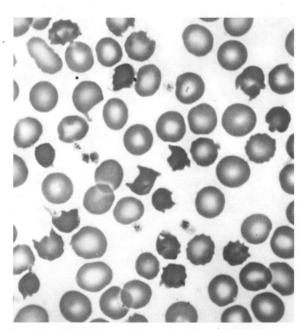

Fig. 7.33 Photomicrograph of a blood film. Haemolytic anaemia caused by an overdose of dapsone. Shows many irregularly-contracted cells.

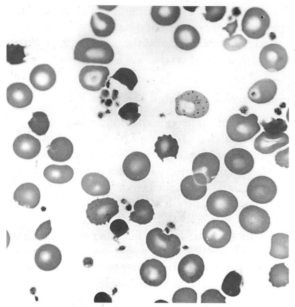

Fig. 7.34   Photomicrograph of a blood film. Haemolytic anaemia caused by an overdose of phenacetin. Shows many markedly and irregularly contracted cells; also punctate basophilia.

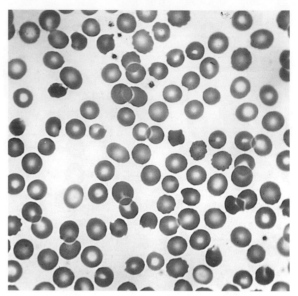

Fig. 7.35   Photomicrograph of a blood film. An unstable haemoglobin haemolytic anaemia (Hb Köln). Shows some moderately contracted cells with somewhat irregular contours.

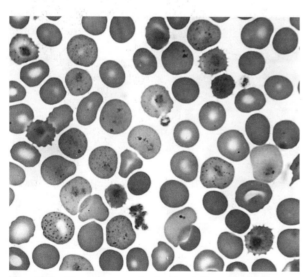

Fig. 7.36   Photomicrograph of a blood film. An unstable haemoglobin haemolytic anaemia (Hb Bristol) after splenectomy. Shows contracted and crenated cells; also punctate basophilia and inclusions (Heinz bodies and Pappenheimer bodies).

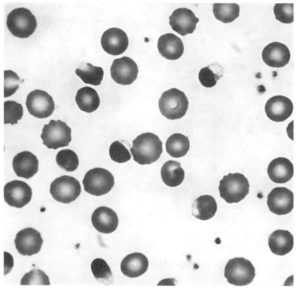

Fig. 7.37   Photomicrograph of a blood film. Favism. Shows numerous markedly contracted cells. Note condensation and contraction of haemoglobin from the cell membrane.

of the contracted cells the haemoglobin appears to have contracted away from the cell membrane (Fig. 7.37).

A type of irregular contraction of unknown origin has been described by the term pyknocytosis.[23]

The pyknocytes closely resemble chemically damaged red cells. As already referred to (p. 98), a small number of pyknocytes may be found in the blood of infants in the first few weeks of life, especially in premature infants. The term 'infantile

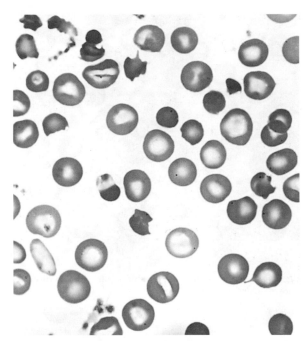

Fig. 7.38   Photomicrograph of a blood film. Infantile pyknocytosis. Shows irregularly-contracted cells similar to those seen in chemical- or drug-induced haemolytic anaemias (cf. Figs. 7.33 and 7.34).

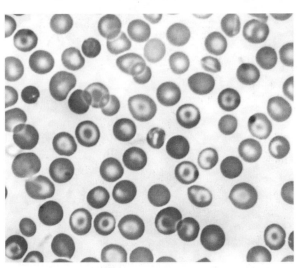

Fig. 7.39   Photomicrograph of a blood film. Chronic liver disease (obstructive jaundice). Shows many target cells.

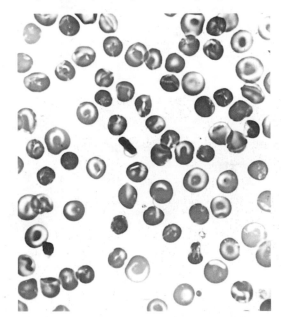

Fig. 7.40   Photomicrograph of a blood film. Hb CC disease. Shows many target cells and an extracellular crystal.

pyknocytosis' refers to a transient haemolytic anaemia of obscure origin affecting infants in which many pyknocytes are present (Fig. 7.38).[12,23]

MISCELLANEOUS CHANGES

Leptocytosis (λεπτός, thin)

This term has been used to describe unusually thin red cells, as in severe iron deficiency or thalassaemia in which the cells may stain as rings of haemoglobin with large almost unstained central areas (Figs. 7.14 and 7.17). The term *target cell* refers to a leptocyte in which there is a central round stained area in addition to a rim of haemoglobin. Target cells are thought to result from cells having a surface which is disproportionately large compared with their volume. They are seen in films in chronic liver diseases in which the cell membrane may be loaded with cholesterol (Fig. 7.39), and in varying numbers in iron-deficiency anaemia and in thalassaemia. They are often conspicuous in certain haemoglobinopathies, e.g. Hb CC disease (Fig. 7.40), Hb AC trait (Fig. 7.41),

Hb SS disease (Figs. 7.42–7.44), Hb SC disease (Fig. 7.45), Hb S/β-thalassaemia, Hb EE disease (Fig. 7.46) and Hb AE trait (Fig. 7.47). In Hb-CC disease crystals of haemoglobin may be seen (Fig. 7.40).

Target cells appear after splenectomy (Fig. 7.48), even in otherwise healthy subjects whose spleens have been removed because of traumatic rupture.

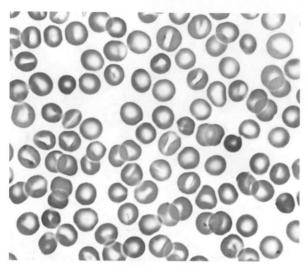

Fig. 7.41   Photomicrograph of a blood film. Hb AC trait.

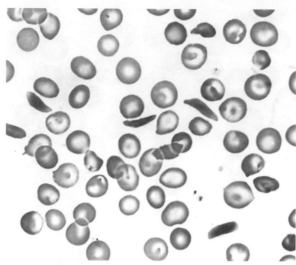

Fig. 7.43   Photomicrograph of a blood film. Hb SS disease. Shows sickled cells and target cells.

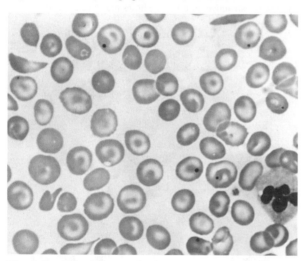

Fig. 7.42   Photomicrograph of a blood film. Hb SS disease. Shows a few sickled cells, target cells and Howell-Jolly bodies.

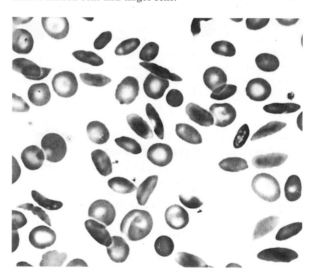

Fig. 7.44   Photomicrograph of a blood film. Hb SS disease. Shows numerous sickled cells.

Splenectomy in thalassaemia may result in an extreme degree of leptocytosis and target cell formation (Fig. 7.49).

Sickle cells (drepanocytes)

The varied film appearances in sickle-cell disease are illustrated in Figs. 7.42–7.44. In homozygous sickle-cell (Hb-SS) disease sickle cells are probably always present in films of freshly withdrawn blood. Sometimes many irreversibly sickled cells are present (Fig. 7.44) and in all cases massive sickling takes place when the blood is subjected to anoxia (see p. 266). In films of fresh blood the sickled cells vary in shape between elliptical forms, oat-shaped cells and sickles. Target cells are also often a feature (Figs. 7.42, 7.43). and Howell-Jolly bodies are found when there is splenic atrophy.

Crenation

This term describes the process by which red cells develop many or numerous projections from their surface (Fig. 7.50). First described by Ponder[17]

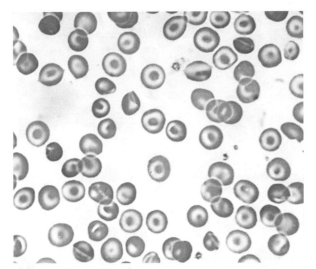

Fig. 7.45 Photomicrograph of a blood film. Hb SC disease. Shows numerous target cells.

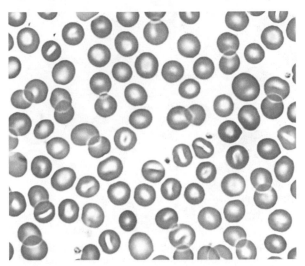

Fig. 7.47 Photomicrograph of a blood film. Hb AE trait.

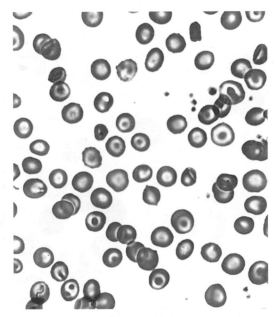

Fig. 7.46 Photomicrograph of a blood film. Hb EE disease.

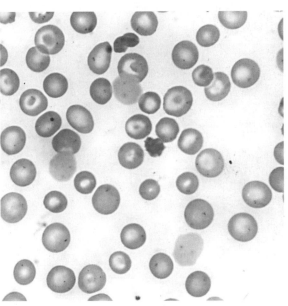

Fig. 7.48 Photomicrograph of a blood film. Pyruvate-kinase deficiency, after splenectomy. Shows macrocytosis, target cells and a markedly crenated cell.

as disc–sphere transformation, crenation can result from many causes, e.g. by washing red cells free from plasma and suspending them in 9 g/l NaCl between glass surfaces, particularly at a raised pH, from the presence of traces of fatty substances on the slides on which films are made and from the presence of traces of chemicals which at higher concentrations cause lysis. The end stages of crenation are the 'finely crenated sphere' and the 'spherical form' which closely resemble spherocytes (Figs. 7.51 and 7.52). The disc–sphere transformation may be reversible, e.g. that produced by washing cells free from plasma, and in this respect the contracted 'spherical form' (which has not lost surface) is quite distinct from the 'spherocyte' (which has lost surface), although they may closely resemble one another in stained films.

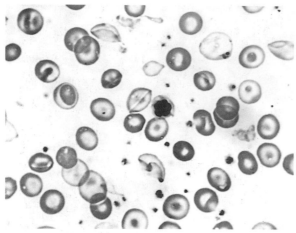

Fig. 7.49 Photomicrograph of a blood film. β-Thalassaemia major, after splenectomy. Shows many target cells and cells grossly deficient in haemoglobin. The relatively deeply staining target cells are normal cells that have been transfused. Normoblasts are present.

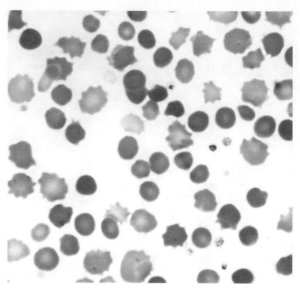

Fig. 7.51 Photomicrograph of a blood film. Hereditary spherocytosis. Shows marked spherocytosis and an unusual degree of crenation.

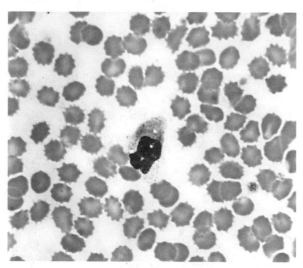

Fig. 7.50 Photomicrograph of a blood film. Normal blood after 18 h at *c* 20°C. Shows a marked degree of crenation.

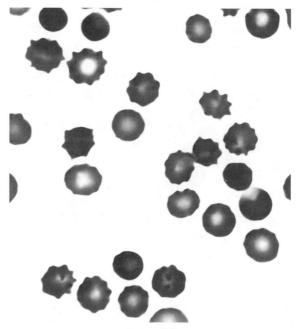

Fig. 7.52 Photomicrograph of a blood film. Acute renal failure following multiple bee stings. Shows crenation leading to finely-crenated spheres.

A few crenated cells may be seen in many blood films, even in those from healthy subjects. Crenation regularly develops if blood is allowed to stand overnight at 20°C before films are made (Fig. 7.50). It may be a marked feature, for obscure and probably diverse reasons, in freshly made blood films made from patients suffering from a variety of illnesses, especially uraemia. It is also seen in films from patients undergoing cardiopulmonary bypass. When crenation is superimposed on an underlying abnormality, the red cells may appear bizarre in the extreme (Fig. 7.29).

Acanthocytosis (άκανθα, spine)

The term 'acanthocytosis' was introduced to describe an abnormality of the red cell associated with abnormal phospholipid metabolism (Fig. 7.53).[7,15,18] Characteristically, the majority of the red cells are coarsely crenated (acanthocytes), the size and number of the projections varying. Some cells have moderate numbers of small regularly arranged projections from their surface, others have smaller numbers of less regularly arranged finer projections with sharper points. Morphologically, rather similar irregularly crenated cells (perhaps acanthocytes) are to be seen, often in quite large numbers, in blood films made from splenectomized patients (Fig. 7.54); and somewhat similar cells may be seen in the films of some patients with anaemia and chronic liver disease ('spur cell' anaemia).[20] Yet another cause of acanthocytosis is the McLeod phenotype, caused by lack of the Kell precursor (Kx) (Fig. 7.55).[27] The cause of these phenomena is obscure, but they may reflect an abnormality in the phospholipid content or phospholipid-cholesterol ratio of the red cell membrane.

In another type of acanthocytosis, a proportion of the red cells bear small numbers of irregularly situated but often quite large projections with rounded tips (Fig. 7.56). Although usually less than 10% of the cells are affected, the appear-

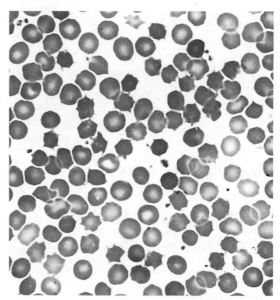

Fig. 7.54 Photomicrograph of a blood film. Hereditary spherocytosis; 11 yr after splenectomy. Show spherocytosis and crenation (cf. Fig. 7.62 for other features of splenic atrophy or post-splenectomy blood films).

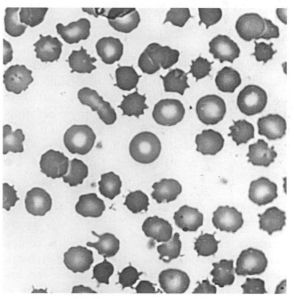

Fig. 7.55 Photomicrograph of a blood film. McLeod phenotype associated with chronic haemolytic anaemia. Acanthocytes are conspicuous.

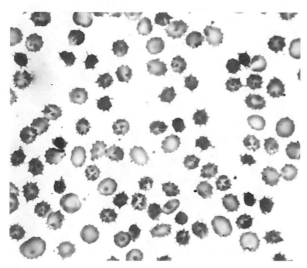

Fig. 7.53 Photomicrograph of a blood film. Acanthocytosis. Many cells show marked crenation and contraction.

ances are unusual and distinctive. The cause of the abnormality is obscure; the phenomenon is not rare and its relationship, if any, to other types

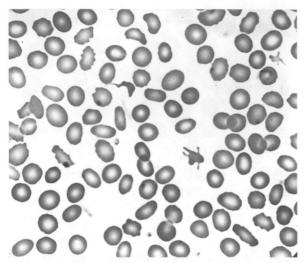

Fig. 7.56 Photomicrograph of a blood film. Acanthocytosis. Shows some bizarre-shaped acanthocytes and cell fragments; also moderate anisocytosis and ovalocytosis.

of acanthocytosis has not been determined. The change has not been found to correlate with any particular type of illness, and in some instances the patients have not been anaemic.

Burr cells

The 'burr' abnormality was described by Schwartz and Motto[19] in the blood films of patients suffering from a variety of disorders, but particularly in uraemia. Burr cells are small cells or cell fragments bearing one or a few spines. They are probably damaged or fragmented cells which have undergone a type of crenation (Figs. 7.29 and 7.30).

Stomatocytosis (στόμα, mouth)

Stomatocytes are red cells in which the central biconcave area appears slit-like in dried films. The term was first used to describe the appearance of some of the cells in a rare type of haemolytic anaemia.[13] In 'wet' preparations, the stomatocyte is a cup-shaped red cell. The slit-like appearance of the cell's concavity, as seen in dried films, is thus to some extent an artefact. Subsequently, stomatocytes have been recognized in small numbers in many films and occasionally many or even the majority of the cells present are

stomatocytes (Fig. 7.57). They have been reported in alcoholism.[5] Their presence in large numbers has been attributed to a genetic factor, stomatocytes having been described as being particularly frequent in films of Australians of Mediterranean origin.[6,16] There is a suspicion that in some films the occurrence of stomatocytosis may be an artefact and it is known that the change can be produced by decreased pH and as the result of exposure to cationic detergent-like compounds and non-penetrating anions.[25] However, it remains to be explained, if the stomatocytic change is usually an artefact, why the change is seen in some films and not in others and why some cells are affected and not others.

The advent of the scanning electron microscope provided the stimulus and the means for a critical re-examination of red cell morphology (see p. 118).

Bessis and his co-workers have published excellent photographs of pathological red cells and proposed a new nomenclature to describe what they have seen.[2,3,25] They use the term echinocyte (ἐχινος, sea urchin) for the crenated cell and clearly differentiate the echinocyte from the acanthocyte. (The normal cell is referred to as a discocyte.) Echinocytes (e.g. crenated red cells as produced by adding oleic acid or lysolecithin to plasma) have 10–30 evenly distributed spicules,

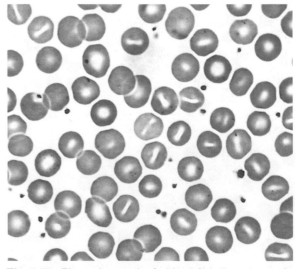

Fig. 7.57 Photomicrograph of a blood film. Stomatocytosis. Many of the cells have slit-like central unstained areas.

while acanthocytes (in congenital abetalipoprotein-aemia) have 5–10 spicules of varying length which are irregularly distributed. Acanthocytes can undergo crenation, the product being termed an 'acantho-echinocyte'. Bessis and his co-workers stressed how the echinocytic and stomatocytic change can be superimposed on other pathological forms. Thus, they illustrated 'sickle-stomatocytes' and 'stomato-acanthocytes'. They also discussed the difficult question of the in-vivo significance of crenation (echinocytic change) observed in vitro. It seems that neither echinocytosis nor acanthocytosis is necessarily associated with increased haemolysis. It cannot be concluded, either, that crenation is occurring in vivo, when the phenomenon is markedly evident in films made on glass slides. To ensure that cells are crenated in any blood sample as it is withdrawn, Brecher and Bessis recommended that the blood be examined immediately between plastic instead of glass cover-slips or slides, to avoid the known 'echinocytogenic' effect of glass surfaces, probably due to alkalinity.[3] Marked echinocytosis has been reported in premature infants following exchange transfusion or transfusion of normal red cells.[8]

CHANGES ASSOCIATED WITH COMPENSATORY ERYTHROPOIESIS

Polychromasia (πολύς, many)

This term suggests that the red cells are being stained many colours. In practice, it denotes that some of the red cells stain shades of bluish grey (Fig. 7.58)—these are the reticulocytes. Cells staining shades of blue, 'blue polychromasia', are unusually young reticulocytes. 'Blue polychromasia' is most often seen when there is extra-medullary erythropoiesis, as, for instance, in myelosclerosis or carcinomatosis.

Punctate basophilia

Punctate basophilia (or basophilic stippling) is a variant of diffuse basophilia, in which numerous granules are distributed throughout the cell (Figs. 7.59 and 7.60); they do not give a positive Perls's reaction for ionized iron, in contrast to Pappenheimer bodies (see below) which do. Punctate

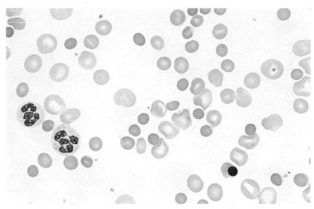

Fig. 7.58 Photomicrograph of a blood film. Polychromasia. Some red cells stain shades of bluish-grey.

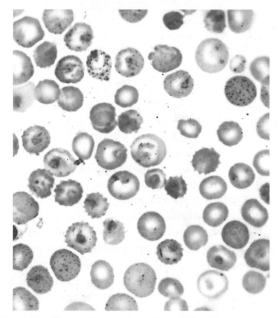

Fig. 7.59 Photomicrograph of a blood film. Unstable haemoglobinopathy (Hb Hammersmith); after splenectomy. There is a remarkable degree of punctate basophilia. Also shows Pappenheimer bodies and circular bodies corresponding to Heinz bodies.

basophilia is indicative of disturbed erythropoiesis. It occurs in many blood diseases: thalassaemia, megaloblastic anaemias, infections, liver disease, poisoning by lead and other heavy metals, unstable haemoglobins, pyrimidine- 5'-nucleotidase deficiency.

Erythroblastaemia

Erythroblasts may be found in the blood films of

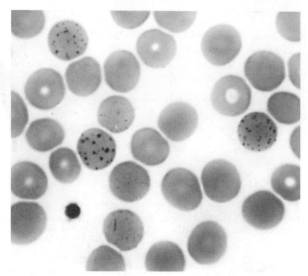

Fig. 7.60   Photomicrograph of a blood film. Punctate basophilia. Pyrimidine-5'-nucleotidase deficiency.

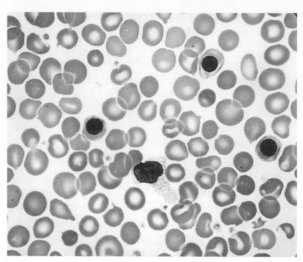

Fig. 7.61   Photomicrograph of a blood film. Myelosclerosis, after splenectomy. Shows three normoblasts and moderate anisocytosis and poikilocytosis.

almost any patient with a severe anaemia; they are, however, very unusual in aplastic anaemia. They are more common in children than in adults and large numbers are a very characteristic finding in haemolytic disease of the newborn. Small numbers can be found in the cord blood of normal infants at birth and quite large numbers in that of premature infants.

When large numbers of erythroblasts are present, many of them are probably derived from extramedullary foci of erythropoiesis, e.g. in the liver and spleen. This seems likely to be true, for instance, in haemolytic disease of the newborn, leukaemia, myelosclerosis and carcinomatosis. In carcinomatosis the number of erythroblasts is often disproportionately high for the degree of anaemia, and a few immature granulocytes are usually present also (so-called leuco-erythroblastic anaemia).

Erythroblasts can usually be found in the peripheral blood after splenectomy and in the presence of extramedullary erythropoiesis many may be present (Fig. 7.61). Large numbers are frequently seen in the blood films of Hb-SS disease patients in painful crises. Small numbers of erythroblasts are not uncommon in blood from patients suffering from cyanotic heart failure or septicaemias.

Howell–Jolly bodies

These are nuclear remnants and (usually singly) may be seen in a small percentage of red cells in pernicious anaemia. Cells containing them are regularly present after splenectomy and where there has been marked splenic atrophy. Usually only a few such cells are present, but they may be numerous in cases of steatorrhoea in which there is splenic atrophy and sometimes deficiency of folate (Fig. 7.62).

EFFECTS OF SPLENECTOMY

Some of the changes have already been mentioned, namely, the occurrence of target cells, 'acanthocytes' (Figs. 7.48 and 7.54) and Howell-Jolly bodies. Pappenheimer bodies are also regularly found. These are granules, staining black with Romanowsky dyes; in size they are usually minute and usually are only present singly or in pairs. Not infrequently they may be found in the majority of circulating red cells (Fig. 7.63). They correspond to the siderotic granules of siderocytes and are never distributed in large numbers throughout the cells as in classical punctate basophilia.

Rouleaux and auto-agglutination

The differences between rouleaux and auto-

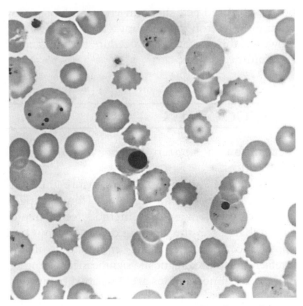

Fig. 7.62 Photomicrograph of a blood film. Steatorrhoea. Shows Howell-Jolly bodies, target cells and crenation, all consequences of splenic atrophy.

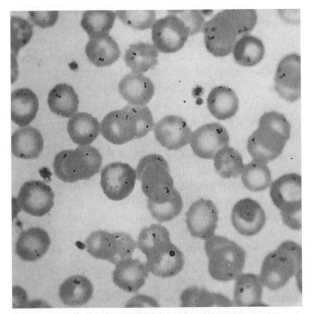

Fig. 7.63 Photomicrograph of a blood film. Pyruvate-kinase deficiency; after splenectomy. Shows many macrocytes, the majority containing Pappenheimer bodies.

in which there is intense rouleaux formation the rouleaux may simulate auto-agglutination. Even so, if the film, apparently showing auto-agglutination, is carefully scanned, an area in which rouleaux can be clearly seen will almost certainly be found. Rouleaux occur to some extent in all films, and their presence adds point, as has been mentioned, to the importance of careful selection of the area of film to be examined.

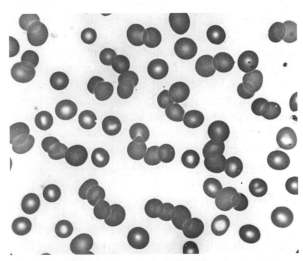

Fig. 7.64 Photomicrograph of a blood film. Shows rouleaux in a normal blood film (cf. Fig. 7.65).

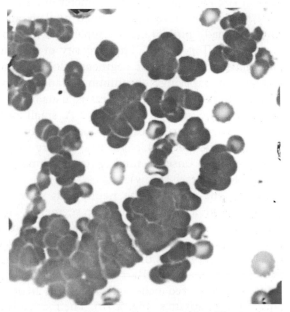

Fig. 7.65 Photomicrograph of a blood film. Shows massive auto-agglutination (cf. Fig. 7.64).

agglutination are described on p. 90 and there is usually no difficulty in determining which is which in stained films (cf. Figs. 7.64 and 7.65). However, in myelomatosis and in other conditions

SCANNING ELECTRON MICROSCOPY

The morphology of red cells, as illustrated in this chapter, may be distorted by spreading and drying films in the traditional way. A more authentic portrayal of red cell shape in vivo can be seen by scanning electron microscopy (Figs. 7.66–7.73). However, this specialized procedure is not practical as a routine.

MORPHOLOGY OF LEUCOCYTES

This section will include a description of the normal leucocytes, some congenital anomalies and reactive changes which are commonly encountered. To describe adequately the various changes found in malignant conditions would require a lengthy text and many illustrations which are beyond the scope of this book. They will be referred to briefly here, but for detailed reference readers should consult an atlas on blood cells. For classification of the acute leukaemias, see the original description by the FAB group;[1] and their subsequent reviews (Chapter 9).

POLYMORPHONUCLEAR NEUTROPHILS

In normal individuals neutrophils account for more than half the circulating leucocytes. They are the main defence of the body against pyogenic bacterial infections. Normal neutrophils are uniform in size, with an apparent diameter of c 13 μm on a film. They have a segmented nucleus and, when stained, pink/orange cytoplasm with fine granulation (Fig. 7.74). The majority of neutrophils have three nuclear segments (lobes) connected by tapering chromatin strands. The chromatin shows clumping and is usually condensed at the nuclear periphery. A small percentage have four lobes, and occasionaly five lobes may be seen. Up to 8% of circulating neutrophils are unsegmented or partly segmented ('band' forms) (see below).

In women, 2–3% of the neutrophils show an appendage at a terminal nuclear segment. This 'drumstick' is about 1.5 μm in diameter and is connected to the nucleus by a short stalk (see Fig. 9.10) It represents the inactive X chromosome, and corresponds to the Barr body of buccal cells.

Occasionally, red cells will adhere to neutrophils, forming rosettes (Fig. 7.75). The mechanism is unknown but it is likely to be an immune mechanism; it appears to be of no clinical significance.

It is extremely important to ensure the consistency of staining of the blood films using a standardized Romanowsky method (see Chapter 6), as changes in the staining density, colour and appearance of cytoplasmic granulation, if not artefact, may have diagnostic significance. Common neutrophil abnormalities are described below.

Granules

'Toxic' granulation is the term used to describe an increase in staining density and possibly number of granules which occurs regularly with bacterial infection, and often with other causes of inflammation (Fig. 7.76). Fractionally larger, coarser granules may be seen in aplastic anaemia and myelofibrosis. Conversely, poorly staining (hypogranular) and agranular neutrophils occur in the myelodysplastic syndromes and some forms of myeloid leukaemia.

There are rare inherited disorders which are manifest by abnormal neutrophils. In the *Alder–Reilly anomaly* the granules are very large, discrete, stain deep red and may obscure the nucleus (Fig. 7.85). Other leucocytes, including some lymphocytes, also show the abnormal granules. In the *Chediak–Higashi syndrome* there are giant but scanty azurophil granules (Fig. 7.77), and the other leucocyte types may also be affected. Alder-Reilly neutrophils function normally, but in Chediak–Higashi syndrome there is a functional defect which is manifest by susceptibility to severe infection.

Vacuoles

In blood films spread without delay the presence of vacuoles in the neutrophils is usually indicative of severe sepsis, when toxic granulation is usually

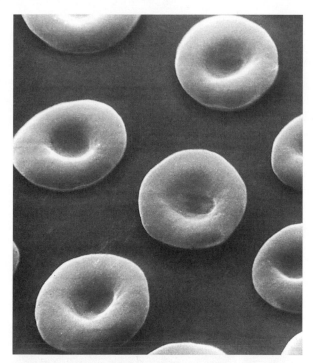

Fig. 7.66 Scanning electron microscope photograph. Normal red cells.

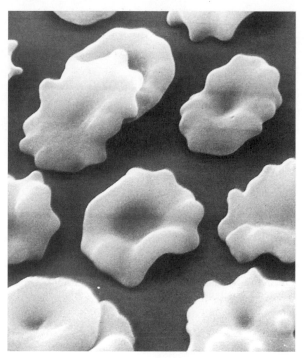

Fig. 7.68 Scanning electron microscope photograph. Normal blood after standing overnight. Note crenation.

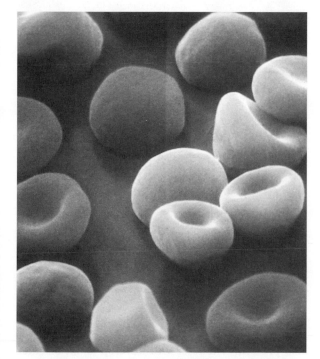

Fig. 7.67 Scanning electron microscope photograph. Hereditary spherocytosis. Note the round shape of spherocytes. Compare with Fig. 7.66; also see blood film appearances as shown in Fig. 7.19.

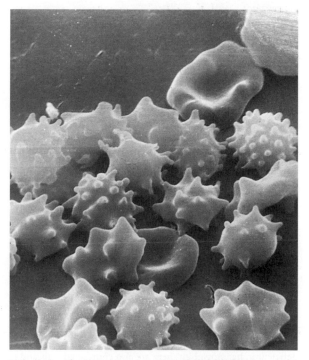

Fig. 7.69 Scanning electron microscope photograph. Acanthocytosis. Some cells also show crenation and contraction. Compare with Fig. 7.68; see also blood film appearances as shown in Fig. 7.53.

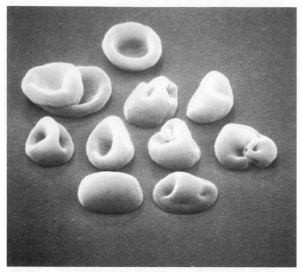

Fig. 7.70   Scanning electron microscope photograph. Drug induced haemolysis; see blood film appearances shown in Fig. 7.33.

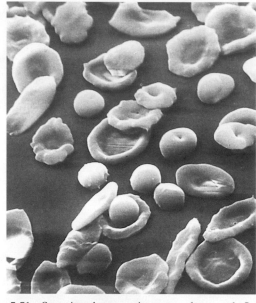

Fig. 7.71   Scanning electron microscope photograph. Iron deficiency anaemia. Compare with Fig. 7.72.

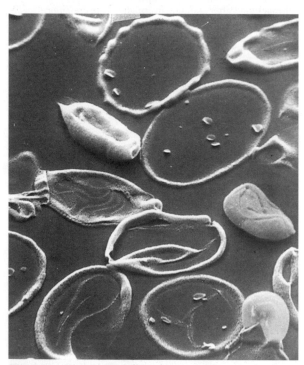

Fig. 7.72   Scanning electron microscope photograph. β-Thalassaemia major, post-splenectomy. Shows cells grossly deficient in haemoglobin; there are also contracted cells and poikilocytes. In the hypochromic cells inclusions are seen, corresponding to Pappenheimer bodies.

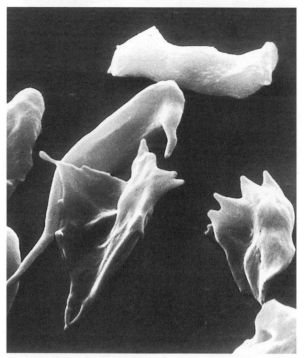

Fig. 7.73   Scanning electron microscope photograph. Hb SS disease. Shows sickled cells.

also present. Vacuoles will develop as an artefact with prolonged standing of the blood before films are made (see Fig. 1.2, p. 5).

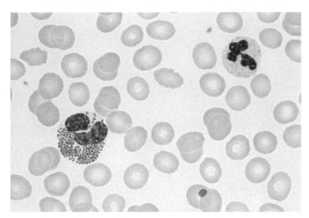

Fig. 7.74 Photomicrograph of a blood film. Normal polymorphonuclear neutrophil and normal eosinophil.

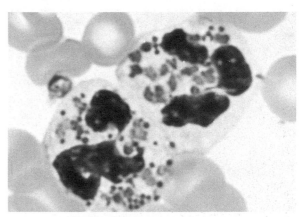

Fig. 7.77 Photomicrograph of a blood film. Chediak-Higashi syndrome. Neutrophils show abnormal granules.

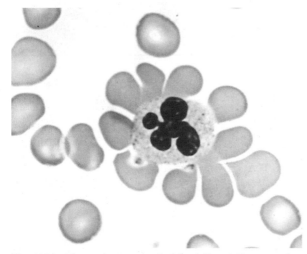

Fig. 7.75 Photomicrograph of a blood film. Adherence of red cells (and two platelets) to a neutrophil. Patient had acquired haemolytic anaemia, with negative direct antiglobulin test.

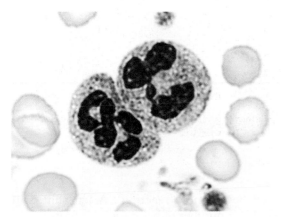

Fig. 7.76 Photomicrograph of a blood film. Severe infection. Neutrophils show toxic granulation.

Bacteria

Very rarely, in the presence of overwhelming septicaemia, bacteria may be seen within vacuoles or lying free in the cytoplasm of neutrophils. When blood is taken from an infected central line clumps of bacteria may be seen scattered in the film as well as in neutrophils (Fig. 7.78).

Döhle bodies

These are small round, or oval pale blue-grey structures, usually found at the periphery of the neutrophil. They consist of decomposed ribosomes and endoplasmic reticulum. They are seen in bacterial infections. There is also a benign inherited condition known as *May–Hegglin anomaly* with a similar morphological structure; in this condition the Döhle bodies occur in all types of leucocyte except lymphocytes.

Nuclei

Segmentation of the nucleus of the neutrophil is a normal event as the cell matures from the myelocyte. With the three-lobed neutrophil as a marker, a shift to the left (less mature) or to the right (hypermature) can be recognised (Table 7.1). A left shift with band forms, metamyelocytes and, perhaps, occasional myelocytes, is common in sepsis (Fig. 7.79), when it is usually accompanied by toxic granulation. If promyelocytes and myeloblasts are also present it is likely to be due

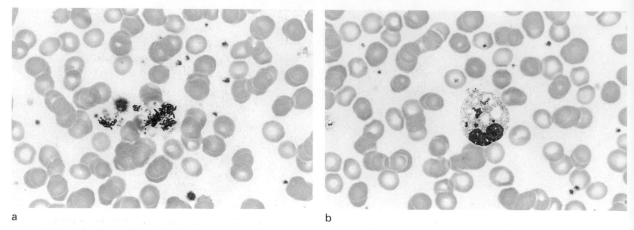

a   b

Fig. 7.78   Photomicrograph of a blood film. Blood collected from infected site, showing bacteria (a) in scattered clumps and (b) in a neutrophil.

Table 7.1   Stages of granulocyte maturation

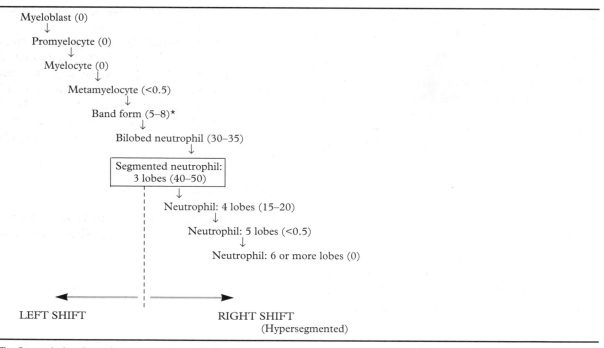

The figures in brackets give an approximate indication of the number per 100 neutrophils in a normal film. They are intended only as a rough guide.
*However, according to the United States Health and Nutrition Examination surveys, the normal band count is lower, *c* 0.5% of the neutrophils.[24]

to leucoerythroblastic anaemia or leukaemia (Fig. 7.80), although occasionally this extreme picture may be seen in very severe infections when it is called 'leukaemoid reaction'. A left shift, with a significant number of band forms, occurs normally in pregnancy.

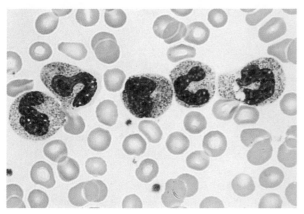

Fig. 7.79 Photomicrograph of a blood film. Infection. Shows left shift of the neutrophils, with toxic granulation.

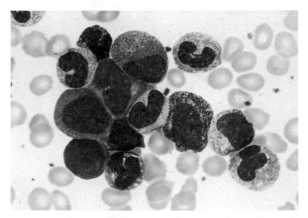

Fig. 7.80 Photomicrograph of a blood film. Chronic granulocytic leukaemia. There is a left shift with band forms, metamyelocytes, myelocytes and one myeloblast.

Hypersegmentation

The presence of hypersegmented neutrophils, with five or more nuclear segments, is an important diagnostic feature of megaloblastic anaemias. In florid megaloblastic states neutrophils are often enlarged and their nuclei may have six or more segments connected by particularly fine chromatin bridges (Fig. 7.81). A right shift with moderately hypersegmented neutrophils may be seen in uraemia and after cytotoxic treatment, especially with methotrexate. Patients undergoing hydroxyurea treatment develop markedly hypersegmented neutrophils.

Pelger cells

The Pelger–Huet anomaly is a benign inherited condition in which neutrophil nuclei fail to segment properly. The majority of circulating neutrophils have only two discrete equal-sized lobes connected by a thin chromatin bridge (Fig. 7.82). The chromatin is coarsely clumped and granular content is normal.

A similar acquired morphological anomaly, known as *Pseudo-Pelger cells* may be seen in myelodysplastic syndromes, acute myeloid leukaemia with dysplastic maturation and occasionally in chronic myeloid leukaemia (Fig. 7.83). In these conditions the neutrophils are often hypogranular and they tend to have markedly irregular nuclear pattern.

Pyknotic neutrophils

Small numbers of dead or dying cells may be found in the blood, especially when there is an

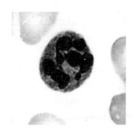

Fig. 7.81 Photomicrograph of a blood film. Pernicious anaemia. Shows a hypersegmented neutrophil.

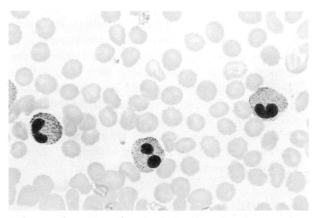

Fig. 7.82 Photomicrograph of a blood film. Pelger-Huet anomaly. Shows three 'Pelger' cells.

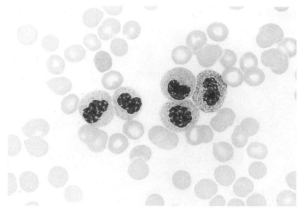

Fig. 7.83 Photomicrograph of a blood film. Chronic granulocytic leukaemia. There are five 'pseudo-Pelger' cells.

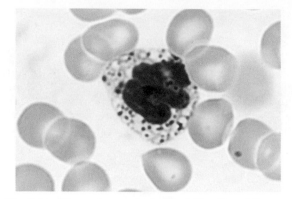

Fig. 7.84 Photomicrograph of a blood film. Basophil. (cf. Fig. 7.85.)

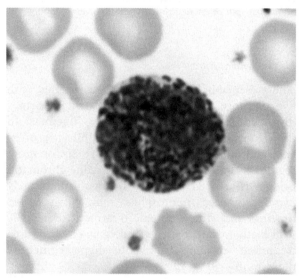

Fig. 7.85 Photomicrograph of a blood film. Alder-Reilly anomaly. The nucleus is obscured by the cytoplasmic granules.

infection. They may also occur in normal blood in-vitro after standing for 12–18 h, even if kept at 4°C. These cells have round, dense, featureless nuclei and their cytoplasm tends to be dark pink (see p. 5). It is important not to confuse these cells with normoblasts.

EOSINOPHILS

Eosinophils are a little larger than neutrophils; 12–17 μm in diameter. They usually have two nuclear lobes or segments, and the cytoplasm is packed with distinctive spherical gold/orange (eosinophilic) granules (Fig. 7.74). The underlying cytoplasm, which is usually obscured by the granules, is pale blue. Prolonged steroid administration causes eosinopenia. Moderate eosinophilia occurs in allergic conditions; more severe eosinophilia ($20–50 \times 10^9$/l) may be seen in parasitic infections, and even greater numbers in hyper-eosinophilia syndromes. These are generally of unknown aetiology, although a few cases have been shown to be associated with T-cell lymphomas, B-cell lymphomas and acute lymphoblastic leukaemias. If true eosinophilic leukaemia does exist it must be extremely rare, although eosinophils with abnormal granules are frequently found in some types of acute myeloid leukaemia, chronic myeloid leukaemia and myelodysplasia.

BASOPHILS

Basophils are the rarest (<1%) of the circulating leucocytes. Their nuclear segments tend to fold up on each other, resulting in a compact irregular dense nucleus resembling a closed lotus flower. The distinctive large, variably-sized blue-black granules of the cytoplasm (Fig. 7.84), often obscure the nucleus; they are rich in histamine, serotonin and heparin-like substances. Basophils tend to form cytoplasmic vacuoles and to degranulate.

Basophils are present in increased numbers in myeloproliferative disorders, and are especially prominent in chronic myeloid leukaemia; in the latter condition, when basophils are >10% of the differential leucocyte count, this is a sign of impending accelerated phase or blast crisis.

MONOCYTES

Monocytes are the largest of the circulating leu-cocytes; 15–18 μm in diameter. They have bluish-grey cytoplasm which contains variable numbers of fine reddish granules. The nucleus is large and curved, often in the shape of a horseshoe, but it may be folded or curled (Fig. 7.86). It never undergoes segmentation. The chromatin is finer and more evenly distributed in the nucleus than in neutrophils. An increased number of monocytes occur in some chronic infections and inflammatory conditions such as tuberculosis and Crohn's disease, in chronic myeloid leukaemia and in acute leukaemias with a monocytic component. In chronic myelomonocytic leukaemia the mature monocyte count may reach as high as $100 \times 10^9/l$. It is occasionally difficult to distinguish mono-cytes from the large activated T-lymphocytes produced in infectious mononucleosis (Fig. 7.87), or from circulating high-grade lymphoma cells.

LYMPHOCYTES

The majority of circulating lymphocytes are small cells with a thin rim of cytoplasm, occasionally containing scanty azurophil granules (Figs. 7.88 and 7.89). Nuclei are remarkably uniform in size (c 9 μm in diameter); This provides a useful guide for estimating red cell size (normally c 7–8 μm) on the blood film. Some 10% of circulating lym-phocytes are larger, with more abundant pale blue cytoplasm containing azurophil granules (Fig. 7.89). The nuclei of lymphocytes have homo-

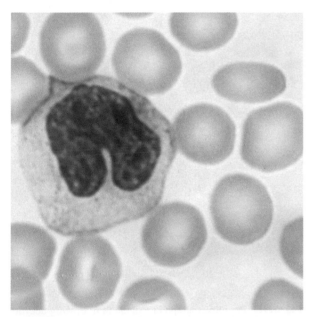

Fig. 7.86 Photomicrograph of a blood film. Healthy adult. Monocyte.

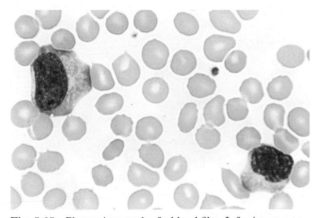

Fig. 7.87 Photomicrograph of a blood film. Infectious mononucleosis. There are two activated lymphocytes.

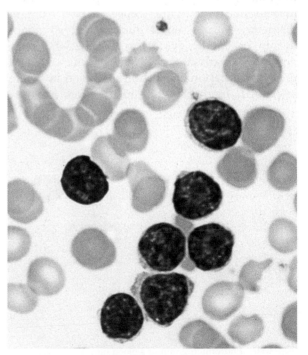

Fig. 7.88 Photomicrograph of a blood film. Chronic lymphocytic leukaemia. The cells are small lymphocytes.

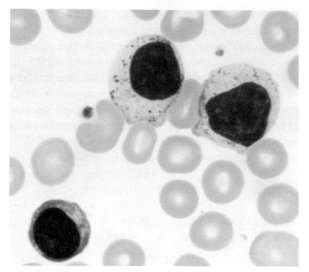

Fig. 7.89 Photomicrograph of a blood film. Shows two large granular lymphocytes with azurophil granules, and a small lymphocyte.

geneous chromatin with some clumping at the nuclear periphery. About 85% of the circulating lymphocytes are T-cells or natural killer (NK) cells.

In infections, both bacterial and viral, transforming lymphocytes may be present. These immunoblasts or 'Türk' cells are 10–15 μm in diameter, with a round nucleus and abundant deeply basophilic cytoplasm (Fig. 7.90). They develop into plasmacytoid and plasma cells and these are occasionally seen in the blood in severe infections. In the absence of infection, multiple

myeloma must be excluded. In viral infection 'reactive lymphocytes' appear in the blood. These have slightly larger nuclei with more open chromatin and abundant cytoplasm which may be irregular. The most extreme examples of these cells are usually found in infectious mononucleosis (Fig. 7.87). These 'glandular fever' cells have irregular nuclei and abundant cytoplasm which is basophilic at the periphery; they have a tendency to adhere to adjacent erythrocytes.

Malignant lymphoid cells vary enormously in their morphology. The commonest malignancy is

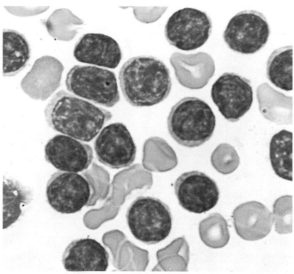

Fig. 7.91 Photomicrograph of a blood film. Prolymphocytic leukaemia. There is a uniform population of prolymphocytes.

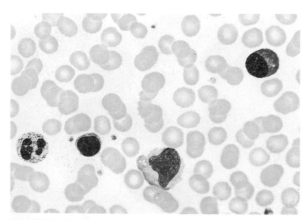

Fig. 7.90 Photomicrograph of a blood film. Viral infection. Shows a Türk cell and a reactive lymphocyte. Compare with Fig. 7.87.

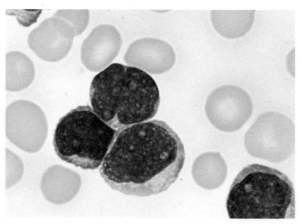

Fig. 7.92 Photomicrograph of a blood film. Acute lymphoblastic leukaemia. L1 type showing lymphoblasts.

chronic lymphocytic leukaemia, composed almost exclusively of small lymphocytes (Fig. 7.88), sometimes with a few larger nucleolated cells. In prolymphocytic leukaemia the majority of cells are a little larger than small lymphocytes with more cytoplasm and usually one distinct nucleolus (Fig. 7.91). Lymphoblasts vary in size from only slightly larger than lymphocytes to cells of 15–17 μm diameter. The nuclei have dense chromatin which is even more condensed in the smaller blasts, and the cytoplasm is deep blue (Fig. 7.92).

Circulating lymphoma cells vary markedly in size, depending on the type of lymphoma. When there is a lymphocytosis, the lymphocytes are usually far less uniform than in chronic lymphocytic leukaemia, and the lymphoma cells frequently have irregular lobed, indented or cleaved nuclei and relatively scanty agranular cytoplasm that varies in its basophilic staining. Lymphocytes with definite lobulation are likely to be an artefact which has developed in blood kept for 18–24 h at room temperature (see p. 5).

Lymphocytes predominate in the blood films of infants and young children. In these, large lymphocytes and reactive lymphocytes tend to be conspicuous, and a small number of lymphoblasts may also be present.

PLATELET MORPHOLOGY

Normal platelets are 1–3 μm in diameter. They are irregular in outline with fine red granules that may be scattered or centralized in the cell. A small number of larger platelets, up to 5 μm in diameter may be seen in normal films. Larger platelets are seen in the blood when platelet production is increased (Fig. 7.93). Thus, for example, in severe immune thrombocytopenia some large platelets will be seen on the film. Very high platelet counts, particularly when associated with myeloproliferative disorders, may show extreme platelet anisocytosis, with some platelets being as large as red cells (Fig. 7.94). These are possibly megakaryocyte cytoplasmic fragments. The platelet count frequently rises with acute inflammatory stress or bleeding, but seldom to more than 1000×10^9/l. Above this, the cause is usually a myeloproliferative disorder.

Characteristic morphological features are seen in two inherited platelet disorders associated with bleeding. These are the *Bernard–Soulier syndrome* in which there are giant platelets with defective ristocetin response, and *grey platelet syndrome* in which the platelets lack granules and have a ghost-like appearance on the stained blood film. Thrombocytopenia may develop in the May-

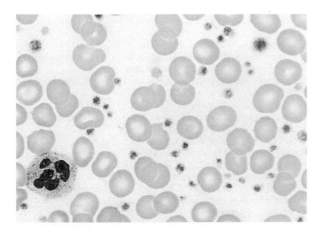

Fig. 7.93 Photomicrograph of a blood film. Essential thrombocythaemia. Shows platelet anisocytosis.

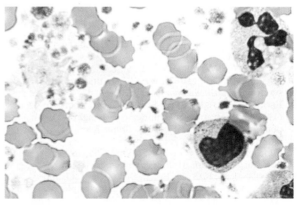

Fig. 7.94 Photomicrograph of a blood film. Myeloproliferative disorder. Shows platelet anisocytosis with some giant platelets.

Hegglin anomaly (see p. 121), where the platelets will appear large and reddish.

In about 1% of individuals EDTA anti-coagulant causes platelet clumping, resulting in pseudo-thrombocytopenia.[10] This phenomenon may be detected when a blood count is performed on a modern blood cell counter by flagging, or identified on the blood film. It is not associated with any coagulation disturbance and platelet function is normal. Occasionally, EDTA may also inhibit the staining of platelets.[22]

Occasionally, platelets may be seen adhering to neutrophils (Fig. 7.95).[4,9,11,21] This has been reported in patients who have demonstrable anti-platelet auto-antibodies,[26] but it is more commonly seen in apparently healthy individuals. It is not seen in films made directly from blood which has not been anticoagulated.

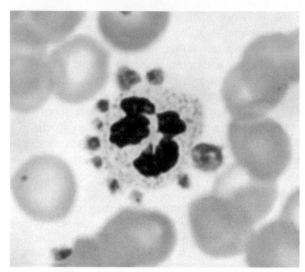

Fig. 7.95   Photomicrograph of a blood film. Idiopathic thrombocytopenic purpura. Shows adhesion of platelets to neutrophil.

REFERENCES

1 BENNETT, J. M., CATOVSKY, D., DANIEL, M. T., FLANDRIN, G., GALTON, D. A. G., GRALNICK, H. R. and SULTAN, C. (1976). Proposals for the classification of the acute leukaemias (FAB cooperative group). *British Journal of Haematology*, **33**, 451.

2 BESSIS, M. (1972). Red cell shapes. An illustrated classification and its rationale. *Nouvelle Revue Française d'Hématologie*, **12**, 721.

3 BRECHER, G. and BESSIS, M. (1972). Present status of spiculated red cells and their relationship to the discocyte-echinocyte transformation: a critical review. *Blood*, **40**, 333.

4 CROME, P. E. and BARKHAN, P. (1963). Platelet adherence to polymorphs. *British Medical Journal*, **ii**, 871.

5 DOUGLASS, C. and TWOMEY, J. (1970). Transient stomatocytosis with hemolysis: a previously unrecognized complication of alcoholism. *Annals of Internal Medicine*, **72**, 159.

6 DUCROU, W. and KIMBER, R. J. (1969). Stomatocytes, haemolytic anaemia and abdominal pain in Mediterranean migrants: some examples of a new syndrome? *Medical Journal of Australia*, **ii**, 1087.

7 ESTES, J. W., MORLEY, T. J., LEVINE, I. M. and EMMERSON, C. P. (1967). A new hereditary acanthocytosis syndrome. *American Journal of Medicine*, **42**, 868.

8 FEO, C. J., TCHERNIA, G., SUBTU, E. and LEBLOND, P. F. (1978). Observation of echinocytosis in eight patients: a phase contrast and SEM study. *British Journal of Haematology*, **40**, 519.

9 FIELD, E. J. and MACLEOD, I. (1963). Platelet adherence to polymorphs. *British Medical Journal*, **ii**, 388.

10 GOWLAND, E., KAY, H. E. M., SPILLMAN, J. C. and WILLIAMSON, J. R. (1969). Agglutination of platelets by a serum factor in the presence of EDTA. *Journal of Clinical Pathology*, **22**, 460.

11 GREIPP, P. R. and GRALNICK, H. R. (1976). Platelet to leucocyte adherence phenomena associated with thrombocytopenia. *Blood*, **47**, 513.

12 KEIMOWITZ, R. and DESFORGES, J. F. (1965). Infantile pyknocytosis. *New England Journal of Medicine*, **273**, 1152.

13 LOCK, S. P., SEPHTON SMITH, R. and HARDISTY, R. M. (1961). Stomatocytosis: a hereditary red cell anomaly associated with haemolytic anaemia. *British Journal of Haematology*, **7**, 303.

14 MARSH, G. W. (1966). Abnormal contraction, distortion and fragmentation in human red cells. London University MD Thesis.

15 MIER, M., SCHWARTZ, S. O. and BOSHES, B. (1960). Acanthrocytosis [*sic*], pigmented degeneration of the retina and ataxic neuropathy: a genetically determined syndrome with associated metabolic disorder. *Blood*, **16**, 1586.

16 NORMAN, J. G. (1969). Stomatocytosis in migrants of Mediterranean origin. *Medical Journal of Australia*, **i**, 315.

17 PONDER, E. (1948). *Hemolysis and Related Phenomena*. Grune & Stratton, New York.

18 SALT, H. B., WOLFE, O. H., LLOYD, J. K., FOSBROOKE, A. S., CAMERON, A. H. and HUBBLE, D. V. (1960). On having no beta-lipoprotein. A syndrome comprising a-beta-lipoprotinaemia, acanthocytosis, and steatorrhoea. *Lancet*, **ii**, 325.

19 SCHWARTZ, S. O and MOTTO, S. A. (1949). The diagnostic significance of 'Burr' red blood cells. *American Journal of Medical Sciences*, **218**, 563.

20 SILBER, R., AMOROSI, E. L., HOWE, J. and KAYDEN, H. J. (1966). Spur-shaped erythrocytes in Laennec's cirrhosis. *New England Journal of Medicine*, **275**, 639.

21 SKINNIDER, L. F., MUSCLOW, C. E. and KAHN, W. (1978). Platelet satellitism—an ultrastructural study. *American Journal of Hematology*, **4**, 179.

22 STAVEM, P. and BERG, K. (1973). A macromolecular serum component acting on platelets in the presence of EDTA—'Platelet stain preventing factor'. *Scandinavian Journal of Haematology*, **10**, 202.

[23] TUFFY, P., BROWN, A. K. and ZUELZER, W. W. (1959). Infantile pyknocytosis: a common erythrocyte abnormality of the first trimester. *American Journal of Diseases of Children*, **98,** 227.

[24] VAN ASSSENDELFT, O. W., McGRATH, C., MURPHY, R. S. and SCHMIDT, R. M. (1977). The differential distribution of leukocytes. In *CAP Aspen Conference: Differential Leukocyte Counting.* Ed. J. A. Koepke. College of American Pathologists, Northfield, IL.

[25] WEED, R. I. and BESSIS, M. (1973). The discocyte-stomatocyte equilibrium of normal and pathologic red cells. *Blood,* **41,** 471.

[26] WHITE, L. A., BRUBAKER, L. H., ASTER, R. H., HENRY, P. H. and ADELSTEIN, E. H. (1978). Platelet satellitism and phagocytosis by neutrophils: association with antiplatelet antibodies and lymphoma. *American Journal of Hematology*, **4,** 313.

[27] WINNER, B. M., MARSH, W. L., TASWEL, H. F. and GALEY, W. R. (1977). Haematological changes associated with the McLeod phenotype of the Kell blood group system. *British Journal of Haematology*, **36,** 219.

8. Red cell cytochemistry

Siderocytes and sideroblasts   131
Haemoglobin derivatives   134
  Heinz bodies   134
  Haemoglobin H   136
  Carboxyhaemoglobin   137
  Methaemoglobin   137

Fetal haemoglobin   137
Haemoglobin variants   138
Haemoglobin S   138
Periodic acid Schiff (PAS) reaction   138
Demonstration of G6PD deficiency   139

SIDEROCYTES AND SIDEROBLASTS

Siderocytes are red cells containing granules of non-haem iron; they were originally described by Grüneberg[11] in small numbers in the blood of normal rat, mouse and human embryos, and in large numbers in mice with a congenital anaemia. The granules are formed of a water-insoluble complex of ferric iron, lipid, protein and carbohydrate. This siderotic material (or haemosiderin) reacts with potassium ferrocyanide to form a blue coloured compound, ferriferrocyanide; this reaction is the basis of a positive Prussian blue (Perls's) test. The material also stains by Romanowsky dyes and then appears as basophilic granules which have been referred to as 'Pappenheimer bodies' (Fig. 8.1).[23] By contrast, ferritin, which is a water-soluble non-haem compound of iron with the protein apoferritin, is not detectable by Perls's reaction. Ferritin is normally present in all cells in the body, whereas haemosiderin is mainly found in monocyte-macrophage cells in the bone marrow, liver (Kupffer cells) and spleen, except when the body is overloaded with iron as in haemochromatosis or transfusional haemosiderosis.

Iron is transported in plasma attached to a β-globulin, transferrin, and passes selectively to the bone marrow where, at the surface of the erythroblast, the iron is released and enters the cell. Most of the iron is rapidly converted to haem in the mitochondria. The non-haem residue is in the form of ferritin. Degradation of the ferritin turns some of it into haemosiderin which can be stained by Perls's reaction and visualized under the light microscope as golden-yellow refractile particles in phagocytic cells.

In health, siderotic granules can normally be seen in preparations stained by Perls's reaction in the cytoplasm of many of the normoblasts of human bone marrow and in marrow reticulocytes.[16] However, they are not normally seen in human peripheral-blood red cells. After splenectomy, on the other hand, siderocytes can always be found in the peripheral blood, often in large numbers. The reason for this is probably because reticulocytes, after delivery from the marrow, are normally sequestered for a time in the spleen and there complete haem synthesis and utilize, for this purpose, the iron stored in their cytoplasm within the siderotic granules. After splenectomy, this stage of reticulocyte ripening has to take place in the blood stream, with the result that even in an otherwise healthy person a small percentage of siderocytes can then be found in the peripheral blood. The spleen is also probably

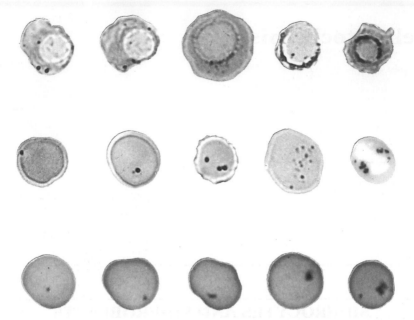

Fig. 8.1   Siderotic granules and 'Pappenheimer bodies'. Photomicrographs of normoblasts and red cells stained by the acid-ferrocyanide method to show siderotic granules (top two rows) and stained by Jenner-Giemsa's stain to demonstrate 'Pappenheimer bodies' (bottom row). ×1000.

able to remove large siderotic granules—as may be found in disease—from red cells by a process of pitting,[5] and in its absence such granules persist in the red cells throughout their life-span in the peripheral blood.

Method of staining siderotic granules

Air-dry films of peripheral blood or bone marrow and fix with methanol for 10–20 min. When dry, place the slides in a solution of 10 g/l potassium ferrocyanide in 0.1 mol/l HCl made by mixing equal volumes of 47 mmol/l (20 g/l) potassium ferrocyanide and 0.2 mol/l HCl immediately before use.

Leave the slides in the solution for about 10 min at *c* 20°C. Wash well in running tap water for 20 min, rinse thoroughly in distilled water and then counterstain with 1 g/l aqueous neutral red or eosin for 10–15 s. Care must be taken to avoid contamination by iron which may have been present on the slides or in staining dishes. Prepare the glassware by soaking in 2 mol/l HCl before washing (see p. 580). For quality control a positive bone marrow film should always be stained together with the test films.

Prussian-blue staining can be applied to films which have previously been stained by Romanowsky dyes, even after years of storage. It is advisable to let the films stand in methanol overnight to remove most of the Romanowsky stain. Sundberg and Bromann described a technique whereby films were stained first by a Romanowsky dye (Wright's stain) and then overstained by the acid-ferrocyanide method.[28] This can give beautiful pictures but the small bluestained iron-containing granules tend to be masked in young erythroblasts by the general basophilia of the cell cytoplasm. Hayhoe and Quaglino described a method for combined PAS and iron staining.[12] This may be helpful in the investigation of abnormal erythropoiesis where the erythroblasts give a positive PAS reaction (see p. 138). A rapid method has been described for demonstrating siderotic granules by staining with 1% bromochlorphenol blue for 1 min.[17] Iron-containing granules stain dark purple.

Significance of siderocytes

Siderocytes contain one or two (rarely many) small iron-containing unevenly distributed granules

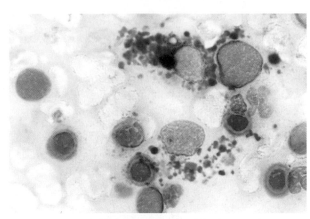

Fig. 8.2   Pathological sideroblasts. Thalassaemia.
There is massive accumulation of iron-containing granules in
normoblasts and phagocytic cells. Perls's acid-ferrocyanide
reaction. ×1000.

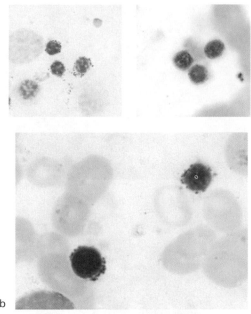

**Fig. 8.3   Pathological sideroblasts. Sideroblastic
anaemias.** Accumulation of iron-containing granules in
normoblasts, arranged characteristically around the nucleus.
(a) Hereditary type; (b) myelodysplastic syndrome. Perls's
acid-ferrocyanide reaction.

which stain a Prussian-blue colour. In about 40%
of polychromatic erythroblasts there are normally
a few very small scattered siderotic granules.[16]
They stain faintly and may be difficult to see by
light microscopy. The percentage of erythroblasts
recognizable as sideroblasts is increased in haemolytic anaemias and megaloblastic anaemias and in
haemochromatosis and haemosiderosis, in proportion to the degree of saturation of transferrin,
i.e. to the amount of iron available. A disproportionate increase in the percentage of erythroblasts that are sideroblasts occurs when the
synthesis of Hb is impaired, in which case the
granules in the sideroblasts are both more numerous and larger than normal. (Fig. 8.2). When
there is a defect in haem synthesis, the granules
are deposited in mitochondria and frequently appear to be arranged in a collar around the nucleus
(Fig. 8.3) giving the 'ring sideroblasts' characteristic
of sideroblastic anaemias. In contrast, the distribution of the granules within the cell tends to be
normal in conditions in which globin synthesis
alone is affected, e.g. in thalassaemia, or when
there is iron overload.

There are several types of sideroblastic
anaemia. These include the primary acquired and
congenital (hereditary) types. Pyridoxine
(vitamin B_6) deficiency also gives rise to a
sideroblastic anaemia, and B_6 antagonists, e.g.
drugs used in anti-tuberculosis therapy, produce
the same effect. Secondary sideroblastic anaemia

can also occur in alcoholism, lead poisoning and
occasionally in rheumatoid arthritis and other
'medical' diseases. Ring sideroblasts are not
uncommonly seen in primary haematological
disorders, notably myelosclerosis, acute myeloid
leukaemias and erythroleukaemia; they are also a
feature of the myelodysplastic syndromes, and
myelodysplastic marrows may contain 15% or
more sideroblasts.[1]

In the primary acquired type, erythroblasts at
all stages of maturity may be loaded with siderotic
granules; whereas in some of the secondary
sideroblastic anaemias and in the hereditary types
the more mature cells seem most affected.

In addition to the siderotic granules within
erythroblasts, haemosiderin can normally be seen
in marrow films as accumulations of small
granules, lying free or in phagocytes in marrow
fragments.[25] The amount of haemosiderin will be
markedly increased in patients with large iron
stores, and reduced or absent in iron-deficiency
anaemias (Fig. 8.4). In infections the iron stores
may be increased, with much siderotic material
in phagocytes but little or none visible in ery-

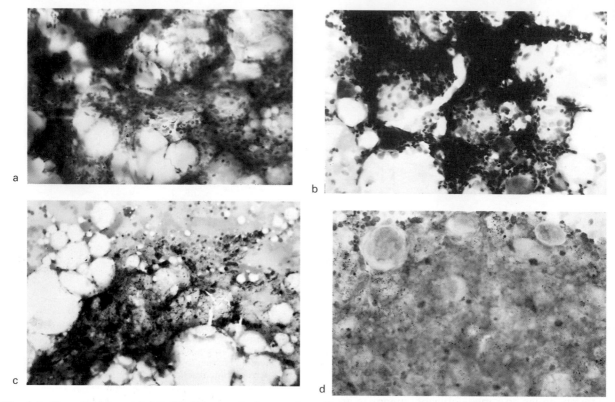

Fig. 8.4   Prussian blue staining (Perls's reaction) on aspirated bone marrow particles to demonstrate iron stores. (a) Normal, (b) absent, (c) increased, (d) grossly increased.

throblasts. Markedly excessive iron in phagocytes is also a feature of some dyserythropoietic anaemias. Conversely, absence of iron is diagnostic of iron deficiency and may be found before anaemia becomes evident. In practice, staining to demonstrate iron stores in marrow fragments and siderotic granules in erythroblasts is a simple and valuable diagnostic procedure and should be applied to marrow films as a routine.

There is no cytochemical method of demonstrating ferritin. Methods of assay are described in Chapter 23.

HAEMOGLOBIN DERIVATIVES

HEINZ BODIES IN RED CELLS

Heinz, in 1890, was the first to describe in detail inclusions in red cells developing as the result of the action of acetylphenylhydrazine on the blood.[14] Now it is known that 'Heinz' bodies can be produced by the action on red cells of a wide range of aromatic nitro- and amino-compounds, as well as by inorganic oxidizing agents such as potassium chlorate. They also occur when one or other of the globin chains of haemoglobin is unstable. In man, the finding of Heinz bodies is a sign of either chemical poisoning, drug intoxication, G6PD deficiency or the presence of an unstable haemoglobin, e.g. Hb Köln. When of chemical or drug origin, Heinz bodies are likely to be visible in red cells only if the patient has been splenectomized previously or when massive doses of the chemical or drug have been taken. When due to an unstable haemoglobin they seem never to be visible in freshly withdrawn red cells except after splenectomy. They nevertheless develop in vitro when pre-splenectomy blood is incubated for 24–48 h.[6]

Heinz bodies are a late sign of oxidative damage, and represent an end-product of the degradation of Hb. Reviews dealing with Heinz bodies include those by Jacob[15] and by White.[36]

DEMONSTRATION OF HEINZ BODIES

Unstained preparations

Heinz bodies may be seen as refractile objects in dry unstained films, if the illumination is cut down by lowering the microscope condenser, and they can be seen by dark-ground illumination or phase-contrast microscopy. However, it is preferable to look for them in stained preparations (see below). In size they vary from 1 to 3 μm. One or more may be present in a single cell. They are usually close to the cell membrane, and in wet preparations may move around within the cells in a slow Brownian movement.

The degradation product of an unstable haemoglobin, e.g. Hb Köln, exhibits green fluorescence when excited by blue light at 370 nm in a fluorescence microscope.[7]

Stained preparations

Methyl violet stains the bodies excellently.

Dissolve c 0.5 g of methyl violet in 100 ml of 9 g/l NaCl and filter. Add 1 volume of blood (in any anticoagulant) to 4 volumes of the methyl violet solution and allow the suspension to stand for c 10 min at c 20°C. Then prepare films and allow them to dry or view the suspension of cells between slide and cover-glass. The Heinz bodies stain an intense purple (Figs. 8.5 and 8.6).

Heinz bodies also stain with other basic dyes. Brilliant green stains them well and none of the stain is taken up by the remainder of the red cell.[26] Rhodanile blue (5 g/l solution in 10 g/l NaCl) stains them rapidly,[27] i.e. within 2 min, at which time reticulocytes are only weakly stained. Compared with methyl violet, Heinz bodies stain less intensely with brilliant cresyl blue or New methylene blue. Nevertheless, they may be readily

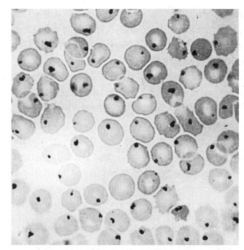

Fig. 8.5 Unstable haemoglobin disease. Hb Köln (after splenectomy). Many of the cells contain large Heinz bodies. Stained supravitally by methyl violet. ×700.

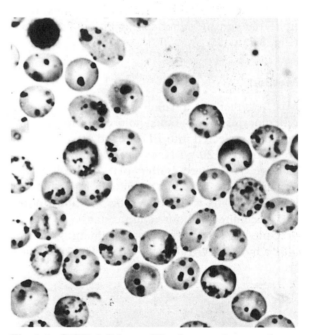

Fig. 8.6 G6PD deficiency. Blood exposed to acetyl phenylhydrazine. The majority of the cells contain several Heinz bodies. Stained supravitally by methyl violet. Reproduced by kind permission from E. Beutler, R. J. Dern and A. S. Alving (1955). The hemolytic effects of primaquine. VI. An in vitro test for sensitivity of erythrocytes to primaquine. *Journal of Laboratory and Clinical Medicine*, **45**, 40.

seen as pale blue bodies in a well-stained reticulocyte preparation, if the preparation is not counterstained.

If permanent preparations are required, fix the vitally stained films by exposure to formalin vapour for 5–10 min. Then counterstain the fixed films with 1 g/l eosin or neutral red, after thoroughly washing in water. If films are fixed in methanol, the bodies are decolourized.

In β-thalassaemia major, methyl violet staining of the bone marrow will demonstrate precipitated α-chains. These appear as large irregular inclusions in late normoblasts, usually single and closely adhering to the nucleus. If such patients are splenectomized, inclusions are also found in reticulocytes and mature red blood cells.

DEMONSTRATION OF HAEMOGLOBIN H

Patients with α-thalassaemia, who form Hb H (β_4), have red cells in which on exposure to brilliant cresyl blue, as in reticulocyte preparations, multiple blue-green spherical inclusions develop[10] (Fig. 8.7).

Method

Mix together in a small tube as for staining reticulocytes (p. 66) equal volumes of fresh blood or blood collected into EDTA and 10 g/l brilliant cresyl blue or 20 g/l New methylene blue in iso-osmotic phosphate buffer pH 7.4. Leave the preparation at 37°C for 1–3 h, and make films at intervals during this time. Allow the films to dry and examine without counterstaining. Hb H precipitates as multiple pale-staining greenish-blue almost spherical bodies of varying size which

can be clearly differentiated from the darker-staining reticulo-filamentous material of reticulocytes (Fig. 8.8 and Fig. 8.9).

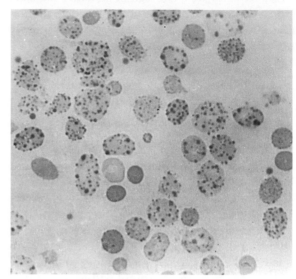

Fig. 8.8   Hb H disease. Almost every erythrocyte is affected. ×900. Compare with Fig. 8.9.

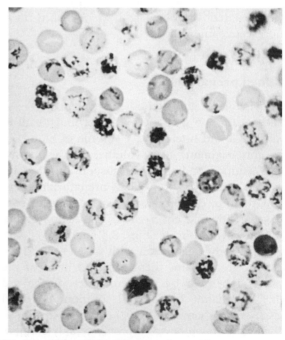

Fig. 8.9   Film of blood from patient with pyruvate kinase deficiency. Postsplenectomy. Almost every erythrocyte is a reticulocyte. Stained supravitally by brilliant cresyl blue. Compare with Fig. 8.8.

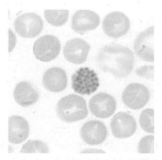

Fig. 8.7   Denaturation of Hb H by brilliant cresyl blue. The round bodies consist of precipitated Hb H. ×900.

The number of cells containing inclusions varies according to the type of α-thalassaemia. In α-thalassaemia-1 trait only 0.01–1% of the red cells contain inclusions, but this finding provides a significant clue to diagnosis. In Hb-H disease (α-thalassaemia-1/α-thalassaemia-2), as a rule at least 10% of the cells develop inclusions and, in some cases, the percentage is considerably greater.

When few cells are affected they will be easier to detect in an enriched preparation.[20] Fill 2–3 capillary tubes with the blood and centrifuge for 5 min in a microhaematocrit centrifuge. Then score the tubes just below the buffy coat layer and also c 1 cm further down; break them at the score marks and transfer the blood from the broken-off segments into a small tube. Add one drop of stain and incubate at 37°C for 3 h before making a film.

CARBOXYHAEMOGLOBIN

HbCO can be demonstrated in the red cells in a blood film. The method is a modification of the methaemoglobin (Hi) elution technique described on p. 139.[2,3] It is based on the fact that HbO_2 is oxidized by nitrite to Hi whereas HbCO is not. The method has, however, only limited practical value.

METHAEMOGLOBIN (Hi)

The peroxidatic capacity of Hi, but not of HbO_2 is reduced by cyanide. The peroxidatic activity prevents elution of haemoglobin by citric acid in the presence of hydrogen peroxide. Thus, normal red cells containing HbO_2 will remain intact and take up a counterstain whereas cells containing Hi will appear as ghosts when subjected to elution. Based on this principle, Kleihauer and Betke devised a simple method for demonstrating Hi in red cells in blood films.[18]

FETAL HAEMOGLOBIN

An acid-elution cytochemical method was introduced by Kleihauer et al in 1957.[19] It is a sensitive procedure which identifies individual cells containing Hb F even when few are present, and their detection in the maternal circulation has provided valuable information on the pathogenesis of haemolytic disease of the newborn.

The identification of cells containing Hb F depends upon the fact that they resist acid-elution to a greater extent than do normal cells; thus, in the technique described below, they appear as isolated darkly-stained cells amongst a background of palely-staining ghost-cells. The occasional cells which stain to an intermediate degree are less easy to evaluate; some may be reticulocytes as these also resist acid-elution to some extent. The following method in which elution is carried out at pH 1.5 is recommended.[21]

Reagents

Fixative. 80% ethanol.

Elution solution. Solution A: 7.5 g/l haèmatoxylin in 90% ethanol. Solution B: $FeCl_3$, 24 g; 2.5 mol/l HCl, 20 ml; doubly-distilled water to 1 litre.

For use, mix well 5 volumes of A and 1 volume of B. The pH is approximately 1.5. The solution can be used for c 4 weeks: if a precipitate forms, the solution should be filtered.

Counterstain. 1 g/l aqueous erythrosin or 2.5 g/l aqueous eosin.

Method

Prepare fresh air-dried films. Immediately after drying, fix the films for 5 min in 80% ethanol in a Coplin jar. Then rinse the slides rapidly in water and stand vertically on blotting paper for about 10 min to dry. Next, place the slides for 20 s in a Coplin jar containing the elution solution. Rinse in tap-water and allow them to dry in the air. Fetal cells stain red and adult ghost-cells stain pale pink (Fig. 8.10). Films prepared from cord blood and from normal adult blood should be stained alongside the test films as positive and negative controls, respectively.

A number of modifications of the Kleihauer method have been proposed. In one, New methylene blue is incorporated in the buffer solution, the reaction time is prolonged and buffer is used for washing the films.[4] The advantage of this technique is that reticulocytes stain blue, whilst cells containing Hb F stain pink.

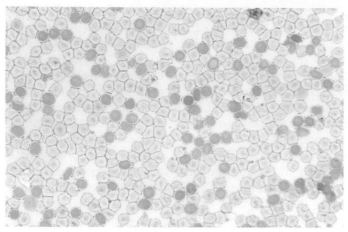

Fig. 8.10   Cytochemical demonstration of fetal haemoglobin.
Acid elution method. The preparation consists of a mixture of cord and
normal adult blood. The darkly staining cells are fetal cells. ×700.

An immunofluorescent staining method has been developed based on the use of a specific antibody against Hb F which does not react with Hb A.[31] By using a double-labelling procedure with rhodamine-labelled antibody against γ-globin and a fluorescein-labelled antibody against β-globin, it is possible to detect the presence of Hb F and Hb A in the same cell.[30]

A sensitive immunochemical method has been described for detecting maternal red cells in the fetal circulation;[35] the preparation is labelled sequentially with Rh immunoglobulin, rabbit anti-human IgG and goat anti-rabbit IgG conjugated to alkaline phosphatase, and is then stained as described.

Hb S AND OTHER HAEMOGLOBIN VARIANTS

Immunodiffusion with specific antibody has been used for the identification of Hb S, Hb A_2 and Hb F in red cells.[13,22] An alternative method is by fluorescent microscopy (flow cytometry) after labelling the cells with fluorescein isothiocyanate (FITC).[13] By a double-labelling method similar to that described above it is possible to identify Hb S as well as another haemoglobin in individual cells.

PERIODIC–ACID–SCHIFF (PAS) REACTION

The PAS reaction is used mainly for leucocyte cytochemistry. The method is described on p. 148. Mature red cells and the cytoplasm of normoblasts at any stage of development do not normally stain.

Erythroblasts may, however, react positively in disease. Deep diffuse staining has been observed in erythroleukaemia[24] and lesser degrees of staining may be seen in thalassaemia, iron-de-ficiency anaemia, cord-blood erythroblasts, sideroblastic anaemia, myelosclerosis, various types of leukaemia and in various types of haemolytic anaemia. Positive reactions have also been recorded in pernicious anaemia, aplastic anaemia, lead poisoning and polycythaemia vera. In acute myeloid leukaemia PAS-positive erythroid precursors have been associated with decreased remission rate.[29]

CYTOCHEMICAL TESTS FOR DEMONSTRATING DEFECTS OF RED CELL METABOLISM

Chemical tests for the recognition of defects of red cell metabolism are described in Chapter 13. Cytochemical methods have been developed by means of which some of these defects can be demonstrated in individual cells. Thus tests have been described for demonstrating red cells deficient in glucose-6-phosphate dehydrogenase (G6PD).[8,9,32] The principle on which the methods are based is that red cells are treated with sodium nitrite to convert their oxyhaemoglobin (HbO$_2$) to methaemoglobin (Hi). In the presence of G6PD, Hi reconverts to HbO$_2$, but in G6PD deficiency Hi persists. The blood is then incubated with a soluble tetrazolium compound (MTT) which will be reduced by HbO$_2$ (but not by Hi) to an insoluble formazan form.[18] Alternatively, the presence of Hi can be demonstrated by converting it to HiCN with potassium cyanide and then adding hydrogen peroxide which elutes HiCN but not HbO$_2$.[9] The cells are then stained, e.g. with eosin, and the HbO$_2$ containing cells can be readily distinguished from unstained ghosts, which had contained the Hi and which do not stain.

Attempts have been made to improve the reliability of the test for detecting heterozygotes, e.g. by controlled slight fixation of the red cells and accelerating the reaction with an exogenous electron carrier (1-methoxyphenazine methosulphate).[33] These cytochemical procedures are not more sensitive in the demonstration of G6PD deficiency than are the simple screening tests described on p. 225. They may, however, be useful in genetic studies and when assessing G6PD activity in women;[34] they may be the only way to detect deficiency in the heterozygous state. The method described below is satisfactory.

DEMONSTRATION OF G6PD DEFICIENCY

Reagents

Sodium nitrite. 0.18 mol/l (12.5 g/l). The solution must be stored in a dark bottle and made up monthly.

Incubation medium. 9 g/l NaCl, 4 ml; 50 g/l glucose, 1.0 ml; 0.3 mol/l phosphate buffer pH 7.0, 2.0 ml; 0.11 g/l Nile blue sulphate, 1.0 ml; water, 2.0 ml.

MTT tetrazolium. 5 g/l of 3-(4,5-dimethyl-thiazolyl-1-2)-2,5-diphenyltetrazolium bromide in 9 g/l NaCl.

Hypotonic saline. 6 g/l NaCl.

Method[8]

Venous blood collected into ACD should be used. The test should be carried out within 8 h of collection and the blood should be kept at 4°C until it is tested. Centrifuge the blood at 4°C for 20 min at 1200–1500g. Discard the supernatant and add 0.5 ml of the packed red cells to 9 ml of 9 g/l NaCl and 0.5 ml of sodium nitrite solution contained in a 15 ml glass centrifuge tube. Incubate at 37°C for 20 min. Centrifuge at 4°C for 15 min at c 500g, then discard the supernatant fluid without disturbing the buffy coat and uppermost layer of red cells. Wash the cells three times in cold saline. After the last washing remove the buffy coat, mix the packed cells well and transfer 50 μl to a glass tube containing 1 ml of the incubation medium. Incubate the suspension undisturbed at 37°C for 30 min. Then add

Fig. 8.11   Cytochemical demonstration of G6PD. Normal blood; positive reaction with formazan granules in the red cells.

0.2 ml of MTT solution, shake gently and incubate at 37°C for 1 h. Resuspend the cells thoroughly. Place one drop adjacent to one drop of hypotonic saline on a glass slide, mix the drops thoroughly and cover with a cover-glass.

Examine the red cells with an oil-immersion objective, noting the presence of formazan granules (Fig. 8.11).

Interpretation

When G6PD activity is normal all the red cells are stained. In G6PD hemizygotes the majority of the red cells are unstained. In heterozygotes mosaicism is usually easily seen, a proportion of cells behaving as normal and the remainder being devoid or almost devoid of stainable material.

REFERENCES

[1] BENNETT, J. M. (1986). Classification of the myelodysplastic syndromes. *Clinics in Haematology*, **15**, 909.

[2] BETHLENFALVAY, N. C. (1971). Cytologic demonstration of carboxyhemoglobin: clinical and in vitro studies in man. *Journal of Laboratory and Clinical Medicine*, **77**, 543.

[3] BETKE, K. and KLEIHAUER, E. (1967). Cytological demonstration of carboxyhaemoglobin in human erythrocytes. *Nature (London)*, **214**, 188.

[4] CLAYTON, E. M., FELHAUS, W. D. and PHYTHYON, J. M. (1963). The demonstration of fetal erythrocytes in the presence of adult red blood cells. *American Journal of Clinical Pathology*, **40**, 487.

[5] CROSBY, W. H. (1957). Siderocytes and the spleen. *Blood*, **12**, 165.

[6] DACIE, J. V., GRIMES, A. J., MEISLER, A., STEINGOLD, L., HEMSTED, E. H., BEAVEN, G. H. and WHITE, J. C. (1964). Hereditary Heinz-body anaemia. A report of studies on five patients with mild anaemia. *British Journal of Haematology*, **10**, 388.

[7] EISENGER, J., FLORES, J., TYSON, J. A. and SHOHET, S. B., (1985). Fluorescent cytoplasm and Heinz bodies of hemoglobin Köln erythrocytes: evidence for intracellular heme catabolism. *Blood*, **65**, 886.

[8] FAIRBANKS, V. F. and LAMPE, L. T. (1968). A tetrazolium-linked cytochemical method for estimation of glucose-6-phosphate dehydrogenase activity in individual erythrocytes: applications in the study of heterozygotes for glucose-6-phosphate dehydrogenase deficiency. *Blood*, **31**, 589.

[9] GALL, J. C., BREWER, G. J. and DERN, R. J. (1965). Studies of glucose-6-phosphate dehydrogenase activity of individual erythrocytes: the methaemoglobin-elution test for identification of females heterozygous for G6PD deficiency. *American Journal of Human Genetics*, **17**, 359.

[10] GOUTTAS, A., FESSAS, Ph., TSEVRENIS, H. and XEFTERI, E. (1955). Description d'une nouvelle variété d'anémie hémolytique congénitale, *Sang*, **26**, 911.

[11] GRÜNEBERG, H. (1941). Siderocytes: a new kind of erythrocytes. *Nature (London)*, **148**, 469.

[12] HAYHOE, F. G. J. and QUAGLINO, D. (1960). Refractory sideroblastic anaemia and erythraemic myelosis: possible relationship and cytochemical observations. *British Journal of Haematology*, **6**, 381.

[13] HEADINGS, V., BHATTACHARYA, S., SHUKLA, S., ANYAIBE, S., EASTON, L., CALVERT, A. and SCOTT, R. (1975). Identification of specific hemoglobins within individual erythrocytes. *Blood*, **45**, 263.

[14] HEINZ, R. (1890). Morphologische Veränderungen der rother Blutkörperchen durche Gifte. *Virchows Archiv*, **122**, 112.

[15] JACOB, H. S. (1970). Mechanisms of Heinz body formation and attachment to red cell membrane. *Seminars in Hematology*, **7**, 341.

[16] KAPLAN, E., ZUELZER, W. W. and MOURIQUAND, C. (1954). Sideroblasts. A study of stainable nonhemoglobin iron in marrow normoblasts. *Blood*, **9**, 203.

[17] KASS, L. and EICKHOLT, M. M. (1978). Rapid detection of ringed sideroblasts with bromchlorphenol blue. *American Journal of Clinical Pathology*, **70**, 738.

[18] KLEIHAUER, E. and BETKE, K. (1963). Elution procedure for the demonstration of methaemoglobin in red cells of human blood smears. *Nature (London)*, **199**, 1196.

[19] KLEIHAUER, E., BRAUN, H. and BETKE, K. (1957). Demonstration von fetalem Hämoglobin in den Erythrocyten eines Blutausstrichs. *Klinische Wochenschrift*, **35**, 637.

[20] LIN, C. K., GAU, J. P., HSU, H. C. and JIANG, M. L. (1990). Efficacy of a modified technique for detecting red cell haemoglobin H inclusions. *Clinical and Laboratory Haematology*, **12**, 409.

[21] NIERHAUS, K. and BETKE, K. (1968). Eine vereinfachte Modifikation der säuren Elution für die cytologische Darstellung von fetalem Hämoglobin. *Klinische Wochenschrift*, **46**, 47.

[22] PAPAYANNOPOULOU, Th., McGUIRE, T. C., LIM, G., GARZEL, E., NUTE, P. E. and STAMATOYANNOPOULOS, G. (1976). Identification of haemoglobin S in red cells and normoblasts, using fluorescent anti-Hb antibodies. *British Journal of Haematology*, **34**, 25.

[23] PAPPENHEIMER, A. M., THOMPSON, K. P., PARKER, D. D. and SMITH, K. E. (1945). Anaemia associated with unidentified erythrocytic inclusions after splenectomy. *Quarterly Journal of Medicine*, **14**, 75.

[24] QUAGLINO, D. and HAYHOE, F. G. J. (1960). Periodic-acid-Schiff positivity in erythroblasts with special reference to Di Guglielmo's disease. *British Journal of Haematology*, **6**, 26.

[25] RATH, C. E. and FINCH, C. A. (1948). Sternal marrow hemosiderin: a method for the determination of available iron stores in man. *Journal of Laboratory and Clinical Medicine*, **33**, 81.

[26] SCHWAB, M. L. L. and LEWIS, A. E. (1969). An improved stain for Heinz bodies. *American Journal of Clinical Pathology*, **51**, 673.

[27] SIMPSON, C. F., CARLISLE, J. W. and MALLARD, L. (1970). Rhodanile blue: a rapid and selective stain for Heinz bodies. *Stain Technology*, **45**, 221.

[28] SUNDBERG, R. D. and BROMANN, H. (1955). The application of the Prussian blue stain to previously stained films of blood and bone marrow. *Blood*, **10**, 160.

[29] SWIRSKY, D. M., DEBASTOS, M., PARISH, S. E.,

REES, J. K. H. and HAYHOE, F. G. J. (1986). Features affecting outcome during remission induction of acute myeloid leukaemia in 619 adult patients. *British Journal of Haematology*, **64**, 435.

[30] THORPE, S. J. and HUEHNS, E. G. (1983). A new approach for the antenatal diagnosis of β-thalassaemia: a double labelling immunofluorescence microscopy technique. *British Journal of Haematology*, **53**, 103.

[31] TOMODA, Y. (1964). Demonstration of foetal erythrocytes by immunofluorescent staining. *Nature (London)*, **202**, 910.

[32] TÖNZ, O. and ROSSI, E. (1964). Morphological demonstration of two red cell populations in human females heterozygous for glucose-6-phosphate dehydrogenase deficiency. *Nature (London)*, **202**, 606.

[33] VAN NOORDEN, C. J. F. and VOGELS, I. M. C. (1985). A sensitive cytochemical staining method for glucose-6-phosphate dehydrogenase activity in individual erythrocytes. *British Journal of Haematology*, **60**, 57.

[34] VOGELS, I. M. C., VAN NOORDEN, C. J. F., WOLF, B. H. M., SAELMAN, D. E. M., TROMP, A., SCHUTGENS, R. B. H. and WEENING, R. S. (1986). Cytochemical determination of heterozygous glucose-6-phosphate dehydrogenase deficiency in erythrocytes. *British Journal of Haematology*, **63**, 402.

[35] WANG, XIN-HUA and ZIPURSKY, A. (1987). Maternal erythrocytes in the fetal circulation: the immuno-cytochemical identification of minor populations of erythrocytes. *American Journal of Clinical Pathology*, **88**, 346.

[36] WHITE, J. M. (1976). The unstable haemoglobins. *British Medical Bulletin*, **32**, 219.

9. Leucocyte cytochemical and immunological techniques

By D. Catovsky

Cytochemical tests   143
Myeloperoxidase reaction   144
  Diaminobenzidene (DAB) method   144
  Fluorenediamine (FDA) method   144
Sudan Black B staining   145
Neutrophil alkaline phosphatase   146
Periodic acid-Schiff (PAS) reaction   148
Acid phosphatase reaction   149
α-naphthol acetate esterase (ANAE)   151
Naphthol AS (or AS-D) acetate esterase   153
Chloracetate esterase   153
Other acid hydrolases   154
Lysozyme activity   154
Practical value of cytochemical reactions   154
Differential diagnosis of acute leukaemias; FAB
  classification   154
  AML   155
  ALL   156
  Chronic myeloproliferative disorders   157

Myelodysplastic syndromes   157
Characterization of chronic lymphoproliferative
  disorders   158
Cell markers   159
Rosette tests   160
Immunofluorescent demonstration of surface
  immunoglobulins   161
Terminal transferase (TdT)   162
  Slide assay   162
Monoclonal antibodies   163
  Cell suspensions   165
  Fixed cells   167
Immunological classification of leukaemia   167
  ALL   167
  T-cell leukaemias   168
  B-cell leukaemias   168
  AML   168
Chromosomes   168
Nuclear sexing of leucocytes   170

CYTOCHEMICAL TESTS

Cytochemical tests applied to haemopoietic cells allow the demonstration of specific enzymes or other substances in individual cells. They are particularly useful for the study of immature cells (e.g. blasts) and lymphocytes because conventional morphology, as seen in Romanowsky-stained films, is not sufficient to identify differentiation features. Most tests are applied to the diagnosis and classification of leukaemia:

1. In distinguishing the patterns of differentiation of early granulocytic and early monocytic cells in the acute leukaemias and in recognizing some types of acute lymphoblastic leukaemia (ALL).

2. In characterizing the cells in chronic lymphoid leukaemias, and, to some extent, in normal lymphocyte subsets.

3. In distinguishing leucocytoses and leukaemoid reactions from genuine myeloproliferative disorders.

4. In studying abnormalities and/or enzyme deficiencies of neutrophils, for example, in the myelodysplastic syndromes.[8]

In special cases, methods of ultrastructural cytochemistry need to be applied, as the resolution of light microscopy may not suffice to demonstrate the localization of the reaction product. One such example is the platelet peroxidase reaction demonstrable in the endoplasmic reticulum and nuclear membrane of mature and immature cells of the megakaryocytic series.[1,14] A number of techniques for enzyme histochemistry can now also be applied to semi-thin sections of plastic-embedded bone-marrow trephine biopsies.

THE MYELOPEROXIDASE REACTION

Myeloperoxidase is a lysosomal enzyme localized in the azurophil granules of neutrophils and monocytes.[3,59] Azurophil granules in granulocytic cells correspond to the relatively large electron-dense (primary) granules seen under the electron microscope.[3,60] The secondary (specific) granules are less electron dense and appear at the myelocyte stage.[3,14] In the monocytic series the azurophil granules are smaller[73] and are not the first to appear during maturation in these cells. Thus the designation primary for them is not appropriate. The lysosomal granules present in early monocytic cells (monoblasts) are very small and have acid phosphatase but lack peroxidase activity.[60]

Myeloperoxidase can also be demonstrated in the specific granules of eosinophils and basophils. In eosinophils the specific granules are not newly formed but derive from primary granules which are also myeloperoxidase positive. The eosinophil peroxidase has been shown by chemical, cyto-chemical and immunological methods to be different from that of neutrophils. The enzyme in eosinophils is cyanide-resistant and, in neutrophils, cyanide-sensitive.[81]

Most of the early methods for the demonstration of peroxidase use benzidine and hydrogen peroxide. The method of Kaplow[47] described in previous editions of this book uses benzidine dihydrochloride, a less carcinogenic compound. As there are difficulties, in some countries, in the use of methods which include benzidine, alternative and probably safer substrates should be considered. These are 3-amino-9-ethyl carbazole, o-tolidine,[38] 2,7-fluorenediamine (FDA)[5] and 3,3'-diaminobenzidine (DAB) tetrahydrochloride.[36]

DAB is the substrate of choice for ultrastructural studies because its oxidized product is electron-dense and can be intensified by post-fixation with osmium tetroxide.[14] DAB is also frequently used to visualize the immunoperoxidase reaction.[14] Hanker et al[36] described a method using DAB that we have found reliable in the diagnosis of acute myeloid leukaemia (AML). This method, as well as one with the alternative substrate (FDA), will be described here.

METHOD WITH DAB

Fixative. A mixture of 1.25% glutaraldehyde and 1% formaldehyde in 0.1 mol/l phosphate buffer (pH 7.3). Mix 50 ml of a 25% solution of glutaraldehyde, 27.8 ml of a 36% solution of formaldehyde and add the buffer up to 1 litre.

Incubation mixture. DAB, 5 mg; tris-HCl buffer, 50 mmol/l, pH 7.6, 10 ml; H_2O_2, 30% (w/v), 0.1 ml. Add the reagents in this order and mix well after each addition. This medium should be prepared just before use.

Enhancer. Dissolve copper sulphate ($CuSO_4$), 0.5 g or copper nitrate ($Cu(NO_3)_2.3H_2O$), 0.5 g in 100 ml of tris-HCl buffer, 50 mmol/l, pH 7.6.

Counterstain. Dissolve 10 g of Giemsa's stain in 100 ml of 66 mmol/l phosphate buffer, pH 6.4.

Method

Fix peripheral-blood or bone-marrow films for 1 min and then rinse in 9 g/l NaCl (saline). Immerse the slides in the incubation mixture for 1 min in a Coplin jar at room temperature (20–25°C). Rinse briefly in tris-HCl buffer (three changes) and then immerse the slides in the reaction enhancer. Rinse in saline and keep in the saline until counterstained. Counterstain for 10 min, dry and mount in DPX (Merck.)

METHOD WITH 2,7-FDA[7]

Fixative. 10% formal-ethanol solution: 9 volumes of 95% ethanol and 1 volume of 40% formaldehyde.

Incubation mixture. Dissolve 40 mg of 2,7-FDA in 40 ml of tris-HCl buffer (pH 8.6) in order to obtain a saturated solution. Stir vigorously for 5 min at room temperature and then filter to remove excess of precipitated substrate. The solution (without H_2O_2) is stable for at least 6 weeks at room temperature. Add just before use 2 drops of 30% H_2O_2 to clear filtrate.

Giemsa counterstain. 10 g of Giemsa stain in 66 mmol/l phosphate buffer (as above).

Method

Fix films for 1 min and rinse in water. Transfer the slides to the incubation mixture in a Coplin jar. Incubate for 5 min at room temperature. Wash for a few seconds and counterstain with Giemsa for 15 min, dry and mount in DPX mountant (Merck).*

Technical considerations

Either reaction works well with films made from freshly withdrawn (uncoagulated) blood or bone marrow. Myeloperoxidase is not inhibited by heparin, oxalate or EDTA and films made from such blood may be stained adequately if the blood is not allowed to stand at c 20°C for more than 6 h. Once films are made they should be left to dry and then fixed; they may then be kept at 4°C for up to 1 week until the reaction is performed. The fixation procedure described above can be interchanged for both cytochemical reactions, and counterstaining may be modified according to individual needs. The methods describe above were tested mainly on cells from cases of acute leukaemia.

Significance

Developing granulocytes always give positive reactions; the reaction is strong in promyelocytes and myelocytes but may be negative in very early myeloblasts. Almost all mature neutrophils give a positive reaction despite the fact that few azurophil granules are visible when the cells are stained with Romanowsky dyes. Eosinophils and basophils give positive reactions, as do promonocytes and monocytes. Monoblasts, lymphocytes and lymphoblasts fail to react.

The main value of the myeloperoxidase reaction is in the distinction between acute myeloid and acute lymphoblastic leukaemia (see below).[6,31,38,39] For practical purposes only immature cells that show myeloperoxidase activity can be confidently referred to as myeloblasts; if the reaction is negative they could be any other type of blast cell. An early myeloblast with negative myeloperoxidase reaction by light microscopy but expressing myeloid antigens is seen in the M0 type of acute myeloblastic leukaemias.[12]

Auer rods nearly always react positively in leukaemic myeloblasts, and the reaction permits a better identification of these characteristic rods than the May-Grünwald-Giemsa stain. An interesting difference has been observed when using the above methods in AML cells. The method with DAB demonstrates a significantly higher percentage of positive rods than techniques with other substrates.[36] In particular, DAB allows the visualization of the so-called Phi bodies,[36] small fusiform-shaped rods, which appear to derive from catalase-containing granules, whilst Auer rods derive from primary granules. Thus the apparent greater sensitivity of the method with DAB in samples of AML may result from the known property of DAB to demonstrate catalase in microperoxisomes as well as myeloperoxidase activity. Phi bodies are not seen using the reaction with 2,7-FDA but Auer rods are easily seen (Fig. 9.1). The latter give a clear brown reaction product without crystals or precipitates, which facilitates the morphological recognition of the cells reacting positively.

The enzyme myeloperoxidase can now be demonstrated by a monoclonal antibody[17] with greater sensitivity than the cytochemical methods (see p. 167).

SUDAN BLACK B STAINING

Sudan Black B was used by Sheehan[71] and later by others to stain the granules of neutrophils, many of which appear to contain phospholipids. The close parallelism observed between sudanophilia and myeloperoxidase activity relates to the fact that both cytochemical reactions are positive in the azurophil granules of neutrophils and monocytes and in the specific eosinophil granules. The biochemical basis for the sudanophilia in these cells is poorly understood.[38] One possible view is that Sudan Black B stains the lipid membrane of the granules which contain the enzyme myeloperoxidase. Another is that the dye stains through an enzymatic mechanism, perhaps linked to myeloperoxidase, and not just by physical solution in the lipids.[38] Both reactions are positive in mature and immature myeloid cells

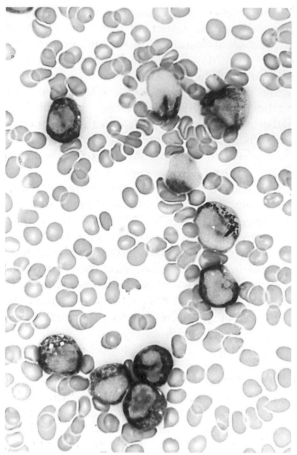

Fig. 9.1 Myeloperoxidase reaction (2,7-FDA method). Bone marrow cells from a case of acute myeloblastic leukaemia with maturation (M2). The cells are myeloperoxidase-positive. Note two blast cells with positive Auer rods.

and thus are useful in the differential diagnosis and classification of the acute leukaemias.[31,38,39] The simplicity of the Sudan Black B reaction makes its use mandatory in routine haematology laboratories. The method of Sheehan and Storey[72] which has been in use, almost unchanged, for more than 40 years, is given below.

Reagents

Fixatives. 40% formaldehyde.

Staining solution. This is a mixture of two solutions, A and B.

(A) Sudan Black B. 0.3 g in 100 ml of absolute ethanol. Shake well to dissolve the stain and filter to remove particles.

(B) Buffer. 16 g of crystalline phenol in 30 ml of absolute ethanol. Add the phenol–ethanol mixture to 100 ml of water in which 0.3 g of disodium hydrogen phosphate ($Na_2HPO_4.12H_2O$) has been dissolved. Stir vigorously until all the phenol has dissolved and filter. Add 30 ml (or 60 ml) of solution A to 20 ml (or 40 ml) of solution B and filter. The mixture can be kept at 4°C for 2–3 months.

Counterstain. May-Grünwald-Giemsa (p. 86), preferably, or safranin.

Method

Fix air-dried films of blood or bone marrow for 10 min in formalin vapour. This can be done by soaking filter paper in formalin and placing inside a 37°C incubator*. Wash gently in water for 5–10 min; longer periods (e.g. 1 h) may result in stronger staining. Wash in 70% ethanol by waving the slides in the alcohol in a Coplin jar for 3–5 min. Wash with water for 2 min, dry, counterstain for 5 min and mount.

The reaction product in the cytoplasm is black; the nuclei stain blue (or red) depending on the counterstain used.

NEUTROPHIL ALKALINE PHOSPHATASE (NAP)

Alkaline-phosphatase activity can be demonstrated cytochemically in the cytoplasm of mature neutrophils, typically in segmented forms and only rarely in band forms. The enzyme is not demonstrable in other blood leucocytes, but fibroblast-like reticulum cells, part of the bone-marrow stroma, react strongly.

NAP was thought initially to be localized in the specific (secondary) granules, by analogy with the findings in rabbit neutrophils,[3] or in late-appearing tertiary granules. Studies by Rustin et al.[66] have shown that NAP is associated with a membranous component of the cytoplasm identified as an irregularly-shaped tubular structure

---

*Alternatively, immerse the films for 5 min in a solution of 9 volumes of absolute ethanol and 1 volume of 40% formaldehyde.

distinct from primary or secondary granules or other cytoplasmic organelles.

Early cytochemical methods for the demonstration of NAP were based upon the hydrolysis of the substrate α-naphthyl phosphate at pH 9.0–10.0 and the coupling of the liberated naphthol to a diazotized amine to form an insoluble coloured precipitate. The intensity of the precipitate is a rough measure of the enzyme content of individual neutrophils. Later methods have used substituted naphthols as substrates,[49] e.g. naphthol AS,[67] AS-BI or AS-MX[47] phosphate; they all give highly chromogenic and insoluble reaction products which are superior to those developed in previously described methods. We describe here below the method of Rutenburg et al.[67] which is simple and highly reproducible and gives an easily recognizable blue reaction product. This method can also be applied to tissue sections. For the technical aspects of the preparation and storage of films and the effects of fixation on NAP activity, refer to the detailed review by Kaplow.[49]

Reagents

Fixative. Absolute methanol, 9 volumes; neutral formalin (40% formaldehyde), 1 volume. The mixture should be kept at −20°C, or in the ice compartment of a refrigerator, and may be used for up to 2–3 weeks.

Stock substrate solution. Dissolve 30 mg of naphthol AS phosphate in 0.5 ml of N,N-dimethylformamide and add 0.3 mol/l Tris buffer, pH 9 (p. 579) to make the volume up to 100 ml. This solution is stable for several months at 2–4°C, but its pH should be checked before use.

Diazonium salt. Fast Blue BB or BBN.

Counterstain. 1 g/l aqueous neutral red.

Control. Each batch of slides to be stained should include two controls, a normal blood film and a blood film giving a strong reaction, e.g. from a patient with a polymorphonuclear leucocytosis due to infection.

Method

Make films, if possible from freshly withdrawn blood (no anticoagulant). Films from blood collected into EDTA are less satisfactory, and if anticoagulated blood has to be used, films should be made as soon as possible, and in any case within 30 min of collection.

When made, fix the films without delay for 30 s in the formal-methanol fixative at 0–5°C. Then wash the slides in running tap-water for 10–15 s, drain off excess water and allow to dry. If staining has to be delayed for more than 5–6 h, store the fixed films at −20°C.

Prepare the incubation mixture by dissolving 10 mg of the diazonium salt in 10 ml of the stock substrate solution. Then filter this on to the slides and allow the reaction to continue for 15 min at *c* 20°C. Then rinse the slides in four changes of tap-water, allow them to dry and counterstain the films with neutral red for 6 min. After drying, place a drop of neutral mountant on the slide, and cover the film with a cover-slip.

Scoring results

Alkaline phosphatase activity is indicated by a precipitate of bright blue granules; the cell nuclei are stained red. Based on the intensity of staining and the number of blue granules in the cytoplasm of the neutrophils, individual cells are rated as follows:

0: negative, no granules
1: positive but very few blue granules
2: positive with few to a moderate number of granules
3: strong positive with numerous granules
4: very strong positive with cytoplasm crowded with granules.

The score in an individual film consists of the sum of the scores of 100 consecutive neutrophils. As this mode of assessment is subjective, each laboratory should establish its own normal range.

Significance

The normal range of NAP is wide, 35–100 in our laboratory. In a few normal individuals occasional neutrophils score 3, none 4. The score is higher in women and children than in men, and in newborn infants the range is 150–300.

High scores are found in the neutrophilia of

infections, in leukaemoid reactions, liver cirrhosis, Down's syndrome and polycythaemia vera. The enzyme seems to be influenced by oestrogens and corticosteroids, which may explain the gradual rise in score in pregnancy. High scores are found in active Hodgkin's disease but they are uncommon in non-Hodgkin's lymphomas; in Hodgkin's disease, however, the determination of NAP has no apparent advantage over simpler tests such as the ESR in the assessment of the activity of the disease.[61] Low scores are found in chronic granulocytic leukaemia in relapse and in myeloblastic leukaemias while the scores in lymphocytic leukaemias are normal or high. Intermediate scores, more often than not rather high, are found in monocytic and myelomonocytic leukaemias.

Low scores are found in paroxysmal nocturnal haemoglobinuria[52] and high scores in aplastic anaemia.[61] The development of PNH in a patient with aplastic anaemia is associated with a falling score.

The value of the NAP reaction in the differential diagnosis of the chronic myeloproliferative disorders is discussed later (see p. 157).

PERIODIC ACID–SCHIFF (PAS) REACTION

The PAS reaction depends on the liberation of carbohydrate radicals from combination with protein and their oxidation to aldehydes by the Schiff reagent. A positive reaction usually denotes the presence of glycogen. This can be confirmed by demonstrating that the positive reaction disappears when the film is treated with saliva or diastase before it is stained. Other PAS-positive material is unchanged by diastase digestion.

Developing granulocytes react positively at all stages of development. Mature polymorphonuclear neutrophils react most strongly (Fig. 9.2) and their cytoplasm contains large amounts of positively-staining material in the form of small granules. Myeloblasts and myelocytes contain fewer positively-staining granules but the cytoplasm stains diffusely pale pink. In eosinophils the background cytoplasm is PAS-positive but the large specific granules are PAS-negative.

Lymphocytes normally contain much less staining material than granulocytes, but a few fine or even coarse granules may often be demon-

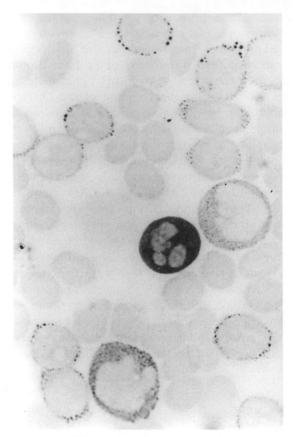

Fig. 9.2 PAS reaction in cells from a peripheral-blood film. Chronic lymphocytic leukaemia. Most of the lymphoid cells are PAS-positive with medium size granules; two large cells with fine granules are monocytes and in the centre there is a neutrophil showing a diffuse positive reaction.

strated. Monocytes contain a small amount of fine, scattered, positively-staining material. The cytoplasm of normoblasts does not normally stain at any stage of development.

Lymphocytes in the B-lymphoproliferative disorders (e.g. chronic lymphocytic leukaemia and prolymphocytic leukaemia) often contain an increased number of positively-staining granules (Fig. 9.2); in lymphoblasts, 'blocks' of staining material may be present.[38,39] This is the typical reaction in the common type of childhood lymphoblastic leukaemia (Fig. 9.3); in the less common T-cell variant the PAS reaction is, however, either weakly positive or negative.[21]

Erythroblasts may react positively in disease. Deep diffuse staining has been observed in erythroleukaemia[63] and in thalassaemia; and lesser

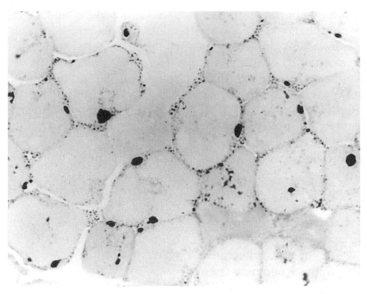

Fig. 9.3   PAS reaction in cells from cerebrospinal fluid. Cytocentrifuge preparation; acute lymphoblastic leukaemia. Most of the cells are PAS-positive with medium size granules and single blocks.

degrees of staining may be seen in iron-deficiency anaemia, myelosclerosis, various types of leukaemia and in various types of haemolytic anaemia. Positive reactions have also been recorded in pernicious anaemia, aplastic anaemia, lead poisoning and polycythamia vera.

The reaction is best carried out on fresh blood or bone-marrow films but old methanol-fixed films or films stained by Romanowsky dyes months or years before can be quite satisfactorily stained.

Reagents

Periodic acid ($HIO_4.2H_2O$), 10g/l.

Schiff's reagent (leucobasic fuchsin). Basic fuchsin, 1.0 g, dissolved in 400 ml of boiling water.

Cool the solution to 50°C and then filter. To the filtrate add 1 ml of thionyl chloride ($SOCl_2$) and allow the solution to stand in the dark for 12 h. Then add 2.0 g of activated charcoal and after shaking for 1 min filter the preparation. Store in the dark at 0–4°C.

Rinsing solution. Sodium metabisulphite, 100 g/l, 6 ml; HCl, 1 mol/l, 5 ml; water to 100 ml.

Counterstain. Mayer's haemalum or Harris's aqueous haematoxylin, 2.0 g; water to 100 ml.

Method

Fix the films in methanol for 5–15 min. Then wash in running tap-water for 15 min. Expose the films to digestion in diastase (1 g in litre of 9 g/l NaCl) for 1 h at room temperature. Thereafter, allow both treated and untreated slides to stand in the periodic acid solution for 10 min, then wash and immerse them in Schiff's reagent for 30 min at room temperature in the dark. Rinse the slides three times in the rinsing solution, then wash in distilled water for 5 min, counterstain with haematoxylin for 10 min and then blue in tap-water for 5 min. Finally, dry in the air and mount in a neutral mountant.

ACID PHOSPHATASE REACTION

There are several techniques for the demonstration of acid phosphatase in leucocytes in films and tissue sections. Some utilize the same reagents used for the demonstration of NAP but at pH 5.0. For example, the method of Li et al[54] uses naphthol AS-BI phosphate and Fast Garnet GBC and gives a highly chromogenic reaction product; it is easily reproducible and suitable for demonstrating the enzyme in the granulocytic series. For lymphocytes and monocytes, a method using naphthol AS-BI phosphate coupled with freshly hexazotized pararosanilin buffered to pH 5.0[32] may be better, although its final reaction product is less distinctly granular than when Fast Garnet GBC is used.[38] Another good coupling agent is Fast Red ITR salt.

Acid phosphatase activity is present in the lysosomes of many types of haemopoietic cell, i.e. myelocytes, polymorphonuclear neutrophils, lymphocytes, plasma cells, megakaryocytes, platelets, and all the cells of the mononuclear phagocyte system (monoblasts, promonocytes, monocytes and macrophages). It is one of the acid hydrolases that can be demonstrated in lymphoid cells, and is of diagnostic value in the differential diagnosis of lymphoproliferative conditions (see below). Studies in tissue sections have demonstrated a greater enzyme content in T-cell-dependent areas than in B-cell-dependent areas (e.g. germinal centres) of lymphoid tissues from men and rodents. The activity of acid phosphatase increases after lymphocyte transformation with phytohaemagglutinin and during the transition from monocyte to tissue macrophage. The technique of Goldberg and Barka[32] has been shown, in our hands, to be reliable in the study of lymphocytic and monocytic proliferations.[19,21] For hairy cell leukaemia (HCL) the method of Li et al[54] has been recommended.[73]

Reagents

Fixative. Methanol, 10 ml; acetone, 60 ml; water, 30 ml; citric acid, 0.63 g. This solution should be adjusted to pH 5.4 with 1 mol/l NaOH and controlled weekly.

Stock solutions.

(A) Buffer pH 5.0. Sodium acetate, trihydrate, 19.5 g; sodium barbiturate, 29.5g; water to 1 litre (Michaeli's veronal acetate buffer).

(B) Substrate. Naphthol AS-BI phosphate dissolved in *N,N*-dimethylformamide, 10 mg/ml (i.e. 25 mg in 2.5 ml).

(C) Sodium nitrite ($NaNO_2$). 4% aqueous solution.

(D) Pararosanilin chloride (Sigma). 2 g in 50 ml of 2 mol/l HCl. Heat gently, without boiling; cool down to room temperature and filter.

Solutions A, B and D can be stored at 4°C; solution C should be freshly made each time or can only be stored for up to 1 week at 4°C.

Working solution. Mix together 92.5 ml of solution A, 2.5 ml of solution B, 32.5 ml of water and 4 ml of hexazotized pararosanilin solution. Make the latter by mixing well 2 ml of solution C and 2 ml of solution D; allow to stand for 2 min before adding to the other constituents. Mix well and adjust the pH of the working solution to pH 5.0 with 1 mol/l NaOH.

Counterstain. 1% methyl green in veronal acetate buffer, pH 4.0.

Mounting medium. Glycerol/gelatin. Add 15 g of gelatin to 100 ml of glycerol and 100 ml of water.

Method

Dry the films well before starting the reaction. (It is desirable to leave them for this purpose for at least 24 h at room temperature.) Fix the films for 10 min, then rinse the slides well in water. They can now be kept for 1–2 weeks at –20°C if required.

Incubate the slides for 1 h at 37°C in the working solution; rinse in tap-water, counterstain the films for 1 min, rinse in tap-water and mount whilst still wet. For this, the glycerol/gelatin mixture has to be in liquid phase; i.e. warmed to 37°C or higher.

The cytoplasmic reaction product is bright red; the nuclei stain pale green.

Test of tartrate resistance

This is often carried out in parallel with the above reaction or preferably the method using Fast Garnet GBC[54,73] for the study of hairy cells. Add 375 mg of crystalline L(+)-tartaric acid (Sigma) to 50 ml of the working solution; the final concentration is then 50 mmol/l. Then carry out the cytochemical reaction. Most positively-reacting leucocytes are tartrate-sensitive and fail to react in the presence of tartrate. The majority of hairy cells of HCL react equally positively in both solutions.[82]

Significance

Almost all acute and chronic T-cell lympho-proliferations are characterized by a strong acid phosphatase reaction. In T-ALL (Fig. 9.4)[19,21] the reaction is localized to an area of the cytoplasm which at ultrastructural level corresponds to the Golgi zone. In the chronic T-cell leukaemias the reaction is also positive but with variable consistency. Two thirds of cases with T-cell prolymphocytic leukaemia (PLL) have cells which react strongly positively. The enzyme activity in these cases is tartrate-sensitive.

In normal T-cells, acid phosphatase activity is an early differentiation feature, e.g. the reaction is positive in fetal thymocytes and it persists in some mature T-lymphocytes. In the B-cell disorders the reaction is often weak or negative with the exception of HCL, the cells of which show a strong acid phosphatase activity[54] resistant to inhibition by tartrate in the majority of cases.[82] This enzyme corresponds to a unique isoenzyme 5 found predominantly in hairy cells.[82] Tartrate-resistant cells have not been found in the peripheral blood of normal individuals but a few such cells can be found in the normal bone marrow. In B-cell PLL one-third of the cells show a positive acid phosphatase reaction if tested by the method of Goldberg and Barka[32] and some of these cells have been shown to be tartrate-resistant, as in HCL.[21]

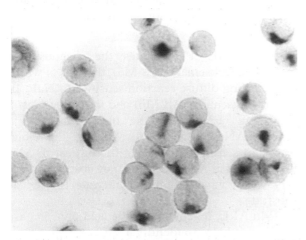

Fig. 9.4   Positive acid phosphatase-reaction in a peripheral-blood film. Acute lymphoblastic leukaemia of T-cell type.

In AML, blasts of the monocyte lineage react more strongly than those of the granulocytic lineage. The reaction in monoblasts is diffuse over the whole cytoplasm and can be seen at ultrastructural level to be localized in small lysosomal granules.[60]

ESTERASES

These are a group of hydrolases with a wide range of pH activity which vary in their localization in cells of different bone-marrow lineages. It is best to consider separately the results obtained with the various substrates used for their cytochemical demonstration. Those currently in use are: α-naphthol acetate, α-naphthol butyrate, naphthol AS acetate (NASA), naphthol AS-D acetate (NASDA) and naphthol AS-D chloracetate.[79]

Li et al described nine esterase isoenzymes in leucocytes:[53] 1, 2, 7, 8 and 9 represent the 'specific' esterase of granulocytes which can be demonstrated by means of naphthol AS-D chloracetate; 3, 4, 5 and 6 represent the so-called 'non-specific' esterases which are sensitive to sodium fluoride (NaF) and are found in monocytes, megakaryocytes and platelets, and are demonstrated by α-naphthol esters (acetate and butyrate). Naphthol AS (or AS-D) reacts with most isoenzymes but is inhibited by NaF in its reaction with the non-specific esterases.

α-NAPHTHOL ACETATE ESTERASE (ANAE)

The cytochemical reaction for ANAE gives distinct patterns in lymphocytes (a dot-like reaction) and in monocytes (a diffuse positive reaction) as illustrated in Fig. 9.5. The localized reaction in lymphocytes is resistant to NaF, whilst that in monocytes is NaF-sensitive. In normal blood there is a good correlation between the proportion of T-cells and the percentage of ANAE-positive lymphocytes. The reaction in immature T-cells (thymocytes) is also localized, but it is weak and seen in only one-third of those cells. The dot-like reaction in peripheral-blood T-lymphocytes is seen mainly in the subset with Fc receptors for IgM.[26] Results with the substrate α-naphthyl butyrate are, in general, very similar to

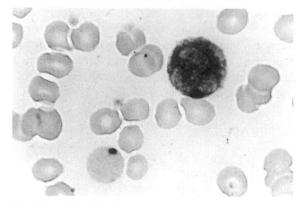

Fig. 9.5   α.-**Naphthyl acetate esterase reaction.** ANAE-positive reaction in normal cells. A lymphocyte (presumably T) has a characteristic single 'dot-like' reaction; a monocyte shows a strong diffuse reaction over the whole cytoplasm.

those obtained with ANAE. Some authors have made a distinction between the ANAE reaction carried out at different pHs, acid or alkaline, the latter favouring the reaction in monocytes and the former being more specific for T-lymphocytes. The method of Yam et al[81] at pH 6.1 permits the adequate demonstration of the distinct reaction in both cell types.

Reagents

Fixative. Phosphate buffered acetone-formaldehyde. Acetone, 40 ml; 35% formaldehyde, 25 ml; Na_2HPO_4, 20 mg, and KH_2PO_4, 100 mg, in 30 ml of water. Filter the solution before use; it must be clear. It will keep at room temperature for 1 month.

Stock solutions.

(A) a-Naphthyl acetate. 50 mg dissolved in 2.5 ml of 2-methoxyethanol.

(B) Phosphate buffer. 0.1 mol/l, pH 7.6, 44.5 ml.

(C). Hexazotized pararosanilin. This is prepared by mixing equal volumes of pararosanilin solution (solution D of the acid phosphatase reaction, see p. 150) and fresh 4% aqueous $NaNO_2$ for 1 min just before use.

Incubation mixture. Mix solutions A and B and add to them the freshly prepared solution C. Adjust the pH to 6.1 with 1 mol/l NaOH. Filter before use; the solution must be clear.

Counterstain and mounting medium. As for acid phosphatase (methyl green and glycerol/gelatin).

Method

Fix the films for 30 s, rinse the slides well in water and allow to dry. Incubate the slides for 45 min in the incubation mixture. After the incubation, wash the slides in tap-water and counterstain for 1 min and mount whilst still wet.

A positive reaction results in dark red granules; the nuclei stain pale green.

Inhibition with sodium fluoride (NaF)

Add 75 mg of NaF to 50 ml of the incubation mixture (concentration 1.5 mg/ml = 37.5 mmol/l).

Carry out the test simultaneously with the ANAE reaction to investigate the NaF sensitivity of a cell population. This may be necessary for the identification of monocytes within a mixture of mononuclear cells or to characterize a particular leukaemic cell type.

Significance [4,26,41,81]

The ANAE cytochemical reaction is often applied to the study of leukaemic cell populations. In normal samples it helps to distinguish between T-lymphocytes and monocytes because of the different pattern of reaction and the different sensitivity to NaF (see above). In leukaemias and lymphoproliferative disorders it has three main applications:

1. In AML it facilitates the diagnosis of monocytic leukaemia (FAB M5), the cells of which give a strong diffuse reaction sensitive to NaF. In erythroleukaemia (FAB M6) and megakaryoblastic leukaemia (FAB M7) the blast cells give a positive ANAE reaction localized to the Golgi zone and sensitive to NaF.[27] In contrast to M5, the reaction in M6 and M7 is not observed (or is very weak) when α-napthyl butyrate is used as substrate.[27]

2. In ALL, together with the acid phosphatase reaction, it helps to identify T-ALL.[4,41]

3. In the chronic B and T lymphoid leukaemias it helps to distinguish T-PLL (positive

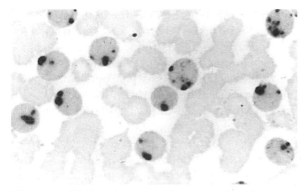

Fig. 9.6 α-**Naphthyl acetate esterase reaction.** Strong localized ANAE reaction in peripheral blood cells of a T-cell prolymphocytic leukaemia. (Photograph by courtesy of Dr. A. D. Crockard.)

or negative in granulocytes. The reaction product with NASDA is often stronger than with NASA and diffuses less; it is thus the substrate of choice. The main value of the reaction is in differentiating between the myeloblastic types (M1 and M2) and the monocytic types (M5a and M5b) of AML[6] In myelomonocytic leukaemia (M4), it helps in assessing the relative size of the monocytic component.[6,9]

CHLORACETATE ESTERASE

The specific esterase present in granulocytes and mast cells is distinct from that in monocytes and megakaryocytes; it can be demonstrated by using naphthol AS-D chloracetate as substrate and Fast Garnet GBC,[57] Fast Red Violet or Fast Blue BB[38] as coupling agents. A method with New Fuchsin has been recommended by the International Committee for Standardization in Haematology.[73] The enzyme is optimally active at pH 7.0–7.6 and is not inhibited by NaF. The positive reaction is found in mature and immature granulocytes and, in general, the reactions parallel those of myeloperoxidase and Sudan Black B in the granulocytic lineage; Auer rods often react positively. Little or no enzyme activity is demonstrable in lymphocytes and monocytes.

One advantage of the chloracetate method is the possibility of demonstrating enzyme activity in paraffin-embedded histological sections of formalin-fixed material. It can be applied as well to material from other tissues, being particularly useful for the diagnosis of granulocytic sarcoma (chloroma).

The chloracetate esterase reaction has been widely used on haematological material in combination with ANAE or α-naphthol butyrate esterase in a single method – the so-called combined or dual esterase reaction.[38,81] The end-result is the demonstration, in the same preparation, of both types of esterase; they can be distinguished by the colour of the reaction products by using different coupling agents, e.g. blue when using Fast Blue BB for the chloracetate esterase and dark red using hexazotized para-rosanilin for ANAE. This procedure simplifies the cytochemical characterization of leukaemic cells. In acute myelomonocytic leukaemia (M4) it

reaction) (Fig. 9.6) from B-PLL (negative reaction). The typical dot-like pattern of normal T-lymphocytes is not observed, however, in large granular lymphocyte (LGL) leukaemias. This probably relates to a similar finding in normal large granular lymphocytes.[26]

Erythroblasts are normally ANAE-negative. However, they can react positively in megaloblastic anaemia. Weak reactions have also been described in thalassaemia and sideroblastic anaemia.

NAPHTHOL AS (OR AS-D) ACETATE ESTERASE

Both substrates are commonly used: naphthol AS acetate (NASA) or naphthol AS-D acetate (NASDA) can demonstrate non-specific esterase activity in monocytic cells. They do not show, as does ANAE, a consistent localized reaction in T-lymphocytes. Fast Blue BB has been recommended as coupling agent.[73] The reaction with both substrates is carried out at pH 6.9.[81] At this pH, however, prolonged incubation can result in hydrolysis of the substrate by the chloracetate esterase of granulocytes,[52] thus making the reaction less specific for monocytes. Therefore, the simultaneous incubation with NaF is needed to improve the recognition of promonocytes and monocytes and to distinguish them from pro-myelocytes and myelocytes. NaF is less necessary with ANAE (or α-naphthol butyrate) because the reaction is strong in monocytic cells and is weak helps to identify both the granulocytic and mono-cytic components.

OTHER ACID HYDROLASES

Two enzymes, β-glucuronidase and β-glucos-aminidase[26] have been shown by histochemical methods to be present in high concentrations in T-cell-dependent areas of lymphoid tissues and to be either absent or present in only small amounts in the B-cell-dependent areas. Both enzymes have now been shown to be markers of leukaemic T-lymphocytes. The reaction product in cells of chronic B-cell leukaemias is usually weak or negative.[26]

LYSOZYME ACTIVITY

A simple cyto-bacterial method for the demon-stration of lysozyme (muramidase) activity based on the technique of Briggs et al,[15] as modified by Syrén and Raeste[75] was described in previous editions of this book. As the method is not often performed nowadays in the characterization of blast cells, we do not reproduce it here.

Normal blood monocytes and neutrophils always give a positive lysis test but lymphocytes do not. In normal bone marrow, lysozyme activity can be demonstrated in granulocytes as far back as the myelocyte stage. In acute leukaemia, myeloblasts and lymphoblasts are lysozyme-negative but promonocytes and monocytes, and sometimes monoblasts, give positive reactions.

Because lysozyme appears relatively late during monocyte maturation, at the promonocyte stage, this reaction is consistently positive in differentiated forms of monocytic leukaemia, i.e. in M4, M5b and CMML of the FAB classification,[6,9] but may be negative in the poorly differentiated type, i.e. M5a. In the former case, a high proportion of leukaemic monocytes (50–90%) are lysozyme-positive. In general, the number of lysozyme-positive cells in the circulation and the serum lysozyme concentration are closely correlated.[22]

PRACTICAL VALUE OF CYTOCHEMICAL REACTIONS

There are four groups of malignancies of haemopoietic cells in which the cytochemical methods described above have been found to be useful for a correct diagnosis and classification:

1. The acute leukaemias, proliferations of immature haemopoietic precursors (blast cells).

2. The chronic myeloproliferative disorders, proliferations of differentiated cells of the myeloid lineage.

3. The chronic lymphoproliferative disorders, proliferations of mature-looking lymphoid cells.

4. The myelodysplastic syndromes,[8] a group of conditions distinct from, but possibly related to, the acute leukaemias should also be consider-ed in the differential diagnosis.

Well-prepared peripheral-blood and bone-marrow films stained with May-Grünwald-Giemsa are the basis for any classification. The cytochemical tests provide clues regarding the type and direction of cellular differentiation, but should be regarded as complementing and not substituting for the morphological analysis. The International Council for Standardization in Haematology has recommended a set of three primary cytochemistry tests which, together with phenotyping procedures (see later), should lead to consistent classification of most acute leukaemias. These are myeloperoxidase, chloro-acetate esterase and α-naphthyl acetate esterase.[42]

DIFFERENTIAL DIAGNOSIS OF THE ACUTE LEUKAEMIAS — THE FAB CLASSIFICATION[6–10,12]

Two main forms of acute leukaemia are recognized: myeloid (AML), more frequent in adults (>20 years), and lymphoblastic (ALL), predominantly found in children (<15 years).

AML

Eight types of AML can be identified by morphology with the help of cytochemistry. The main features of each type (M1–M7) are summarized in Table 9.1. AML M0[12] is characterized by negative cytochemistry, peroxidase, Sudan Black B and esterases. The blast cells of M0, however, express myeloid antigens[28] and have small amounts of peroxidase detected by electron microscopy[56] and occasionally by a monoclonal antibody.[17] Certain cytochemical reactions are essential in distinguishing AML from undifferentiated forms of ALL (e.g. L2). This is particularly so in cases where the cells are immature, e.g. in M1 (myeloblastic leukaemia

without maturation) and M5a (monoblastic leukaemia, poorly differentiated). The peroxidase, Sudan Black B and chloracetate esterase reactions reveal granulocytic differentiation in the M1, M2, M3 and M4 types of AML whilst the non-specific esterases (NASDA and ANAE ± NaF), and the acid phosphatase and lysozyme reactions, demonstrate monocytic differentiation. AML M0 cannot be distinguished from ALL by cytochemical methods but only with immunological techniques (see below) which detect lymphoid antigens in ALL and myeloid antigens in AML, including M0.

Although most cases of hypergranular promyelocytic leukaemia (M3) can be diagnosed in

Table 9.1 Classification and cytochemistry of AML

Reaction	Myeloblastic[@]		Promyelocytic	Myelomonocytic	Monocytic	Erythroleukaemia	Megakaryoblastic[10]
	M1	M2	M3	M4	M5	M6	M7
May-Grünwald-Giemsa stain	Blasts with few or no granules (90%); Auer rods	Blasts (>30%). Maturation beyond pro-myelocytes. Abnormal neutrophils	Hypergranular promyelocytes; faggots. Bilobed nuclei. Hypogranular variant	Blasts (>30%). Evidence of granulocytic and monocytic differentiation	(a) Monoblasts; (b) Monoblasts, promonocytes & monocytes. (a) & (b) >80% monocytic cells.	Over 50% of erythroid cells, often bizarre. Myeloblasts with Auer rods. The % of blasts is >30% by excluding erythroid cells from the differential count.[9]	Blasts (>30%) often dry tap aspirate; bone marrow trephine biopsy required
Peroxidase Sudan Black B	**+ or ++** (>5%) blasts)	++	+++	+ or ++ (2 population)	– or +	+ (blasts)	–
Esterases 1. Chloroacetate	+	++	**+++**	**+ or ++**	– or ±	+	–
2. NASDA	+	+	++	**+ or +++** *	**+++** *	++ *	–
3. ANAE	–	±	±	**+ or ++** *	+++	+ * (erythroid precursors) in Golgi zone	+ +* in Golgi zone
Acid phosphatase	– or +	+	+ or ++	+ or ++	+++	±	++
Lysozyme	–	–	±	+ or ++	± or +++	–	–
PAS	+ diffuse	+ diffuse	++ diffuse	+ or ++ variable	+ or ++ granules	+ (erythroblasts)	+ or ++
Incidence	23%	30%	8%	16%	16%	6%	1%

*NaF sensitive. *Degree of reaction*: –, negative; ±, weak (few positive cells); +, moderate; + +, moderate to strong; + + +, most of the cells strongly positive. Cytochemical reactions that are useful for differential diagnosis are printed in bold type. [@]Cases of myeloblastic leukaemia may give negative cytochemical reactions with peroxidase, Sudan Black B, and also give negative esterase reactions. These forms of AML have been designated as M0;[12] the evidence for the myeloid nature is provided by the presence of myeloid antigens[28,35,69] and by myeloperoxidase activity demonstrated at ultrastructural level,[56] and by a monoclonal antibody anti-MPO.[17]

May-Grünwald-Giemsa-stained films, an M3-variant characterized by having fewer azurophil granules may require for its identification a positive reaction with the cytochemical methods for granulocytic cells (Table 9.1). Because of their (typical) bilobed nuclei, cells of the M3-variant can sometimes be confused with atypical monocytes (as in M4 and M5 leukaemias). However, the non-specific esterase reactions are usually weak or negative in M3.

In erythroleukaemia (M6) the PAS reaction may be strongly positive, with a diffuse or granular pattern being found in erythroblasts and sometimes in erythrocytes, too; the ANAE reaction may also be positive in red-cell precursors and is often localized in the Golgi zone.[27]

A rare form of AML is acute megakaryoblastic leukaemia.[10,14] The blast cells appear undifferentiated, and may resemble lymphoblasts.[1] The cytochemical profile of these cells is similar to that of megakaryocytes: i.e. positive reactions with PAS, acid phosphatase and ANAE (NaF-sensitive as in monocytes).[27] A specific test for megakaryoblasts, the so-called 'platelet peroxidase' reaction, can be demonstrated by electron microscopy in the nuclear membrane and endoplasmic reticulum of these cells although not in the Golgi apparatus.[1,14]

The enzyme content of mature neutrophils in AML, particularly in M2 and M6, can often be shown by negative cytochemical reactions to be deficient. The NAP score is often low in M2 (myeloblastic leukaemia with maturation),[46] especially in M2 cases with the chromosome translocation t(8;21). An interesting difference between the low NAP values seen in CGL and in M2 has been reported by Kamada et al[46] — namely, that if the leukaemic cells are suspended in liquid culture for 1 week the NAP score increases in CGL whilst it remains unchanged in M2. The peroxidase, Sudan Black B and chloracetate reactions may also be negative in variable proportions of neutrophils in AML, more frequently in M2 and M6.[23] In contrast, the neutrophils in CGL and in M5 react positively in these reactions to about the same degree as do normal neutrophils.

ALL

Three morphological types have been described by the FAB group: L1, L2 and L3.[6,7] The differences in age incidence (L1 is more common in children and L2 more frequent in adults), the strong correlation of L3 with B-ALL (with monoclonal membrane immunoglobulins) and the difference in prognosis between L1 and L2 (worse in L2) within similar age-groups together suggest that the three morphological types may reflect biological differences.

L1 lymphoblasts tend to be small and to have scanty cytoplasm; the nucleo-cytoplasmic (N:C) ratio is high in the majority and they have a small and not easily visible nucleolus; the nuclear membrane is often regular. L2 lymphoblasts, in contrast to L1, are larger, have more abundant cytoplasm (low N:C ratio) and have one or more prominent nucleoli; the nuclear outline is irregular in over 25% of cells. The differences between L1 and L2 can be solved in borderline cases by the simple scoring system proposed by the FAB group.[7] L3 cells (or Burkitt type), because of their resemblance to cells of the endemic African lymphoma, are uniformly large, have finely stippled nuclear chromatin and, characteristically, a deep basophilic cytoplasm often associated with prominent vacuolation.[7]

Two cytochemical tests have been used in the study of ALL; the PAS and acid phosphatase reactions. They do not correlate with the L1, L2 or L3 morphological types but they do show some relationship to the immunological subtypes of ALL (Table 9.2). In cases in which the cells are undifferentiated (usually L2 blast cells in adult patients), it is important to exclude AML (usually M1 and M5a). For this, the peroxidase, Sudan Black B and NASDA reactions should be shown to be negative. For the diagnosis of ALL it is nowadays essential to have evidence of the lymphoid nature of the blasts by membrane markers (see below). The PAS reaction is often positive in ALL — at least, in a proportion of blasts, as shown by coarse granules or blocks of positively-reacting material (usually glycogen). This pattern of reaction, particularly with a negative background, is rarely seen in AML. It is more typical of the common form of childhood ALL which can be defined by immunological tests for the ALL antigen (glycoprotein [gp] 100). This form was described initially by Greaves et al[34] as common-ALL and is now

Table 9.2 Cytochemistry and the immunological classification of ALL*

Method	Early-B-ALL	Common-ALL	T-ALL	B-ALL
Morphology	L1–L2	L1–L2	L1–L2	L3
PAS	– or + +	+ or + +	– or +	–
	coarse granules	coarse granules		
Acid phosphatase	– or +	– or +	+ + or + + +	–
Peroxidase ⎫				
Sudan Black B ⎬	–	–	–	–
Lysozyme	–	–	–	–

*For details of the membrane and enzyme markers in ALL, see Table 9.4. Degree of reaction as in Table 9.1.

recognized by monoclonal antibodies (McAb) to the cluster of differentiation 10 (CD10).

In T-ALL (positive T-cell markers), the PAS reaction is negative in two-thirds of cases; in B-ALL it is almost always negative. The differences shown by the PAS reaction probably reflect the different proliferation kinetics of the immuno-logically-defined subtypes of ALL. For example, in B-ALL (PAS-negative) a greater number of cells are in cycle; this is also reflected in the numerous mitotic figures seen in bone marrow with L3 morphology. The acid phosphatase test gives a consistently localized positive reaction in T-ALL and pre-T-ALL blast cells.[4,19,41]

Chronic myeloproliferative disorders

Low NAP scores are typical of untreated chronic granulocytic leukaemia (CGL) and high NAP scores are characteristic of polycythaemia vera, leucocytoses and leukaemoid reactions secondary to infection or neoplasia and of most cases of myelosclerosis. Normal scores are often found in secondary polycythaemia due to hypoxia, 'stress' or renal disorders. In CGL the low scores may change to normal or high during remission; scores become high during severe infections, after splenectomy and in up to 50% of cases under-going blast-cell transformation.

The possibility of characterizing more precisely the type of blast cells seen during the trans-formation of CGL has improved significantly in recent years. CGL blasts are very undifferen-tiated by cytological and cytochemical criteria. Ultrastructural studies, e.g. the platelet-peroxidase reaction, may help in the diagnosis of megakaryo-blastic transformation (15% of cases).[14] Nowadays a number of McAb against platelet glycoproteins can be used to demonstrate the megakaryoblastic nature of the blasts.[27,77] A 'lymphoid' trans-formation occurs in 20% of cases of CGL; most cytochemical tests are negative in this form, but the PAS reaction may show granular positivity. Lymphoblastic transformation can be diagnosed by positive criteria by demonstrating the common ALL-antigen (CD10),[34,43] and other B-lineage antigens (CD19, CD22) and the enzyme ter-minal deoxynucleotidyl transferase (TdT).[13] A mixed population of blast cells is not rare during transformation of CGL; thus mixed lymphoid and myeloid blast crises have been documented.

Myelodysplastic syndromes (MDS)

Precise diagnostic criteria for the MDS were pro-posed by the FAB group.[8] All of them are charac-terized by hypercellular bone marrows. Five conditions are included under the broad term MDS:

1. Refractory anaemia (RA), with erythroid hyperplasia and/or dyserythropoiesis.

2. RA with ring sideroblasts, also designated as acquired idiopathic sideroblastic anaemia (AISA), the main feature being the presence of ring sideroblasts in at least 15% of erythroblasts. (See p. 132 for staining techniques.)

3. RA with excess of blasts (RAEB) which shows dyspoiesis in the three bone-marrow cell lineages, dysgranulopoiesis being always con-spicuous. The percentage of bone-marrow blasts is between 5 and 20%; these cells may have a few or no azurophil granules.

4. Chronic   myelomonocytic   leukaemia

(CMML), with many features of RAEB plus a significant peripheral blood monocytosis (usually over $1 \times 10^9/l$).

5. RAEB in transformation, a group close to AML and defined by the presence of blasts in the peripheral blood (over 5%) and between 20 and 30% in the bone marrow.

In order to distinguish RAEB from AML with more than 50% erythroid cells in the bone marrow the FAB group recommended in those circumstances that erythroid cells be excluded from the differential count and then, if more than 30% of the residual bone marrow cells are blasts, the diagnosis is M6.

In addition to staining for iron, the other cytochemical methods used in AML may be useful for the study of the MDS. They may help to define the monocytic component in CMML or the type of blasts in RAEB and they are particularly useful in demonstrating dysgranulopoiesis, e.g. by the presence of neutrophils negative for peroxidase and/or Sudan Black B reactions or giving extremely low NAP scores.

MDS features can be demonstrated in patients presenting as de-novo AML. When there is evidence that the three bone marrow cell lines are dysplastic, the designation AML with trilineage myelodysplasia has been coined.[16] These patients remit less readily than those with primary AML without MDS changes, and may relapse with pure MDS and without blast cells.[16] Because these patients may have a preceding preleukaemic process and abnormal erythropoiesis they often present with more severe anaemia than other patients with AML without MDS.

CHARACTERIZATION OF CHRONIC LYMPHOPROLIFERATIVE DISORDERS[11,21,26]

Analysis using immunological markers shows that the majority of lymphoproliferative disorders are of the B-cell type (Table 9.3). In the most common of these, chronic lymphocytic leukaemia (CLL), and in prolymphocytic leukaemia (PLL), the PAS reaction is often positive in a granular form.[21] This reaction is variable, often negative, in the chronic T-cell disorders.

The reactions for acid hydrolases (acid phosphatase, ANAE, β-glucuronidase and β-glucosaminidase) are positive in most T-cell disorders and negative in the B-cell types (Table 9.3). The non-specific esterase reaction can also help to diagnose the rare 'true' histiocytic lymphomas within the group of large-cell lymphomas, which are usually of B-cell type. The cells of large-cell lymphomas may occasionally spillover to the peripheral blood and may resemble monoblasts.[2]

Table 9.3 Cytochemistry of chronic lymphoproliferative disorders and relation to membrane phenotype

Disease	Immunological subtype*	Relative incidence@	ANAE	Acid Phosphatase	ß-Glucuronidase ß-Glucosaminidase
CLL[‖]	B	98%	−	−	−
LGLL§	T	2%	− or ±	++	+++
PLL[[]]	B	70%	−	− or +	−
	T	30%	+++	± or ++	+++
Non-Hodgkin's	B	85%	−	− or +	−
lymphomas	T**	15%	++	+ or +++	++
HCL@@	B	100%	− or +	++†	−

B-cell markers: membrane bound and/or cytoplasmic monoclonal immunoglobulins; and B-cell lineage McAb, e.g. CD19, CD20, CD22.
T-cell markers: McAbs to T-cell antigens, e.g. CD2, CD3, CD4, CD7, CD8, etc.
@Based on over 2000 cases studied in the MRC Leukaemia Unit Laboratories by D.C.
**Includes Sézary syndrome and adult T-cell lymphoma-leukaemia (HTLV-1 positive).
†Resistant to tartaric acid.
‖Chronic lymphocytic leukaemia.
[[]]Prolymphocytic leukaemia.
@@Hairy cell leukaemia.
§Large granular lymphocyte leukaemias.

Both cytochemistry and immunological reagents are necessary to establish the correct diagnosis.[2] True histiocytic lymphomas are tumours of mono-cytic lineage and show strong diffuse positivity with NASA, NASDA or ANAE, the reactions being NaF-sensitive. These cytochemical reactions are negative in the majority of B-cell lymphomas. Despite the characteristic cytochemical patterns set out in Table 9.3, the current trend is to classify the lymphoid malignancies on the basis of reactions to immunological reagents, chiefly McAbs, which cover a wide range of differentia-tion antigens demonstrable in the B- and T-cell lineages. These reagents have the additional advantage that they detect antigens which charac-terize early or late stages of lymphoid maturation.

CELL MARKERS

Cells can be identified, not only by their morphology and cytochemistry, but also by the presence of characteristic receptors and antigens on the cell membrane, immunoglobulin molecules on the membrane (SmIg) and/or in the cytoplasm (CyIg) and by enzymes such as terminal de-oxynucleotidyl transferase (TdT) in the nucleus.[13] By this means it is possible to distinguish B- and T-lymphocytes and also subsets within the major types of lymphocytes. Marker studies help in identifying the lineage of immature cells; they have also contributed to the study of early and late stages of lymphoid differentiation, and to the diagnosis and classification of the acute and chronic lymphoid leukaemias.

Separation of mononuclear (MN) cells

For most cell marker studies it is necessary to separate the MN cell fraction containing lympho-cytes, monocytes, blasts and other mononuclear cells (according to the sample) and to exclude neutrophils, eosinophils, basophils and erythrocytes. Methods include density gradient centrifugation with Ficoll-Triosil, Hypaque or Lymphoprep*. The method with Lymphoprep is described below. When necessary, platelets can also be excluded by defibrinating the blood before separation.

Method

Dilute 10 ml of the anticoagulated (e.g. hepa-rinized) blood with an equal volume of 9 g/l

*Nyegaard, Oslo

NaCl (saline). Add the diluted blood drop by drop to 7.5 ml of Lymphoprep and then centri-fuge at $400g$ for 30 min. The MN layer separates from the upper plasma layer and from the red cells and neutrophils (which settle to the bottom of the tube). After separation, take up the MN cell layer into another tube and wash three times with TC 199.

METHODOLOGY FOR THE STUDY OF CELL MARKERS

There are several ways of testing cell markers:

1. In suspensions of viable cells;
2. In cells on cytospin-made slides, or directly using blood or bone-marrow films (immunocytochemistry);
3. In cells in frozen sections of bone marrow or other haemopoietic tissues (immunohistochemistry);
4. In sections of paraffin embedded bone-marrow biopsies or other tissues (immunohistochemistry).

Tests on cell suspensions will only detect membrane antigens while tests on fixed cells will often detect cytoplasmic as well as membrane antigens. Some antigens are expressed first in the cytoplasm of early blasts, e.g. CD3 in early T-cells, CD22 in early B-cells and CD13 in early myeloid cells, and only later on the surface of the cell membrane. Thus tests for markers may be negative when tested on cell suspensions but positive on fixed cells. By fixing cells in sus-pension in 4% p-formaldehyde and using 0.5%

Table 9.4 Immunological classification of ALL

Reactivity against	Marker*	B-lineage**				T-lineage***	
		Early B	cALL	pre-B	B-ALL	pre-T	T-ALL
Precursor cells	HLA-Dr	+	+	+	+	– or ±	–
	TdT	+	+	+	– or ±	+	+
	CD34	+	+	+	–	–	–
B-cell antigens	CD19	+	+	+	+	–	–
	CD22-Cyt	+	+	+	+	–	–
	CD10	–	+	+	– to +	– to +	–
	Cyt μ chain	–	–	+	+@	–	–
T-cell antigens	CD7	–	–	–	–	+	+
	CD3-Cyt	–	–	–	–	+	+
	CD5	–	–	–	–	– to +	+
	CD2	–	–	–	–	–	+
Incidence in children		10%	60%	15%	1%	4%	10%

*Given according to cluster of differentiation (CD) number. The McAbs are listed according to the sequential order in which the corresponding antigens are first expressed in cells of the B- and T-lineages.
**All cases show rearrangement of the Ig heavy chain gene.
***All cases show rearrangement of the T-cell receptor ß and/or γ and/ or δ chain genes
Cyt: Cytoplasmic; negative by membrane staining (in cell suspension).
@ Immunoglobulin heavy and light chain positive in the membrane in B-ALL blasts (L3).

Tween to lyse the membrane it is possible now to detect nuclear and cytoplasmic antigens by flow cytometry with cells still in suspension.

Cells in suspension can be tested by rosetting methods or by staining directly (1 layer) or indirectly (2 or more layers) with antibodies labelled with fluorescent dyes (immunofluorescence, IF). IF labelling is detected using fluorescence microscopes equipped with ultraviolet light or by flow cytometers, like FACS* or EPICS**, which are equipped with a laser source of illumination.[43] Fixed cells can be studied also by direct or indirect IF, or more frequently by peroxidase or alkaline phosphatase labelled reagents.[29,55] The latter methods do not require special microscopy equipment and provide permanent preparations.

ROSETTE TESTS

These are based on the affinity of red cells (RBC) to bind specifically to membrane receptors. This binding can be demonstrated with the RBC of various species (sheep, mouse, ox, etc.) which form rosettes with various types of lymphocytes. There are two types of rosette, immune and spontaneous, depending on whether the RBC are or are not coated by Ig molecules.

Immune rosettes are used to demonstrate receptors for the Fc part of IgG (Fc γ) or IgM (Fc μ) in B- and T-lymphocytes and can also be used to test McAbs. Human RBC (Rh positive) coated with anti-D can also be used to detect high affinity Fc receptors in monocytes.

The formation of sheep red blood cell rosettes (E-rosettes) and mouse red blood cell rosettes (M-rosettes) were described in earlier editions of

Table 9.5 Markers in mature T-cell leukaemias*

Marker (McAb)	LGLL	T-PLL	ATLL	Sézary
CD2	++	++	++	+
CD3	++	++	++	++
CD4	–	+ + to –	++	++
CD5	– to +	++	++	++
CD7	–	++	–	–
CD8	++	+ to –	–	–
CD11b	– to +	–	–	–
CD56/57	– to +	–	–	–
CD16	– to +	–	–	–
CD25	–	–	++	– to +

*All cases TdT –, CD1a –; B-markers (–); HLA-Dr may be positive in some cases.
LGL, large granular lymphocyte leukaemia.

*Becton Dickinson.
**Coulter.

this book. Nowadays, the E-rosette receptor is detected by monoclonal antibodies (McAbs) of the CD2 group. There is no equivalent McAb against the M-rosette receptor, but there are several reagents which fulfil the diagnostic potential of this test in B-cell CLL.

IMMUNOFLUORESCENCE TESTS

In general, to detect cellular antigens, antibodies conjugated with fluorescein *iso*-thiocyanate (FITC) or tetra-ethylrhodamine *iso*-thiocyanate (TRITC) are used. For details of the methods used to demonstrate antigens in immature haemopoietic cells and some blast cells, e.g. the common-ALL antigen, see Janossy[43] and Mason and Erber.[55] A method for SmIg is described below. Most mature B-cells fluoresce with anti-SmIg sera (Table 9.6). In the B-lymphoproliferative disorders, the degree of positivity (intensity of immunofluorescence) can help to distinguish the various conditions.

While the presence of SmIg is looked for with viable cells in suspension, CyIg (cytoplasmic immunoglobulin) is looked for in cells fixed on a slide, usually prepared by means of a cytocentrifuge (Cytospin). A good fluorescence microscope equipped with incident illumination and an appropriate filter system is essential. Currently, many laboratories are equipped with flow cytometers which facilitate the reading and allow more objective assessment of fluorescence intensity.

DEMONSTRATION OF SURFACE MEMBRANE IMMUNOGLOBULINS (SmIg) BY FLUORESCENT ANTIBODY STAINING

Reagents

Acetate buffered saline, pH 5.5. Add 8.8 ml of 0.2 mol/l (12 ml/l) glacial acetic acid to 41.2 ml of 0.2 mol/l (16.4 g/l) anhydrous sodium acetate and make the volume up to 200 ml with water. To each 200 ml add 1.8 g of NaCl and 0.2 g of anhydrous $CaCl_2$. Store in 10-ml volumes at $-20°$ C.

Phosphate buffered saline (PBS). pH 7.4. See p. 579.

Azide. 0.2% sodium azide in PBS. This solution will keep for up to 1 month at 4°C without loss of potency.

Fluorescent antibodies. Preferably, use $F(ab)_2$ reagents, i.e. antibodies which have been treated with papain to destroy the Fc region. Such treatment leaves the $F(ab)_2$ antigen-binding fragment intact. This is essential when using rabbit antisera, although it may not be necessary with goat or sheep immunoglobulins.

Pipettes. Use Eppendorf-type pipettes (e.g. Oxford sampler system) and tips and plastic tubes throughout the test.

Method

Wash the separated lymphocytes in 9 g/l NaCl (saline), and resuspend in acetate buffered saline, e.g. 0.2 ml of cell suspension (containing $1–2 \times 10^6$

Table 9.6 Markers in chronic B-cell leukaemias and lymphomas*

Markers	B-CLL	B-PLL	NHL*	HCL	PCL**
M-rosettes	++	−	− to +	− to +	−
SmIg (intensity)	±	++	++	++	−
CD23	++	− to +	− to +	−	−
CD19/CD20 } CD24/CD37 }	++	++	++	++	−
CD5	++	− to +	− to +	−	−
CD10	−	−	+ to −	−	− to +
CD22/FMC7	− to +	++	++	++	−
CD25/CD11c	−	−	−	++	−
anti-HC2	−	−	−	++	−
CD38	−	−	−	−	++

*Non-Hodgkin's lymphomas: included here are disorders which often evolve into a leukaemia phase: follicular lymphoma (FL), mantle-cell NHL and splenic lymphoma with circulating villous lymphocytes (SLVL). In general all these have similar markers except that FL cells are usually CD5−, CD10+ and mantle-cell lymphoma cells are CD5+, CD10−.
**Plasma cell leukaemia B-cells lose B-cell antigens at the plasma cell stage, but express strongly CyIg.

cells) in 2 ml of buffer. Incubate the mixture at 37° C for 15 min.

Wash the cells twice in PBS and then incubate the deposited cells in 5 ml of TC 199 at 37°C for 1 h to remove cytophilic antibodies.

Centrifuge the cells, remove the supernatant and resuspend the cells in 0.2 ml of the azide solution. (The cell concentration should be $10–15 \times 10^6$/ml.)

Add 0.2 ml of diluted (usually 1 in 20) anti-Ig fluorescent conjugated antiserum. Mix the cell suspension well and allow to stand at 4°C or (preferably) in crushed ice for 30 min. Then top up the tube containing the cell suspension with TC 199 and centrifuge for 5 min at 40*g* (to remove unbound conjugates). Discard the supernatant and wash the deposited cells twice in PBS.

Remove the supernatant and add to the deposited cells 1 drop of a mixture of equal volumes of PBS and glycerol*. Resuspend the cells and place 1 drop on a slide; cover with a cover-slip and seal with nail varnish.

Examine under the fluorescence microscope.

TERMINAL TRANSFERASE (TdT)

This remarkable DNA polymerase can be demonstrated by a biochemical assay but is usually now demonstrated by an immunofluorescence test.[13,43] Both these methods give similar results[13,25] but the demonstration of TdT in cell nuclei by immunofluorescence or by the APAAP method[29,55] is to be preferred because of its simplicity and sensitivity to low numbers of cells. As shown in Table 9.4, tests for TdT are positive in all types of ALL with the exception of the rare B-ALL. It should be noted that 15–30% of cases of AML, particularly immature forms, may show TdT activity.[18,44,62] By combining TdT with other lymphoid markers (B or T) the majority of cases of ALL can be diagnosed confidently. If the tests for the common ALL antigen (CD10) and TdT are positive the likelihood of a case being AML is low. In our experience two sorts of AML cases may show TdT activity: in biphenotypic ALL/AML cases the test for TdT is positive in blasts[18] and in 30–50% of AML cases of M1 (peroxidase positive) and M0 (peroxidase negative) TdT activity persists in myeloblasts.

Three other situations in which the TdT assay gives useful information are:

1. In blast crisis of CGL, in which the TdT test is almost always positive in the lymphoblastic type of transformation (20% of cases).

2. In T-lymphoblastic lymphoma, which is the only non-Hodgkin's lymphoma with positive TdT activity.[13]

3. In the chronic (mature) T-cell proliferations (Table 9.5), in which TdT activity is always absent, contrasting with the positive findings in acute (immature) T-cell proliferations (T-ALL, pre-T-ALL and T-lymphoblastic lymphoma).[43]

SLIDE ASSAY FOR TERMINAL DEOXYNUCLEOTIDYL TRANSFERASE (TdT)

Reagents

*Anti-TdT***. For use, dilute 1 in 10 in phosphate buffered saline (PBS), pH 7.4 (p. 579).

Fluorescent-conjugated (FITC) goat anti-rabbit Ig serum. For use, dilute 1 in 10 in phosphate buffered saline. (Rhodamine-conjugated antibodies and porcine anti-rabbit Ig may be used instead of the goat antiserum.)

Mounting medium. Glycerol 48 ml, PBS 48 ml, formalin 4 ml.

Method

Make cytocentrifuge (Cytospin) preparations, using 250 µl of a 1×10^6/ml cell suspension per slide. Centrifuge for 1 min at 300 rpm (*c* 7*g*) and allow the film to dry in the air. Ring the deposited cells with a wax pencil.

Such slides may be stored at room temperature for up to a week but it is preferable to carry out the test as soon as possible.

Fix the film in methanol for 15 min at 4°C. Then wash in PBS for 10 min in a jar provided

---

*To reduce fading during examination the following alternative mixture has been recommended.[45] Add 10 ml of PBS containing 10 mg of *p*-phenylenediamine to 90 ml of glycerol. Adjust the pH to 8.0 with 0.5 mol/1 carbonate bicarbonate buffer, pH 9.0.
**This can be purchased from Bethesda Research Laboratories In. (USA) or Sera Lab (UK).

with a magnetic stirrer. Wipe off the excess PBS around the ring of cells and cover the ring with 10 μl of the diluted anti-TdT serum. Leave for 10 min at room temperature in a moist chamber.

Wash the slides in PBS for a further 15 min using a magnetic stirrer as before.

Wipe off the excess PBS around the ring of cells and cover the cells with 10 μl of the diluted fluorescent-conjugated anti-rabbit Ig serum. Allow to stand for 30 min at room temperature in a moist chamber.

Wash the slide in PBS for 15 min at room temperature, as before; then cover the ring of cells with a cover-glass, using as mountant the glycerol/PBS/formalin mixture.

Examine under the fluorescence microscope. A positive reaction is denoted by nuclear fluorescence. Using the appropriate filters, this will be bright yellow with fluorescein conjugation and bright red with rhodamine conjugation.

The APAAP method[55] appears to be more sensitive than the immunofluorescence test described above. Therefore a higher percentage of cases of AML may be found to be TdT positive.[18] Currently it is possible to detect nuclear TdT by flow cytometry methodology and to combine TdT with the detection of membrane or cytoplasmic antigens (Fig. 9.7).

Controls

Negative. Carry out the test leaving out the anti-TdT and also on cells known not to react (e.g. B-CLL cells).

Positive. Use a common-ALL cell line (e.g. NALM-1) or cells from a patient with known common-ALL who is not in remission

MONOCLONAL ANTIBODIES (McAbs)

A significant development in the last decade has been the possibility of producing antibodies of great purity by means of the hybridoma technology. A great number of reagents reactive with antigens present on haemopoietic cells are now available. Their major applications have been in defining the stages of T- and B-cell differentiation, from early T- and B-cells to mature (peripheral-blood) lymphocytes. The order of appearance of antigens (on the cell membrane unless specified) in the T-cell lineage is as follows: CD3 (cytoplasm), CD7, CD5, CD2 (E-rosette receptor), CD1a (cortical thymocyte antigen), CD4, CD8 and CD3 (membrane).[43,64] Equivalent findings in the B-cell lineage are as follows: CD19, CD22 (cytoplasm), CD24, CyIg (μ chain only), CD10, CD20, M-rosette receptor, SmIg (heavy and light chains), CD22 (membrane) and FMC7.[34,43,58] When applied to the diagnosis of acute lymphoblastic leukaemia (ALL) of B- and T-cell lineage (Table 9.4), the combined findings with McAbs characterize certain types of ALL and also indicate both the direction (B or T) and the stage of differentiation of the lympho-blasts. For example, the presence of the common-ALL antigen, a glycoprotein of 100 kD demonstrable by McAb of the CD10 group[34,43] is used to define common-ALL (Fig. 9.7). On the other hand, the presence of the antigen demonstrable by CD1a characterizes cortical thymocytes and the cells of T-lymphoblastic lymphoma which arise from that particular stage of thymic maturation.

Recently it has been possible to develop McAbs with specificity for myeloid cells which are useful for the study of early AML. Thus, early myeloid antigens are characterized by McAbs of the CD13[28,31,35] and CD33[28,31] groups (Table 9.7, Fig. 9.8). In addition, McAbs with specificity for platelet glycoproteins[77] are used to characterize megakaryoblasts and other platelet-precursor cells.[27]

Instructions for using McAbs are usually provided by the manufacturers. The antigens are demonstrated by direct or indirect IF (fluorescence microscopy or flow cytometry) or by staining fixed cells by the immunoperoxidase (IP)[28] or alkaline phosphatase anti-alkaline phosphatase

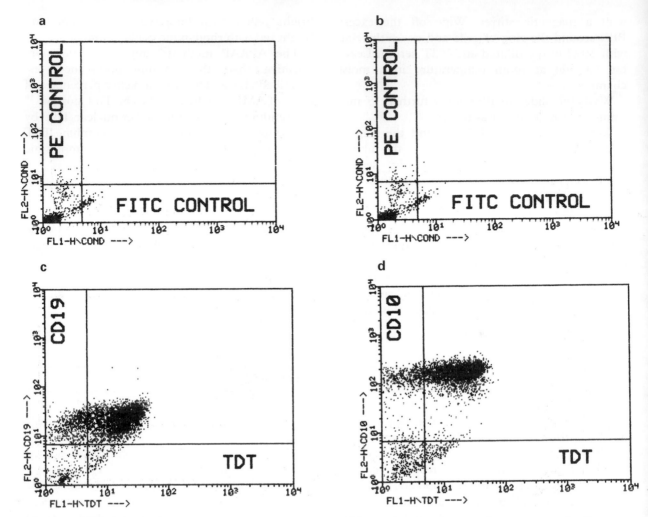

Fig. 9.7　FACS scan analysis of a case of common-ALL (TdT+, CD10+, CD19+). (a, b) The isotypic controls using the fluorescence reagents fluorescein (FITC) and phycoerythrin (PE). (c) Co-expression of TdT and CD19 using directly labelled antibodies. (d) Co-expression of TdT and CD10 (cALL antigen).

Table 9.7　Cell markers in AML

McAb	M0*	M1	M2/M3	M4/M5	M6	M7
CD34	+	+	± to −	± to −	−	±
CD13**	+	+	+	+	+	+
CD33	±	+	+	+	±	+
CD11b	−	−	+	±	−	−
CD14	−	−	−	+	−	−
Anti-MPO[17]	− to +	+	+	+	±	−
Glycoph/Gero	−	−	−	−	+	−
CDw41/42	−	−	−	−	−	+
TdT***	− to +	− to +	−	−	−	−

*Minimally differentiated myeloblastic leukaemia with negative light microscopy cytochemistry for AML, absence of lymphoid antigens, and positive peroxidase by electron microscopy.
**More sensitive when tested on fixed cells (cytoplasmic expression).[28]
***Positive in up to 50% of M0 and M1 cases, and in less than 10% in other types (M2 to M7).[62]

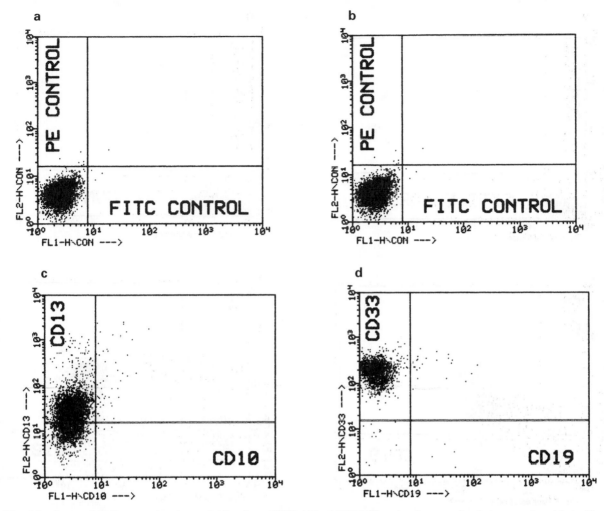

Fig. 9.8 A case of AML expressing the myeloid antigens CD13 (c) and CD33 (d) and at the same time being negative with the B-lineage markers CD10 (c) and CD19 (d) using double fluorescence staining with PE and FITC; isotypic controls in (a) and (b).

(APAAP)[29,55] methods. The APAAP method is suitable for use on blood and bone-marrow films and allows good preservation of cell morphology. The IF methods are quicker and simpler and flow cytometry allows rapid and accurate counting of thousands of cells. Directly labelled McAbs can be used in the FACS system to demonstrate co-expression of two antigens on the same cell (Figs 9.7–9.9). The McAb, a mouse antibody of IgG or IgM class, is used as the first layer, the second layer is an FITC or TRIC conjugated anti-mouse Ig, prepared in goats or rabbits. The use of $F(ab_2)$ fragments of antibody in the second layer is recommended in order to

prevent non-specific binding of the Fc portion of the Ig molecule to high affinity Fc receptors. When testing myeloid cells it is also important to block non-specific binding of the Fc portion of the McAb (first layer) by pre-incubation of the cells in 0.5% of human AB serum.[28,56] The method we use for the demonstration of membrane antigens by IF with McAb is given below.

METHOD FOR DEMONSTRATION OF McAb ON CELL SUSPENSIONS BY IF

1. Isolate mononuclear cells using Lymphoprep (see p. 159).

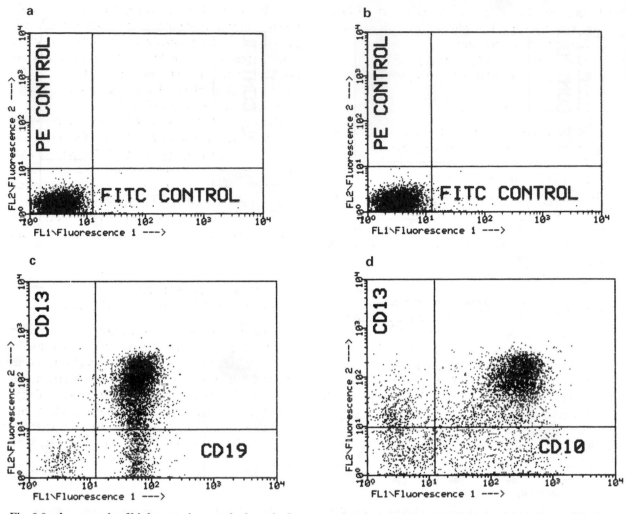

Fig. 9.9   An example of biphenotypic acute leukaemia demonstrating the co-expression of the myeloid antigen (CD13) and lymphoid antigens (CD19 and CD10) on the same cells. (a, b) Isotypic controls; (c) CD13+ and CD19+ (right upper quadrant); (d) CD13+, CD10+ (right upper quadrant). In (d) it is possible to see those blasts which are only CD10+ (right lower quadrant) and others which are only CD13+ (left upper quadrant).

2. Wash twice in phosphate buffer saline (PBS) (p. 579) or Hanks solution.

3. Remove all supernatant.

4. Resuspend the cells in the buffer: PBS containing 0.2% sodium azide (azide) and 0.2% bovine serum albumin (BSA) or Hanks solution.

5. Place in small tube: 50 μl of cells (total 2×10^6); add first layer of McAb (the amount varies with each McAb)*.

6. Keep for 30 min at 4°C or 10 min at room temperature (c 20°C).

7. Wash twice in PBS-azide-BSA (see 4 above).

8. Remove all supernatant.

9. Add 50 μl of PBS-azide-BSA and as second layer 50 μl of FITC $F(ab_2)$ fragment of goat antimouse IgG**.

---

*McAb-Mouse Ig against specific antigenic determinants. The amount of McAb to be used will depend on the reagent tested.
**The reagent for the second layer is usually conjugated with fluorescein (FITC); rhodamine (TRITC) labelled antibodies may, however, also be used. The use of $F(ab_2)$ fragments, as opposed to whole antibody molecules, is to prevent non-specific binding of the second layer to cells with high affinity Fc receptors (e.g. monocytes), thus resulting in a false positive test which could be detected by a positive control when the McAb (first layer) is omitted.

10 Keep for 30 min at 4°C or 10 min at *c* 20°C.
11. Wash twice in PBS-azide-BSA.
12. Remove all supernatant.
13. Add 1 drop of PBS/glycerol (50:50).
14. Mount on glass slide and cover with cover-slip.
15. Seal with nail varnish.

For the analysis by flow cytometry the cells are kept in suspension, usually resuspended in Isoton II (Coulter), and read according to the manufacturer's recommended specifications.

It is important to set up a control with the McAb and preferably also with mouse ascitic fluid (without antibody activity against human antigens) of the same Ig isotype as that of the McAb used.

TESTS ON FIXED CELLS

Ig, McAb and TdT can be stained for on fixed cells by immunocytochemical methods. Those most commonly used are the immunoperoxidase (IP)[28] and the APAAP techniques.[29,55] They are more elaborate and slower than IF on cell suspensions but have, on the other hand, several practical advantages. Films (Cytospin or hand-spread) can be stored unfixed at -20°C (the slides being covered in foil) and the tests can be performed in batches immediately or days or even weeks after the sample is obtained, if that is required. They also provide permanent preparations and allow good comparison with the equivalent film stained with May-Grünwald-Giemsa. Thus with mixed preparations of cells, e.g. blasts and normal cells, it is possible to identify which cells are positive or negative.

IP is simpler than APAAP and is useful for the study of lymphoid cells (mature and immature) but it may present problems when studying bone-marrow samples that contain myeloid cells with endogenous peroxidase, which may give a false positive reaction unless precautions to inhibit its activity are taken. These measures often affect cell morphology and thus defeat one of the purposes of the test. The IP method can be carried out with directly labelled antibodies (e.g. anti-human Ig) or more often by indirect methods using two or three layers. The first layer is a McAb (mouse Ig); the second layer is an anti-mouse Ig antibody conjugated with horse-radish peroxidase; a third layer, a complex of peroxidase anti-peroxidase which binds to the second layer, can be used to reinforce the reaction. The reaction is completed by testing for peroxidase using diaminobenzidine (DAB).

The APAAP method involves several steps but the end results are quite satisfactory for peripheral blood and bone-marrow films. The stages include: incubation with the McAb, incubation with a rabbit anti-mouse Ig, and incubation with immune complexes of alkaline phosphatase and anti-alkaline phosphatase (APAAP). The second and third steps can be repeated to reinforce the reaction.

THE IMMUNOLOGICAL CLASSIFICATION OF LEUKAEMIA

The use of immunological methods, in particular McAbs, has improved the possibility of classifying more objectively the acute leukaemias in which the cells are too poorly differentiated to be characterized by morphology and cytochemistry. It has also enabled the lymphoproliferative disorders to be classified more precisely because B- and T-cells and their subsets can be defined by marker studies.

ALL

The immunological classification of ALL is summarized in Table 9.4. It is important to remember that some antigens appear first in the cytoplasm (CD3 in T-blasts and CD22 in B-lineage blasts) and will not be detected when testing the cells in suspension. Similarly, in early myeloid cells CD13 is expressed first in the cytoplasm before the membrane.[28]

There are two major lineages in the lymphoid system and lymphoblastic leukaemias will therefore arise from early B- or T-precursor cells. Table 9.4 illustrates that only a few McAbs react positively with the most immature lymphoblasts; with maturation, however, more McAbs react. Thus to demonstrate all cases of a particular lineage it is important to include in the battery of McAbs used those which will detect the most immature cells. In B-lineage ALL these are CD19 and CD22 (cytoplasmic), in T-lineage ALL they are CD7 and CD3 (cytoplasmic) and with myeloid cells CD13 (cytoplasmic) and CD33. The expression of the antigens reacting with the two anti-myeloid reagents often correlates with the expression of myeloperoxidase detectable at the ultrastructural level.[17,56] Several reagents are particularly needed in cases with mixed lymphoblastic and myeloblastic proliferations and in the so-called biphenotypic acute leukaemias in which antigens denoting one lineage are found in the cells of another (Fig. 9.9). Both types of apparent lineage infidelity may represent the proliferation of multipotent stem cells[18,33] with potential for differentiation in several directions.

T-cell leukaemias (Tables 9.3 and 9.5)

Proliferating mature T-lymphocytes are always TdT and CD1a negative. Cells with these characteristics are found in large granular lymphocyte leukaemia, in T-PLL (prolymphocytes) and with so-called leukaemia-lymphoma syndromes like Sézary syndrome and adult leukaemia/lymphoma (ATLI), a disorder associated with the human retrovirus HTLV-1. These disorders share common antigens (markers), but there are differences that can be exploited for differential diagnosis.

B-cell leukaemias (Table 9.6)

The malignant proliferations of mature (differentiated) B-lymphocytes are the chronic B-cell leukaemias: B-CLL, B-PLL and HCL and non-Hodgkin lymphomas (NHL) which often evolve with peripheral blood and/or bone marrow involvement (leukaemic phase). As stated above, the membrane phenotype of B-CLL is different from that of the other B-cell disorders and this facilitates the more precise characterization of this disease which is the most common form of leukaemia in adults over the age of 50 years. The immunophenotype of CLL is unique within the B-cell leukaemias: CD5+, CD23+, weak SmIg and CD22 (membrane) and negative FMC7.

AML (Table 9.7)

In recent years a number of McAbs with specificity for myeloid cells have become available, namely, CD13,[28] CD33[35] and anti-MPO.[17] When used in combination with some of the lymphoid markers (to exclude ALL), they show a pattern which may be characteristic of some types of AML and which may complement the FAB classification. For example antibodies to glycophorin A or the Gerbich blood group (McAb Ge) help to characterize the immature erythroblasts of M6; and McAbs against platelet glycoproteins[77] are useful for the diagnosis of M7 (megakaryoblastic) leukaemia and megakaryoblastic blast crisis in CGL. CD34 reacts with early precursor cells, the antigen being expressed in immature AML (M0, MI) and B-lineage but not T-lineage ALL.

In general, it is not necessary to apply all the tests suggested in Tables 9.4 to 9.7, but it is useful to select combinations of three reagents which are useful for immature B-cells (CD19, CD10, CD22), T-cells (CD7, CD3 cyt., CD2), mature T-cells (CD3, CD4, CD8), mature B-cells (SmIg, CD20, CD37) and, depending on the findings, to extend the number of tests as required, according to the diagnostic problem.

DEMONSTRATION OF CHROMOSOMES

The demonstration of human chromosome abnormalities has become a subject of increasing importance in clinical haematology. Description of how to obtain adequate mitosis and of the various methods of chromosome banding (Q: quinacrine mustard; G: Giemsa stain; R: reverse banding pattern) are beyond the scope of this book. Details can be found in the references at the end of this chapter.[68,76,80,83]

For analysis, chromosomes are usually studied in mitoses arrested at metaphase by the addition of colchicine, demecolcine or vinblastine. Bone-marrow aspirates provide the best material for study in cases of leukaemia; peripheral blood may be adequate when the leucocyte count is very high, particularly in CGL. Blood lymphocytes should be studied simultaneously to define the normal constitutional karyotype. This is done by short-term culture with the mitogen phyto-haemagglutinin (PHA).

Since the discovery of the Philadelphia (Ph) chromosome, due to the translocation of material from the long arm (q) of chromosome 22 (22q–) to the long arm of chromosomes 9 (9q+), known also as t(9;22), numerous haemopoietic malignancies have been found to be associated with specific abnormalities. These are summarized in Table 9.8.

The abnormalities in a karyotype may be numerical, e.g. trisomy (an extra chromosome) or monosomy (only one chromosome of the pair), or structural. The modal number of chromosomes, 46 in man, may be less than 46 (hypodiploid) or more than 46 (hyperdiploid).

For example, a hyperdiploid karyotype (47 chromosomes or more) is seen in 23% of children with ALL.[78,80] A modal chromosome number greater than 50 is associated with the best prognosis in childhood ALL.[80]

Marker chromosomes are structurally abnormal chromosomes in banded or unbanded karyotypes. When the banding pattern can be recognized it should be described by the standard nomenclature.[65] Non-random abnormalities refer to consistent changes seen in a particular cell population which are unlikely to have occurred by chance. A clone refers to a population of cells, presumably derived from a single progenitor cell, which is characterized by the same marker chromosome(s).

The karyotype of the bone-marrow cells of a particular leukaemia (e.g. AML) may show that all the metaphases are abnormal (AA), or that some are normal and others abnormal (AN), or that all the metaphases are normal (NN). AA suggests that no normal cells are present and has

Table 9.8   Non-random* acquired+ chromosome abnormalities in haemopoietic malignancies[31,69,70,78,80,85]

Disease	Abnormality
I. Acute leukaemia	
(i) ALL	
B-lineage	t(9;22)**; t(4;11); 6q –; t(1;19)
Burkitt type (L3, B-ALL)	t(8;14); t(2;8); t(8;22)
T-lineage	t or del (9); t(11;14) 6q–
(ii) AML	+8
M2	t(8;21)
M3 and M3-variant	T(15;17)
M4***	inv or del (16q)
M5	t or del (11q)
M2 with basophilia	t(6;9)
II. Chronic leukaemias/NHL	
(i) Lymphoid	
B-CLL	+12; 13q–
B-PLL	t(11;14)
Follicular NHL	t(14;18)
Mantle cell NHL	t(11;14)
T-PLL	inv (14q)
(ii) CGL	t(9;22)
Blast crisis	iso(17); +8; +9
III. MDS/RAEB****	–5,5q–, –7,7q–

*Present in the majority of the abnormal metaphases.
+ Present in the leukaemic cell population but not in normal cells (e.g. T-lymphocytes, fibroblasts, etc.).
**Ph[1] + ALL.
***Myelomonocytic leukaemia with bone marrow eosinophilia (10%).
****Refractory anaemia with excess of blasts.
t: translocation; del: deletions; inv: inversions.

usually a bad prognosis.[68,70] AN represents a mixture of normal and leukaemic cells; recent studies suggest that examination of mitotic figures after 24–48 h culture may yield more abnormal metaphases compared with direct preparations of the same material.[84] NN indicates that there are no gross abnormalities; this might mean that the method is insensitive or that only the karyotype of normal cells is being analysed rather than that of the leukaemic population.

The more sensitive techniques for the study of human chromosomes (long chromosomes, prometaphase banding) that are now becoming available may be expected to provide more information. For example, finely banded chromosome preparations can be obtained by high-resolution techniques, in particular those using culture techniques, and cell synchronization with amethopterin.

Abnormalities in the chronic lymphoid leukaemias can be obtained by stimulating the cells with specific (B or T) mitogens or non-specific mitogens (e.g. phorbol ester TPA). Peripheral blood samples from patients with these leukaemias are usually sufficient to document abnormalities. In the acute leukaemias the material of choice is bone marrow.

Major technical advances are taking place in this field. One is the availability of image analysis equipment, e.g. Cytoscan, that facilitates the documentation of abnormalities in leukaemia. Second, the technique of fluorescence in-situ hybridization (FISH) which, using specific probes, enables one to detect changes in chromosome numbers and to clarify complex translocations.

NUCLEAR SEXING OF LEUCOCYTES

Sex chromosome anomalies are not uncommon and they can usually be identified readily by nuclear sexing. Buccal mucosa is the material usually examined but in experienced hands valuable information can also be gained by inspection of the neutrophil leucocytes. The feature to be identified is a nuclear appendage, the drumstick, which is present in a proportion of the neutrophils of normal females but not of normal males. The drumstick represents one X chromosome and is equivalent to the single Barr body which may be seen in normal (XX) female cell nuclei.

METHOD

Make blood films, stain them and cover with a cover-glass in the usual way. They scan them systematically with an oil-immersion lens for drumsticks of the correct size and staining quality. The use of a micrometer ocular may be necessary to measure the drumsticks.

The drumsticks are pedunculated nuclear appendages, with a spherical or oval head of between 1.4 and 1.6 μm in diameter, formed of densely staining chromatin attached by a thread-like neck to the rest of the nucleus (Fig. 9.10). Very often a small space or chink can be seen in the chromatin of the head of the drumstick. These sex drumsticks have to be distinguished from non-specific nodules which may be of smaller or larger size, irregular in shape, and sometimes deficient in chromatin. Sessile chromatin sex nodules of the same size as drumsticks may also be seen; they stain densely and project by more than half their diameter beyond the nuclear membrane (Fig. 9.10). They also occur only in females, but they are less easily distinguished from other non-specific nodules and appendages which have no diagnostic significance.

As a screening test, scrutinize at least 50 neutrophils for drumsticks (and sessile nodules). In females, three or more definite sessile nodules and one or more drumsticks are usually seen in the first 50 cells. On the other hand, in males no drumsticks and no definite sessile nodules should be seen. If there is any doubt, examine further cells, and if at least two definite drumsticks and

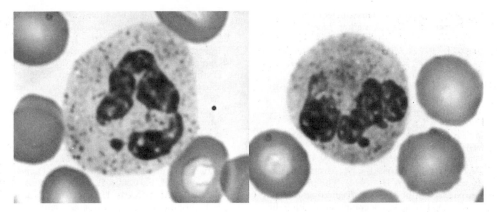

Fig. 9.10   Nuclear sexing of neutrophils. Photomicrographs of neutrophils showing female sex appendages. The left-hand cell has a 'drumstick'; the right-hand cell has a sessile nodule.

accompanying sessile nodules are identified in the first 500 cells, it can reliably be assumed that the cells are chromatin-positive and the subject female (XX). Usually at least six definite drumsticks are found in less than 200 neutrophils. If neither drumsticks nor sessile nodules are seen in the first 200 neutrophils, the cells can be regarded as chromatin-negative and the subject male (XY) or XO. When there is a shift to the left in the segmentation of the neutrophil nuclei it is more difficult to arrive at a clear-cut answer, and it may be necessary to examine many more cells.

REFERENCES

1 BAIN, B. J., CATOVSKY, D., O'BRIEN, M., PRENTICE, H. G., LAWLOR, E., KUMARAN, T. O., McCANN, S. R., MATUTES, E. and GALTON, D. A. G. (1981). Megakaryoblastic leukemia presenting as acute myelofibrosis. A study of four cases with the platelet-peroxidase reaction. *Blood*, **58**, 206.

2 BAIN, B., MATUTES, E., ROBINSON, D., LAMPERT, I. A, BRITO-BABAPULLE, V., MORILLA, R. and CATOVSKY, D. (1991). Leukaemia as a manifestation of large cell lymphoma. *British Journal of Haematology*, **77**, 301.

3 BAINTON, D. F., ULLVOT, J. L. and FARQUHAR, M. G. (1971). The development of neutrophilic polymorphonuclear leukocytes in human bone marrow. *Journal of Experimental Medicine*, **134**, 907.

4 BASSO, G., COCITO, M. G., POLETTI, A., MESSINA, C., COLLESELLI, P. and ZANESCO, L. (1980). Study of cytochemical markers ACP and ANAE in childhood lymphoma and leukaemia. *British Journal of Cancer*, **41**, 835.

5 BENAVIDES, I. and CATOVSKY, D. (1978). Myeloperoxidase cytochemistry using 2,7-fluorenediamine. *Journal of Clinical Pathology*, **31**, 1114.

6 BENNETT, J. M., CATOVSKY, D., DANIEL, M. T., FLANDRIN, G., GALTON, D. A. G., GRALNICK, H. R. and SULTAN, C. (1976). Proposals for the classification of the acute leukaemias. *British Journal of Haematology*, **33**, 451.

7 BENNETT, J. M., CATOVSKY, D., DANIEL, M. T., FLANDRIN, G., GALTON, D. A. G., GRALNICK, H. R. and SULTAN, C. (1981). The morphological classification of acute lymphoblastic leukaemia — concordance among observers and clinical correlations. *British Journal of Haematology*, **47**, 553.

8 BENNETT, J. M., CATOVSKY, D., DANIEL, M. T., FLANDRIN, G., GALTON, D. A. G., GRALNICK, H. R. and SULTAN, C. (1982). Proposals for the classification of the myelodysplastic syndromes. *British Journal of Haematology*, **51**, 189.

9 BENNETT, J. M., CATOVSKY, D., DANIEL, M. T., FLANDRIN, G., GALTON, D. A. G., GRALNICK, H. R. and SULTAN, C. (1985). Proposed revised criteria for the classification of acute myeloid leukemia. *Annals of Internal Medicine*, **103**, 620.

10 BENNETT, J. M., CATOVSKY, D., DANIEL, M. T., FLANDRIN, G., GALTON, D. A. G., GRALNICK, H. R. and SULTAN, C. (1985). Criteria for the diagnosis of acute leukemia of megakaryocyte lineage (M7). A report of the French–American–British Cooperative Group. *Annals of Internal Medicine*, **103**, 460.

11 BENNETT, J. M., CATOVSKY, D., DANIEL, M.-T., FLANDRIN, G., GALTON, D. A. G., GRALNICK, H. R. and SULTAN, C. (1989). The French–American–British (FAB) Cooperative Group. Proposals for the classification of chronic (mature) B and T lymphoid leukaemias. *Journal of Clinical Pathology*, **42**, 567.

12 BENNETT, J. M., CATOVSKY, D., DANIEL, M.-T., FLANDRIN, G., GALTON, D. A. G., GRALNICK, H. R. and SULTAN, C. (1991). Proposals for the recognition of minimally differentiated acute myeloid leukaemia (AML-M0). *British Journal of Haematology*, **78**, 325.

[13] BOLLUM, F. J. (1979). Terminal deoxynucleotidyl transferase as a hematopoietic cell marker. *Blood*, **54**, 1203.

[14] BRETON-GORIUS, J. (1991). Ultrastructure of the leukemic cell. In *The Leukemic Cell*. Ed. D. Catovsky, Chap. 4, pp. 91. Churchill Livingstone, Edinburgh.

[15] BRIGGS, R. S., PERILLIE, P. E. and FINCH, S. C. (1966). Lysozyme in bone marrow and peripheral blood cells. *Journal of Histochemistry and Cytochemistry*, **14**, 167.

[16] BRITO-BABAPULLE, F., CATOVSKY, D. and GALTON, D. A. G. (1987). Clinical and laboratory features of de novo acute myeloid leukaemia with trilineage myelodysplasia. *British Journal of Haematology*, **66**, 445.

[17] BUCCHERI, V., SHETTY, V., YOSHIDA, N., MORILLA, R., MATUTES, E. and CATOVSKY, D. (1992). The role of an anti-myeloperoxidase antibody in the diagnosis and classification of acute leukaemia: a comparison with light and electron microscopy cytochemistry. *British Journal of Haematology*, **80**, 62.

[18] BUCCHERI, V., MATUTES, E., DYER, M. J. S. and CATOVSKY, D. (1993). Lineage commitment in biphenotypic leukemia. *Leukemia*, **7**, 919.

[19] CATOVSKY, D., CHERCHI, M., GREAVES, M. F., PAIN, C., JANOSSY, G. and KAY, H. E. M. (1978). The acid phosphatase reaction in acute lymphoblastic leukaemia. *Lancet*, **i**, 749.

[20] CATOVSKY, D., CHERCHI, M., OKOS A., HEGDE, U. and GALTON, D. A. G. (1976). Mouse red cell rosettes in B-lymphoproliferative disorders. *British Journal of Haematology*, **33**, 173

[21] CATOVSKY, D., GALETTO, J., OKOS, A., MILLANI, E. and GALTON, D. A. G. (1974). Cytochemical profile of B and T leukaemic lymphocytes with special reference to acute lymphoblastic leukaemia. *Journal of Clinical Pathology*, **27**, 767.

[22] CATOVSKY, D. and GALTON, D. A. G. (1973). Lysozyme activity and nitroblue-tetrazolium reduction in leukaemic cells. *Journal of Clinical Pathology*, **26**, 60.

[23] CATOVSKY, D., GALTON, D. A. G. and ROBINSON, J. (1972). Myeloperoxidase-deficient neutrophils in acute myeloid leukaemia. *Scandinavian Journal of Haematology*, **9**, 142.

[24] CHERCHI, M. and CATOVSKY, D. (1980). Mouse RBC rosettes in chronic lymphocytic leukaemia — different expression in blood and tissues. *Clinical and Experimental Immunology*, **39**, 411.

[25] CIBULI, M. L., COLEMAN, M. S., NELSON, O., HUTTON, J. J., GORDON, D. and BOLLUM, F. J. (1982). Evaluation of methods of detecting terminal deoxynucleotidyl transferase in human hematologic malignancies. *American Journal of Clinical Pathology*, **77**, 420.

[26] CROCKARD, A. D., CHALMERS, D., MATUTES, E. and CATOVSKY, D. (1982). Cytochemistry of acid hydrolases in chronic B and T cell leukemias. *American Journal of Clinical Pathology*, **78**, 437.

[27] DE OLIVEIRA, M. S. P., GREGORY, C., MATUTES, E., PARREIRA, A. and CATOVSKY, D. (1987). Cytochemical profile of megakaryoblastic leukaemia: a study with cytochemical methods, monoclonal antibodies, and ultrastructural cytochemistry. *Journal of Clinical Pathology* **40**, 663.

[28] DE OLIVEIRA, M. S. P., MATUTES, E., RANI, S., MORILLA, R. and CATOVSKY, D. (1988). Early expression of MCS2 (CD13) in the cytoplasm of blast cells from acute myeloid leukaemia. *Acta Haematologica (Basel)*, **80**, 61.

[29] ERBER, W. N., MYNHEER, L. C. and MASON, D. Y. (1986). APAAP labelling of blood and bone-marrow samples for phenotyping leukaemia. *Lancet*, **i**, 761.

[30] FAIRBANKS, V. F. and LAMPE, L. T. (1968). A tetrazolium-linked cytochemical method for estimation of glucose-6-phosphate dehydrogenase activity in individual erythrocytes: applications in the study of heterozygotes for glucose-6-phosphate dehydrogenase deficiency. *Blood*, **31**, 589.

[31] FIRST MIC COOPERATIVE STUDY GROUP (1986). Morphologic, immunologic and cytogenetic (MIC) working classification of acute lymphoblastic leukemias. *Cancer Genetics and Cytogenetics*, **23**, 189.

[32] GOLDBERG, A. F. and BARKA, T. (1962). Acid phosphatase activity in human blood cells. *Nature (London)*, **195**, 297.

[33] GREAVES, M. F., CHAN, L. C., FURLEY, A. J. W., WATT, S. M. and MOLGAARD, H. V. (1986). Lineage promiscuity in hemopoietic differentiation and leukemia. *Blood*, **67**, 1.

[34] GREAVES, M. F., HARIRI, G., NEWMAN, R. A., SUTHERLAND, D. R., RITTER, M. A. and RITZ, J. (1983). Selective expression of the common acute lymphoblastic leukemia (gp 100) antigen on immature lymphoid cells and their malignant counterparts. *Blood*, **61**, 628.

[35] GRIFFIN, J. D., LINCH, D., SABBATH, K., LARCOM, P. and SCHLOSSMAN, S. F. (1984). A monoclonal antibody reactive with normal and leukaemic human myeloid progenitor cells. *Leukemia Research*, **8**, 521.

[36] HANKER, J. S., AMBROSE, W. W., JAMES, C. J., MANDELKORN, J., YATES, P. E., GALL, S. A., BOSSEN, E. H., FAY, J. W., LAZLO, J. and MOORE, J. O. (1979). Facilitated light microscopic cytochemical diagnosis of acute myelogenous leukemia. *Cancer Research*, **39**, 1635.

[37] HAYHOE, F. G. J. and QUAGLINO, D. (1960). Refractory sideroblastic anaemia and erythraemic myelosis: possible relationship and cytochemical observations. *British Journal of Haematology*, **6**, 381.

[38] HAYHOE, F. G. J. and QUAGLINO, D. (1980). *Haematological Cytochemistry*. Churchill Livingstone, Edinburgh.

[39] HAYHOE, F. G. J., QUAGLINO, D. and DOLL, R. (1964). *The Cytology and Cytochemistry of Acute Leukaemias: A Study of 140 Cases*. Her Majesty's Stationery Office, London.

[40] HAYHOE, F. G. J., QUAGLINO, D. and FLEMANS, R. J. (1960). Consecutive use of Romanowsky and periodic-acid-Schiff techniques in the study of blood and bone-marrow cells. *British Journal of Haematology*, **6**, 23.

[41] HUHN, D., THIEF, E., RODT, H. and ANDREEWA, P. (1981). Cytochemistry and membrane markers in acute lymphatic leukaemia (ALL). *Scandinavian Journal of Haematology*, **26**, 311.

[42] INTERNATIONAL COUNCIL FOR STANDARDIZATION IN HAEMATOLOGY (1993). Recommended procedures for the classification of the leukaemias. *Leukemia and Lymphoma*, **11**, 37.

[43] JANOSSY, G. (1991). Monoclonal antibodies in the diagnosis of acute leukaemia. In *The Leukaemic Cell*. Ed. D. Catovsky, Chap. 6, pp. 168. Churchill Livingstone, Edinburgh.

[44] JANOSSY, G., HOFFBRAND, A. V., GREAVES, M. F., GANESHAGURU, K., PAIN, C., BRADSTOCK, K. F., PRENTICE, W. G., RAY, H. E. M. and LISTER, T. A. (1980). Terminal transferase enzyme assay and immunological membrane markers in the diagnosis of leukaemia — a multiparameter analysis of 300 cases. *British Journal of Haematology*, **44**, 221.

[45] JOHNSON, G. D. and NOQUEIRA ARAUJO, G. M. DE C.

(1981). A simple method of reducing the fading of immunofluorescence during microscopy. *Journal of Immunological Methods*, **43**, 349.

[16] KAMADA, N., DOHY, H., OKADA, K. OGUMA, N., KURAMOTO, A., TANARA, A. and UCHINO, H. (1981). In vivo and in vitro activity of neutrophil alkaline phosphatase in acute myelocytic leukemia with 8;21 translocation. *Blood*, **58**, 1213.

[47] KAPLOW, L. S. (1963). Cytochemistry of leukocyte alkaline phosphatase. Use of complex naphthol AS phosphates in azo dye-coupling technics. *American Journal of Clinical Pathology*, **39**, 439.

[48] KAPLOW, L. S., (1965). Simplified myeloperoxidase stain using benzidine dihydrochloride. *Blood*, **26**, 215.

[49] KAPLOW, L. S. (1968). Leukocyte alkaline phosphatase cytochemistry: applications and methods. *Annals of New York Academy of Sciences*, **155**, 911.

[50] KUNG, P, C., GOLDSTEIN, G., REINHERZ, E. L. and SCHLOSSMAN, S. F. (1979). Monoclonal antibodies defining distinctive human T cell surface antigens. *Science*, **206**, 347.

[51] LENNOX, B. and DAVIDSON, W. M. (1964). Nuclear sexing. *Association of Clinical Pathologists Broadsheet No. 47.*

[52] LEWIS, S. M. and DACIE, J. V. (1965). Neutrophil (leucocyte) alkaline phosphatase in paroxysmal nocturnal haemoglobinuria. *British Journal of Haematology*, **11**, 549.

[53] LI, C, Y., LAM, K. W. and YAM, L. T. (1973). Esterases in human leukocytes. *Journal of Histochemistry and Cytochemistry*, **21**, 1.

[54] LI, C. Y., YAM, L. T. and LAM, K. W. (1970). Acid phosphatase isoenzyme in human leukocytes in normal and pathologic conditions. *Journal of Histochemistry and Cytochemistry*, **8**, 473.

[55] MASON D. Y and ERBER W. N. (1991). Immunocytochemical labeling of leukemia samples with monoclonal antibodies by the APAAP procedure. In *The Leukemic Cell*. Ed. D. Catovsky. Chap. 7, pp. 196. Churchill Livingstone, Edinburgh.

[56] MATUTES, E., DE OLIVEIRA, M. P., FORONI, L., MORILLA, R. and CATOVSKY, D. (1988). The role of ultrastructural cytochemistry and monoclonal antibodies in clarifying the nature of undifferentiated cells in acute leukaemia. *British Journal of Haematology*, **69**, 205.

[57] MOLONEY, W. C., MCPHERSON, K. and FLIEGELMAN, L. (1960). Esterase activity in leukocytes demonstrated by the use of naphthol AS-D chloracetate substrate. *Journal of Histochemistry and Cytochemistry*, **8**, 200.

[58] NADLER, L. M., KORSMEYER, S. J., ANDERSON, K. C., BOYD, A. W., SLAUGHENHOUPT, B., PARK, E., JENSEN, J., CORAL, F., MAYER, B. J., SALLAN, S. E., RITZ, J. and SCHLOSSMAN, S. F. (1984). B cell origin of non T cell acute lymphoblastic leukemia: a model for discrete stages of neoplastic and normal pre B-cell differentiation. *Journal of Clinical Investigation*, **74**, 332.

[59] NICHOLS, B. A., BAINTON, D. F. and FARQUHAR, M. G. (1971). Differentiation of monocytes — origin, nature and fate of their azurophil granules. *Journal of Cell Biology*, **50**, 498.

[60] O'BRIEN, M., CATOVSKY, D. and COSTELLO, C. (1980). Ultrastructural cytochemistry of leukaemic cells: characterization of the early small granules of monoblasts. *British Journal of Haematology*, **45**, 201.

[61] OKUN, D. B. and TANAKA, K. R. (1978). Leukocyte alkaline phosphatase. *American Journal of Hematology*, **4**, 293.

[62] PARREIRA, A., DE OLIVEIRA, M. S. P., MATUTES, E.,

FORONI, L., MORILLA, R. and CATOVSKY, D. (1988). Terminal deoxynucleotidyl transferase positive acute myeloid leukaemia: an association with immature myeloblastic leukaemia. *British Journal of Haematology*, **69**, 219.

[63] QUAGLINO, D. and HAYHOE, F. G. J. (1960). Periodic-acid-Schiff positivity in erythroblasts with special reference to Di Guglielmo's disease. *British Journal of Haematology*, **6**, 26.

[64] REINHERZ, E. L., KUNG, P. C., GOLDSTEIN, G., LEVEY, R. H. and SCHLOSSMAN, S. F. (1980). Discrete stages of human intrathymic differentiation: analysis of normal thymocytes and leukemia lymphocytes of T cell lineage. *Proceedings of the National Academy of Sciences, USA*, **77**, 1588.

[65] REPORT OF THE STANDING COMMITTEE ON HUMAN CYTOGENETIC NOMENCLATURE (1978). An international system for human cytogenic nomenclature: ISCN, 1978. *Cytogenetics and Cell Genetics*, **21**, 309.

[66] RUSTIN, G. J. S., WILSON, P. D. and PETERS, T. J. (1979). Studies on the subcellular localisation of human neutrophil alkaline phosphatase. *Journal of Cell Science*, **36**, 401.

[67] RUTENBURG, A. B., ROSALES, C. L. and BENNETT, J. M. (1965). An important histochemical method for the demonstration of leukocyte alkaline phosphatase activity: clinical application. *Journal of Laboratory and Clinical Medicine*, **65**, 698.

[68] SANDBERG, A. A. (1990). *The Chromosomes in Human Cancer and Leukemia*, 2nd edn. Elsevier, New York.

[69] SECOND MIC COOPERATIVE STUDY GROUP (1988). Morphologic, immunologic and cytogenetic (MIC) working classification of the acute myeloid leukaemias. *British Journal of Haematology*, **68**, 487.

[70] SECOND INTERNATIONAL WORKSHOP ON CHROMOSOMES IN LEUKEMIA — 1979 (1980). Cytogenetic, morphologic and clinical correlations in acute non-lymphocytic leukaemia with t(8q −; 21q+). *Cancer Genetics and Cytogenetics*, **2**, 99

[71] SHEEHAN, H. L. (1939). The staining of leucocyte granules by Sudan Black B. *Journal of Pathology and Bacteriology*, **49**, 580.

[72] SHEEHAN, H. L. and STOREY, G. W. (1974). An improved method of staining leucocyte granules with Sudan Black B. *Journal of Pathology and Bacteriology*, **59**, 336.

[73] SHIBATA, A., BENNETT, J. M., CASTOLDI, G. L., CATOVSKY, D., FLANDRIN, C., JAFFE, E. S., KATAYAMA, I., NANBA. K, SCHMALZL, F., YAM, L. T. and LEWIS, S. M. [International Committee for Standardization in Haematology (ICSH)] (1985). Recommended methods for cytological procedures in haematology. *Clinical and Laboratory Haematology*, **7**, 55.

[74] SIMPSON, C. F., CARLISLE, J. W. and MALLARD, L. (1970) Rhodanile blue: a rapid and selective stain for Heinz bodies. *Stain Technology*, **45**, 221.

[75] SYRÉN, E and RAESTE, A-M. (1971). Identification of blood monocytes by demonstration of lysozyme and peroxidase activity. *Acta Haematologica* (Basel), **45**, 29.

[76] TESTA, J. R. and ROWLEY, J. D. (1981). Chromosomes in leukaemia and lymphoma with special emphasis on methodology. In *The Leukaemic Cell*. Ed. D. Catovsky. Chap. 6. Churchill Livingstone, Edinburgh.

[77] TETTEROO, P. A. T., LANSDORP, P. M., LEEKSMA, O. C. and VON DEM BORNE, A. E. G. Kr. (1983). Monoclonal antibodies against human platelet glycoprotein IIIa. *British Journal of Haematology*, **55**, 509.

[78] THIRD INTERNATIONAL WORKSHOP ON CHROMOSOMES IN LEUKEMIA — 1980 (1981). *Cancer Genetics and Cytogenetics*, **4**, 95.

[79] WACHSTEIN, M. and WOLF, G. (1958). The histochemical demonstration of esterase activity in human blood and bone marrow smears. *Journal of Histochemistry and Cytochemistry*, **6**, 457.

[80] WILLIAMS, D. L. (1991). Cytogenetics of acute leukemia. In *The Leukemic Cell*. Ed. D. Catovsky. Chap. 11, pp. 288. Churchill Livingstone, Edinburgh.

[81] YAM, L. T., LI, C. Y. and CROSBY, W. H. (1971). Cytochemical identification of monocytes and granulocytes. *American Journal of Clinical Pathology*, **55**, 283.

[82] YAM, L. T., LI, C. Y. and LAM, K. W. (1971). Tartrate-resistant acid phosphatase isoenzyme in the reticulum cells of leukemic reticuloendotheliosis. *New England Journal of Medicine*, **284**, 357.

[83] YUNIS, J. J. (1981). Chromosomes and cancer: new nomenclature and future directions. *Human Pathology*, **12**, 494.

[84] YUNIS, J. J. (1981). New chromosome techniques in the study of human neoplasia. *Human Pathology*, **12**, 540.

[85] YUNIS, J. J., OKEN, M. M., KAPLAN, M. E. ENSRUD, K. M., Howe, R. R. and THEOLOGIDES, A. (1982). Distinctive chromosomal abnormalities in histologic subtypes of non-Hodgkin's lymphoma. *New England Journal of Medicine*, **307**, 1231.

10. Bone-marrow biopsy

Needle (aspiration) biopsy   176
    Ilium   176
    Sternum   176
    Spine   177
Needle biopsy in children   177
Marrow puncture needles   177
Bone-marrow aspiration for transplantation   178
Examination of aspirated bone marrow   178

Quantitative cell counts   180
Differential cell counts; the myelogram   180
Reporting on bone-marrow films   181
Preparation of sections of aspirated bone marrow   183
Percutaneous trephine biopsy   185
Preparation of sections of bone marrow obtained by trephine
    biopsy   185
Staining of bone-marrow sections   187

Biopsy of bone marrow is an indispensible adjunct to the study of diseases of the blood and may be the only way in which a correct diagnosis can be made. Marrow can be obtained by needle aspiration, percutaneous trephine biopsy or surgical biopsy. *Needle biopsy* is simple, safe and relatively painless, and it can be repeated many times and performed on out-patients. It seems to be safe in almost all circumstances, even in thrombocytopenic purpura. However, it should never be attempted when there is a major disorder of coagulation as in haemophilia without appropriate cover and checking by coagulation factor assay. *Trephine biopsy*, using a 'microtrephine', is a little less simple, but it too can be performed on out-patients.

The disadvantage of aspiration biopsy is that the arrangement of the cells in the marrow and the relationship between one cell and another are more or less destroyed by the process of aspiration, and in fibrotic marrows little but blood may be aspirated. On the other hand, when marrow is aspirated, individual cells are perfectly preserved in well made films and, after staining, subtle differences between cells can be recognized usually to a far greater degree than is possible with sectioned material. If present, particles of aspirated marrow can be concentrated and subsequently sectioned and this allows the structure of small pieces of marrow to be studied. The great value of microtrephine biopsy is that it can provide a perfect view of the structure of relatively large pieces of marrow — that is, if the material obtained by the biopsy has been skilfully processed. At the same time morphological features of individual cells may be identified by making an imprint or a smear from the material obtained.

Studies on large numbers of cases have demonstrated that, whereas microtrephine-biopsy specimens are superior to films of aspirated material in some circumstances, e.g. for diagnosing marrow involvement by lymphoma or non-haematological neoplastic diseases, the simple procedure of aspiration marrow biopsy seldom fails to provide important information in patients who have a blood disease.[10,42] Both techniques have an important and complementary role in their investigation.

NEEDLE (ASPIRATION) BIOPSY OF THE BONE MARROW

Satisfactory samples of bone marrow can usually be aspirated from the sternum, iliac crest or anterior or posterior iliac spines. The iliac spines have the advantage that if no material is aspirated a microtrephine biopsy can be performed immediately. These sites may, however, be difficult in obese subjects, and puncture of the sternum may occasionally be necessary. However, the sternum is no longer favoured, and aspiration from this site should only be carried out by an experienced person; unless the needle is correctly inserted there is a danger of perforating the inner cortical layer and damaging the underlying large blood vessels and right atrium with serious consequences.

The sternum should never be used in children. The preferred site in children of all ages is the posterior iliac spine. In children aged below 2 years the upper end of the tibia may also be used, but with caution, as it is vulnerable to fractures and laceration of the adjacent major blood vessels.

Puncture of the ilium

The usual site for puncture in adults is the iliac crest. If serial punctures are being performed, a different site should be selected for each, in order to avoid marrow possibly disorganized by haemorrhage resulting from previous punctures.

Only needles designed for the purpose should be used (see below). They should be stout and made of hard stainless steel, about 7–8 cm in length, with a well-fitting stilette, and must be provided with an adjustable guard. The point of the needle and the edge of the bevel must be kept well sharpened. The patient's overlying skin is cleaned with 70% alcohol (e.g. ethanol) or 0.5% chlorhexidine (5% diluted 1 in 10 in ethanol). The skin, subcutaneous tissue and periosteum overlying the site selected for the puncture are carefully infiltrated with a local anaesthetic such as 2% lignocaine.

With a boring movement, pass the needle perpendicularly into the cavity of the ilium at a point just posterior to the anterior superior iliac spine or 2 cm posterior and 2 cm inferior to the anterior superior iliac spine. When the bone has been penetrated remove the stilette and with a well-fitting 2 or 5 ml syringe suck up not more than 0.3 ml of marrow contents — bone marrow diluted with a variable amount of blood. As a rule, material can be sucked into the syringe without difficulty; occasionally it may be necessary to re-insert the stilette and to push the needle in a little further and to suck again.

The anterior superior iliac spine can also be punctured. It may be easier to locate in very obese individuals and the bone overlying it is said to be thinner than that of the iliac crest.[33]

The posterior iliac spine overlies a large marrow-containing area and relatively large volumes of marrow can be aspirated from this site.[7] An advantage of puncturing the ilium rather than the sternum is that the patient can lie on his side and cannot see what is happening, and several attempts at puncture and aspiration can be made, if necessary, in the same anaesthetized area. Posterior iliac puncture can be carried out with the patient lying prone or on his side.

Make films from some of the aspirated material without delay (see p. 178). The remainder of the material may then be delivered into a suitable fixative for the preparation of histological sections (see p. 184). Fix some of the films in absolute methanol as soon as they are dry for subsequent staining by a Romanowsky method or by PAS or for iron. Further films should be fixed in formal-ethanol if other cytochemical staining is to be carried out (p. 143). If there has been a 'dry tap', insert the stilette into the needle and push any material in the lumen of the needle on to a slide; in lymphomas and carcinomas, especially, sufficient material may be obtained to make a diagnosis.[11]

Puncture of the sternum

As stated above, this must be performed with great care and only by a trained person. The usual site for puncture is the manubrium or the first or second pieces of the body of the sternum. The manubrium is formed of rather denser bone than the body of the sternum, and, in elderly subjects at least, it tends to contain more fatty marrow than is found elsewhere in the sternum. It is also sometimes less easy to be certain that the needle point has reached the cavity of the bone. However, completely satisfactory samples are obtained more often than not from the manubrium.

If the manubrium is selected, the site of the puncture should be about 1 cm above the sternomanubrial angle and slightly to one side of the mid-line; if the body of the bone is to be punctured, this should be done opposite the second or third intercostal spaces slightly to one side of the mid-line.

It is essential to use a guard on the needle. After piercing the skin and subcutaneous tissues, when the needle-point reaches the periosteum, adjust the guard on the needle to allow it to penetrate for about 5 mm further, and fix the guard tightly in position. Then push the needle with a boring motion into the cavity of the bone. The amount of force required varies, but may need to be considerable. It is usually easy to appreciate when the cavity of the bone has been entered. Aspiration is then carried out as described above.

Puncture of spinous processes

Good samples of marrow may be obtained from adults by puncturing the spines of lumbar vertebrae.[36] Puncture is not difficult since the bones lie superficially, but rather more pressure is required than for ilium or sternal puncture.

Pass the needle into the spine of a lumbar vertebra slightly lateral to the mid-line in a direction at right angles to the skin surface, with the patient either sitting up or lying on his side as for a lumbar puncture.

Comparison of the different sites for needle puncture

There is considerable variation in the composition of cellular marrow withdrawn from adjacent or different sites. Aspiration from only one site may give misleading information;[22] especially is this true in aplastic anaemia as the marrow may be affected patchily.[13,35] In general, however, the overall cellularity and type of maturity of haemopoiesis and the balance between erythropoiesis and leucopoiesis are similar.[2,12] In practice, it is a distinct advantage to have a choice of several sites for puncture, particularly when puncture at one site results in a 'dry tap' or when blood alone is withdrawn. Aspiration at a different site may yield cellular marrow or strengthen suspicion of a widespread change affecting the bone marrow, such as fibrosis or hypoplasia. In aplastic anaemia several punctures may be necessary in order to arrive at the diagnosis.

NEEDLE BIOPSY OF THE BONE MARROW IN CHILDREN

In very young children, from birth to 2 yr, the medial aspect of the upper end of the tibia just below the level of the tibial tubercle may be punctured and active marrow withdrawn. In older children the tibial cortical bone is usually too dense and the marrow within is normally less active. Iliac puncture, particularly in the region of the posterior crest, is then the method of choice.

Occasionally, in an older child who is obese the posterior iliac spine cannot be felt. In this case a satisfactory sample can usually be obtained from the anterior ilium.

It must be remembered that sternal puncture is hazardous for the bone is thin and the marrow cavities are small.

MARROW PUNCTURE NEEDLES

The most commonly used needles are the Salah and Klima needles (Fig. 10.1). A slightly larger needle with a T-bar handle at the proximal end has been developed by Islam* (Fig. 10.2). It is said to provide a better grip and to be more manoeuverable.[27]

A modified version of the Islam needle has multiple holes in the distal portion of the shaft in addition to the opening at the tip, in order to overcome sampling error when the marrow is not uniformly involved in a pathological lesion.[26]

---

* Downs Surgical, 32 New Cavendish Street, London W1M 8BU, UK.

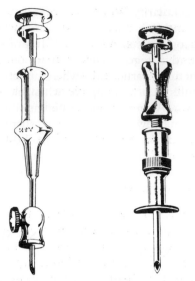

Fig. 10.1   Marrow-puncture needles. Salah (left) and Klima (right) (reduced × 0.75).

ASPIRATION OF BONE MARROW FOR TRANSPLANTATION

Bone-marrow grafting has led to the introduction of techniques suitable for obtaining large volumes (0.5–1 litre or even more) of bone marrow from a donor. The method in general use is the multiple puncture technique which was described by Thomas and Storb.[48] They devised a special needle with a 45° bevel to avoid plugging of the lumen during aspiration, but ordinary marrow puncture needles can be used satisfactorily.

Selection and preparation of a donor and the technique for harvesting the bone marrow and its storage for transplantation have been described by Jones and Burnett.[29]

EXAMINATION OF ASPIRATED BONE MARROW

Quite large volumes of marrow (plus blood) can be aspirated, but the more material aspirated the greater is the proportion of contaminating blood. There is little if any advantage in aspirating more than 0.3 ml of marrow fluid. The material aspirated can be dealt with in at least four ways: films can be made of the material as aspirated; films can be made after it has been concentrated; 'particle smears' can be made, and histological sections can be cut.

Bone-marrow films

Careful preparation is essential and it is desirable, if possible, to concentrate the marrow cells at the expense of the blood in which they are diluted.

The following simple manoeuvre is generally satisfactory. Deliver single drops of aspirate on to slides about 1 cm from one end and then quickly suck off most of the blood with a fine Pasteur pipette applied to the edge of each drop. Alternatively, place the slides on a slope to allow the blood to drain away. The irregularly shaped marrow fragments tend to adhere to the slide and most of them will be left behind. Then make films, 3–5 cm in length, of the marrow fragments and the remaining blood using a smooth-edged glass spreader of not more than 2 cm in width (Fig. 10.3). The marrow fragments are dragged behind the spreader and leave a trail of cells behind them. (It is in these cellular trails that differential counts should be made, commencing from the marrow fragment and working back towards the head of the film; in this way smaller

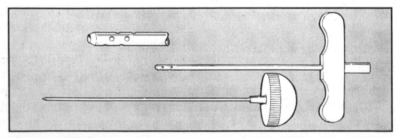

Fig. 10.2   Islam's bone-marrow aspiration needle. The dome-shaped handle and T-bar are intended to provide stability and control during operation.

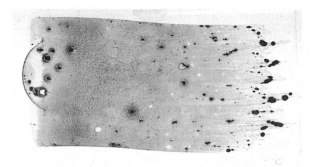

Fig. 10.3   Film of aspirated bone marrow. The marrow particles are easily visible, mostly at the tail of the film (×1.5).

numbers of cells from the peripheral blood become incorporated in a differential count.)

The preparation can be considered satisfactory only when marrow particles as well as free marrow cells can be seen in stained films, as is usual with the above technique. No attempt should be made to squash the marrow particles. Their structure — whether hypocellular or hypercellular — can be readily appreciated without recourse to squashing.

Fix the films of bone marrow and stain them with Romanowsky dyes as for peripheral blood films (p. 86). However, a longer fixation time (at least 20 min in methanol) is essential for high quality staining. Films should be stained by Perls's method as a routine to demonstrate iron (see p. 132).

Some workers add the aspirated marrow routinely to an anticoagulant, e.g. dried EDTA, in a tube and prepare films on return to the laboratory. While this is convenient, it is all too easy to use an excess of anticoagulant. When films of marrow containing a gross excess of anti-coagulant are spread (as when a few drops of marrow are added to a tube containing sufficient EDTA to prevent the clotting of 5 ml of blood) masses of pink-staining amorphous material may be seen and some of the erythroblasts and reticulocytes may clump together.

Concentration of bone marrow by centrifugation

Centrifugation can be used to concentrate the marrow cells and to assess the relative proportions of marrow cells, peripheral blood and fat in as-pirated material. While concentration of poorly cellular samples is useful, especially when an abnormal cell is present in small numbers,[14] it is unnecessary when the aspirated material is of average or increased cellularity. Volumetric data, too, are of little value in individual patients because of the wide range of values encountered even in health.

Methods for separation of marrow cells are described on p. 91.

'Particle smears'

Some workers deliberately isolate aspirated marrow particles and make 'smears' of them on slides or between two cover-slips using slight pressure. While this technique undoubtedly gives pre-parations of authentic marrow cells, squashing and smearing out of the particle causes disruption and distortion of cells, and the resultant thick preparations are difficult to stain really well. The authors feel that this technique has no advantages over the method described on p. 178.

Imprints

One or two glass slides are gently touched in several places by the exposed marrow at the surface of the specimen. These imprints are allow-ed to dry; the slides are then fixed and stained in the same manner as films. When there is a dry tap on aspiration the biopsy core should be gently rolled on a slide before putting it into fixative (see below). The slide should then be fixed and stained as before.

Preparation of films of post-mortem bone marrow

Films made of bone marrow obtained post mortem are seldom satisfactory. When the marrow is spread in the ordinary way the majority of the cells tend to break up and appear as smears. Berenbaum described how the blood cells are much better preserved if the marrow is suspended in albumin before the films are made.[4] He recommended that a small piece of marrow be suspended in 1–2 ml of 5% bovine albumin (1 volume 30% albumin, 5 volumes 9 g/l NaCl). The suspension is then centrifuged and the deposited marrow cells are resuspended in a volume of supernatant approximately equal to, or slightly less than, that of the deposit. Films are made of this suspension in the usual way. Berenbaum also pointed out that the addition of albumin to blood so as to give a 5% concentration improves the preservation of lymphocytes in cases of lymphocytic leukaemia in which many 'smear cells' are often seen in films of peripheral blood prepared in the ordinary way.

The rate and pattern of cellular autolysis during the first 15 h after death has been studied and the differences between the changes of post-mortem autolysis and those which occur in life as a result of blood diseases have been defined.[24]

QUANTITATIVE CELL COUNTS ON ASPIRATED BONE MARROW

A number of values for the cell content of aspirated normal bone marrow have been given in the literature.[41,50] The percentage marrow that is cellular rather than fatty in the sternum of healthy adults was given by Berman and Axelrod as 48–79%.[6] But quantitation of the cell content of aspirated marrow is not reliable in view of the tendency of the marrow to be aspirated in the form of particles of varying size as well as free cells and the uncontrollable factor of dilution with peripheral blood, which according to some authors may amount to 40–100% in 0.25–0.5 ml bone-marrow samples.[5]

For the above reasons quantitative cell counts on aspirated marrow seem hardly worth carrying out; instead, the degree of cellularity can be assessed within broad limits as increased, normal or reduced by inspection of a stained film containing marrow particles, and for practical purposes this is all that is usually necessary. As a rough guide, if less than 25% of the particle is occupied by haemopoietic cells it is probably hypocellular, and if more than 75–80% it is hypercellular.

Less subjective quantitative measurement can be obtained by 'point counting' of sections;[21,30] a normal range of 30–80% has been reported in the anterior iliac crest.[21]

Physiological variation in the cell content has to be taken into account. The cellularity of the marrow is affected by age. In adults, a smaller proportion of the marrow cavity is occupied by haemopoietic marrow than in children and the proportion of fat cells to cellular marrow is increased. In one study, by means of point counting of sections from the iliac crest, the range of cellularity in children under 10 years was reported as 59–95% with a mean of 79%; at 30 years the mean was 50%, and at 70 years it was 30% with a range of 11–47%.[21] The decrease in cellularity in elderly subjects is even more marked in the manubrium sterni. The marrow undergoes slight to moderate hyperplasia in pregnancy.[37]

DIFFERENTIAL CELL COUNTS ON ASPIRATED BONE MARROW; THE 'MYELOGRAM'

Many workers perform differential counts on marrow films and by presenting the data in the form of a myelogram express the incidence of the various cell types as percentages. Such figures are not as accurate as they might appear. Films made from aspirated material inevitably include cells from the peripheral blood as well as from the bone marrow, and the variable dilution with blood involves an error for which no compensation is possible. In addition, the more fixed and primitive cells may resist aspiration or, if aspirated, tend to remain embedded in marrow fragments. Megakaryocytes in particular are most irregularly distributed and tend to be carried to the tail of the film.

Ideally, differential counts should be performed on sectioned material. However, difficulties in identification make this impractical, although methacrylate embedding offers a better opportunity for correctly identifying cells. Fadem and Yalow recommended that differential counts be done on preparations made by the particle-smear technique.[12] As mentioned above, a fairly reliable method is to count the cells in the trails of cells left behind the marrow particles as they are carried to the tail during spreading.

Because of the naturally variegated pattern of the bone marrow and the irregular distribution of the marrow cells when spread in films, differential cell counts on marrow aspirated from normal subjects are likely to vary widely in health — so widely that minor degrees of deviation from the normal occurring in disease are difficult to establish. Lymph follicles occur in the bone marrow as a normal constituent, and chance aspiration at the site of such a follicle would result in a film with an unusually high proportion of lymphocytes. Follicles have been reported to occur especially in infants, although in one large study they were reported to be quite rare in children and more common in middle-aged and elderly people.[38]

The normal values given in Table 10.1 can be taken only as an approximate guide. Glaser et al gave figures for the cellular composition of the bone marrow in normal infants, children and young adults, based on 151 samples.[18] Variation is marked in the first year, particularly so in the first month. The percentage of erythroblasts falls from birth, and at 2–3 weeks they constitute only c 10% of the nucleated cells. Myeloid cells (granulocyte presursors) increase during the first two weeks of life, following which a sharp fall occurs at about the third week, but by the end of the first month c 60% of the cells are myeloid.

Table 10.1 Normal ranges for differential counts on aspirated bone marrow

	Range (%)
Reticulum cells	0.1–2
Myeloblasts	0.1–3.5
Promyelocytes	0.5–5
Myelocytes:	
neutrophil	5–20
eosinophil	0.1–3
basophil	0–0.5
Metamyelocytes	10–30
Polymorphonuclears:	
neutrophil	7–25
eosinophil	0.2–3
basophil	0–0.5
Lymphocytes	5–20
Monocytes	0–0.2
Megakaryocytes	0.1–0.5
Plasma cells	0.1–3.5
Proerythroblasts	0.5–5
Normoblasts*:	
polychromatic	2–20
pyknotic**	2–10

* Or erythroblasts.

** The term 'pyknotic' is preferred to 'orthochromatic' as a description of the most mature normoblasts. Cells with fully ripened cytoplasm (orthochromatic in the strict sense) are rarely found in normal bone marrow.

Lymphocytes constitute up to 40% of the nucleated cells in the marrow of small infants; the mean value at 2 yr is c 20%, falling to c 15% during the rest of childhood. The percentage of plasma cells is especially low from infancy up to the age of 5 yr.[47]

The hyperplasia which occurs in pregnancy affects both erythropoiesis and granulopoiesis, the latter proportionately less, though with some increase in the relative proportion of immature cells.[37] The hyperplasia is maximal in the third trimester; a return to normal begins in the puerperium but is not completed until at least 6 weeks *post partum*.

Ratios

Ratios based on a count of 200–500 cells provide useful qualitative information without recourse to more time-consuming differential counts.

The myeloid:erythroid ratio has been widely used. Leucocytes of all types and stages of maturation are counted together. The very wide normal range, 2.5–15:1, reflects the variegated pattern of normal marrow.

As an alternative, the leuco-erythrogenetic ratio can be calculated; for this mature leucocytes are excluded. The normal ratio has been reported as 0.56–2.67:1.[43]

The myeloid:lymphoid ratio varies widely, 1–17:1, and the lymphoid:erythroid ratio is similarly a wide one, 0.2–4.0:1.[16]

REPORTING ON BONE-MARROW FILMS

The first thing to do is to look with the naked eye at a selection of slides and to choose from them several of the best spread films containing easily visible marrow particles. The particles should then be examined with a low-power (×10) objective with particular reference to their cellularity, and an estimate of whether the marrow is hypoplastic, normoplastic or hyperplastic can usually be made without much difficulty, if sufficient particles are available for study (Fig. 10.4). The next step is to select for detailed examination — still using the ×10 objective — a highly cellular area of the film where the nucleated cells are well stained and well spread. Areas such as these can

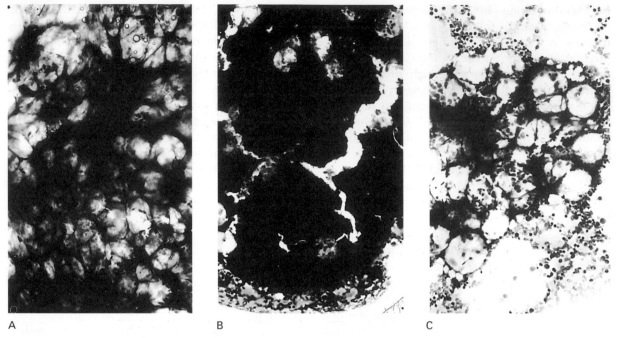

A   B   C

Fig. 10.4   Film of aspirated bone marrow. Photomicrographs of particles illustrating cellularity: (A) normal; (B) hypercellular; (C) hypocellular.

usually be found towards the tails of films in the vicinity of marrow particles. The cells in these cellular areas should be examined first with a higher power (e.g. ×40) objective and subsequently, if necessary, with the ×100 oil-immersion objective. Megakaryocytes should be looked for at this stage of the examination; they are most often found towards the tail of the film.

Systematic examination, backed by a knowledge of the patient's peripheral blood count and his history, will usually enable a diagnosis to be made without recourse to a differential count. A detailed 'myelogram' is, in fact, not often required in clinical practice. A description of the general cellularity of the marrow and the type of erythropoiesis (e.g. whether normoblastic, megaloblastic or dyserythropoietic) and of the general maturity of the erythropoietic and leucopoietic cells, and perhaps an estimate of the myeloid:erythroid ratio, are all that are usually needed when reporting on bone-marrow films for diagnostic purposes.

This is not to say that detailed differential counts are never useful and need never be done.

Thus, changes in the proportion of primitive to maturing myeloid cells reflect response to treatment in leukaemia or recovery from agranulocytosis, and the actual percentage of blast cells may be of significance in the differentiation of refractory anaemias and myelodysplasia.

The proportion of lymphoid cells is an important indicator of prognosis in chronic lymphocytic leukaemia.[45] On the other hand, time is often much better spent in examining a series of slides than in performing a detailed differential count as a routine on the first few hundred cells looked at in the marrow film of each patient. A wide search may, for instance, in a case of obscure anaemia, settle the diagnosis by revealing isolated groups of metastatic carcinoma cells. In addition, a film should always be stained and examined for iron.

Other features of possible diagnostic value include the presence of erythrophagocytosis, abnormal numbers of phagocytic reticulum cells, excess plasma cells, non-haemopoietic cells and degenerate or necrotic cells. Bone-marrow necrosis is a not uncommon complication of sickle-cell disease; it also occurs occasionally in lymphomas, lymphoblastic and chronic lymphocytic leukaemia, myeloproliferative diseases and metastatic carcinoma as well as in septicaemia, tuberculosis and anorexia nervosa.[8,31,39,46,51]

In marrow necrosis cells stain irregularly, with blurred outlines, cytoplasmic shrinkage and nuclear pyknosis. In anorexia there may be gelatinous transformation of ground substance of the marrow.[46]

It is helpful in reporting on bone-marrow films to have a printed form on which the report and conclusion can be set out in an ordered fashion (Fig. 10.5). Where a computerized report system is in use, a list of the various descriptive comments which may be used should be provided in coded form to facilitate data entry.

PREPARATION OF SECTIONS OF ASPIRATED BONE MARROW

Sections give a better picture of the marrow architecture than can be deduced from films. In a

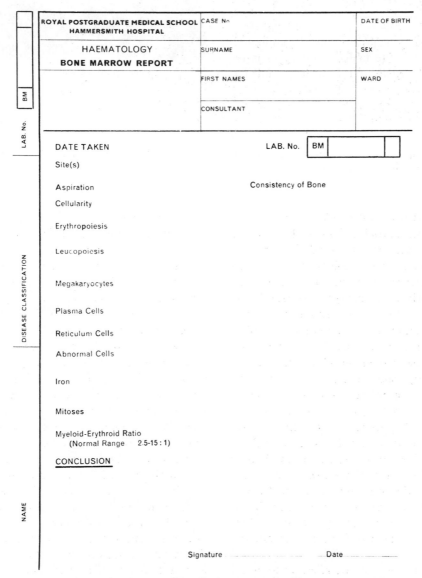

Fig. 10.5 Example of report form for bone-marrow films.

good preparation the relationship between cellular marrow and fat spaces is preserved, hypoplasia or hyperplasia can be recognized, and tumour cells and granulomata can be seen. However, for cytological detail sectioned material is usually less satisfactory, especially when it has had to be decalcified and is paraffin embedded. The subtle differences between cells such as normoblasts and megaloblasts, which are usually easy to appreciate in well stained films, are difficult to recognize in sections and it may sometimes be difficult even to differentiate erythroblasts from leucocytes with complete certainty.

The fragments obtained by aspirating bone marrow are small, rarely greater than 1 mm in size, and a careful technique in handling them is required. They are usually free from bone and the marrow architecture is well preserved, but their usefulness it limited because their small size makes it uncertain how representative of the bone marrow they are. A more serious disadvantage of the aspiration technique is that fragments are often not obtained by suction in just those patients — with perhaps marrow hypoplasia, myelosclerosis or invasion by tumour — in whom histological evidence of any marrow abnormality is particularly required. In these patients trephine biopsy may be necessary.

A number of methods of dealing with aspirated fragments have been published which differ in the details of handling and concentrating the fragments, fixation and embedding.[10,44] The following method gives adequate concentration of the marrow particles and is simple to carry out (Fig. 10.6) Fixation is good and sections may be successfully stained by a Romanowsky method as well as by other dyes.

Preparation of sections of aspirated bone-marrow particles[44]

Fixative

Absolute ethanol is diluted with an equal volume of 15% formalin (150 ml/l of 40% formaldehyde). The specific gravity of the mixture is 0.93, almost exactly the same as that of human fat. When a marrow aspirate is added to this fixative, the blood remains in suspension while the marrow particles

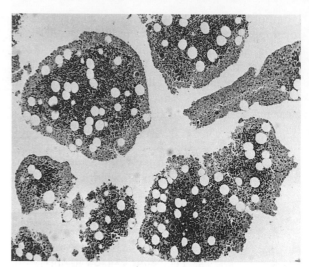

Fig. 10.6   Section of aspirated bone-marrow particles. See text for method of preparation.

rapidly sediment. Even fatty marrow settles down in a few seconds.

Method

Add 0.25 ml of bone-marrow aspirate to 20 ml of the fixative in a stoppered container and mix thoroughly. Allow it to fix overnight at room temperature.

The following morning, resuspend the sediment by inversion. With a Pasteur pipette provided with a teat, pick out the coarser marrow fragments after they have re-settled to the bottom of the bottle, which usually takes only a few seconds. Then transfer them to a round-bottomed test-tube, provided with a rubber bung, containing 70% (v/v) ethanol. Leave for at least 15 min, then dehydrate with two changes of absolute ethanol, leaving the particles for 1 h in each. Then drain off the ethanol and replace with toluene. After 1 h decant off the toluene and replace it by a toluene-paraffin wax mixture and then by two changes of paraffin wax. Free the block by breaking the tube when the wax has cooled and hardened. The marrow fragments will have settled as a small mass at the bottom of the block and little or no trimming will be required. Cut sections of 4–5 μm thickness, the thinner the better.

PERCUTANEOUS TREPHINE BIOPSY OF THE BONE MARROW

Several types of trephines have been used. Türkel and Bethell described a microtrephine of about 2 mm bore which could be passed through a hollow introducing needle only slightly larger than a marrow aspirating needle.[49] No skin incision was necessary and the instrument could be used on the sternum and the procedure carried out in the ward. However, the cylinders of bone and underlying marrow obtained with the Türkel and Bethell trephine were small, and they were apt to break up while being prepared for sectioning. Needles of the Vim-Silverman type[9] are suitable for use in posterior iliac-crest punctures; but they yield smaller specimens of marrow than most other needles. However, the specimens are as a rule free from bone dust.

A disadvantage of most marrow trephines is that not infrequently the specimen is crushed and its architecture altered. The Jamshidi needle[28] which has a tapering end was designed to overcome this problem (Fig. 10.7). The trephine should be inserted by to-and-fro rotation through approximately 90°. It should not be continuously rotated as this tends to distort and twist the core of marrow. Sometimes, however, the sample fractures while being extracted from the needle and in other cases the specimen does not detach readily from its base and efforts to detach it by movement of the needle result in it being crushed. These disadvantages have been overcome by having a core-securing device, as in the Islam trephine*.[25] This makes it possible to obtain a long uniform core of marrow-containing bone without the marrow architecture being distorted (Fig. 10.8). With these trephines biopsies are usually performed at the anterior or posterior superior iliac spine. The latter site is said to provide samples that are longer and larger, while the aspiration is less uncomfortable for the patient.[23]

A larger trephine is sometimes of value as it may provide sufficient material for an accurate diagnosis when the result of a smaller and perhaps less representative biopsy is inconclusive.

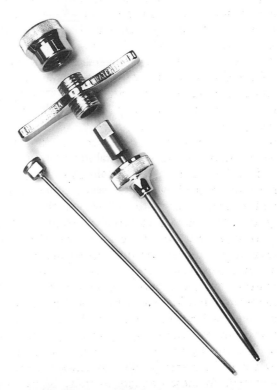

Fig. 10.7   Jamshidi trephine for bone-marrow biopsy.

Trephines have been developed which have bores of 4–5 mm.[32,52] They can safely be used on the iliac crest, under local anaesthesia, but as a small skin incision is necessary the biopsy should be performed in the operating theatre where full aseptic precautions can be taken. Full-scale bone biopsy involving, for instance, removal of a piece of rib ('surgical biopsy') is nowadays seldom carried out.

PREPARATION OF SECTIONS OF BONE MARROW OBTAINED BY TREPHINE BIOPSY

Fix the specimen in 10% formal saline, buffered to pH 7.0, or preferably in Helly's fluid (potassium dichromate 2.5 g, mercuric chloride 5 g, formalin (40% formaldehyde) 5 ml, water 100 ml) for 12–48 h. Then wash in running water overnight before decalcifying, dehydrating and embedding

* Downs Surgical, 32 New Cavendish Street, London W1M 8BU, UK.

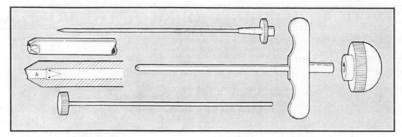

Fig. 10.8   Islam trephine for bone-marrow biopsy. The distal cutting edge is shaped to hold the core secure during extraction of the material.

in paraffin wax by the usual histological procedures. Then cut and stain 4–5 μm thick sections. The relatively thick sections prepared in this way, together with cell shrinkage and the distortion produced by decalcification, make it difficult to interpret cellular detail. Almost all these disadvantages can be overcome by methyl methacrylate ('plastic') embedding.[17] In this process the undecalcified biopsy specimen is fixed in the usual way. It is then embedded in glycol or methyl methacrylate. Sections 1–2 μm thick can

then be obtained using a tungsten carbide knife and a purpose-built microtome, e.g. Reichert-Jung Autocut.[17,20] Not only does this provide clearer detail of cell morphology but cell and tissue relationships are maintained and the embedding procedure is less damaging to the tissue than paraffin-wax embedding. Aspirated marrow can also be processed in this way after special fixation to separate the marrow particles from blood and precipitated protein.[19]

Before staining plastic-embedded sections, the

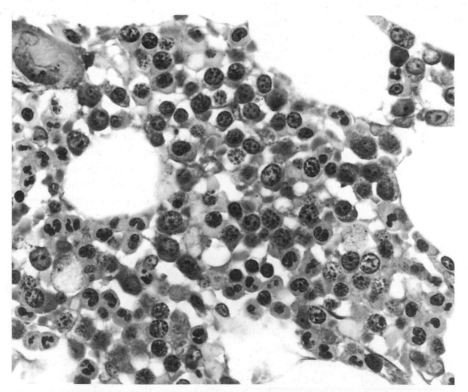

Fig. 10.9   Photomicrograph of section of normal bone marrow. Iliac crest biopsy. Methacrylate embedding. Stained by May-Grünwald-Giemsa (×300).

methyl methacrylate must be dissolved from the sections by passing them sequentially through benzol or acetone, methanol, methanol-ammonia solution and water.[17]

Sections of marrow should be stained as a routine by haematoxylin and eosin (H & E) and by a reticulin impregnation method. It is worthwhile also to stain sections by a Romanowsky stain, and for iron by Perls's reaction. H & E staining is excellent for demonstrating the cellularity and pattern of the marrow and for revealing pathological changes such as fibrosis or the presence of granulomata or carcinoma. Haemopoietic cells, on the other hand, may be more easily identified in a Romanowsky-stained preparation (Figs. 10.9 and 10.10). In Fig. 10.11 is shown the extent to which the cellularity of the marrow varies in health. Sections can also be stained for various cytochemical reactions; however, specimens which have been embedded in plastic are unsuitable for immunohistology.[1]

Silver impregnation stains the glycoprotein matrix which is associated with connective tissue. The bone marrow always contains a small amount of this material which is referred to as 'reticulin' and which is actually collagen.[3] The reticulin content of normal iliac bone marrow is shown in Fig. 10.12.

The term myelofibrosis strictly refers to an increase in fine fibres and myelosclerosis to the condition when there is an increase in coarse

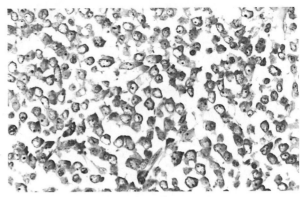

Fig. 10.10 Photomicrograph of section of bone marrow. Iliac crest biopsy. Methacrylate embedding. Myeloblastic leukaemia. Stained by May-Grünwald-Giemsa (×300).

fibres (Fig. 10.12). The latter type predominates in chronic ('idiopathic') myelofibrosis. Increased reticulin also occurs in other myeloproliferative disorders, particularly in cases associated with proliferation of megakaryocytes and in lymphoproliferative disorders, secondary carcinoma with marrow infiltration, osseous disorders such as hyperparathyroidism and Paget's disease, and in inflammatory reactions.[15,34,40]

Staining of sections of bone marrow by May-Grünwald-Giemsa

The many techniques which have been re-

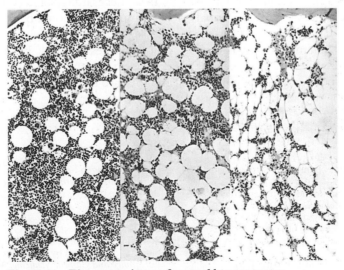

Fig. 10.11 Biopsy specimen of normal bone marrow. Photomicrographs of sections of iliac-crest bone marrow illustrating range of cellularity in heath (x100).

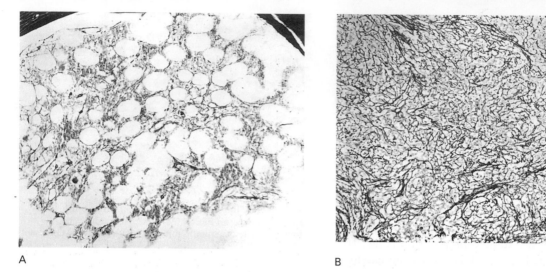

A   B

Fig. 10.12   Photomicrographs of sections of bone marrow. Iliac crest biopsy. Stained for reticulin by silver impregnation method: (A) normal; (B) chronic myelofibrosis (×100).

commended for staining sectioned bone marrow by Romanowsky dyes are evidence of the real difficulty in obtaining good results. The following method is fairly satisfactory. It may be applied to aspirated marrow fragments, trephine or post-mortem material.

Place the cut sections which have been processed, as described on p. 185, in Lugol's iodine (5 g iodine crystals and 10 g potassium iodide in 100 ml of water) for 2 min. Then wash in several changes of water and finally rinse in water buffered to pH 6.8. Stain the sections for 1 h in May-Grünwald's stain diluted with an equal volume of buffered water. Then stain for a further 2 h in a fresh solution of Giemsa's stain diluted with 19 volumes of buffered water. The sections become grossly over-stained and deep blue in colour. Rinse in buffered water (pH 6.8) before differentiation.

Differentiate the sections by covering with a small volume of glycerin-ether, freshly diluted with four volumes of absolute ethanol. Differentiation takes place quickly and is usually adequate in a few seconds. Next dehydrate the sections by a rapid dip in absolute ethanol, clear them in xylol and finally mount them in a xylol-miscible mounting medium. The use of glycerin-ether helps to prevent 'blueing' of the section during dehydration.

In a successfully stained section the cytoplasm of primitive cells should be blue, that of myelocytes and segmented neutrophils pale pink, the eosinophil granules should be bright red and the cytoplasm of the red cells orange. Neutrophil granules are not as a rule easily seen.

REFERENCES

[1] BARTL, R., FRISCH, B., BUCHENRIEBER, B., SOMMERFELD, W., MUTHMANN, H., JÄGER, K., HOFFMAN-FEZER, G. and BURKHARDT, R. (1984). Multiparameter studies on 650 bone marrow biopsy cores. *Bibliotheca Haematologica*, **50**, 1.

[2] BENNIKE, T., GORMSEN, H. and MØLLER, B. (1956). Comparative studies of bone marrow punctures of the sternum, the iliac crest and the spinous process. *Acta Medica Scandinavica*, **155**, 377.

[3] BENTLEY, S. A., ALABASTER, O. and FOIDART, J. M. (1981). Collagen heterogeneity in normal human bone marrow. *British Journal of Haematology*, **48**, 287.

[4] BERENBAUM, M. C. (1956). The use of bovine albumin in the preparation of marrow and blood films. *Journal of Clinical Pathology*, **9**, 381.

[5] BERLIN, N. I., HENNESSY, T. G. and GARTLAND, J. (1950). Sternal marrow puncture: the dilution with peripheral blood as determined by P³² labelled red cells. *Journal of Laboratory and Clinical Medicine*, **36**, 23.

[6] BERMAN, L. and AXELROD, A. R. (1950). Fat, total cell and megakaryocyte content of sections of aspirated marrow of normal persons. *American Journal of Clinical Pathology*, **20**, 686.

[7] BERMAN, H. R. and KELLY, K. H. (1956). Multiple marrow aspiration in man from the posterior ilium. *Blood*, **11**, 370.

[8] CONRAD, M. E. and CARPENTER, J. T. (1979). Bone marrow necrosis. *American Journal of Haematology*, 7, 181.

[9] CONRAD, M. E. and CROSBY, W. H. (1961). Bone marrow biopsy: modification of the Vim-Silverman needle. *Journal of Laboratory and Clinical Medicine*, **57**, 642.

[10] DEE, J. W., VALDIVIESO, M. and DREWINKO, B. (1976). Comparison of the efficacies of closed trephine needle biopsy, aspirated paraffin-embedded clot section and smear preparation in the diagnosis of bone-marrow involvement by lymphoma. *American Journal of Clinical Pathology*, **65**, 183.

[11] ENGESET, A., NESHEIM, A. and SOKOLOWSKI, J. (1979). Incidence of 'dry tap' on bone marrow aspirations in lymphomas and carcinomas. Diagnostic value of the small material in the needle. *Scandinavian Journal of Haematology*, **22**, 417.

[12] FADEM, R. S. and YALOW, R. (1951). Uniformity of cell counts in smears of bone marrow particles. *American Journal of Clinical Pathology*, **27**, 541.

[13] FERRANT, A. (1980). Selective hypoplasia of pelvic bone marrow. *Scandinavian Journal of Haematology*, **25**, 12.

[14] FILLOLA, G. M., LAHARRAGUE, P. F. and CORBERAND, J. X. (1992). Bone marrow enrichment technique for detection and characterization of scarce abnormal cells. *Nouvelle Revue Française d'Hématologie*, **34**, 337.

[15] FRISCH B. and BARTL., R. (1985). Histology of myelofibrosis and osteomyelosclerosis. In *Myelofibrosis: Pathophysiology and Clinical Management*. Ed. S. M. Lewis, p. 51–86. Marcel Dekker, New York.

[16] FRISCH B. and LEWIS, S. M. (1974). The bone marrow in aplastic anaemia: diagnostic and prognostic features. *Journal of Clinical Pathology*, **27**, 231.

[17] FRISCH B., LEWIS, S. M., BURKHARDT, R. and BARTL, R. (1985). *Biopsy Pathology of Bone and Bone Marrow*. Chapman & Hall, London.

[18] GLASER, K., LIMARZI, L. R. and PONCHER, H. G. (1950). Cellular composition of the bone marrow in normal infants and children. *Pediatrics*, **6**, 789.

[19] GREEN, G. H. (1970). A simple method for histological examination of bone marrow particles using hydroxyethyl methacrylate embedding. *Journal of Clinical Pathology*, **23**, 640.

[20] GREEN, G. H. and KURREIN, F. (1981). Glycol methacrylate embedding in general histopathology, *ACP Broadsheet No. 97*. Association of Clinical Pathologists, London.

[21] HARTSOCK, R. J., SMITH, E. B. and PETTY, C. S. (1965). Normal variations with aging of the amount of hematopoietic tissue in bone marrow from the anterior iliac crest. *American Journal of Clinical Pathology*, **43**, 326.

[22] HASHIMOTO, M. (1960). The distribution of active marrow in the bones of normal adults. *Kyushu Journal of Medical Science*, **11**, 103.

[23] HERNÁNDES-GARCIÁ, M. T., HERNÁNDEZ-NIETO. L., PÉREZ-GONZÁLEZ, E. and BRITO-BARROSO. M. L. (1993). Bone marrow trephine biopsy: anterior superior iliac spine versus posterior superior iliac spine. *Clinical and Laboratory Haematology*, **15**, 15.

[24] HOFFMAN, S. B., MORROW, G. W. Jnr, PEASE, G. L. and STROEBEL, C. F. (1964). Rate of cellular autolysis in postmortem bone marrow. *American Journal of Clinical Pathology*, **41**, 281.

[25] ISLAM, A. (1981). A new bone marrow biopsy needle with core securing device. *Journal of Clinical Pathology*, **35**, 359.

[26] ISLAM, A. (1983). A new bone marrow aspiration needle to overcome the sampling errors inherent in the technique of bone marrow aspiration. *Journal of Clinical Pathology*, **36**, 954.

[27] ISLAM, A. (1991). New sternal puncture needle. *Journal of Clinical Pathology*. **44**, 690.

[28] JAMSHIDI, K. and SWAIM, W. R. (1971). Bone marrow biopsy with unaltered architecture: a new biopsy device. *Journal of Laboratory and Clinical Medicine*, 77, 335.

[29] JONES, R. and BURNETT, A. K. (1992). How to harvest bone marrow for transplantation. *Journal of Clinical Pathology*, **45**, 1053.

[30] KERNDRUP, G., PALLESEN, G., MELSEN, F. and MOSEKILDE, L. (1980). Histological determination of bone marrow cellularity in iliac crest biopsies. *Scandinavian Journal of Haematology*, **24**, 110.

[31] KIRALY, J. F. and WHEBY, M. S. (1976). Bone marrow necrosis. *American Journal of Medicine*, **60**, 361.

[32] LANDYS, K. (1980). A new trephine for closed bone marrow biopsy. *Acta Haematologica*, **64**, 216.

[33] LEFFLER, R. J. (1957). Aspiration of bone marrow from the anterior superior iliac spine. *Journal of Laboratory and Clinical Medicine*, **50**, 482.

[34] LENNERT, K., NAGAI, K. and SCHWARZE, E. W. (1975). Patho-anatomic features of the bone marrow. *Clinics in Haematology*, **4**, 331.

[35] LEWIS, S. M. (1965). Course and prognosis in aplastic anaemia. *British Medical Journal*, **i**, 1027.

[36] LOGE, J. P. (1948). Spinous process puncture. A simple clinical approach for obtaining bone marrow. *Blood*, **3**, 198.

[37] LOWENSTEIN, L. and BRAMLAGE, C. A. (1957). The bone marrow in pregnancy and the puerperium. *Blood*, **12**, 261.

[38] MAEDA, K., HYUN, B. H. and REBUCK, J. W. (1977). Lymphoid follicles in bone marrow aspirates. *American Journal of Clinical Pathology*, **67**, 41.

[39] MACFARLANE, S. D. and TAURO, G. P. (1986). Acute lymphocytic leukaemia in children presenting with bone marrow necrosis. *American Journal of Hematology*, **22**, 341.

[40] MCCARTHY, D. M. (1985) Fibrosis of the bone marrow; content and causes. *British Journal of Haematology*, **59**, 1.

[41] OSGOOD, E. E. and SEAMAN, A. J. (1944). The cellular composition of normal bone marrow as obtained by sternal puncture. *Physiological Reviews*, **24**, 46.

[42] PASQUALE, D. and CHIKKAPPA, G. (1981). Comparative evaluation of bone marrow aspirate particle smears, biopsy imprints, and biopsy sections. *American Journal of Hematology*, **22**, 381.

[43] PONTONI, L. (1936). Su alcuni rapporti citologici ricavati dal mielogramma; metodica e valutazione fisopatognostica generale. *Haematologica*, **17**, 833.

[44] RAMAN, K. (1955). A method of sectioning aspirated bone-marrow. *Journal of Clinical Pathology*, **8**, 265.

[45] ROZMAN, C., MONTSERRAT, E., RODRIGUEZ-FERNANDEZ, J. M. et al (1984). Bone marrow histologic pattern — the best single prognostic parameter in chronic lymphocytic leukemia; a multivariate survival analysis of 329 cases. *Blood*, **64**, 642.

[46] SMITH, R. R. L. and SPIVAK, J. L. (1985). Marrow cell

necrosis in anorexia nervosa and involuntary starvation. *British Journal of Haematology*, **60**, 525.

[47] STEINER, M. L. and PEARSON, H. A. (1966). Bone marrow plasmacyte values in childhood. *Journal of Pediatrics*, **68**, 562.

[48] THOMAS, E. D. and STORB, R. (1970). Technique for human marrow grafting. *Blood*, **36**, 507.

[49] TÜRKEL, H. and BETHELL, F. H. (1943). Biopsy of bone marrow performed by a new and simple instrument.

Journal of Laboratory and Clinical Medicine, **28**, 1246.

[50] VAUGHAN, S. L. and BROCKMYRE, F. (1947). Normal bone marrow as obtained by sternal puncture. *Blood*, Special Issue No. 1, p. 54.

[51] VESTERBY, A. and JENSEN, O. M. (1985). Aseptic bone/bone marrow necrosis in leukaemia. *Scandinavian Journal of Haematology*, **35**, 354.

[52] WILLIAMS, J. A. and NICHOLSON, G. I. (1963). A modified bone-biopsy drill for outpatient use. *Lancet*, **1**, 1408.

11. Diagnosis of blood cell disorders

Revised by J. Parker-Williams

Screening for an abnormality   191
Diagnosis of a blood cell disorder   192
Anaemia   192

Leucocyte disorders   193
Other disorders   195

Haematology is a rapidly changing discipline. Over the last quarter century it has experienced a dramatic shift from dependence on simple laboratory observations into the field of basic science. However, for the great majority of patients with a blood disorder, reliance on simple laboratory techniques is still relevant and adequate.

The diagnosis of blood disorders will continue to require correlation of both the clinical and laboratory evidence. The history and clinical examination of the patient is central to the diagnostic process, as is consideration of the patient's age, sex and geographical location. The clinical aspects are beyond the scope of this book and will not be discussed further.

The laboratory has two major roles. First, to provide a screening service both for the general health of the patient and to determine fitness for an operation. Second, to provide a provisional diagnosis of a blood disorder, which may subsequently have to be investigated in much greater detail using more complex tests. The haematologist has at his disposal an ever increasing array of sophisticated tests involving immunological, genetic and molecular biological techniques. Tests involving other disciplines may also be required before arriving at a definitive diagnosis.

The haematologist occupies a crucial position in the provision of a diagnostic service for his colleagues. Changes in the constituents of the blood may be a reflection of virtually any organic disorder, and do not necessarily imply an underlying blood disorder. The effects of other therapy, particularly cytotoxic drugs, may have to be considered. Being at the interface of a clinical and laboratory discipline the haematologist has to interpret the differences between a primary haematological disorder and a 'secondary' or symptomatic effect of other disease processes, and achieve the maximum return as economically and efficiently as possible; value for money is a major consideration.

SCREENING FOR AN ABNORMALITY

There are probably few laboratories which today rely solely on haemoglobin and haematocrit measurements and blood film examination for diagnosing blood disorders. Electronic blood cell counters are widely available; many are fully automated and are able to provide a five-part differential leucocyte count. This technology at a time of increasing workload, and often accompanied by diminishing personnel and financial resources, has brought about changes in laboratory practice. Intelligent use of cell counters is a vital component of the screening process.

The ideal of examining a blood film for unsuspected blood disorders on all samples analysed by the laboratory is no longer practical. With the aid of modern technology and selective blood film examination, a much more effective screening service is available. The automated counter provides the screening, and this is supplemented by selective blood film examination of those samples where an abnormal parameter is 'flagged' up; an abnormality may be occasionally missed, but it is unlikely to be a serious omission. The well-stained blood film, for so long the cornerstone of haematology, continues to provide an essential input into haematological diagnosis. It is important to file blood films so that they are available for re-examination should an abnormality be detected at a later date. All bone marrow films should have a peripheral blood film filed with them.

APPROACH TO THE DIAGNOSIS OF BLOOD CELL DISORDERS

For the majority of cases, the diagnosis of a blood disorder will be indicated by the history and clinical examination. This is confirmed by the screening procedures and blood film examination, supplemented by simple tests such as the reticulocyte count, erythrocyte sedimentation rate, or direct antiglobulin test. A bone-marrow aspirate or a trephine biopsy is only required for those in whom the diagnosis is not immediately obvious. The need for trephine biopsies is particularly important for the diagnosis of malignant blood disorders. The resin-embedding techniques, in addition to paraffin sections and the use of monoclonal antibodies, have become major contributors to the diagnosis of these diseases. The extension of investigational procedures into other areas of haematology (serological, haemoglobin disorders and coagulation) will be directed by the initial history, clinical examination and screening procedures, and will be considered in other chapters. Non-haematological procedures such as urine examination, biochemistry, ultrasound, computerized tomography (CT) and magnetic resonance imaging (MRI) may also be critical for the diagnosis of a blood disorder. However, the indiscriminate use of tests is uneconomical and unnecessary.

A logical sequence of haematological investigations should be followed, with the more valuable and informative procedures being undertaken first, and only when necessary, followed by the more complicated tests. These sequences are illustrated in the flow charts.

ANAEMIA

In anaemia, the clinical history may be a suffi-cient clue to the diagnosis. The type of anaemia should be established on a morphological basis. The automated blood cell counter will provide an accurate measurement of the red cell indices, including the red cell distribution width (RDW).

Three groups are distinguished:

1. Microcytic, hypochromic (MCV <78 fl).
2. Normocytic, normochromic.
3. Macrocytic (MCV >100 fl).

These are clear-cut distinctions. However, there will be instances when the morphological characterization of the anaemia is not clear, the changes depending on the stage in the evolution of the anaemic process. For example, the anaemia of chronic disease may be normocytic and normochromic, or, if the time-scale is more prolonged, microcytic and hypochromic. These diagnostic problems are often resolved by a thorough assessment of the morphological appearances of the red cells; consideration of any leucocyte and platelet changes may provide critical clues on the nature of the anaemia. Most anaemias are due to a single cause, but there are occasions when the anaemia is due to several factors, and secondary or symptomatic anaemias will usually fall into this category. A multifactorial anaemia may not 'obey' the rules and will not fit into a specific category.

The flow charts (Figs. 11.1–11.3) indicate those tests which are most likely to provide a rapid diagnosis. If these fail to provide a diagnosis, additional tests become necessary. These are discussed below. Selection of the most useful procedures will depend on the preliminary results, and on the facilities available in the laboratory. The aim in the flow charts and in the text is to highlight, first, the most informative and valuable tests, then to include the more complex and more specific tests.

Microcytic hypochromic anaemias

Measurement of serum iron, total iron-binding capacity and ferritin; bone marrow aspirate with staining for iron; stools for occult blood; blood loss studies with ^{51}Cr labelled red cells; tests for malabsorption; endoscopic examination with biopsy. If thalassaemia is suspected, haemoglobin electrophoresis plus Hb A_2 and Hb F measurements; 'H' body preparation; family studies; tests for unstable haemoglobin; globin chain synthesis; recombinant DNA technology.

Macrocytic anaemias

Recognition of the morphological red cell changes of alcohol excess and liver disease is vital, as is the increased polychromasia of a reticulocytosis. Where macrocytic, megaloblastic erythroid maturation is demonstrated, further investigations should be undertaken as described on p. 417.

'Secondary anaemias'

The haematologist's principal task is to exclude a primary haematological disorder or a disorder, such as secondary tumour, directly involving the marrow. These anaemias may be complicated by other factors such as blood loss or folate deficiency which will further confuse the picture.

Aplastic anaemia

Bone marrow aspirate and trephine biopsy; Ham's test for PNH; urine for haemosiderin; neutrophil alkaline phosphatase; vitamin B_{12} and folate levels; chromosome studies; radiology of hands and forearms if Fanconi's anaemia is suspected; viral studies; ^{59}Fe (or ^{52}Fe scan if available) to study red cell production; HLA typing if bone marrow transplantation is a consideration; colony cultures.

Haemolytic anaemias

A haemolytic process may be suspected by the presence of red cell abnormalities, a reticulocytosis and an increased unconjugated bilirubin level. For further investigations, see p. 197.

LEUCOCYTE DISORDERS

The blood may appear entirely normal in some patients with lymphoma, myelomatosis, immune deficiency, neutrophil dysfunction, whether lymphadenopathy and/or splenomegaly is present or not. However, changes in leucocyte numbers or morphology may occur rapidly in response to local or systemic disorders. Leucocyte abnormalities are more likely to require marrow examination, especially in the diagnosis of a primary marrow disorder, and although in chronic leukaemias it adds little to the diagnosis, the pattern of infiltration may have prognostic significance as in chronic lymphocytic leukaemia. The distribution of leucocytes is better appreciated in trephine biopsies, which are particularly important in lymphomas.

Neutropenia

Bone marrow aspirate and trephine biopsy; serial neutrophil counts for cyclic neutropenia; tests for anti-neutrophil antibodies; auto-antibody screen; vitamin B_{12} and folate levels; Ham's test; bone marrow colony cultures.

Acute leukaemia

Bone marrow aspirate; cytochemical stains; blood and marrow immunological cell marker studies (fluorescence microscopy, alkaline phosphatase anti-alkaline phosphatase (APAAP), flow cytometry); chromosome studies; gene rearrangement studies.

Chronic granulocytic leukaemia

Bone marrow aspirate; neutrophil alkaline phosphatase; chromosome studies.

Chronic lymphocytic leukaemia

Bone marrow aspirate and trephine biopsy (for lymphocyte distribution); cell marker studies; serum protein electrophoresis and immunoglobulin levels; lymph node biopsy (fine needle or surgical).

Myelomatosis

Bone marrow aspirate; serum protein electrophoresis and immunoglobulin levels, serum albumin and Ca measurements; β_2-microglobulin level; urine (random and 24 h) for Bence-Jones protein quantitation; tests of renal function; radiological skeletal survey; plasma cell labelling index.

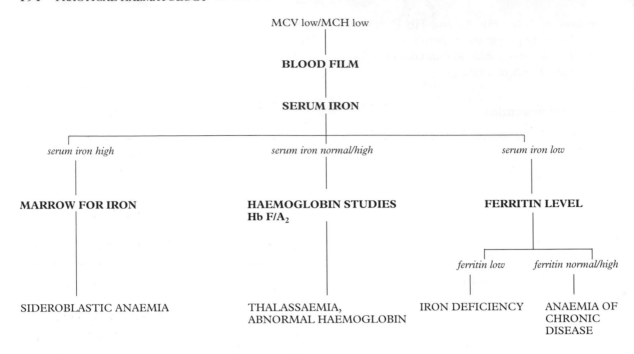

Fig. 11.1   Investigation of a microcytic hypochromic anaemia.

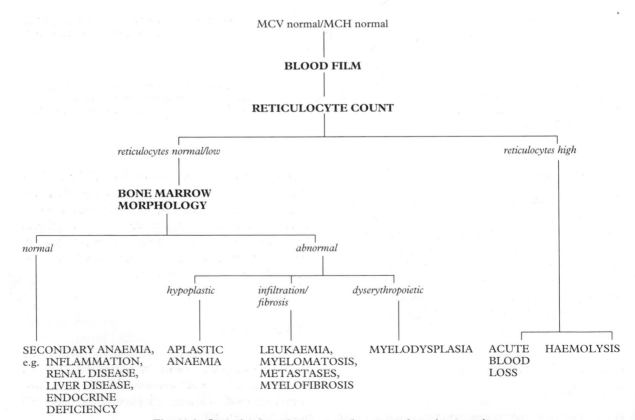

Fig. 11.2   Investigation of a normocytic, normochromic anaemia.

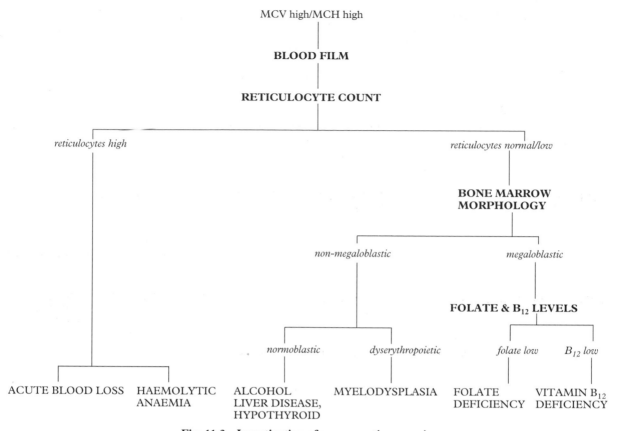

Fig. 11.3   Investigation of a macrocytic anaemia.

The flow charts provide an orderly sequence of investigation for the different types of anaemia as distinguished by the red cell indices. Tests are in bold capitals, results are in italics, and the diagnosis is in capitals. The key to all three flow charts is examination of the blood film, which will suggest the quickest route to the diagnosis. Confirmation may require the more specific tests, which are given in the text.

Lymphadenopathy

Serological screening for infectious mononucleosis, cytomegalovirus and toxoplasmosis; serum protein electrophoresis; lymph node biopsy (fine needle or surgical); bone marrow aspirate and trephine biopsy; serum urate level; serum calcium; serum lactate dehydrogenase (LDH); radiological studies (X-ray, ultrasonography, lymphangiography, CT scan, MRI); lymphocyte subsets; HIV screening.

OTHER DISORDERS

Polycythaemia

Blood volume measurement; bone marrow aspirate and trephine biopsy; neutrophil alkaline phosphatase; vitamin B_{12} level (or B_{12}-binding capacity); serum urate level; abdominal ultrasound; arterial oxygen saturation; carboxyhaemoglobin level; haemoglobin electrophoresis; erythropoietin assay; erythroid colony formation, spleen scan and red cell pool measurement.

Myelofibrosis

Bone marrow trephine biopsy; folate level; urate level; ferrokinetic (^{59}Fe or ^{52}Fe) and ^{51}Cr labelled red cell survival studies; neutrophil alkaline phosphatase; blood volume; spleen scan and red cell pool measurement.

Pancytopenia with splenomegaly

Bone marrow aspirate and trephine biopsy; bacterial culture of marrow; marrow examination for parasites, e.g. Leishmania; biopsy of palpable lymph nodes (aspiration or surgical); vitamin B_{12} and folate levels; liver biopsy; splenic aspirate; Ham's test; serum rheumatoid factor; autoantibody screen; laparotomy and splenectomy.

12. Laboratory methods used in the investigation of the haemolytic anaemias

Investigation of haemolytic anaemia: a summary   197
Plasma haemoglobin   199
Serum haptoglobins   201
Examination for methaemalbumin   203
　　Schumm's test   203
　　Quantitative estimation   204
Haemosiderin in urine   204
Serum haemopexin   205
Chemical tests of haemoglobin catabolism   205
Serum bilirubin   206

Urobilin and urobilinogen   206
Porphyrins   207
　　Red cell porphyrins   207
　　Porphobilinogen in urine   207
　　Porphyrins in urine   208
Abnormal haemoglobin pigments   210
　　Methaemoglobin   210
　　Sulphaemoglobin   211
　　Carboxyhaemoglobin   212
Myoglobin in urine   212

Normally, effete red cells undergo lysis at the end of their life-span of 100–120 days within cells of the reticulo-endothelial (RE) system in the spleen, liver and bone marrow (extravascular haemolysis) and haemoglobin is not liberated into the plasma in appreciable amounts. In a haemolytic anaemia the red cell life-span is, by definition, shortened (accelerated haemolysis). In some types of haemolytic anaemia the increased haemolysis is predominantly extravascular and the plasma haemoglobin concentration is barely raised: in other disorders a major degree of haemolysis takes place within the blood stream (intravascular haemolysis): the plasma haemoglobin rises substantially, and in some cases the amount of haemoglobin so liberated may be sufficient to lead to haemoglobin being excreted in the urine (haemoglobinuria).

The clinical and laboratory phenomena of increased haemolysis reflect the nature of the haemolytic mechanism, where the haemolysis is taking place and the response of the bone marrow to the anaemia resulting from the increased haemolysis, namely, erythroid hyperplasia and reticulocytosis.

INVESTIGATION OF HAEMOLYTIC ANAEMIA: A SUMMARY

The two pathways by which haemoglobin derived from effete red cells is metabolized are illustrated in Fig. 12.1.

The investigation of patients suspected of suffering from a haemolytic anaemia comprises several distinct stages: recognizing the existence of increased haemolysis; determining the type of haemolytic mechanism; making the precise diagnosis; and, if facilities are available, carrying out tests of scientific rather than of immediate diagnostic or prognostic value. In practice, the procedures are often telescoped, for the diagnosis in some instances may be obvious to the experienced observer from a glance down the microscope at the patient's blood film.

The following practical scheme of investigation is recommended. The tests are arranged 1, 2, 3 and 4 in order of importance and practicability.

Is there evidence of increased haemolysis?

1. Hb estimation; reticulocyte count; inspection of a stained blood film for the presence of sphero-

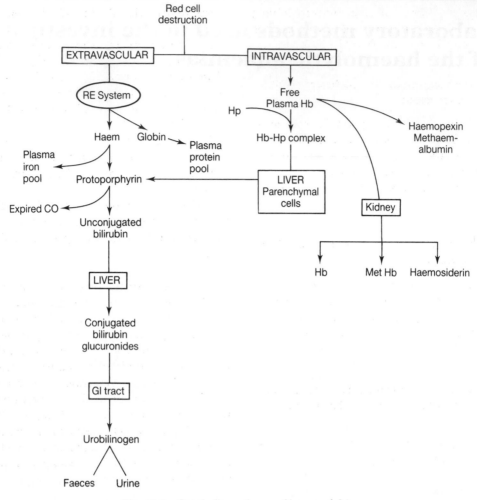

Fig. 12.1   Catabolic pathway of haemoglobin.

cytes, elliptocytes, irregularly-contracted cells, schistocytes or auto-agglutination (see Chapter 7).

2. Osmotic-fragility test or glycerol lysis test; serum bilirubin estimation.

3. Measurement of life-span of patient's red cells (^{51}Cr method); demonstration of haptoglobins; test for increased urinary urobilinogen excretion.

What is the type of haemolytic mechanism?

1. Direct antiglobulin test (DAT) with broad spectrum serum.

2. Test for haemosiderin and Hb in urine; estimation of plasma Hb; Schumm's test.

What is the precise diagnosis?

Which test should be done depends upon the results of the tests which have already been carried out. Not all are appropriate in every case.

1. If a hereditary haemolytic anaemia is suspected:

Osmotic-fragility determination after 24 h incubation at 37°C; autohaemolysis test ± the addition of glucose; red-cell instability at 45°C; screening test for red cell G6PD deficiency; red cell pyruvate kinase assay; assay of other red cell enzymes involved in glycolysis; estimation of red cell glutathione.

Electrophoresis for abnormal haemoglobins; estimation of Hb A$_2$; estimation of Hb F; tests for sickling; tests for heat-labile Hb (Hb Köln, etc.).

2. If an auto-immune acquired haemolytic anaemia is suspected:

Direct antiglobulin test using anti-Ig and anti-complement (C) sera; tests for auto-antibodies in the patient's serum; titration of cold agglutinins; Donath-Landsteiner test; electrophoresis of serum proteins; demonstration of thermal range of auto-antibodies.

3. If the haemolytic anaemia is suspected of being drug-induced:

Screening test for red cell G6PD; glutathione stability test; staining for Heinz bodies; identification of methaemoglobin (Hi) and sulphaemoglobin (SHb); tests for drug-dependent antibodies.

4. In all instances of haemolytic anaemia of obscure type (and in all cases of aplastic anaemia):

Acidified serum test (Ham's test) for paroxysmal nocturnal haemoglobinuria (PNH); sucrose lysis test, etc.

Tests primarily of scientific interest

1. Elution of auto-antibodies and determination of antibody specificity (of practical but not diagnostic importance); tests for agglutination and/or lysis of enzyme-treated cells by auto-antibodies; tests for lysis of normal cells by auto-antibodies.

2. Determination of sites of haemolysis by radionuclide scan or surface counting (may be of practical importance if splenectomy is contemplated).

3. Demonstration of the proteins of the red-cell membrane and cytoskeleton (spectrin, etc.) by gel electrophoresis and by specific radio-immune assay.

In this and subsequent chapters, descriptions will be given of most of the tests which have been referred to. This chapter will include tests of general importance in providing evidence of increased haemolysis. The investigation of hereditary haemolytic anaemias is described in Chapter 13, haemoglobinopathies in Chapter 14, PNH in Chapter 15 and auto-immune acquired haemolytic anaemias in Chapter 27. Some relevant tests, which are normally carried out in clinical chemistry laboratories, will not be described in detail. Instead, recommended methods are referred to.

ESTIMATION OF PLASMA HAEMOGLOBIN

The technique described below is adapted from Crosby and Furth's[8] modification of Wu's original peroxidase method.[43] The catalytic action of haem-containing proteins brings about the oxidation of benzidine by hydrogen peroxide to give a green colour which changes to blue and finally to reddish violet. The intensity of reaction may be compared in a photoelectric colorimeter or spectrophotometer with that produced by solutions of known Hb content. Methaemalbumin and Hb are measured together.

Benzidine is a recognized carcinogen, and in many countries its use is prohibited without a special licence. Tetramethylbenzidine is an analogue which is more readily available as it is considered to be less hazardous; *it should, however, be handled with great care.*

When the plasma Hb concentration is >50 mg/l it can be measured by means of a spectrophotometer at 540 nm by a modification of the whole-blood haemiglobincyanide method.[21] A pink tinge to the plasma is detectable by eye when the Hb concentration is about 200 mg/l or more.

Sample collection

Every effort must be made to prevent haemolysis during the collection and manipulation of the blood. A clean venepuncture is essential; a relatively wide-bore needle should be used and the syringe, first rinsed with sterile 9 g/l NaCl (saline), should fill spontaneously with blood. When the required amount of blood has been withdrawn, the needle should be detached and 9 volumes of blood added to 1 volume of 32 g/l sodium citrate. All glassware must be scrupulously clean.

In order to reduce haemolysis to a minimum, Hanks and his colleagues recommended that blood should be collected through a wide-bore needle direct into a siliconized centrifuge tube containing heparin.[15] The blood is then lightly centrifuged and the supernatant recentrifuged after being transferred to a clean tube. With this technique, the upper limit for plasma Hb in health was found to be as low as 6 mg/l.

PEROXIDASE METHOD[31]

Reagents

Benzidine reagent. Dissolve 1 g of 3,3',5,5'-tetramethylbenzidine in 90 ml of glacial acetic acid and make up to 100 ml with water. The solution will keep for several weeks in a dark bottle at 4°C.

Hydrogen peroxide. Dilute 1 volume of 3% ('10 vols') H_2O_2 with 2 volumes of water before use.

Acetic acid. 100 g/l glacial acetic acid.

Standard. A blood sample of known Hb content is diluted with water to a final concentration of 200 mg/l. It is convenient to use a HiCN standard solution (p. 51) as the source of Hb.

Method

Add 20 µl of plasma to 1 ml of the benzidine reagent in a large glass tube. At the same time set up a control tube, in which 20 µl of water are substituted for the plasma, and a standard tube, containing 20 µl of the Hb standard. Add 1 ml of the H_2O_2 solution to each tube and mix the contents well.

Allow the mixture to stand at *c* 20°C for 20 min and then add 10 ml of the acetic acid solution to each tube and, after mixing, allow the tubes to stand for a further 10 min. Compare the coloured solutions at 600 nm or in a photoelectric colori-meter provided with an orange (e.g. Ilford 607) filter, using the colour developed by the control tube as a blank. If the Hb content of the plasma to be tested is abnormally high, the plasma should be diluted with saline until it is just visibly tinged red.

Normal range

10–40 mg/l;[7] up to 6 mg/l.[15]

Significance of raised plasma-haemoglobin concentrations

Haemoglobin liberated from the intravascular or extravascular breakdown of red cells interacts with the plasma haptoglobins to form a haemoglobin–haptoglobin complex[19] which, because of its size, does not undergo glomerular filtration, but it is removed from the circulation by, and degraded in, RE cells. Hb in excess of the capacity of the haptoglobins to bind it passes into the glomerular filtrate; it is then partly excreted in the urine in an uncomplexed form, resulting in haemoglobinuria, and partly reabsorbed by the proximal glomerular tubules where it is broken down into haem, iron and globin. The iron is retained in the cells and eventually excreted in the urine (haemosiderin). The haem and globin are reabsorbed into the plasma.

The haem complexes with albumin forming methaemalbumin (see p. 203) and with haemopexin (see p. 205); the globin competes with Hb to form a complex with haptoglobin. In effect, the plasma-haemoglobin level is significantly raised in haemolytic anaemias when haemolysis is sufficiently severe for the available haptoglobin to be fully bound. The highest levels are found when haemolysis takes place predominantly in the blood stream (intravascular haemolysis). Thus marked haemoglobinaemia, with or without haemoglobinuria, may be found in paroxysmal nocturnal haemoglobinuria, paroxysmal cold haemoglobinuria, the cold-haemagglutinin syndrome, blackwater fever, and in march haemoglobinuria and in other mechanical haemolytic anaemias, e.g. that after cardiac surgery. In warm-type auto-immune haemolytic anaemias, sickle-cell anaemia and severe Mediterranean anaemia, the plasma-haemoglobin level may be slightly or moderately raised, but in hereditary spherocytosis, in which haemolysis occurs predominately in the spleen, the levels are normal or only very slightly raised.

Haem within the proximal tubular epithelium undergoes further degradation to bilirubin with liberation of iron, some of which is retained intra-cellularly bound to proteins as ferritin and hae-mosiderin. When haemolysis is severe the excess of haemoglobin which occurs in the glomerular filtrate will lead to an accumulation of intra-cellular haemosiderin in the glomerular tubular cells; when these cells slough haemosiderin will appear in the urine (see p. 204).

It cannot be over-emphasized that the presence of excess Hb in the plasma is a reliable sign of intravascular haemolysis only if the observer can be sure that the lysis has not been caused during or after the withdrawal of the blood.

Increased levels may occur as a result of violent exercise,[6,40] but not, apparently, with prolonged exercise such as in long distance runners.[3]

ESTIMATION OF SERUM HAPTOGLOBINS

Haptoglobin is a glycoprotein which is synthesized in the liver. It consists of two pairs of α-chains and two pairs of β-chains. Free haemoglobin readily dissociates into dimers of α- and β-chains; the α-chains bind avidly with the β-chains of haptoglobin in plasma or serum to form a complex which can be differentiated from free haemo-globin by column chromatographic separation[26] or by its altered rate of migration on electro-phoresis. For electrophoretic separation, paper,[19] cellulose acetate,[4,36] starch gel,[30] agar gel[27] and acrylamide gel[13] have been used.

Methods for direct measurement of haptoglobins by turbidimetry[41] or nephelometry,[39] and by radial immunodiffusion[9,35] have also been developed. The methods described below are cellulose-acetate electrophoresis and radial immunodiffusion.

ELECTROPHORESIS METHOD

Principle. A known amount of haemoglobin is added to serum. The Hb-haptoglobin complex is separated by electrophoresis on cellulose acetate, and the relative amounts of bound and free Hb are estimated by scanning the electrophoresis strips after staining. The concentration of haptoglobin can then be expressed as mg Hb-binding capacity per litre serum.

Reagents

Buffer (pH 7.0, ionic strength 0.05). Na_2HPO_4. H_2O 7.1 g/l, 2 volumes; $NaH_2PO_4.H_2O$ 6.9 g/l, 1 volume. Store at 4°C.

Haemolysate. Prepare as described on p. 257. Adjust the Hb concentration to 35–40 g/l with water. This solution is stable at 4°C for several weeks.

Stain. Dissolve 0.5 g of o-dianisidine (3,3'-dimethoxybenzidine) in 70 ml of 95% ethanol; prior to use add together 10 ml of acetate buffer, pH 4.7 (sodium acetate 2.92 g, glacial acetic acid 1 ml, water to 1 litre), 2.5 ml of 3% (10 vol) H_2O_2 and water to 100 ml.

Clearing solution. Glacial acetic acid 25 ml, 95% ethanol 75 ml.

Acetic acid rinse. Glacial acetic acid, 50 ml/l.

Method

Serum is obtained from blood allowed to clot un-disturbed at 37°C. As soon as the clot starts to retract, remove the serum by pipette and centri-fuge it to rid it of suspended red cells. The serum may be stored at −20°C until used.

Mix well 1 volume of haemolysate with 9 vol-umes of serum. Allow to stand for 10 min at room temperature.

Impregnate cellulose acetate membrane filter-strips (12 × 2.5 cm) in buffer solution and blot to remove all obvious surface fluid. Apply 0.75 µl samples of the serum haemolysate mixture across the strips as thin transverse lines, and electro-phorese at 0.5 mA/cm width. Good separation patterns about 5–7 cm in length should be obtained in 30 min (Fig. 12.2).

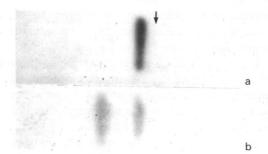

Fig. 12.2   Demonstration of serum haptoglobins.
(a) Serum from case of haemolytic anaemia with added haemoglobin; there is a Hb band in β-globulin position but no haptoglobin is present.
(b) Normal serum with added haemoglobin, showing bands in β-globulin (Hb) and α_2-globulin (Hb-haptoglobin complex) positions, respectively.
The line of origin is indicated by the arrow.

After electrophoresis is completed, immerse the membranes in freshly prepared *o*-dianisidine stain for 10 min. Then rinse with water and immerse in 50 ml/l acetic acid for 5 min. Remove the membranes and place in 95% ethanol for exactly 1 min. Transfer the membranes to a tray containing freshly prepared clearing solution and immerse for exactly 30 s. While still in the solution, position the membranes over a glass plate placed in the tray. Remove the glass plate with the membranes on it, drain the excess solution from the membranes, transfer the glass plate to a ventilated oven preheated to 100°C, and allow the membranes to dry for 10 min.

After the plate has cooled, scan the membranes by a densitometer at 450 nm with a 0.3 mm slit width.

Calculation

Calculate the density of the haptoglobin band as a fraction of the total Hb in the electrophoretic strip:

$$\text{Haptoglobin (g/l)} = \text{Haptoglobin fraction} \times \text{Hb conc (g/l)}$$

RADIAL IMMUNODIFFUSION (RID) METHOD

Principle. The test serum samples and reference samples of known haptoglobin concentra-tion are dispensed into wells in a plate of agarose gel containing a monospecific antiserum to human haptoglobin. Precipitation rings form by the re-action of haptoglobin with the antibody; the diameter of each ring is proportional to the con-centration of haptoglobin in the sample.

Reagents

Single diffusion plates. Dissolve agarose (20 g/l) in boiling phosphate buffered water pH 7.4 (p. 578). Allow to cool to 60°C. Add 5% sheep or goat anti-human haptoglobin antiserum diluted in buffered water, pH 7.4, and heated to 55°C. Mix well but without creating bubbles. Pour the gel onto thin plastic trays (plates) to a thickness of less than 1 mm. After the gel has set, cut out a series of wells *c* 1 cm in diameter, about 2 cm apart. Cover the plates with fitted lids and store in sealed packets at 4°C until used.

Plates of agarose gel containing the antiserum are available commercially.

Reference sera. Preparations of human serum with stated haptoglobin concentration are avail-able commercially. They should be stored at 4°C.

Test serum. This can be kept at 4°C for 2–3 days, but if not used within this time store at −20°C. Thaw completely and mix well im-mediately before use.

Method

Allow the plate (in its sealed packet) and the sera to equilibrate at room temperature for 15 min. Remove the lid from the plate. Check for moisture; if present, allow to evaporate. Add 5 µl of each serum into one of the wells in the plate. Stand for about 10 min to ensure that the serum is com-pletely absorbed into the gel. Then cover the plate, return it to its container and reseal the packet. Leave on a level surface at room tempera-ture for 18 h. From measurements of the reference sera construct a reference curve on log-linear graph paper by plotting haptoglobin con-centration on the vertical axis (logarithmic scale) and the diameter of the rings on the horizontal scale (linear scale). Measure the diameter of the precipitation ring formed by the test serum and express concentration in g/l (Fig. 12.3).

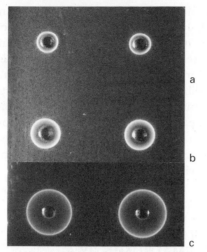

Fig. 12.3 Demonstration of serum haptoglobins. Radial immunodiffusion: (a) low; (b) normal; (c) increased concentrations.

Significance of haptoglobin levels

By direct measurement results are expressed as haptoglobin concentration; slightly different normal reference values have been reported for the different methods:[25,33,39,41]

RID	0.8–2.7 g/l
Nephelometry	0.3–2.2 g/l
Turbidimetry	0.5–1.6 g/l.

When measured as Hb binding capacity, in normal sera haptoglobins will bind 0.3–2.0 g of Hb/l; levels are higher in men than in women.[25]

Haptoglobins begin to be depleted when the daily Hb turnover exceeds about twice the normal.[4] This occurs irrespective of whether the haemolysis is predominantly extravascular or intravascular; but rapid depletion, often with the formation of methaemalbumin, occurs as a result of small degrees of intravascular haemolysis, even when the daily total Hb turnover is not increased appreciably above normal. Low concentrations of haptoglobins, in the absence of increased haemolysis, may be found in hepatocellular disease, and are characteristic of congenital ahaptoglobinaemia which occurs in about 2% of Caucasians and a larger number of Blacks.[24] Low concentrations may also be found in megaloblastic anaemias probably because of increased haemolysis, and following haemorrhage into tissues.

The haptoglobin-haemoglobin complex is cleared by the RE system, mainly in the liver. The rate of removal is influenced by the concentration of free haemoglobin in the plasma: at levels below 10 g/l the clearance $T_{1/2}$ is 20 min; at higher concentrations clearance is considerably slower.

Increased haptoglobin concentrations may be found in pregnancy, chronic infections, malignancy, tissue damage, Hodgkin's disease, rheumatoid arthritis, systemic lupus erythematosus, biliary obstruction and as a consequence of steroid therapy or the use of oral contraceptives. Under these circumstances a normal haptoglobin concentration does not exclude increased haemolysis.

EXAMINATION OF PLASMA (OR SERUM) FOR METHAEMALBUMIN

A simple but not very sensitive method is to examine the plasma using a hand spectroscope.

Free the plasma from suspended cells and platelets by centrifuging at 1200–1500g for 15–30 min. Then view it in bright daylight with a hand spectroscope using the greatest possible depth of plasma consistent with visibility. Methaemalbumin gives a rather weak band in the red (at 624 nm) (Fig. 12.4). As HbO_2 is usually present as well, its characteristic bands in the yellow-green may also be visible. The position of the methaemalbumin absorption band in the red can be readily differentiated from that of methaemoglobin (Hi) by means of a reversion spectroscope.

Presumptive evidence of the presence of small quantities of methaemalbumin, giving an absorption band too weak to recognize, can be obtained by extracting the pigment by ether and then converting it to an ammonium haemochromogen which gives a more intense band in the green (Schumm's test).

SCHUMM'S TEST

Method

Cover the plasma (or serum) with a layer of ether.

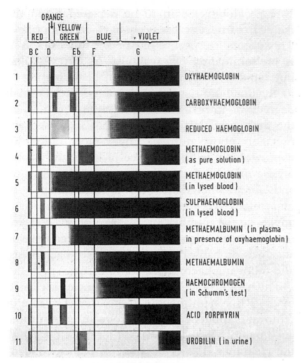

Fig. 12.4 Absorption spectra of derivatives of human haemoglobin. The absorption bands are shown in relation to the Fraunhofer lines, the positions of which are as follows: B at 686.7 nm, C at 656.3 nm, D at 589 nm, E at 527 nm, b at 518.4 nm, F at 486.1 nm and G at 430.8 nm.

Add a one-tenth volume of saturated yellow ammonium sulphide and mix it with the plasma. Then view it with a hand spectroscope. If methaemalbumin is present, a relatively intense narrow absorption band will be seen in the green (at 558 nm) (Fig. 12.4).

Significance of methaemalbuminaemia

Methaemalbumin is found in the plasma when haptoglobins are absent in haemolytic anaemias in which lysis is predominantly intravascular. It was first observed by Fairley and Bromfield in black-water fever.[12] It is a haem-albumin compound formed subsequent to the degradation of Hb liberated into plasma. In contrast to haptoglobin-bound Hb and haemopexin-bound haem, the haem-albumin complex is thought to remain in circulation until the haem is transferred from albumin to the more highly avid haemopexin.[23]

QUANTITATIVE ESTIMATION OF METHAEMALBUMIN BY A SPECTROPHOTOMETRIC METHOD

To 2 ml of plasma (or serum) add 1 ml of iso-osmotic phosphate buffer, pH 7.4. Centrifuge the mixture for 30 min at 1200–1500g and measure its absorbance in a spectrophotometer at 569 nm. Add c 5 mg of solid sodium dithionite to the supernatant diluted plasma. Shake the tube gently to dissolve the dithionite and leave for 5 min to allow complete reduction of the methaemalbumin. Remeasure the absorbance. The difference between the two readings represents the absorbance due to methaemalbumin; its concentration can be read off from a calibration graph.

The calibration graph is constructed as follows: solutions containing 10–100 mg/l methaemalbumin are obtained by dissolving appropriate amounts of haemin (bovine or equine) in a minimum volume of 40 g/l human serum albumin. The absorbance of each solution is measured in a spectrophotometer at 569 nm, and a graph drawn from the figures obtained.

DEMONSTRATION OF HAEMOSIDERIN IN URINE

Method

Centrifuge 10 ml of urine at 1200g for 10–15 min. Transfer the deposit to a slide, spread out to occupy an area of 1–2 cm and allow to dry in the air. Fix by placing the slide in methanol for 10–20 min and then stain by the method used to stain blood films for siderocytes (p. 132). Haemosiderin, if present, appears in the form of isolated or grouped blue-staining granules, usually from 1 to 3 μm in size (Fig. 12.5). If haemosiderin is present in small amounts, and especially if distributed irregularly on the slide, or if the findings are difficult to interpret, the test should be

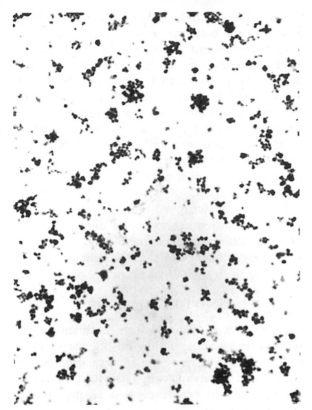

Fig. 12.5 Photomicrograph of urine deposit stained by Perls's reaction.

repeated on a fresh sample of urine collected into an iron-free container and centrifuged in an iron-free tube. (For the preparation of iron-free glassware, see p. 580).

Significance of haemosiderinuria[10]

Haemosiderinuria is a sequel to the presence of Hb in the glomerular filtrate. It is a valuable sign of chronic intravascular haemolysis, for the urine will be found to contain iron-containing granules even if there is no haemoglobinuria at the time. However, haemosiderinuria is not found in the urine at the onset of a haemolytic attack even if this is accompanied by haemoglobinaemia and haemoglobinuria, as the haemoglobin has first to be absorbed by the cells of the renal tubules. The intracellular breakdown of Hb liberates iron which is then re-excreted. Haemosiderinuria may persist for several weeks after a haemolytic episode.

DEMONSTRATION OF SERUM HAEMOPEXIN

Haem derived from Hb, which fails to bind to haptoglobins, complexes with either albumin or haemopexin. The latter has a much higher affinity, and when complexed the haem is eliminated from the circulation, e.g. by the liver Kupffer cells.

Haemopexin is a haem-binding (but not Hb-binding) serum glycoprotein of molecular weight 70 000. In normal adults of both sexes its concentration is 0.5–1 g/l;[23] in newborn infants there is much less, c 0.3 g/l, but adult levels are reached by the end of the first year of life. In severe intravascular haemolysis haemopexin levels are low or zero when haptoglobins are depleted. With less severe haemolysis, although haptoglobins are likely to be reduced or absent, haemopexin may be normal or only slightly lowered, and it has been suggested that the haemopexin level gives a more reliable measure of haemolysis than does the haptoglobin level. Haem binds in a 1:1 molar ratio to haemopexin; 6 μg/ml of free haem is required to deplete the normal binding levels of haemopexin. Haemopexin seems to be disproportionately low in thalassaemia major, and low levels may be found in certain pathological conditions other than haemolytic disease, namely, renal and liver diseases. The concentration is raised in diabetes mellitus, infections and carcinoma.[23]

Haemopexin can be measured by starch-gel electrophoresis[17] or immunochemically by radial immunodiffusion.[16]

CHEMICAL TESTS OF HAEMOGLOBIN CATABOLISM

Measurement of serum bilirubin, urinary urobilin and faecal urobilinogen can provide important information in the investigation of haemolytic anaemias. As these tests come within the province of the clinical chemist, they are, nowadays, seldom performed in a haematological laboratory. Accordingly, the principles of the tests and their interpretation will be described, but for details of the techniques readers are referred to text books of clinical chemistry, e.g. that by N. W. Tietz.[33]

SERUM BILIRUBIN

Bilirubin is present in serum in two forms: as unconjugated prehepatic bilirubin and bilirubin conjugated to glucuronic acid. Normally, the serum-bilirubin concentration is <17 μmol/l (10 mg/l), and is mostly unconjugated.

In haemolytic anaemias the serum bilirubin usually lies between 17 and 50 μmol/l (10–30 mg/l) and most is unconjugated. Sometimes the level may be normal, despite a considerable increase in haemolysis. Levels >85 μmol/l (50 mg/l) and/or a large proportion of conjugated bilirubin suggest liver disease. Tisdale et al, who reported on the concentration of direct-reacting (conjugated) pigment in haemolytic jaundice, concluded that some of this type of bilirubin may often be regurgitated into the blood stream from the bile when the excretion of pigment is high, even in the absence of overt liver disease.[34]

In haemolytic disease of the newborn (HDN) the bilirubin level is an important factor in determining whether an exchange transfusion should be carried out, as high values of unconjugated bilirubin are toxic to the brain and can lead to kernicterus. In normal newborn infants the level may often reach 85 μmol/l, whilst in HDN infants levels of 350 μmol/l are not uncommon and need to be urgently lowered by exchange transfusion.

Moderately raised serum-bilirubin levels are frequently found in dyshaemopoietic anaemias, e.g. pernicious anaemia, where there is ineffective erythropoiesis. Although part of the bilirubin comes from red cells which have circulated, a major proportion is derived from red cell precursors in the bone marrow which have failed to complete maturation.

Total bilirubin can be measured by direct reading spectrophotometry at 454 (or 461) and 540 nm; the former are the selected wavelengths for bilirubin whilst the latter automatically corrects for any interference by free haemoglobin. The instrument can be standardized with bilirubin solutions of known concentration or with a coloured glass standard. Another direct reading method is by reflectance photometry on a drop of serum which is added to a reagent film.

An alternative 'wet chemistry' method is by the reaction with aqueous diazotized sulphanilic acid.

A red colour is produced which is compared in a photoelectric colorimeter with that of a freshly prepared standard or read in a spectrophotometer at 600 nm. Only conjugated bilirubin reacts directly with this aqueous reagent; unconjugated bilirubin, which is bound to albumin, requires the addition of ethanol to free it from albumin to enable it to react or the action of an accelerator such as methanol or caffeine. The method of Michaelson et al[20] in which caffeine benzoate is used as the accelerator is said to have advantages.[42]

Bilirubin is destroyed by exposure to direct sunlight or any other source of ultraviolet light, including fluorescent lighting. Solutions are stable for 1–2 days if kept at 4°C in the dark.

UROBILIN AND UROBILINOGEN

Urobilin and its reduced form urobilinogen are formed by bacterial action on bile pigments in the intestine. The excretion of faecal urobilinogen is increased in patients with a haemolytic anaemia. Estimations are best expressed as mg of urobilinogen per 100 g of circulating Hb. In health this amounts to 18–35 μmol (11–21 mg) per 100 g Hb per day.[42]

Quantitative measurement of faecal urobilinogen should, in theory, provide an estimate of the total rate of bilirubin production. This is, however, a crude method of assessing rates of haemolysis, and minor degrees are more reliably demonstrated by red cell life-span studies. Urobilinogen excretion is also increased in dyshaemopoietic anaemias such as pernicious anaemia because of ineffective erythropoiesis.

The amount of urobilinogen in the urine is a still less reliable index of haemolysis, for excessive urobilinuria can be a consequence of liver dysfunction as well as of increased red cell destruction.

For estimation in the faeces the bile-derived pigments (stercobilin) are reduced to urobilinogen which is extracted with water. The solution is then treated with Ehrlich's dimethylaminobenzaldehyde reagent to produce a pink colour which can be compared with either a natural or an artificial standard in a quantitative assay.

QUALITATIVE TEST FOR UROBILINOGEN AND UROBILIN IN URINE

Schlesinger's zinc test

To 5 ml of urine, add 2 drops of 0.5 mol/l iodine to convert urobilinogen to urobilin. After mixing and standing for 1–2 min, add 5 ml of a 100 g/l suspension of zinc acetate in ethanol and centrifuge the mixture. A green fluorescence becomes apparent in the clear supernatant if urobilin or urobilinogen is present.

If a spectroscope is available the fluid may be examined for the broad absorption band (due to urobilin) at the green-blue junction (Fig. 12.4).

Urobilinogen can also be detected in freshly voided urine by commercially available reagent strip methods.

PORPHYRINS

Deranged haem synthesis results in alteration in the quantities of porphyrin synthesized and excreted by the body. The three porphyrins of clinical importance in man are: protoporphyrin, uroporphyrin and coproporphyrin together with their precursor δ-aminolaevulinic acid. Protoporphyrin is widely distributed in the body and, in addition to its main role as a precursor of haem in Hb and myoglobin, it is a precursor of cytochromes and catalase. Uroporphyrin and coproporphyrin, which are precursors of protoporphyrin, are normally excreted in small amounts in urine and faeces; and red cells, too, normally contain a small amount of free protoporphyrin and coproporphyrin (Fig. 12.6).

ESTIMATION OF RED CELL PORPHYRINS

Principle. Porphyrins are extracted from washed red cells by a mixture of ethyl acetate and acetic acid. The preparation is treated with ether. Coproporphyrin is extracted from the ethereal solution by 0.1 mol/l HCl and protoporphyrin by 1.5 mol/l HCl. The porphyrin concentration in each extract is determined by a spectrophotometric method. Details of the procedure are given by Moore.[22]

DEMONSTRATION OF PORPHOBILINOGEN IN URINE

Principle. Ehrlich's dimethylaminobenzaldehyde reagent reacts with porphobilinogen to produce a pink aldehyde compound which can be differentiated from that produced by urobilinogen by the fact that the porphobilinogen compound is insoluble in chloroform.

Ehrlich's reagent. Dissolve 0.7 g of p-dimethylaminobenzaldehyde in a mixture of 150 ml of 10 mol/l HCl and 100 ml of water.

Method

The test is best carried out on a freshly passed specimen of urine. Mix a few ml of urine and an equal volume of Ehrlich's reagent in a large test-tube. Add 2 volumes of a saturated solution of sodium acetate. The urine should then have a pH of about 5.0, giving a red reaction with Congo red indicator paper.

If a pink colour develops in the solution, add a few ml of chloroform and shake the mixture thoroughly to extract the pigment. The colour due to urobilinogen or indole will be extracted by the chloroform, whereas that due to porphobilinogen will not, and remains in the supernatant aqueous fraction. When present, the concentration of porphobilinogen in the urine may be estimated quantitatively by a spectrophotometric method at 555 nm.[22]

Aminolaevulinic acid (ALA)

When ALA is present in the urine it can be concentrated with acetyl acetone. It then reacts with Ehrlich's reagent in the same way as porphobilinogen to give a red solution with an absorbance maximum at 553 nm. It can be separated from porphobilinogen by ion exchange resins and estimated quantitatively by a spectrophotometric method.[22]

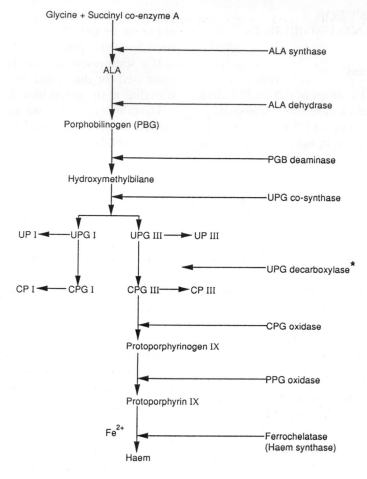

Fig. 12.6 Biosynthesis of porphyrin. See Table 12.1 for explanation of abbreviations.

DEMONSTRATION OF PORPHYRINS IN URINE

Principle. Porphyrins exhibit pink-red fluorescence when viewed by UV light (at 405 nm). Uroporphyrin can be distinguished from coproporphyrin by the different solubilities of the two substances in acid solution.

Method

Mix 25 ml of urine with 10 ml of glacial acetic acid in a separating funnel and extract twice with 50 ml volumes of ether. Set the aqueous fraction (Fraction 1) aside. Wash the ether extracts in a separating funnel with 10 ml of 1.6 mol/l HCl

and collect the HCl fraction (Fraction 2). View both fractions in UV light (at 405 nm) for pink-red fluorescence. Its presence in Fraction 1 indicates uroporphyrin; in Fraction 2, coproporphyrin. The presence of the porphyrins should be confirmed spectroscopically (see below).

If uroporphyrin has been demonstrated, the reaction can be intensified by the following procedure. Adjust the pH of Fraction 1 to 3.0–3.2 with 0.1 mol/l HCl and extract the fraction twice with 50 ml volumes of ethyl acetate. Combine the extracts and extract three times with 2 ml volumes of 3 mol/l HCl. View the acid extracts for pink-red fluorescence in UV light and spectroscopically for acid porphyrin bands.

Table 12.1   Distribution of porphyrins in red cells, urine and faeces in different forms of porphyria

Disease	Enzyme defect*	Red cells	Urine	Faeces
Acute intermittent porphyria	PBG deaminase		PBG ALA	
Congenital erythropoietic porphyria	UPG III cosynthase	UP I CP I	UP I CP I	UP I CP I
Acquired cutaneous hepatic porphyria ('cutanea tarda')	UPG decarboxylase		UP I CP III	
Hereditary coproporphyria	CPG oxidase		CP III	CP III
Variegate porphyria	PPG oxidase		PBG** ALA**	CP III PP
Erythropoietic protoporphyria	Ferrochelatase	PP		PP

*See Fig. 12.6.
**Mainly during acute attacks
ALA, δ-aminolaevulinic acid; PBG, Porphobilinogen; UP, Uroporphyrin; CP, Coproporphyrin; PP, Protoporphyrin; UPG, Uroporphyrinogen; CPG, Coproporphyrinogen; PPG, Protoporphyrinogen.

SPECTROSCOPIC EXAMINATION OF URINE FOR PORPHYRINS

This is carried out on extracts, made as described above, or on urine which is acidified with a few drops of 10 mol/l HCl. If porphyrins are present, a narrow band will appear in the orange at 596 nm and a broader band in the green at 552 nm (Fig. 12.4).

Qualitative tests are adequate for screening purposes. Accurate determinations require spectrophotometry or fluorimetry.

Significance of porphyrins in blood and urine

Normal red cells contain <650 nmol/l of protoporphyrin and <64 nmol/l of coproporphyrin.[22] Increased amounts are present during the first few months of life. At all ages there is an increase in red cell protoporphyrin in iron-deficiency anaemia or latent iron deficiency, in lead poisoning, thalassaemia, some cases of sideroblastic anaemia and the anaemia of chronic infection.

Normally, a small amount of coproporphyrin is excreted in the urine (<430 nmol/day). This is demonstrable by the qualitative test described above, the intensity of pink-red fluorescence being proportional to the concentration of copro-porphyrin. The excretion of coproporphyrin is increased when erythropoiesis is hyperactive, e.g. in haemolytic anaemias, polycythaemia and in pernicious anaemia, sideroblastic anaemias, etc. It is exceptionally high in lead poisoning and it is also high in liver disease; renal impairment results in diminished excretion.

Normally, porphobilinogen cannot be demonstrated in urine, and only traces of uroporphyrin (<50 nmol/day[22]), not detectable by the qualitative test described above, are present. Amino-laevulinic acid excretion is <40 μmol/day;[22] it is increased in lead poisoning.

The increase in urinary coproporphyrin excretion occurring in the above conditions is known as 'porphyrinuria'. There is no increase in uroporphyrin excretion. The porphyrias, on the other hand, are a group of disorders associated with abnormal porphyrin metabolism.

There are several forms of porphyria, due to specific enzyme defects, each with a different clinical and biochemical manifestation.[2,14] The effects are predominantly either hepatic or erythropoietic. The commonest hepatic type is *porphyria cutanea tarda*; which results in photosensitivity, dermatitis and, often, hepatic siderosis; it is due to a defect in uroporphyrinogen decarboxylase. There are two erythropoietic types, *congenital erythropoietic porphyria*, due to defective uroporphyrinogen cosynthase and *erythropoietic protoporphyria*, due to defective ferrochelatase (Table 12.1). In the former, uroporphyrin and coproporphyrin are present in red cells and urine in increased amounts; in the latter, increased protoporphyrin is found in the red cells, but the urine is normal. In erythropoietic porphyria haemolytic anaemia may occur. The patterns of excretion of porphyrin and precursors in the different types of porphyria are shown in Table 12.1.

RECOGNITION AND MEASUREMENT OF ABNORMAL HAEMOGLOBIN PIGMENTS

Methaemoglobin (Hi), sulphaemoglobin (SHb) and carboxyhaemoglobin (HbCO) are of clinical importance, and each has a characteristic absorption spectrum demonstrable by simple spectroscopy or, more definitely, by spectrophotometry. If the absorbance of a dilute solution of blood (e.g. 1 in 200) is measured at wavelengths between 400 and 700 nm, characteristic absorption spectra are obtained (Fig. 12.7). In practice, the abnormal substance represents usually only a fraction of the total Hb (except in coal-gas poisoning), and its identification and accurate measurement may be difficult. Hi can be measured more accurately than SHb.

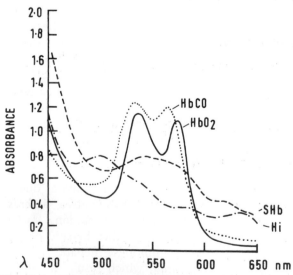

Fig. 12.7   Absorption spectra of various haemoglobin pigments. HbCO, carboxyhaemoglobin; HbO₂, oxyhaemoglobin; SHb, sulphaemoglobin; Hi, methaemoglobin.

SPECTROSCOPIC EXAMINATION OF BLOOD FOR METHAEMOGLOBIN AND SULPHAEMOGLOBIN

Method

Dilute blood 1 in 5 or 1 in 10 with water and then centrifuge. Examine the clear solution, if possible in daylight, using a hand spectroscope. It is important that the greatest possible depth or concentration of solution consistent with visibility should be examined and that a careful search should be made (with varying depths or concentrations of solution) for absorption bands in the red part of the spectrum at 620–630 nm. If bands are seen in the red, add a drop of yellow ammonium sulphide to the solution. A band due to Hi, but not that due to SHb, will disappear. For comparison, lysed blood may be treated with a few drops of potassium ferricyanide (50 g/l) solution which will cause the formation of Hi. SHb may be prepared by adding to 10 ml of a 1 in 100 dilution of blood 0.1 ml of a 1 g/l solution of phenylhydrazine hydrochloride and a drop of water which has been previously saturated with hydrogen sulphide. The spectra of the unknown and the known pigments may then be compared in a reversion spectroscope. The absorption band in the red due to Hi is at 630 nm (cf. methaemalbumin at 624 nm) (Fig. 12.4).

Hi and SHb are formed intracellularly; they are not found in plasma except under very exceptional circumstances, e.g. when their formation is associated with intravascular haemolysis.

MEASUREMENT OF METHAEMOGLOBIN IN BLOOD

Principle. Hi has a maximum absorption at

630 nm. When cyanide is added this absorption band disappears and the resulting change in absorbance is directly proportional to the concentration of Hi. Total Hb in the sample is then measured after complete conversion to HiCN by the addition of ferricyanide-cyanide reagent. The conversion will measure HbO_2 and Hi but not SHb. Thus, the presence of a large amount of SHb will result in an erroneously low measurement of total Hb.

The method described below is based on that of Evelyn and Malloy.[11] Turbidity of the haemolysate can be overcome by the addition of a non-ionic detergent such as Nonidet P40[38] (see p. 50).

Reagents

Phosphate buffer: 0.1 mol/l, pH 6.8.
Potassium cyanide: 50 g/l.
Potassium ferricyanide: 50 g/l.
Non-ionic detergent (see p. 50): 10 ml/l.

Method

Lyse 0.2 ml of blood in a solution containing 4 ml of buffer and 6 ml of detergent solution. Divide the lysate into two equal volumes (A and B). Measure the absorbance of A in a spectrophotometer at 630 nm (D_1). Add 1 drop of KCN solution and measure the absorbance again, after mixing (D_2). Add 1 drop of potassium ferricyanide solution to B, and after 5 min, measure the absorbance at the same wavelength (D_3). Then add 1 drop of KCN solution to B and after mixing make a final reading (D_4). All the measurements are made against a blank containing buffer and detergent in the same proportion as present in the sample.

Calculation

$$\text{Methaemoglobin (\%)} = \frac{D_1 - D_2}{D_3 - D_4} \times 100$$

The test should be carried out within 1 h of collecting the blood. After dilution, the buffered lysate can be stored for up to 24 h at 2–4°C without significant auto-oxidation of Hb to Hi.

SCREENING METHOD FOR DETERMINATION OF SULPHAEMOGLOBIN IN BLOOD

Principle. An absorbance reading at 620 nm measures the sum of the absorbance of HbO_2 and SHb in any blood sample. In contrast to HbO_2, the absorption band due to SHb is unchanged by the addition of cyanide. The residual absorbance, as read at 620 nm, is therefore proportional to the concentration of SHb.

The absorbance of the HbO_2 alone at 620 nm can only be inferred from a reading at 578 nm, and a conversion factor,[38] A^{578}/A^{620}, has to be determined experimentally for each instrument on a series of normal blood samples. The absorbance of SHb is obtained by subtracting the absorbance of the HbO_2 from that of the total Hb. This provides an approximation only, but it may be regarded as adequate for clinical purposes in the absence of a more reliable method.

Method

Mix 0.1 ml of blood with 10 ml of a 20 ml/l solution of a non-ionic detergent (Sterox SE or Nonidet P40). Record the absorbance (A) at 620 nm (total Hb). Add 1 drop of 50 g/l KCN and after standing for 5 min, record A at 620 nm and at 578 nm.

Calculation

$$\text{Sulphaemoglobin (SHb) (\%)} = 2 \times \frac{A^{620}\text{SHb}}{A^{620}\text{HbO}_2}$$

where

$$A^{620}\text{HbO}_2 = \frac{\text{Absorbance read at 578 nm}}{\text{Conversion factor}}$$

and $A^{620}\text{SHb} = A^{620}$ total Hb $- A^{620}\text{HbO}_2$.

Significance of methaemoglobin and sulphaemoglobin in blood

Hi is present in small amounts in normal blood, and constitutes 1–2% of the total Hb. Its concentration is very slightly higher in infants, especially in premature infants, than in older children and adults.[18] Excessive formation of Hi occurs as the result of oxidation of Hb by drugs and chemicals such as phenacetin, sulphonamides, aniline dyes, nitrates and nitrites, etc.

The Hi produced by drugs is chemically normal and the pigment can be reconverted to HbO_2 by reducing agents such as methylene blue.

Other (rare) types of methaemoglobinaemia are caused by inherited deficiency of the enzyme NADH-methaemoglobin reductase and by inherited haemoglobin abnormalities (types of Hb M). The absorption spectra of the Hb Ms differ from that of normal Hi and they react slowly and incompletely with cyanide; their concentration cannot be estimated by the method of Evelyn and Malloy.[11]

Methaemoglobinaemia leads to cyanosis which becomes obvious with as little as 15 g Hi per litre, i.e. c 10%.

SHb is usually formed at the same time as Hi; it represents a further and irreversible stage in Hb degradation. It is present as a rule at a much lower concentration than is Hi.

DEMONSTRATION OF CARBOXYHAEMOGLOBIN

Principle. HbO_2, but not HbCO, is reduced by sodium dithionite and the percentage of HbCO in a mixture can be determined by reference to a calibration graph.

Calibration graph

Dilute 0.1 ml of normal blood in 20 ml of 0.4 ml/l ammonia and divide into two parts. To each add 20 mg of sodium dithionite. Then bubble pure CO into one for 2 min, so as to provide a 100% solution of HbCO.

Add various volumes of the HbCO solution to the reduced Hb solution to provide a range of concentrations of HbCO. Within 10 min of adding the dithionite, measure the absorbance of each solution at 538 nm and 578 nm. Plot the quotient A^{538}/A^{578} on arithmetical graph paper against the % HbCO in each solution.

Method[37,38]

Dilute 0.1 ml of blood in 20 ml of 0.4 ml/l ammonia and add 20 mg of sodium dithionite. Measure the absorbance in a spectrophotometer at 538 nm and 578 nm within 10 min. Calculate the quotient A^{538}/A^{578} and read the % HbCO in the blood from the calibration curve[38] or calculate it from the equation:[37]

$$\% \, HbCO = \left\{ 2.44 \times \frac{A^{538}}{A^{578}} \right\} - 2.68$$

Significance of carboxyhaemoglobin in circulating blood

Carbon monoxide has an affinity for Hb c 200 times that of oxygen. This means that even low concentrations of CO rapidly lead to the formation of HbCO. Less than 1% of HbCO is present in normal blood and up to 10% in smokers.[28,29] A high concentration in blood causes tissue anoxia and may lead to death. Recovery can take place, as HbCO dissociates in time in the presence of high concentrations of oxygen.

IDENTIFICATION OF MYOGLOBIN IN URINE

Myoglobin is the principal protein in muscle, and may be released into the circulation when there is cardiac or skeletal muscle damage. Some may be excreted in the urine where its concentration can be measured by a specific and relatively sensitive radio-immune assay.[32] As the absorption spectra of myoglobin and Hb are similar, although not identical, it is not possible to distinguish them readily by spectroscopy or even by spectrophotometry. But they can be separated by column chromatography.[5] The following is a simple screening test for identifying the presence of myoglobin in urine; it is based on the fact that Hb and myoglobin are precipitated in urine at different degrees of ammonium sulphate saturation. First, it is necessary to demonstrate by precipitation with sulphosalicylic acid that the pigment in the urine is a protein.

Method[1]

Add 3 ml of a 30 g/l solution of sulphosalicylic acid to 1 ml of urine. Mix well and filter. If the pigment is a protein, it will be precipitated. (If the filtrate retains the abnormal colour, this must be due to a non-protein pigment, perhaps a porphyrin.) If the pigment has been shown to be protein, add 2.8 g of ammonium sulphate to 5 ml of urine (= 80% saturation). Shake the mixture to dissolve the ammonium sulphate, then filter or centrifuge. In myoglobinuria the filtrate will be abnormally coloured; in haemoglobinuria the filtrate will be of normal colour and the precipitate coloured.

Normal range[33]

Men, <80 µg/l; women, <60 µg/l; increasing slightly in older age. Children have very low values.

REFERENCES

[1] BLODHEIM, S. H., MARGOLIASH, E. and SHAFRIR, E. (1958). A simple test for myohemoglobinuria (myoglobinuria). *Journal of American Medical Association*, **167**, 453.

[2] BOTTOMLEY, S. S. and MULLER-EBERHARD, U. (1988). Pathophysiology of heme synthesis. *Seminars in Hematology*, **25**, 282.

[3] BROTHERHOOD, J., BROZOVIC, B. and PUGH, L. G. C. (1975). Haematological status of middle- and long-distance runners. *Clinical Science and Molecular Medicine*, **48**, 139.

[4] BRUS, I. and LEWIS, S. M. (1959). The haptoglobin content of serum in haemolytic anaemia. *British Journal of Haematology*, **5**, 348.

[5] CAMERON, B. F., AZZAM, S. A., KOTITE, L. and AWAD, E. S. (1965). Determination of myoglobin and hemoglobin. *Journal of Laboratory and Clinical Medicine*, **65**, 883.

[6] CHAPLIN, H. Jnr, CASSELL, M. and HANKS G. E. (1961). The stability of the plasma hemoglobin level in the normal human subject. *Journal of Laboratory and Clinical Medicine*, **57**, 612.

[7] CROSBY, W. H. and DAMESHEK, W. (1951). The significance of hemoglobinemia and associated hemosiderinuria, with particular reference to various types of hemolytic anemia. *Journal of Laboratory and Clinical Medicine*, **38**, 829.

[8] CROSBY, W. H. and FURTH, F. W. (1956). A modification of the benzidine method for measurement of hemoglobin in plasma and urine. *Blood*, **11**, 380.

[9] CROWLE, A. J. (1973). *Immunodiffusion*. 2nd edn. Academic Press, New York.

[10] DACIE, J. (1985). *The Haemolytic Anaemias: Volume I: The Hereditary Haemolytic Anaemias*, 3rd edn, p. 45. Churchill Livingstone, Edinburgh.

[11] EVELYN, K. A. and MALLOY, H. T. (1938). Microdetermination of oxyhemoglobin, methemoglobin and sulfhemoglobin in a single sample of blood. *Journal of Biological Chemistry*, **126**, 655.

[12] FAIRLEY, N. H. and BROMFIELD, R. J. (1934). Laboratory studies in malaria and blackwater fever. Part III. A new blood pigment in blackwater fever and other biochemical observations. *Transactions of the Royal Society of Tropical Medicine and Hygiene*, **28**, 307.

[13] FERRIS, T. G., EASERLING, R. E., NELSON, K. J. and BUDD, R. E. (1966). Determination of serum-hemoglobin binding capacity and haptoglobin-type by acrylamide gel electrophoresis. *American Journal of Clinical Pathology*, **46**, 385.

[14] GOLDBERG, A., MOORE, M. R., McCOLL, K. E. L. and BRODIE, M. J. (1987). Porphyrin metabolism and the porphyrias. In *Oxford Textbook of Medicine*, 2nd edn. Eds. D. J. Weatherall, J. G. G. Ledingham and D. A. Warrell, p. 9. 136. Oxford University Press, Oxford.

[15] HANKS, G. E., CASSELL, M., RAV, R. N. and CHAPLIN, H. Jnr (1960). Further modifications of the benzidine method for measurement of hemoglobin in plasma: definition of a new range of normal values. *Journal of Laboratory and Clinical Medicine*, **56**, 486.

[16] HANSTEIN, A. and MULLER-EBERHARD, U. (1968). Concentration of serum hemopexin in healthy children and adults and in those with a variety of hematological disorders. *Journal of Laboratory and Clinical Medicine*, **71**, 232.

[17] HEIDE, K., HAUPT, H., STÖRIKO, K. and SCHULTZE, H. E. (1964). On the heme-binding capacity of hemopexin. *Clinica Chimica Acta*, **10**, 460.

[18] KRAVITZ, H., ELEGANT, L. D., KAISER, E. and KAGAN, B. M. (1956). Methemoglobin values in premature and mature infants and children. *American Journal of Diseases of Children*, **91**, 1.

[19] LAURELL, C. B. and NYMAN, N. (1957). Studies on the serum haptoglobin level in hemoglobinemia and its influence on renal excretion of hemoglobin, *Blood*, **12**, 493.

[20] MICHAELSSON, M., NOSSLIN, B. and SJÖLIN, S. (1965). Plasma bilirubin determination in the new born infant. A methodological study with special reference to the influence of haemolysis. *Paediatrica*, **35**, 925.

[21] MOORE, G. L., LEDFORD, M. E. and MERYDITH, A. (1981). A micromodification of the Drabkin hemoglobin assay for measuring plasma hemoglobin in the range of 5 to 2000 mg/dl. *Biochemical Medicine*, **26**, 167.

[22] MOORE, M. R. (1983). Laboratory investigation of disturbances of porphyrin metabolism. *Association of Clinical Pathologists, Broadsheet No. 109*. British Medical Association, London.

[23] MULLER-EBERHARD, U. (1970). Hemopexin. *New England Journal of Medicine*, **283**, 1090.

[24] NAGEL, R. L. and GIBSON, Q. H. (1971). The binding of hemoglobin to haptoglobin and its relation to subunit dissociation of hemoglobin. *Journal of Biological Chemistry*, **246**, 69.

[25] NYMAN, M. (1959). Serum haptoglobin: methodological and clinical studies. *Scandinavian Journal of Clinical and Laboratory Investigation*, **11**, Suppl 39.

[26] RATCLIFF, A. P. and HARDWICKE, J. (1964). Estimation of serum haemoglobin-binding capacity (haptoglobin) on Sephadex G 100. *Journal of Clinical Pathology*, **17**, 676.

[27] ROWE, D. S. (1961). A rapid method for the estimation of serum haptoglobin. *Journal of Clinical Pathology*, **14**, 205.

[28] RUSSELL, M. A. H., WILSON, C., COLE, P. V. and IDLE, M. (1973). Comparison of increases in carboxyhaemoglobin after smoking 'extra mild' and 'non mild' cigarettes. *Lancet*, **ii**, 687.

[29] SHIELDS, C. E. (1971). Elevated carbon monoxide level from smoking in blood donors. *Transfusion (Philadelphia)*, **11**, 89.

[30] SMITHIES, O. (1959). An improved procedure for starch-gel electrophoresis: further variations in the serum proteins of normal individuals. *Biochemical Journal*, **71**, 585.

[31] STANDEFER, J. C. and VANDERJOGT, D. (1977). Use of

tetramethyl benzidine in plasma hemoglobin assay. *Clinical Chemistry*, **23**, 749.

[32] STONE, M. J., WILLERSON, J. T. and WATERMAN, M. R. (1982). Radioimmunoassay of myoglobin. *Methods in Enzymology*, **84**, 172.

[33] TIETZ, N. W. (1986). *Textbook of Clinical Chemistry*. W B Saunders, Philadelphia.

[34] TISDALE, W. A., KLATSKIN, G. and KINSELLA, E. D. (1959). The significance of the direct-reacting fraction of serum bilirubin in hemolytic jaundice. *American Journal of Medicine*, **26**, 214.

[35] VAERMAN, J. P. (1981). Single radial immunodiffusion. *Methods in Enzymology*, **73**, 291.

[36] VALERI, C. R., BOND, J. C., FLOWER, K. and SOBUCKI, J. (1965). Quantitation of serum hemoglobin-binding capacity using cellulose acetate membrane electrophoresis. *Clinical Chemistry*, **11**, 581.

[37] VAN ASSENDELFT, O. W. (1970). *Spectrophotometry of Haemoglobin Derivatives*. Royal VanGorcum Ltd, Assen, The Netherlands.

[38] VAN KAMPEN, E. J. and ZIJLSTRA, W. G. (1965). Determination of hemoglobin and its derivates. *Advances in Clinical Chemistry*, **8**, 141.

[39] VAN LENTE, F., MARCHAND, A. and GALEN, R. S. (1979). Evaluation of a nephelometric assay for haptoglobin and its clinical usefulness. *Clinical Chemistry*, **25**, 2007.

[40] VANZETTI, G. and VALENTE, D. (1965). A sensitive method for the determination of hemoglobin in plasma. *Clinica Chimica Acta*, **11**, 442.

[41] VIEDMA, J. A. (1987). Immunoturbidimetry of haptoglobin and transferrin in the EPOS 5060 analyzer. *Clinical Chemistry*, **33**, 1257.

[42] WOOTTON, I. D. P. and FREEMAN, H. (1982). *Micro-Analysis in Medical Biochemistry*, 6th edn. Churchill Livingstone, Edinburgh.

[43] WU, H. (1923). Studies on hemoglobin: ultra-method for determination of hemoglobin as peroxidase. *Biochemical Journal*, **2**, 189.

13. Investigation of the hereditary haemolytic anaemias: membrane and enzyme abnormalities

Revised by L. Luzzatto and D. Roper

Osmotic fragility, as measured by lysis in hypotonic saline   216
Osmotic fragility after incubating the blood at 37°C for 24 hours   217
Factors affecting osmotic-fragility tests   218
Recording the results of osmotic-fragility tests   219
　Alternative methods of recording osmotic fragility   219
　Interpretation of results   219
Acidified glycerol lysis-time tests   221
Autohaemolysis   222
　Significance of increased autohaemolysis   222
Detection of enzyme deficiencies in hereditary haemolytic anaemias   225
Screening tests for G6PD deficiency and other defects of the pentose phosphate pathway   225
　Fluorescent screening test for G6PD deficiency   227
　Methaemoglobin reduction test   228
Detection of heterozygotes for G6PD deficiency   229

Methaemoglobin elution test   229
Pyrimidine-5'-nucleotidase screening test   230
Red cell enzyme assays   231
　General points of technique   231
G6PD assay   233
　Interpretation of results   234
Identification of G6PD variants   235
Pyruvate kinase assay   235
　Interpretation of results   236
Estimation of reduced glutathione (GSH)   236
　The glutathione stability test   238
2,3-Diphosphoglycerate (DPG)   239
　Measurement of red cell DPG   239
　Significance of DPG concentration   240
The oxygen dissociation curve   241
　Measurement   241
Abbreviations used in this chapter   245

The various initial steps to be taken in the investigation of a patient suspected of having a haemolytic anaemia are outlined in Chapter 12 and the changes in red cell morphology which may be found in haemolytic anaemias are illustrated in Chapter 7. In this chapter are described procedures useful in the investigation of patients thought to have haemolytic anaemias based on defects within the red cell membrane or defective enzymes important in red cell metabolism.

The technical expertise required to identify precisely the defect in a particular instance of hereditary haemolytic anaemia is beyond the scope of most haematological laboratories. The precise identification of an enzyme defect, for example, depends upon the isolation and purification of the enzyme and the characterization of its kinetic and structural uniqueness. In a service laboratory it is sufficient to identify the general nature of the defect, whether it be in the membrane or the metabolic pathways of the red cell. With metabolic defects an attempt should be made, where possible, to pin-point the enzyme involved. Most of the enzyme assays have been standardized by the International Council for Standardization in Haematology (ISCH). A number of commercial kits are also available for the assay of various enzymes and for 2,3-diphosphoglycerate (DPG). In the first part of this chapter are described screening tests for spherocytosis, including hereditary spherocytosis (HS), and for glucose 6-phosphate dehydrogenase (G6PD) deficiency. In the later sections specific enzyme assays are described and the measurement of DPG and reduced glutathione (GSH).

OSMOTIC FRAGILITY, AS MEASURED BY LYSIS IN HYPOTONIC SALINE

The osmotic fragility test gives an indication of the surface area/volume ratio of erythrocytes. Its greatest usefulness is in the diagnosis of hereditary spherocytosis. The test may also be used in screening for thalassaemia. Red cells that are spherocytic, for whatever cause, take up less water in a hypotonic solution before rupturing than normal red cells.

Principle. The method to be described is based upon that of Parpart and co-workers.[37]

Small volumes of blood are mixed with a large excess of buffered saline solutions of varying concentration. The fraction of red cells lysed at each saline concentration is determined colorimetrically. The test is normally carried out at room temperature (15–25°C).

Reagents

Prepare a stock solution of buffered sodium chloride (AR), osmotically equivalent to 100 g/l (1.71 mol/l) NaCl, as follows: dissolve NaCl, 90 g; Na_2HPO_4, 13.65 g[*] and $NaH_2PO_4.2H_2O$, 2.34 g in water and adjust the final volume to 1 litre. This solution will keep for months at 4°C in a well stoppered bottle. Salt crystals may form on storage and must be thoroughly redissolved before use.

In preparing hypotonic solutions for use it is convenient to make first a 10 g/l solution from the 100 g/l NaCl stock solution by dilution with water. Dilutions equivalent to 9.0, 7.5, 6.5, 6.0, 5.5, 5.0, 4.0, 3.5, 3.0, 2.0 and 1.0 g/l are convenient concentrations. Intermediate concentrations such as 4.75 and 5.25 g/l are useful in critical work and an additional 12.0 g/l dilution should be used for incubated samples.

It is convenient to make up 50 ml of each dilution. The solutions keep well at 4°C if sterile, but they should be inspected for moulds each time they are used and discarded if moulds develop.

Method

Heparinized venous blood or defibrinated blood

may be used: oxalated or citrated blood is not suitable because of the additional salts added to it. The test should be carried out within 2 h of collection with blood stored at room temperature or within 6 h if the blood has been kept at 4°C.

1. Deliver 5.0 ml of each of the 11 saline solutions into 1×12 cm test-tubes. Add 5.0 ml of water to tube 12.

2. Add to each tube 50 µl of well mixed blood, and mix immediately by inverting the tubes several times avoiding foam.

3. Leave the suspensions for 30 min at room temperature. Mix again, and then centrifuge for 5 min at 1200*g.*

4. Remove the supernatants and estimate the amount of lysis in each using a spectrophotometer[**] at a wavelength setting of 540 nm or a photoelectric colorimeter provided with a yellow-green (e.g. Ilford 625) filter. Use as a blank the supernatant from tube 1 (osmotically equivalent to 9 g/l NaCl).

5. Assign a value of 100% lysis to the reading with the supernatant of tube 12 (water) and express the readings from the other tubes as percent of the value of tube 12. Plot the results against the NaCl concentration (Fig. 13.1).

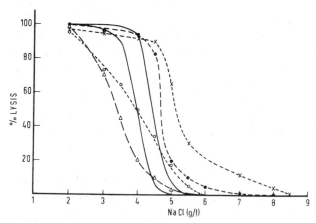

Fig. 13.1   Osmotic-fragility curves. Osmotic fragility curves of patients suffering from: (a) sickle cell anaemia Δ — — Δ, (b) β-thalassaemia major O – – – O, (c) hereditary spherocytosis ● – – – ●, and (d) 'idiopathic' warm auto-immune haemolytic anaemia X – – – X. The normal range is indicated by the unbroken lines.

---

[*]Or $Na_2HPO_4.2H_2O$, 17.115 g.
[**]See footnote on p. 50.

Notes

1. The measurement of osmotic fragility (OF) is a simple procedure which requires a minimum of equipment. It will yield gratifying results if carried out carefully.

2. The blood must be delivered into the 12 tubes with great care. The critical point is not that the amount be exactly 50 μl, but rather that the amount added to each tube must be the same. Two methods are recommended:

(a) Using an automatic pipette (e.g. a Pipetman with a yellow tip). After aspirating the blood gently, the outside should be wiped with tissue paper taking care not to suck out any blood from the inside of the tip by capillary action. The blood is then delivered into the saline solution and the pipette rinsed in and out several times until no blood is visible inside its tip.

The tip has to be changed before moving on to the next tube. This procedure takes time and may result in an increased exposure for the first few tubes. It is therefore advisable to start the timing on the addition of the sample to the first tube.

(b) Using a Pasteur pipette with a perfectly flat end, 1 mm in diameter. About 1 ml of blood should be sucked up, avoiding any bubbles, and the outside of the pipette wiped. With the pipette held vertically above tube 1, a single drop (about 50 μl) is delivered without the blood touching the wall of the tube. Further single drops are then delivered into the remaining 11 tubes.

Method (b) appears to be primitive, but with practice it is perfectly satisfactory; it is also more economical and much faster than method (a). With either method, the best way to test its accuracy is to do a preliminary test by delivering the blood into several tubes all containing the same saline solution (e.g. either 3.0 or 1.0 g/l). The readings with the supernatants should be all within 5% of each other.

3. If the amount of blood available is limited (e.g. from babies), and the spectrophotometer takes 1 ml cuvettes, the volumes can be scaled down to 1 ml of saline solution and 10 μl of blood. However, to deliver reproducibly 10 μl of blood is not easy. With method (b) a Pasteur pipette or capillary pipette with a much smaller diameter,

calibrated to give 10 μl drops of blood would have to be used. It is then more difficult to maintain accuracy. Method (a) may be preferable in this case.

4. With the method using 50 μl of blood and with non-anaemic blood the reading for 100% lysis will be about 0.7. With a modern spectrophotometer any figure between 0.5 and 1.5 is acceptable. If the value is below 0.5, the test should be repeated using more blood or less saline (the reverse if the reading is above 1.5). With photoelectric colorimeters values above 0.5 are often not very accurate.

5. When transferring the supernatant from a tube to the spectrophotometer cuvette, care has to be taken not to disturb the pellet. If it is well packed, the supernatant can be simply poured from the tube into the cuvette; with a spectrophotometer provided with an automatic suction device, this is usually satisfactory. Alternatively, a Pasteur pipette should be used (fitted with a little plastic tubing at the end in order not to scratch the cuvette).

6. Even when a normal range has been established, it is essential always to run a normal control sample along with that of the patients to be tested in order to check, for example, the saline solutions.

The sigmoid shape of the normal osmotic fragility curve indicates that normal red cells vary in their resistance to hypotonic solutions. Indeed, this resistance varies gradually (osmotically) as a function of red cell age, with the youngest cells being the most resistant and the oldest cells the most fragile. The reason for this is that old cells have a higher sodium content and a decreased capacity to pump out sodium.

OSMOTIC FRAGILITY AFTER INCUBATING THE BLOOD AT 37°C FOR 24 HOURS

Method

Defibrinated blood should be used, care being taken to ensure that sterility is maintained.

Incubate 1 ml or 2 ml volumes of blood in sterile 5 ml screw-capped bottles. It is advisable to set up the samples in duplicate in case one bottle has become infected, as indicated by gross lysis and change in colour.

After 24 h, if no infection is evident, pool the contents of the duplicate bottles after thoroughly mixing the sedimented red cells in the overlying serum and estimate the fragility as previously described.

As the fragility may be markedly increased (Fig. 13.2), set up additional hypotonic solutions containing 7.0 g/l and 8.0 g/l NaCl. In addition, use a solution equivalent to 12.0 g/l NaCl, for sometimes, as in hereditary spherocytosis (HS), lysis may take place in 9.0 g/l NaCl. In this case use the supernatant of the tube containing 12.0 g/l NaCl as the blank in the colorimetric estimation.

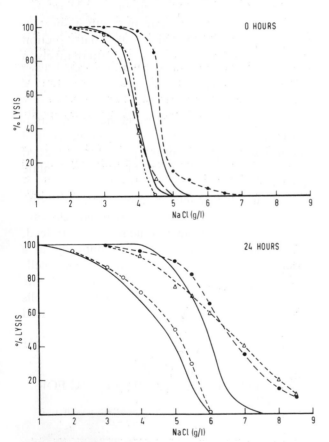

Fig. 13.2 Osmotic-fragility curves before and after incubating blood at 37°C for 24 hours. From patients suffering from: (a) hereditary spherocytosis ● – – – ●, (b) pyruvate-kinase deficiency △ – – – △, and (c) hereditary non-spherocytic haemolytic anaemia of undiagnosed type O – – – O. The normal range is indicated by the unbroken lines.

The incubation fragility test is conveniently combined with the estimation of the amount of spontaneous autohaemolysis (see p. 222).

Factors affecting osmotic-fragility tests

In carrying out osmotic-fragility tests by any method three variables capable of markedly affecting the results must be controlled, quite apart from the accuracy with which the saline solutions have been made up. These are:

1. The relative volumes of blood and saline.
2. The final pH of the blood in saline suspension.
3. The temperature at which the tests are carried out.

A proportion of 1 volume of blood to 100 volumes of saline is chosen because the concentration of blood is so small that the effect of the plasma on the final tonicity of the suspension is negligible. When weak suspensions of blood in saline are used it is necessary to control the pH of the hypotonic solutions and it is for this reason that phosphate buffer is added to the saline. Even so, small differences will be found between the fragility of venous blood and maximally aerated (i.e. oxygenated) blood. For the most accurate results it is recommended that the blood should be mixed until bright red. Finally, it is ideal for tests to be carried out always at the same temperature, although for most purposes room temperature is sufficiently constant.

The extent of the effect of pH and temperature on osmotic fragility was well illustrated in the paper of Parpart and co-workers.[37] The effect of pH is more important: a shift of 0.1 of a pH unit is equivalent to altering the saline concentration by 0.1 g/l, the fragility of the red cells being increased by a fall in pH. A rise in temperature decreases the fragility, a rise of 5°C being equivalent to an increase in saline concentration of about 0.1 g/l.

Lysis is virtually complete at the end of 30 min at 20°C and the hypotonic solutions may be centrifuged at the end of this time.

Further details of the factors which affect and control haemolysis of red cells in hypotonic solutions were given by Murphy.[36]

Recording the results of osmotic-fragility tests

In the past, osmotic fragility most often has been expressed in terms of the highest concentration of saline at which lysis is just detectable (initial lysis or minimum resistance) and the highest concentration of saline in which lysis appears to be complete (complete lysis or maximum resistance). It is however, useful also to record the concentration of saline causing 50% lysis, i.e. the median corpuscular fragility (MCF), and to inspect the entire fragility curve (Fig. 13.1). The findings in health are summarized in Table 13.1.

Alternative methods of recording osmotic fragility

Two simple alternative methods of recording the results quantitatively are available: the data may be plotted on probability paper or increment-haemolysis curves can be drawn (see below). Both methods emphasize heterogeneity of the cell population with respect to osmotic fragility. If the observed amounts of lysis of normal blood are plotted on the probability scale against concentrations of saline, an almost straight line can be drawn through the points, there being skewness only where lysis is becoming almost complete. This method enables the MCF to be read off with ease.

In disease, tailed curves result in varying degrees of skewness at the other end of the probability plot as well. In order to obtain increment-haemolysis curves, the differences in lysis between adjacent tubes are plotted against the corresponding saline concentrations. Definitely bimodal curves may be obtained during recovery from a haemolytic episode.[42]

Interpretation of results

The osmotic fragility of freshly taken red cells reflects their ability to take up a certain amount of water before lysing. This is determined by their volume to surface area ratio. The ability of the normal red cell to withstand hypotonicity results from its biconcave shape which allows the cell to increase its volume by about 70% before the surface membrane is stretched: once this limit is reached lysis occurs.[27] Spherocytes have an increased volume to surface area ratio; their ability to take in water before stretching the surface membrane is thus more limited than normal and they are therefore particularly susceptible to osmotic lysis. The increase in osmotic fragility is a property of the spheroidal shape of the cell and is independent of the cause of the spherocytosis. Characteristically, osmotic fragility curves from patients with HS who have not been splenectomized show a 'tail' of very fragile cells (Fig. 13.3). When plotted on probability paper the graph indicates two populations of cells, the very fragile and the normal or slightly fragile. After splenectomy the red cells are more homogeneous, the osmotic-fragility curve indicating a more continuous spectrum of cells, from fragile to normal.

Decreased osmotic fragility indicates the presence of unusually flattened red cells (leptocytes) in which the volume to surface area ratio is decreased. Such a change occurs in iron-defi-

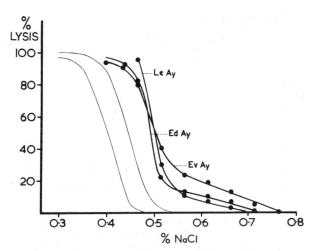

Fig. 13.3 Osmotic-fragility curves of three HS patients belonging to the same family (brother, sister and uncle (Le Ay)). The area between the thin lines represents the normal range.

Table 13.1 Osmotic fragility in health (at 20°C and pH 7.4)

	Fresh blood (g/l NaCl)	Blood incubated for 24 h at 37°C (g/l NaCl)
Initial lysis	5.0	7.0
Complete lysis	3.0	2.0
MCF (50% lysis)	4.0–4.45	4.65–5.9

ciency anaemia and thalassaemia in which the red cells with a low MCH and MCV are unusually resistant to osmotic lysis (Fig. 13.1). Reticulocytes and red cells from splenectomized patients also tend to have a greater amount of membrane compared with normal cells and are osmotically resistant. In liver disease, target cells may be produced by passive accumulation of lipid and these cells, too, are resistant to osmotic lysis.[15]

The osmotic fragility of red cells after incubation for 24 h at 37°C is also a reflection of their volume to surface area ratio but the factors which alter this ratio are more complicated than in fresh red cells. The increased osmotic fragility of normal red cells which occurs after incubation (Fig. 13.2) is mainly caused by swelling of the cells associated with an accumulation of sodium which exceeds loss of potassium. Such cation exchange is determined by the membrane properties of the red cell which control the passive flux of ions and the metabolic competence of the cell which determines the active pumping of cations against concentration gradients. During incubation for 24 h the metabolism of the red cell becomes stressed and the pumping mechanisms tend to fail, one factor being a relative lack of glucose in the medium.

The osmotic fragility of red cells which have an abnormal membrane, such as those of HS and hereditary elliptocytosis (HE), increases abnormally after incubation (Fig. 13.2). The results with red cells with a glycolytic deficiency, such as those of pyruvate kinase (PK) deficiency, are variable. In severe deficiencies, osmotic fragility may increase substantially (Fig. 13.2) but in other cases the fragility may decrease due to a greater loss of potassium than gain of sodium. In thalassaemia major and minor, osmotic fragility is frequently markedly reduced after incubation, again due to a marked loss of potassium.[23] A similar, though usually less marked, change is seen in iron-deficiency anaemia.

To summarize, measurement of red cell osmotic fragility provides a useful indication as to whether a patient's red cells are normal, for an abnormal result invariably indicates abnormality. The reverse is, however, not true, i.e. a result that is within the normal range does not mean that the red cells are normal. The findings in some important haemolytic anaemias are summarized in Table 13.2.

Table 13.2   Osmotic fragility in haemolytic anaemias: a summary

Condition	Notes
A. Associated with increased OF Hereditary spherocytosis (HS)	Entire curve may be 'shifted to the right', or most of it may be within the normal range, but with a 'tail' of fragile cells. Curve within normal range in 10–20% of cases. After incubation for 24 h abnormalities usually more marked, but still some 'false-negative'. Splenectomy does not affect MCF, but reduces the tail of fragile cells
Hereditary elliptocytosis (HE)	As in HS, but in general changes less marked. Abnormal OF usually correlates with severity of haemolysis, i.e. OF is normal in non-haemolytic HE
Other inherited membrane abnormalities	Results variable; with milder disorders curve more likely to be abnormal after incubation for 24 h
Auto-immune haemolytic anaemia	Tail of fragile cells roughly proportional to number of spherocytes; rest of curve normal (or even left-shifted on account of high reticulocytosis)
B. Associated with decreased OF Thalassaemia	MCF decreased in all forms of thalassaemia, except in some α-thal heterozygotes; usually the entire curve is left-shifted
Enzyme abnormalities	OF usually normal (anaemia originally referred to as hereditary non-spherocytic), but tail of highly resistant cells may be seen on account of high reticulocytosis. After incubation for 24 h there may be a tail of fragile cells

GLYCEROL LYSIS-TIME TESTS

The osmotic-fragility test is somewhat cumbersome and requires 2 ml or more of whole blood. It is thus not suitable for use in newborn babies nor as a population screening test. In 1974 Gottfried and Robertson[21] introduced a glycerol lysis-time (GLT) test, a one-tube test, to measure the time taken for 50% haemolysis of a blood sample in a buffered hypotonic saline-glycerol mixture. The original method had greater sensitivity in the osmotic resistant range but could also identify most patients with HS by a shorter GLT_{50}. Better identification of HS blood from normal was obtained by 24 h incubation of samples and by modifying the glycerol reagent.[20] Zanella and colleagues modified the original test further by decreasing the pH.[51] There is some loss of specificity for HS with the acidified compared with the original method but in practice this loss is unimportant.

ACIDIFIED GLYCEROL LYSIS-TIME TEST[51]

Principle. Glycerol present in a hypotonic buffered saline solution slows the rate of entry of water molecules into the red cells so that the time taken for lysis may be more conveniently measured. Like the osmotic-fragility test, differentiation can be made between spherocytes and normal red cells.

Reagents

Phosphate buffered saline (PBS). Add 9 volumes of 9.0 g/l (154 mmol/l) NaCl to 1 volume of 100 mmol/l phosphate buffer (2 volumes of Na_2HPO_4, 14.9 g/l added to 1 volume of KH_2PO_4, 13.61 g/l). Adjust the pH to 6.85 ± 0.05 at room temperature (15–25°C). This adjustment must be accurate.

Glycerol reagent (300 mmol/l). Add 23 ml of glycerol (27.65 g AR grade) to 300 ml of PBS and bring the final volume to 1 litre with water.

Method

Add 20 μl of whole blood, anticoagulated with EDTA, to 5.0 ml of PBS, pH 6.85. Mix the suspension carefully.

Transfer 1.0 ml to a standard 4 ml cuvette of a spectrophotometer equipped with a linear-logarithmic recorder. Fix the wavelength at 625 nm and start the recorder. Add 2.0 ml of the glycerol reagent rapidly to the cuvette with a 2.0 ml syringe pipette and mix well.

The rate of haemolysis is measured by the rate of fall of turbidity of the reaction mixture. The results are expressed as the time required for the optical density to fall to half the initial value ($AGLT_{50}$). The test can also be carried out using a colorimeter and stop-watch.

Results

Normal blood takes more than 1800 s (30 min) to reach the $AGLT_{50}$. The time taken is similar for blood from normal adults, newborn infants and cord samples. In patients with HS the range of the $AGLT_{50}$ is 25–150 s. A short $AGLT_{50}$ may also be found in chronic renal failure, chronic leukaemias, auto-immune haemolytic anaemia and in some pregnant women.

Significance of the AGLT

The same principles apply as with the osmotic-fragility test. Cells with a high volume to surface area ratio resist swelling for a shorter time than normal cells. This applies to all spherocytes, whether the spherocytosis is caused by HS or other mechanisms. The test is particularly useful in screening family members of patients with HS where morphological changes are too small to indicate clearly whether the disorder is present or not.

AUTOHAEMOLYSIS (SPONTANEOUS HAEMOLYSIS DEVELOPING IN BLOOD INCUBATED AT 37°C FOR 48 HOURS)

The autohaemolysis test is useful as an initial screen in suspected cases of haemolytic anaemia. It provides information about the metabolic competence of the red cells and helps to distinguish membrane and enzyme defects if the results of the tests are taken together with other observations such as morphology, inheritance and the presence or absence of associated clinical disorders.

Principle. Aliquots of blood are incubated both with and without sterile glucose solution at 37°C for 48 hours. After this period the amount of spontaneous haemolysis is measured colorimetrically.

Method

It is essential to use aseptic techniques in setting up the autohaemolysis test in order to maintain sterility throughout the incubation period.

Use sterile defibrinated blood and deliver four 1 ml or 2 ml samples into sterile 5 ml screw-capped bottles. Retain a portion of the original sample; separate and store this as the pre-incubation serum.

Add to two of the bottles 50 or 100 µl of sterile 100 g/l glucose solution so as to provide a concentration of glucose in the blood of at least 30 mmol/l. Make sure that the caps of the bottles are tightly closed and place the series of bottles in the incubator at 37°C. A sample from a known normal individual should be run in parallel as a control.

After 24 h, thoroughly mix the content by gentle swirling. After incubating for 48 h, inspect the samples for signs of infection, thoroughly mix again, then from each bottle remove a sample for the estimation of the PCV and Hb and centrifuge the remainder to obtain the supernatant serum.

Estimate the spontaneous lysis by means of a colorimeter or in a spectrophotometer at 540 nm.

As a rule it is convenient to make a 1 in 10 dilution of the incubated serum in cyanide-ferricyanide (Drabkin's) solution, unless there is marked haemolysis when a 1 in 25 or 1 in 50 dilution is more suitable. A corresponding dilution of the pre-incubation serum is used as a blank and a 1 in 100 or 1 in 200 dilution of the whole blood in Drabkin's solution indicates the total amount of Hb present and serves as a standard.

Calculate the percentage lysis, allowing for the change in PCV resulting from the incubation as follows:[41]

$$\text{Lysis (\%)} = \frac{R_t}{R_o} \times \frac{D_o}{D_t} \times (1 - PCV_t) \times 100,$$

where, R_o = reading in colorimeter of diluted whole blood; R_t = reading in colorimeter of diluted serum at 48 h; PCV_t = packed cell volume at time T; D_o = dilution of whole blood (e.g. 1 in 200 = 0.005), and D_t = dilution of serum (e.g. 1 in 10 = 0.1).

The reading at time T is multiplied by $(1 - PCV_t)$ so as to give the concentration which would be found if the liberated haemoglobin was dissolved in whole blood, i.e. in both plasma and red cell compartments, not in the plasma compartment alone.

Normal range of autohaemolysis

Lysis at 48 h. Without added glucose 0.2–2.0%; with added glucose 0–0.9%.

The results obtained are sensitive to slight differences in technique and each laboratory should use a carefully standardized procedure and establish its own normal range. It is more accurate (although more time consuming) to measure lysis by a chemical method rather than by a direct photometric method, particularly if the amount of liberated haemoglobin is small.[22]

Significance of increased autohaemolysis

Little or no lysis takes place when normal blood is incubated for 24 h under sterile conditions and the amount present after 48 h is small.[41] If glucose is added so that it is present throughout the incubation the development of lysis is markedly slowed. The amount of autohaemolysis which occurs after 48 h with and without glucose is determined by the properties of the membrane and the metabolic competence of the red cell. In membrane disorders such as HS the rate of glucose consumption is increased to compensate for an increased cation leak through the membrane.[16a] During the 48 h incubation glucose is therefore used up relatively rapidly so that energy production fails more quickly than normal unless glucose is added. This is one factor which contributes to the increased rate of autohaemolysis in HS. Usually, but not always, the addition of glucose to the blood decreases the rate of autohaemolysis in HS (Fig. 13.4). This was referred to as Type-1 autohaemolysis.[41] When the utilization of glucose via the glycolytic pathway is impaired, as in PK deficiency, the rate of autohaemolysis at 48 h is usually increased and glucose fails to correct or may even aggravate lysis (Type-2 autohaemolysis, Fig. 13.5). Although a similar result may be seen in severe HS (Type B), in the absence of spherocytosis failure of glucose to diminish autohaemolysis is a strong indication of a glycolytic

block. Blood from patients with G6PD deficiency or other disorders of the pentose phosphate pathway may undergo a slight increase in autohaemolysis (without additional glucose) which is corrected by the addition of glucose. Commonly the result is normal but examination of the incubated blood may show an increase in methaemoglobin (Hi) (see below). Not all glycolytic enzyme deficiencies give a Type 2 reaction so that a Type 1 result does not exclude the possibility of such a defect.

In the acquired haemolytic anaemias the results of the autohaemolysis test are variable and generally not very helpful in diagnosis. In the autoimmune haemolytic anaemias lysis may be increased in the absence of additional glucose but the effect of added glucose is unpredictable. In paroxysmal nocturnal haemoglobinuria (PNH) the autohaemolysis of aerated defibrinated blood is usually normal.

Autohaemolysis may be increased in haemolytic anaemias caused by oxidant drugs or when there

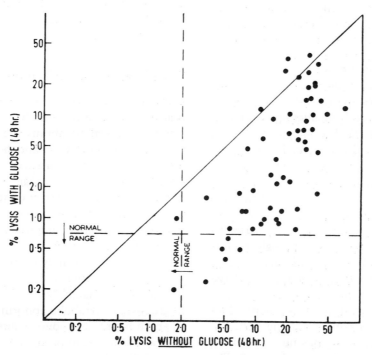

Fig. 13.4   **Autohaemolysis after 48 hours' incubation at 37°C of sterile defibrinated blood derived from 57 patients suffering from hereditary spherocytosis, with and without the addition of glucose.** Points lying near or on the diagonal line indicate that glucose had little or no effect on the rate of haemolysis (a Type-B result). This pattern was subsequently referred to as Type-1 autohaemolysis. (Reproduced from *The Hereditary Haemolytic Anaemias* by J. V. Dacie, Davidson Lecture, 1967. Publication No. 34 of the Royal College of Physicians of Edinburgh.)

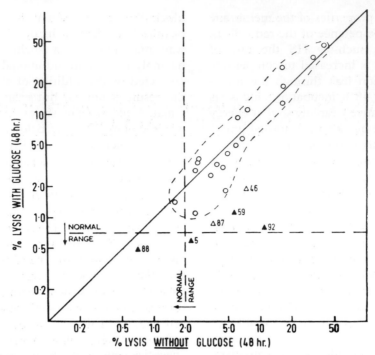

Fig. 13.5   Autohaemolysis after 48 hours' incubation at 37°C of sterile defibrinated blood derived from 19 patients suffering from pyruvate-kinase deficiency with and without the addition of glucose (hollow circles). Data from six other patients suffering from other types of hereditary non-spherocytic haemolytic anaemia have been added for comparison. Points lying near or on the diagonal line indicate that glucose had little or no effect on haemolysis. This pattern was originally referred to as Type-2 autohaemolysis. (For reference see Fig. 13.4.)

are defects in the reducing power of the red cell. Heinz bodies and/or Hi will be detectable at the end of incubation. Normally, red cells produce less than 4% Hi after 48 h incubation and Heinz bodies are not seen. Red cells containing an unstable haemoglobin also contain Heinz bodies at the end of the incubation period and increased amounts of Hi.

The nucleosides adenosine, guanosine and inosine, like glucose, diminish the rate of auto-haemolysis when added to blood. Remarkably, adenosine triphosphate (ATP) strikingly retards haemolysis in PK deficiency, although glucose itself is ineffective.[17] ATP does not pass the red cell membrane.

The autohaemolysis test lacks specificity. This has drawn much criticism upon the test, including the suggestion that it has no place in the screening of blood for inherited defects.[6] The best way to detect metabolic defects in red cells is undoubtedly to measure glucose consumption, lactate production and the contribution to metab-

olism of the pentose phosphate pathway. These measurements are, unfortunately, difficult and are likely to be undertaken only by specialized laboratories. The autohaemolysis test does provide some information about the metabolic competence of the red cells and helps to distinguish membrane defects from enzyme defects.

In summary, we feel that the autohaemolysis test is still useful in the investigation of patients who have or who may have *chronic haemolytic anaemia* for the following reasons:

1. If the result is entirely normal, an intrinsic red cell abnormality is unlikely.
2. If abnormal haemolysis is fully corrected by glucose, a metabolic abnormality is unlikely and a membrane abnormality is likely.
3. If abnormal haemolysis shows little or no correction by glucose, a metabolic abnormality is very likely, *provided* obvious features of spherocytosis are not present on the blood film.

Thus, in our experience a combination of red cell morphology with the results of the auto-haemolysis tests makes it possible to sort out membrane abnormalities from enzyme abnormalities in the vast majority of cases.

DETECTION OF ENZYME DEFICIENCIES IN HEREDITARY HAEMOLYTIC ANAEMIAS

It should be possible for most haematological laboratories to identify the commoner enzyme deficiencies, i.e. of G6PD and PK, and to indicate where the probable defect lies in the rarer disorders. Detailed investigation of the aberrant enzymes and of the metabolism of the abnormal cells is probably best done in specialized laboratories. Comprehensive accounts of methods available for studying red cell metabolism are to be found in *Red Cell Metabolism, a Manual of Biochemical Methods*, by Beutler[5] and the ICSH recommendations.[9]

There are two stages in the diagnosis of red cell enzyme defects: first, screening procedures and, secondly, specific enzyme assays. The simple non-specific screening procedures such as the osmotic-fragility and autohaemolysis tests, which have already been described, may indicate the presence of a metabolic disorder and simple biochemical tests are available to show whether the disorder is in the pentose phosphate or the Embden-Meyerhof pathways; these intermediate stages of glycolysis are illustrated in Fig. 13.6.

SCREENING TESTS FOR G6PD DEFICIENCY AND OTHER DEFECTS OF THE PENTOSE PHOSPHATE PATHWAY

Many variants of the red cell enzyme, G6PD, have been detected and the methods used to identify variants have been standardized.[48] Inheritance is sex-linked as the enzyme is controlled by one gene locus in the X chromosome. Variants which have deficient activity produce one of several types of clinical disorder. The two most common variants are the Mediterranean type which has very low activity and which may lead to favism, i.e. acute intravascular haemolysis following the ingestion of broad beans, and the A-type found in black populations in West Africa and the USA which leads to primaquine sensitivity. Both groups are susceptible to haemolysis produced by oxidant drugs and infections.

Much less frequently a chronic, non-spherocytic haemolytic anaemia is produced by rare variants of the enzyme. Severe neonatal jaundice with anaemia occurs in about 5% of patients who have major deficiencies of enzyme activity.

G6PD deficiency in hemizygous (male) or homozygous (female) individuals may be readily detected by screening tests but it is more difficult to detect heterozygous (female) carriers. Other defects of the pentose phosphate pathway (see p. 226) also lead to deficiency in the reducing power of the red cell. The clinical syndromes associated with these defects include intravascular haemolysis, with or without methaemoglobinaemia, in response to oxidative drugs.

G6PD catalyses the oxidation of glucose-6-phosphate (G6P) to 6-phosphogluconate (6PG) with the simultaneous reduction of nicotine adenine dinucleotide phosphate (NADP) to reduced NADP (NADPH):

$$G6P + NADP \xrightarrow{G6PD} 6PG + NADPH$$

In a second, consecutive, oxidative reaction 6PG is converted to 6-phosphogluconolactone, with reduction of a further molecule of NADP to NADPH. The lactone then undergoes decarboxylation to ribulose 5-phosphate through a reaction catalysed by a specific lactonase, but which can also take place spontaneously. Thus the overall reaction catalysed by 6PG dehydrogenase (6PGD), can be written as:

$$6PG + NADP \xrightarrow{6PGD} Ru5P + CO_2 + NADPH$$

The release of CO_2 drives the reaction to the right so that in practice the pathway is not reversible.

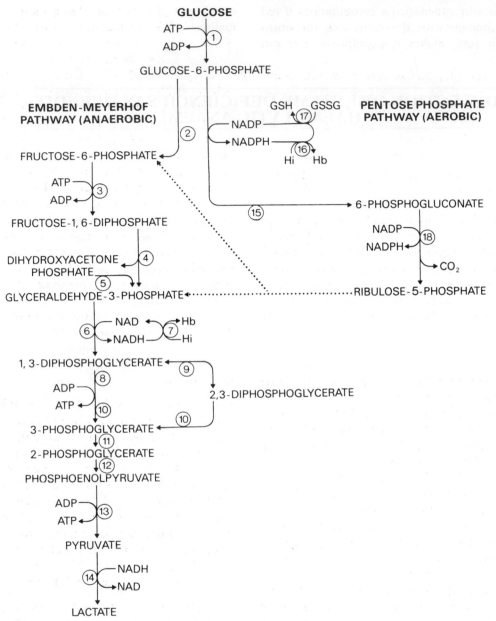

Fig. 13.6 Schematic representation of red cell glycolytic pathways. The enzymes are indicated as follows: (1) hexokinase; (2) glucosephosphate isomerase; (3) phosphofructokinase; (4) aldolase; (5) triose phosphate isomerase; (6) glyceraldehyde-3-phosphate dehydrogenase; (7) NADH-methaemoglobin reductase; (8) phosphoglycerate kinase; (9) diphosphoglyceromutase; (10) diphosphoglycerate phosphatase; (11) phosphoglyceromutase; (12) enolase; (13) pyruvate kinase; (14) lactate dehydrogenase; (15) glucose-6-phosphate dehydrogenase; (16) NADPH-methaemoglobin reductase; (17) glutathione reductase; (18) 6-phosphogluconate dehydrogenase. For explanation of abbreviations, see p. 245.

NADPH is an important reducing compound for the conversion of oxidized glutathione (GSSG) to glutathione (GSH) (see Fig. 13.6) and, under conditions of stress, the reconversion of Hi to Hb. Screening tests for G6PD deficiency depend upon the inability of cells from deficient subjects to convert an oxidized substrate to a reduced state. The substrates used may be the natural one of the enzyme, NADP, or other naturally oc-curring substrates linked by secondary reactions to the enzyme, for example GSSG or Hi or artificial dyes.

Which screening test is used in any particular laboratory will depend upon a number of factors such as cost, time required, temperature and humidity and availability of reagents. Two specific tests are described here.

FLUORESCENT SCREENING TEST FOR G6PD DEFICIENCY

The method is that of Beutler and Mitchell[11] modified on the recommendation of the ICSH.[9]

Principle. NADPH, generated by G6PD present in a lysate of blood cells, fluoresces under long-wave UV light. In G6PD deficiency there is an inability to produce sufficient NADPH; this results in a lack of fluorescence.

Reagents

D-*Glucose-6-phosphate*, 10 mmol/l. Dissolve 305 mg of the disodium salt, or an equivalent amount of the potassium salt, in 100 ml of water.

NADP⁺, 7.5 mmol/l. Dissolve 60 mg of $NADP^+$, disodium salt, in 10 ml of water.

Saponin. 750 mmol/l (10 g/l).

Tris-HCl buffer. pH 7.8. See p. 579.

Oxidized glutathione (GSSG), 8 mmol/l. Dissolve 49 mg of GSSG in 10 ml of water.

Mix the reagents in the following proportion: 2 volumes of G6P; 1 volume of $NADP^+$; 2 volumes of saponin; 3 volumes of buffer; 1 volume of GSSG; 1 volume of water.

The combined reagent is stable at –20°C for 2 or more years and for 2 months at least if kept at 4°C. Azide may be added to prevent growth of contaminants without loss of activity. 100 μl volumes of the reagent may be placed in appropriate small tubes and kept at –20°C ready to use.

Method

Thaw out sufficient tubes to set up test and controls. Allow reagent to reach room temperature before use.

Add 10 μl of whole blood, either anticoagulated (EDTA, heparin, ACD or CPD) or added before clotting, to 100 μl of the reagent mixture and keep at room temperature (15–25°C).

Apply 10 μl of the reaction mixture on to a Whatman No. 1 filter paper at the beginning of the reaction and after 5–10 min. A shorter interval may be appropriate at a high ambient temperature (*c* 25–30°C). Allow to air dry thoroughly before examining the spots under UV light. Always set up samples of normal blood and known G6PD-deficiency blood in parallel.

If the samples are to be collected away from the laboratory, place about 10 μl of blood on Whatman No. 1 filter paper and allow it to dry. Cut out the disc of dried blood in the laboratory and add it to the reaction mixture. A control sample should be tested as a reference.

The test can be carried out on blood stored in ACD (provided it is sterile) for up to 21 days at 4°C and for about 5 days at 25°C.

Interpretation

Fluorescence is produced by NADPH formed from $NADP^+$ in the presence of G6PD. Some of the NADPH produced is oxidized by GSSG, but this reaction, catalysed by glutathione reductase, is normally slower than the rate of NADPH production. Red cells with less than 20% of normal G6PD activity do not cause fluorescence.

Like all screening tests, this method is useful when large numbers of samples are to be tested but the result must be interpreted with caution in an individual patient. The main causes of erroneous inferences are as follows:

1. *False-normal.* If there is reticulocytosis, a vivid fluorescence may be seen with a genetically G6PD-deficient blood sample, because young red cells have more G6PD activity.

2. *False-deficient.* If the patient is anaemic, very little fluorescence may be seen despite the G6PD being genetically normal, simply because there are relatively few red cells in the 10 μl of blood used. Although it is possible to correct for either or both of these contingencies, it is best, if in doubt, to proceed directly to a quantitative enzyme assay (see below).

The test is meant to give only a + or − (normal or deficient) result, by comparison with the controls, and it does not make sense to grade by the eye the intensity of fluorescence. If a control G6PD-deficient sample is not available, the appearance of the 'zero time' spot can be used for reference. The threshold for a 'deficient' result can be worked out by making dilutions of a normal blood sample in saline, and is best set by regarding as deficient the fluorescence obtained when G6PD activity is 20% of normal or less (corresponding to a 1 in 5 dilution of normal blood). This means that very mildly deficient variants, and a substantial proportion of heterozygotes (see p. 229), will be missed. However, clinically important haemolysis is unlikely to occur in subjects who have more than 20% G6PD activity, and therefore this seems an appropriate (though arbitrary) threshold for a diagnostic laboratory. Because the test depends on visual inspection, it is best to select the time of incubation in relation to ambient temperature in preliminary trials. NADPH production is a cumulative process. Therefore, given enough time, a G6PD-deficient sample will fluoresce! The time allowed for the reaction should be one at which the contrast in fluorescence between a G6PD-normal and a G6PD-deficient sample is maximal.

METHAEMOGLOBIN REDUCTION TEST

The method was developed by Brewer et al in 1962.[13]

Principle. Sodium nitrite converts Hb to Hi. When no methylene blue is added methaemoglobin persists, but incubation of the samples with methylene blue allows stimulation of the pentose phosphate pathway in subjects with normal G6PD levels. The Hi is reduced during the incubation period. In G6PD-deficient subjects the block in the pentose phosphate pathway prevents this reduction.

Reagents

Sodium nitrite. 180 mmol/l.

Dextrose. 280 mmol/l. Dissolve 5 g of AR dextrose and 1.25 g of $NaNO_2$ in 100 ml of water.

Methylene blue. 0.4 mmol/l. Dissolve 150 mg of methylthionine chloride (methylene blue chloride, Sigma) in 1 litre of water.

Nile blue sulphate. 22 mg in 100 ml of water. This may be used as an alternative to methylene blue. It is the better reagent if the test is to be combined with the Hi elution test (see p. 229).

The reagents may be used in a variety of ways to suit the convenience of the laboratory. A batch of tubes may be prepared in advance of use by mixing equal volumes of the reagents (sodium nitrite with methylene blue or Nile blue sulphate) and pipetting 0.2 ml of the combined reagent into individual glass tubes. Glass tubes must be used because plastic may adsorb some reagents. The contents of the tubes are allowed to evaporate to dryness at room temperature (15–25°C) or in an oven at a temperature not exceeding 37°C. The tubes must then be tightly stoppered. The reagent will keep for 6 months at room temperature. The reagents may, however, be used fresh, without drying.

Method

Use anticoagulated blood (EDTA, heparin or ACD) and test the samples preferably within 1 h of collection. Blood in ACD, however, can be stored for up to 1 week. With blood from severely anaemic patients adjust the PCV to 0.40 ± 0.05.

Add 2 ml of blood to the tube containing 0.2 ml of the combined reagent either freshly prepared or dried. Close the tube with a stopper and gently mix the contents by inverting it 15 times.

Prepare control tubes by adding 2 ml of blood to a similar tube without reagents (normal reference tube) and to a tube containing 0.1 ml of sodium nitrite-dextrose mixture without methylene blue ('deficient' reference tube).

Incubate the samples at 37°C for 3 h.

After the incubation, pipette 0.1 ml volumes from the test sample, the normal reference tube and the deficient reference tube into 10 ml of water in separate, clear glass test-tubes of identical diameter. Mix the contents gently. Compare the colours in the different tubes (see below).

Interpretation

Normal blood yields a colour similar to that in

the normal reference tube—a clear red. Blood from deficient subjects gives a brown colour similar to that in the deficient reference tube. Heterozygotes give intermediate reactions.

The advantages of this method include the fact that it is extremely cheap, and that the only equipment required is a water-bath. In addition, the test can be complemented by cytochemical analysis which lends itself to detecting G6PD deficiency in patients with reticulocytosis and in heterozygotes.

The only disadvantage is the time taken to perform the test.

DETECTION OF HETEROZYGOTES FOR G6PD DEFICIENCY

Females heterozygous for G6PD deficiency have two populations of cells, one with normal G6PD activity and the other deficient. This is the result of inactivation of one of the two X chromosomes in individual cells early in the development of the embryo. All progeny cells (i.e. somatic cells) in females will have the characteristics of only the active X chromosome.[33] The total G6PD activity of blood in the female will depend on the proportion of normal to deficient cells. In most cases the activity will be between 20 and 80% of the normal. However, a few heterozygotes (about 1%) may have almost only normal or almost only G6PD-deficient cells.

Screening tests for G6PD deficiency fail to demonstrate most heterozygotes. The deficient red cells may, however, be identified in blood films by a cytochemical elution procedure based on the methaemoglobin reduction test[19] (see also p. 139).

METHAEMOGLOBIN ELUTION TEST

Principle. HbO_2 cannot be eluted from red cells in the presence of H_2O_2 presumably because of its peroxidase activity. HiCN has no peroxidase activity and is eluted. This property has been adapted for use in a differential staining technique so that individual cells retaining HbO_2 in the methaemoglobin elution test are stained and Hi-containing cells appear as ghosts.[19]

Reagents

Potassium cyanide. 400 mmol/l. Dissolve 260 mg of KCN in 10 ml of water. Under no circumstances should this solution be pipetted by mouth.

Elution fluid. Mix 80 ml of ethanol (96% v/v, 16 ml of 200 mmol/l citric acid (3.84 g in 100 ml of water) and 5 ml of H_2O_2 (30% v/v). The solution is only active for 1 day.

Staining fluid. Haematoxylin, 7.5 g/l in 96% (v/v) ethanol.

Counterstain. Aqueous erythrosin, 1 g/l or aqueous eosin, 20 g/l.

Method

Use the incubated samples from the reduction test (see p. 228). For preference use samples incubated with Nile blue sulphate rather than methylene blue. Ideally the samples should be oxygenated during incubation by bubbling 95% O_2–5% CO_2 mixtures through them continously. However, it is equally adequate to blow air gently through the samples with a pipette from time to time.

After 2–3 h add 20 µl of KCN solution to 1 ml of the incubated mixture and mix gently. Make blood films on clean, dry glass slides.

Dry the films quickly in air. Immerse the slides in the elution fluid and agitate them up and down for 1 min.

Wash the slides first in methanol and then in water for 3 s each.

Stain the films for 2 min with haematoxylin, rinse in tap water, then counterstain with the erythrosin for 2 min.

Rinse the slides in tap water and allow to dry in the air.

Examine the films under the microscope and count the proportion of stained (HbO_2) cells to ghosts (Hi cells).

Interpretation and comments

In females heterozygous for G6PD deficiency the proportion of G6PD-deficient (ghost) cells varies from case to case: while usually 40–60% of the cells are deficient, the proportion may be much less and in extreme cases even only as few as

2–3% are deficient. Apparently normal subjects may, in a few instances, have a small residue of Hi-containing cells after the Hi reduction test, but this rarely exceeds 5% of the cells. Nearly all heterozygotes can be reliably detected if Nile blue sulphate is used and there is good oxygenation of the samples in the initial incubation. Nile blue sulphate increases the sensitivity of the test because the reduced form of the dye, which is produced in any normal cells that are present, diffuses less readily out of these cells than reduced methylene blue. An artefactual reduction of Hi in G6PD deficient cells from inward diffusion of an extrinsic reducing compound is thus less likely.

PYRIMIDINE-5'-NUCLEOTIDASE SCREENING TEST

Pyrimidine-5'-nucleotidase (P5N) was first described by Valentine et al[45] as a cytosolic enzyme in human red cells. Inheritance of P5N deficiency is autosomal recessive. Heterozygotes are clinically and haematologically normal and typically have about half the normal red cell P5N activity. In homozygotes, levels of 5–15% of normal have been reported; deficiency results in a chronic non-spherocytic haemolytic anaemia. This is characterized by mild to moderate haemolysis, pronounced basophilic stippling of the red cells and marked increase in both red cell glutathione and pyrimidine nucleotides. Osmotic fragility is normal. The rate of autohaemolysis is increased with little or no reduction in lysis by added glucose.[16b]

P5N deficiency appears to be one of the more common causes of HNSHA. It may also be important in the pathogenesis of the anaemia of lead intoxication. The ultimate diagnostic test is a quantitative assay of P5N activity; but the finding of supranormal levels of red cell nucleotides (mostly pyrimidines) is strongly suggestive, and can be used for screening.

Activity of P5N may be quantitatively measured by a colorimetric method[45] or by a radiometric method.[44] For the screening of P5N deficiency, the method recommended by ICSH is the determination of the UV spectra of a blood extract. This is described here.[26]

Principle. The nucleotide pool of normal red cells consists largely (>96%) of purine (adenine and small amounts of guanine) derivatives. The levels of pyrimidine derivatives (cytidine and uridine) are normally extremely low. However, in P5N deficient cells, more than 50% of this pool consists of pyrimidine nucleotides.

In acidic solutions, cytidine nucleotides have an absorbance maximum at approximately 280 nm, while adenine, guanine and uridine nucleotides absorb maximally at 260 nm. The ratio of absorbance at 260 nm to absorbance at 280 nm reflects the relative abundance of cytidine nucleotide; the absorbance ratio is lower when pyrimidine derivatives are higher.

Reagents

Sodium chloride solution, NaCl, 9 g/l.

Perchloric acid, 4%. 28.6 ml of a 70% perchloric acid solution are diluted to a final volume of 500 ml with water.

Glycine buffer. 1 mol/l pH 3.0. 7.51 g of glycine are dissolved in about 80 ml of water, the pH is adjusted to 3.0 with concentrated HCl and the solution made up to a final volume of 100 ml with water.

Method

Sample preparation. Centrifuge blood freshly collected in EDTA at 3000g for 5 min, remove the plasma, and wash the cells three times with ice-cold 9 g/l NaCl solution. Add 1 ml of a 50% suspension of the washed red cells to 4 ml of ice-cold 4% perchloric acid (PCA) solution and then shake vigorously for 30 s. Transfer the clear supernatant obtained after centrifugation at 3000g for 15 min to a small test-tube. Prepare a sham extract by adding 1 ml of 9 g/l NaCl to 4 ml of 4% PCA solution.

Add 500 µl of water and 300 µl of 1 mol/l glycine buffer to each of two cuvettes. In order to correct for optical differences between the cuvettes, read the sample cuvette against the blank at 260 and at 280 nm, giving readings B_{260} and B_{280}. Add 200 µl of the red cell extract to the sample cuvette and 200 µl of the sham extract to the blank cuvette. With the spectrophotometer zeroed at 260 nm on the blank cuvette, read the sample cuvette to obtain the value S_{260}. Repeat the process at 280 nm to obtain the reading S_{280}.

The A_{260}/A_{280} absorbance ratio (R) is calculated by subtracting the cuvette blank readings (positive or negative) at 260 and 280 nm from the readings obtained on the red cell extract when blanked against the sham extract:

$$R = \frac{S_{260} - B_{260}}{S_{280} - B_{280}}$$

Interpretation

The A_{260}/A_{280} absorbance ratio of freshly collected washed red cells has been reported to be 3.22 ± 0.10 (mean ± SD). Absorbance ratios of less than 2.29 imply that the concentration of cytidine nucleotide is increased and suggest a reduced level of pyrimidine 5'-nucleotidase.

RED CELL ENZYME ASSAYS

As is illustrated in Fig. 13.6, a large number of enzymes play a part in the metabolism of glucose in the red cell, and genetically-determined variants of almost all the enzymes are known to occur. This means that in investigating a patient suspected of suffering from a hereditary enzyme-deficiency haemolytic anaemia, multiple enzyme assays may be needed to identify the defect. In practice, however, G6PD deficiency and pyruvate kinase (PK) deficiency should be excluded first, because of the relative frequency (common in the case of G6PD, not rare in the case of PK) with which variants of these enzymes are associated with deficiency and increased haemolysis.

Many methods are available for assaying each enzyme, and for this reason the *International Council for Standardization in Haematology* has produced simplified methods suitable for diagnostic purposes.[8] These methods are not necessarily the most appropriate for detailed study of the kinetic properties of the variant enzymes but they are relatively simple to set up and allow comparison of results between different laboratories.

GENERAL POINTS OF TECHNIQUE

Collection of blood samples

Blood samples may be anticoagulated with heparin (10 IU/ml blood), EDTA (1.5 mg/ml blood) or acid-citrate-dextrose (for formulae and volumes see p. 575). In any of these anticoagulants all normal enzymes are stable for 6 days (and most for 20 days) at 4°C and 24 h at 25°C. However, enzyme variants in samples from patients may be less stable. Therefore, we recommend that ACD is used as anticoagulant and that the samples are tested promptly. Ideally, samples of blood should be transferred to central laboratories in tubes surrounded by wet ice (4°C). Frozen samples are unsuitable because the cells are lysed by freezing. Further details of enzyme stability were given by Beutler.[5] Approximately 1 ml of blood is required for each enzyme assay.

Separation of red cells from blood samples

Leucocytes and platelets generally have higher enzyme activities than red cells. Moreover, with abnormalities causing enzyme deficiency, the decrease in enzyme activity may be much less pronounced in leucocytes and platelets than in red cells, as for example in PK deficiency. It is, therefore, necessary to prepare red cells as free from contamination as possible. Various methods are suitable (see ICSH[8]); two are described below.

Washing the red cells

Centrifuge the anticoagulated blood at 1200–1500g for 5 min and remove the plasma together with the buffy coat layer.

Resuspend the cells in 9 g/l NaCl (saline) and repeat the procedure three times. This will remove about 80–90% of the leucocytes.

This simple method is adequate in most instances when more complicated manoeuvres are impracticable, but it has the disadvantage that some of the reticulocytes and young red cells are lost together with the buffy coat. In addition, the remaining leucocytes may still be sufficient to cause misleading results, for instance in PK deficiency. Therefore, ideally the method below should be adopted.

Filtration through microcrystalline cellulose mixtures

Pure red cell suspensions can be made from whole blood by filtering the blood through a mixed bed of microcrystalline cellulose (mean size 50 μm) and α-cellulose. Mix approximately 0.5 g of each type of cellulose with 20 ml of ice-cold saline; this gives sufficient slurry for 3–5 columns. The barrel of a 5 ml syringe is used as a column. The outlet of the syringe is blocked with absorbent cotton wool, equal in volume to the 1 ml mark on the barrel. Pour the well-shaken slurry into the column to give a bed volume of 1–2 ml after the saline has run through. Wash the bed with 5 ml of saline to remove any 'fines'. When the saline has run through, pipette 1–2 ml of whole blood onto the column, taking care not to disturb the bed. Collect the filtrate, and once the blood has completely run into the bed, wash the column through with 5–7 ml of saline. The column should be made freshly for each batch of enzyme assays and used promptly.

By this method, about 99% of the leucocytes and about 90% of the platelets are removed. About 97% of the red cells are recovered and reticulocytes are not removed selectively. The procedure should not alter the age or size of distribution of the recovered red cells compared to native blood. This should be checked with each new batch of cellulose by counting reticulocytes.

Wash the cells collected from the column twice in 10 volumes of ice-cold saline and finally resuspend them in the saline to give a 50% suspension.

Determine the haemoglobin and/or red cell count in a sample of the suspension.

Preparation of haemolysate

Mix 1 volume of the washed or filtered suspension with 9 volumes of lysing solution consisting of 2.7 mmol/l EDTA, pH 7.0 and 0.7 mmol/l 2-mercapto-ethanol (100 mg of EDTA disodium salt and 5 μl of 2-mercapto-ethanol in 100 ml of water); adjust the pH to 7.0 with HCl or NaOH.

Ensure complete lysis by freeze-thawing. Rapid freezing is achieved using a dry-ice acetone bath or methanol which has been cooled to –20°C. Thawing is achieved in a water-bath at 25°C or simply in water at room temperature. Usually the haemolysate is ready for use without further centrifugation, but a 1-min spin in a microfuge is preferable in order to remove any turbidity (this may be unsuitable for some red cell enzymes which are stroma-bound!). Dilutions, when necessary, are carried out in the lysing solution. The haemolysate should be prepared freshly for each batch of enzyme assays. Most enzymes in haemolysates are stable for 8 h at 0°C, but it is best to carry out assays immediately. G6PD is one of the least stable enzymes in this haemolysate and its assay should be conducted within 1 or 2 hours of the lysate being prepared. The storing of frozen cells or haemolysates is not recommended; it is much better to store whole blood in ACD.

Control samples

Control samples should always be assayed at the same time as the test samples even when a normal range for the various enzymes has been established.

Take the control samples of blood at the same time as the test samples and treat them in the same way. When receiving samples from outside sources, always ask for a normal 'shipment control' to be included.

Reaction buffer

The ICSH recommendation is for a Tris-HCl/EDTA buffer which is appropriate for all the common enzyme assays. The buffer consists of 1 mol/l Tris-HCl and 5 mmol/l Na_2EDTA, the pH being adjusted to 8.0 with HCl.

Dissolve 12.11 g of Tris (hydroxymethyl) methylamine and 186 mg of Na_2EDTA in water; adjust the pH to 8.0 with 1 mol/l HCl and bring the volume to 100 ml at 25°C.

Only two assays will be described in detail—those for G6PD and PK. However, the principles of these assays apply to all other enzyme assays. The assays are carried out in a spectrophotometer at a wavelength of 340 nm unless otherwise indicated. A final reaction mixture of 1.0 ml (or 3.0 ml) is suitable, the quantities given in the text being for 1.0 ml reaction mixtures unless otherwise stated. All dilutions of auxiliary enzymes are made in the lysing solution and all working materials should be kept in an ice-bath until ready for use. The assays are carried out at a controlled temperature, 30°C being the most appropriate. Cuvettes loaded with the assay reagents should be pre-incubated at this temperature for 10 min before starting the reaction. In most cases the reaction is started by the addition of substrate. Nowadays many spectrophotometers have a built-in or attached recorder, by which the absorbance changes can be conveniently measured. If no recorder is available, visual readings should be made every 60 s. In any case, the reaction should be followed for 5 to 10 min, and it is essential to ensure that during this time the change in absorbance is linear with time.

G6PD ASSAY

The reactions involving G6PD have already been described (p. 225). The activity of the enzyme is assayed by following the rate of production of NADPH which, unlike NADP, has a peak of ultraviolet light absorption at 340 nm.

Method

Assay conditions. The assays are carried out at 30°C, the cuvettes containing the first five reagents being incubated for 10 min before starting the reaction by adding the substrate, as shown in Table 13.3.

The change in absorbance following the addition of the substrate is measured over the first 5 min of the reaction. The value of the blank is subtracted from the test reaction, either automatically or by calculation.

In the 6th edition of this book (p. 166) the recommended method for G6PD measurement included an assay for G6PD + 6PGD activity,

Table 13.3   G6PD assay

Reaction	Assay (µl)	Blank (µl)
Tris-HCl EDTA buffer, pH 8.0	100	100
MgCl$_2$, 100 mmol/l	100	100
NADP, 2 mmol/l	100	100
1:20 Haemolysate	20	20
Water	580	680
Start reaction by adding: G6P, 6 mmol/l	100	–

with G6PD activity being calculated by subtraction. Although this assay can be regarded as more accurate for certain research purposes, it is not necessary for diagnostic purposes. Indeed, in G6PD deficiency it tends to introduce an error greater than the one it is meant to correct for.

Calculation of enzyme activity

The activities of the enzymes in the haemolysate are calculated from the initial rate of change of NADPH accumulation:

G6PD activity in the lysate (in mol/ml)
$$= \Delta A/min \times \frac{10^3}{6.22}$$

where 6.22 is the mmol extinction coefficient of NADPH at 340 nm and 10^3 is the factor appropriate for the dilutions in the reaction mixture. Results are expressed per 10^{10} red cells, per ml red cells or per g haemoglobin by reference to the respective values obtained with the washed red cell suspension. However, the ICSH recommendation is to express values per g haemoglobin, and it is ideal to determine the haemoglobin concentration of the haemolysate directly. When doing this, use a haemolysate to Drabkin solution ratio of 1:25.

G6PD is very stable and with most variants venous blood may be stored in ACD for up to 3 weeks at 4°C without loss of activity.

Some enzyme-deficient variants lose activity more rapidly, and this will cause deficiency to appear more severe than it is. Therefore, for diagnostic purposes a delay in assaying well-conserved samples should not be a deterrent.

Normal values

The normal range for G6PD activity should be

determined in each laboratory. If the ICSH method is used, values should not differ widely from those given by that panel. Results are expressed in enzyme units (eu) which are the µmoles of substrate converted per min.

For adults these values are 8.83 ± 1.59 eu/g haemoglobin at 30°C. However, newborns and infants may have enzyme activity which deviates appreciably from the adult value.[8] Comparison of the activities of red cell enzymes in adults and newborns has been published elsewhere.[28]

Interpretation of results

In assessing the clinical relevance of a G6PD assay three important facts must be borne in mind.

1. As already stated (p. 225), the gene for G6PD is on the X-chromosome, and therefore males, having only one G6PD gene, can be only either normal or deficient hemizygotes. By contrast, females, who have two allelic genes, can be either normal homozygotes or heterozygotes with 'intermediate' enzyme activity or deficient homozygotes.

2. Red cells are likely to haemolyse on account of G6PD deficiency only if they have less than about 20% of the normal enzyme activity.

3. G6PD activity falls off markedly as red cells age. Therefore, whenever a blood sample has a young red cell population G6PD activity will be higher than normal, sometimes to the extent that a genetically deficient sample may yield a value within the normal range. This will be usually but not always associated with a high reticulocytosis.

In practice, the following notes may be useful.

1. In males, diagnosis does not present difficulties in most cases, because the demarcation between normal and deficient subjects is sharp. There are very few acquired situations in which G6PD activity is decreased (one is pure red cell aplasia where there is reticulocytopenia); whereas an increased G6PD activity is found in all acute and chronic haemolytic states. Therefore a G6PD value below a well-established normal range always indicates G6PD deficiency. A value in the low-normal range in the face of reticulocytosis should also raise the suspicion of G6PD deficiency, because with reticulocytosis G6PD activity should

be *higher* than normal. In such suspicious cases G6PD deficiency can be confirmed by repeating the assay when the reticulocytosis has subsided, or by assaying older red cells after fractionation by density, or by family studies.

2. In females, all the same criteria apply, with the added consideration that heterozygosity can *never* be rigorously ruled out by a G6PD assay: for this purpose, the cytochemical test described on p. 229 is more useful than a spectrophotometric assay, and a counsel of perfection is to use the two in conjunction with each other and with family studies. However, in most cases, a normal value in a female means that she is a normal homozygote, and a value below 10% of normal means that she is a deficient homozygote (see Table 13.4): but a few heterozygotes may fall in either of these ranges, because of the 'extreme phenotypes' that can be associated with an unbalanced ratio of the mosaicism consequent on X-chromosome inactivation. Any value between 10 and 90% of normal usually means a heterozygote, except for the complicating effect of reticulocytosis. As far as the clinical significance of heterozygosity for G6PD deficiency is concerned, it is important to remember that, because of mosaicism, a fraction of red cells in heterozygotes (on the average, 50%) are as enzyme-deficient as in a hemizygous male, and therefore susceptible to haemolysis. The severity of potential clinical complications is roughly proportional to the fraction of deficient red cells. Therefore, within the heterozygote range, the actual value of the assay (or the proportion of

Table 13.4   G6PD in various clinical situations (activity in enzyme units (eu) per g haemoglobin)

Male genotypes Female genotypes	Gd^+ Gd^+/Gd^+	Gd^- Gd^-/Gd^-	Gd^+/Gd^-
In health	7–10	<2	2–7
In increased haemolysis: Unrelated to			
G6PD deficiency	15	4	4–9
During recovery from			
G6PD-related anaemia	–	6.5	6–10

The values quoted are examples.
Gd^+ designates a gene encoding normal G6PD; Gd^- designates a gene encoding a variant associated with G6PD deficiency.

deficient red cells estimated by the cytochemical test) correlates with the risk of haemolysis.

IDENTIFICATION OF G6PD VARIANTS

There are many variants of G6PD in different populations with enzyme activities ranging from nearly zero to 400–500% of normal activity (see full details in ref. 32). Classification and provisional identification of variants are based on their physico-chemical and enzymic characteristics.[50] Criteria were laid down by a WHO scientific group in 1967[48] for the minimum requirements for identification of such variants and these re-commendations have been revised recently.[49] The tests are carried out on male hemizygotes and are:

Red cell G6PD activity
Electrophoretic migration
Michaelis constant (K_m) for G6PD
Relative rate of utilization of 2-deoxyG6P (2dG6P)
Thermal stability.

Recently the full amino-acid sequence of G6PD has been established and definitive identification can be made by sequence analysis at the DNA level.[47] The provisional data have been confirmed in general but with some exceptions.[7]

PYRUVATE KINASE ASSAY

Many variants of PK have deficient enzyme activity in vivo.[34,35] In most cases deficient activity can be identified by simple enzyme assay. However, PK activity is subject in red cells to regulation by a number of effector molecules. With some PK variants the maximum velocity (V_{max}) of the enzyme is normal or nearly so, but at the low substrate concentrations found in vivo PK activity may be sufficiently low to cause haemolysis, either because affinity for the substrates, phos-phoenolpyruvate (PEP) and ADP, is low or be-cause binding of the important allosteric ligand, fructose-1,6-diphosphate, is altered. Some of these unusual variants can be identified by carrying out the enzyme assay not only under standard con-ditions but also at low substrate concentrations. Functional PK deficiency can also be identified by finding high concentrations of the substrates immediately above the block in the glycolytic pathway, particularly DPG.[25] (For measurement of DPG, see p. 239.)

Pyruvate kinase deficiency is inherited as an autosomal recessive condition.

Method

The preparation of haemolysate, buffer and lysing solution are exactly the same as for the G6PD assay. In the PK assay it is particularly important to remove as many contaminating leucocytes and platelets as possible because these cells may be unaffected by a deficiency affecting the red cells and contain high activities of PK. The principle of the assay is as follows:

$$PEP + ADP \xrightleftharpoons{PK} pyruvate + ATP$$

The pyruvate so formed is reduced to lactate in a reaction catalysed by lactate dehydrogenase with the conversion of NADH to NAD:

$$pyruvate + NADH \xrightleftharpoons{LDH} lactate + NAD$$

In order to ensure that this secondary reaction is not rate-limiting, LDH is added in excess to the reaction mixture and the PK activity is measured by the rate of fall of absorbance at 340 nm.

The reaction conditions are established in a 1 ml cuvette at 30°C by adding all the reagents except the substrate PEP to the cuvette and in-cubating them at 30°C for 10 min before starting the reaction by the addition of the PEP.

The amounts to be added for low-substrate conditions are also shown in Table 13.5.

Reagents (Table 13.5)

The change in absorbance (A) is measured over the first 5 min and the activity of the enzyme in micromoles of NADH reduced/min/ml haemolysate is calculated as follows:

Table 13.5   Reagents

Reaction	Assay (µl)	Blank (µl)	Low-S (µl)
Tris-HCl EDTA buffer, pH 8.0	100	100	100
KCl 1 mol/l	100	100	100
MgCl$_2$ 100 mmol/l	100	100	100
NAD, 2 mmol/l	100	100	100
ADP, neutralized. 30 mmol/l	50	–	20
LDH 60 u/ml	100	100	100
1:20 haemolysate	20	20	20
Water	330	380	455
PEP 50 mmol/l	100	100	5

Low-S, low-substrate conditions.

$$\frac{\Delta A/\text{min}}{6.22} \times 10$$

where 6.22 is the millimolar extinction coefficient of NADH at 340 nm.

Express results as for G6PD.

A blank assay should be carried out to be certain that the LDH is free of PK activity. Use the 2-mercapto-ethanol-EDTA stabilizing solution (p. 232) in place of haemolysate for both the blank and system mixtures. If no change in absorbance is observed, indicating that the LDH is free of contaminating PK it is unnecessary to re-check on subsequent assays. Otherwise, the blank rate must be subtracted in computing the true enzyme activity each time.

Normal values

As with all enzyme assays, a normal range should be determined for each laboratory. Values should, however, not be widely different between laboratories if the ICSH methods are used. The normal range of PK activity at 30°C is 10.3 ± 2 eu/g Hb. At a low substrate concentration the normal activity is $15 \pm 3\%$ of that at the high substrate concentration.

Interpretation of results

PK, like G6PD, is a red cell age-dependent enzyme. But unlike G6PD deficiency, PK deficiency is usually associated with chronic haemolysis. Therefore, patients in whom PK deficiency is suspected almost invariably have a reticulocytosis, and if their PK level is below the normal range they can be considered to be PK-deficient. Thus, once the technique and normal values are well established in a laboratory, and provided shipment controls are always included, the main problem is of underdiagnosis rather than of overdiagnosis of PK deficiency. One way to pick up abnormal variants has been included in the method recommended, i.e. the use of low substrate concentrations. Even so, PK deficiency may be missed because high reticulocytosis may increase PK activity quite markedly. This means that a PK activity in the normal range in the presence of a high reticulocytosis is highly suspicious of inherited PK deficiency (because with reticulocytosis the activity ought to be *higher* than normal). In such cases the importance of family studies cannot be over-emphasized. Heterozygotes have about 50% of the normal PK activity, sometimes less; but they do not suffer from haemolysis. Therefore, the heterozygous parents of a patient may well have a red cell PK activity lower than that of their homozygous PK-deficient offspring. This finding may clinch the diagnosis.

ESTIMATION OF REDUCED GLUTATHIONE (GSH)[10]

The red cell has a high concentration of this sulphydryl-containing tripeptide. An important function of GSH in the red cell is the detoxification of low levels of hydrogen peroxide which may form spontaneously or as a result of drug administration. GSH may also function in maintaining the integrity of the red cell by reducing sulphydryl groups of haemoglobin, membrane proteins and enzymes which may have become oxidized. Maintenance of normal levels of GSH is a major preoccupation of the hexose monophosphate shunt. Reduction of GSSG (oxidized glutathione) back to the functional GSH is linked to the rate of reduction of NADP$^+$ in the initial step of the shunt.

Principle. The method described is based on

the development of a yellow colour when 5,5'-dithiobis(2-nitrobenzoic acid) (Ellman's reagent, DTNB) is added to sulphydryl compounds. The colour which develops is fairly stable for about 10 min and the reaction is little affected by variation in temperature.

The reaction is read at 412 nm. GSH in red cells is relatively stable and venous blood samples anticoagulated with ACD maintain GSH levels for up to 3 weeks at 4°C. GSH is slowly oxidized in solution, so only fresh lysates should be used for the assay.

Reagents

Lysing solution. Disodium EDTA, 1 g/l.

Precipitating reagent. Metaphosphoric acid (sticks), 1.67 g; disodium EDTA 0.2 g; NaCl 30 g; water to 100 ml.

Solution is more rapid if the reagents are added to boiling water and the volume made up after cooling.

This solution is stable for at least 3 weeks at 4°C. If any EDTA remains undissolved the clear supernatant should be used.

Disodium hydrogen phosphate, 300 mmol/l: $Na_2HPO_4.12H_2O$, 107.4 g/l, or $Na_2HPO_4.2H_2O$, 53.4 g/l or anhydrous Na_2HPO_4, 42.6 g/l.

DTNB reagent. Dissolve 20 mg of DTNB in 100 ml of buffer, pH 8.0. Trisodium citrate, 34 mmol/l (10 g/l) or Tris/HCl (p. 579), are suitable buffers.

The solution is stable for up to 3 months at 4°C.

Glutathione standards. When standard curves are constructed, suitable dilutions are made from a 1.62 mmol/l (50 mg/dl) stock solution of GSH.

The stock solution should be made freshly with degassed (boiled) water or saline for each run as GSH oxidizes slowly in solution.

Method

Add 0.2 ml of well mixed, anticoagulated blood, of which the PCV, red cell count and haemoglobin have been determined, to 1.8 ml of lysing solution and allow to stand at room temperature for no more than 5 min for lysis to be completed.

Add 3 ml of precipitating solution, mix the solution well and allow to stand for a further 5 min.

After remixing, filter through a single thickness Whatman No. 42 filter paper.

Add 1 ml of clear filtrate to 4 ml of freshly made Na_2HPO_4 solution. Record the absorbance at 412 nm (A_1). Then add 0.5 ml of the DTNB reagent, and mix well by inversion.

The colour develops rapidly and remains stable for about 10 min. Read its development at 412 nm in a spectrophotometer (A_2).

A reagent blank is made using saline or plasma instead of whole blood.

Standard curves. If assays are carried out frequently, it is not necessary to construct standard curves for each batch. They are, however, essential initially to calibrate the apparatus used and should be done regularly to check the suitability of the reagents. Suitable dilutions of GSH are achieved by substituting 5, 10, 20 and 40 µl of the 1.62 mmol/l stock solution, made up to 0.2 ml with lysing solution, for the blood in the reaction.

Calculation

Determination of extinction coefficient (ε). The molar extinction coefficient of the chromophore at 412 nm is 13 600. This only applies when a narrow band wave length is available. When a broader wave band is used, the extinction coefficient is lower.

The system may be calibrated by comparing the extinction absorbance in the test system (D_2) with that obtained in a spectrophotometer with a narrow band at 412 nm (D_1). The derived correction factor, E_1, is given by D_1/D_2 and is constant for the test system.

Calculation of GSH concentration

The amount of GSH in the cuvette sample (GSH_c) is given by:

$$\Delta A^{412} \times \frac{E_1}{\epsilon} \times 5.5 \ \mu mol$$

The concentration of GSH in the whole blood sample is:

$$\frac{GSH_c \times 5}{0.2} \ \mu mol/ml$$

The unit is often expressed in terms of mg/dl of red cells. The molecular weight of GSH is 307. Thus, GSH in mg/dl packed red cells is given by:

$$GSH_c \times \frac{5}{0.2} \times \frac{1}{PCV} \times 307 \times 100$$

Normal range

The normal range may be expressed in a number of ways, e.g. 6.57 ± 1.04 µmol/g Hb or 223 ± 35 µmol (or 69 ± 11 mg)/dl packed red cells.

Significance

Glutathione replenishment in mature red cells is accomplished through the consecutive action of two enzymes; γ-glutamylcysteine synthetase and glutathione synthetase. Although very rare, hereditary deficiency of either enzyme virtually abolishes the synthesis of GSH. The deficient cells are very prone to oxidative destruction and are short lived, resulting in a non-spherocytic haemolytic anaemia.

Increases in GSH have been described in various conditions such as dyserythropoiesis, myelofibrosis, pyrimidine-5'-nucleotidase deficiency and other rare congenital haemolytic anaemias of unknown aetiology.

THE GLUTATHIONE STABILITY TEST

Principle. In normal subjects incubation of red cells with the oxidizing drug acetylphenylhydrazine has little effect on the GSH content, since its oxidation is reversed by glutathione reductase, which in turn relies on G6PD for a supply of NADPH. Therefore, in G6PD deficient subjects the stability of GSH is significantly lowered.

Reagents

Acetylphenylhydrazine, 670 mmol/l. Dissolve 100 mg in 1 ml of acetone.

Transfer 0.05 ml volumes (containing 5 mg of acetylphenylhydrazine) by pipette to the bottom of 12×75 mm glass tubes.

Dry the contents of the tubes in an incubator at 37°C, stopper with rubber bungs and store in the dark until used.

Method

Venous blood, anticoagulated with EDTA, heparin or ACD may be used; it may be freshly collected or previously stored at 4°C for up to 1 week.

Add 1 ml to a tube containing acetylphenylhydrazine and place a further 1 ml in a similar tube not containing the chemical. Invert the tubes several times and then incubate them at 37°C.

After 1 h mix the contents of the tubes once more and incubate the tubes for a further 1 h. At the end of this time determine and compare the GSH concentration in the test sample and in the control sample.

Interpretation

In normal adult subjects red cell GSH is lowered by not more than 20% by incubation with acetylphenylhydrazine. In G6PD-deficient subjects it is lowered by more than this: in heterozygotes (females) the fall may amount to about 50% whilst in hemizygotes (males) the fall is often much greater and almost all may be lost.

The test is not specific for G6PD deficiency and other rare defects of the pentose phosphate pathway may give abnormal results.

GSH and GSH stability in infants

During the first few days after birth the red cells have a normal or high content of GSH. On the addition of acetylphenylhydrazine the GSH is unstable in both normal and G6PD-deficient infants. In normal infants, however, the instability can be corrected by the addition of glucose and by the time the normal infant is 3–4 days old the cells behave like adult cells.[31,52]

2,3-DIPHOSPHOGLYCERATE (DPG)

The importance of the high concentration of DPG in the red cells of man was recognized at about the same time by Chanutin and Curnish[14] and Benesch and Benesch.[4] DPG binds to a specific site in the β-chain of haemoglobin and it decreases its oxygen affinity by shifting the balance of the so-called T and R conformations of the molecule. The higher the concentration of DPG the greater the partial pressure of oxygen (pO_2) needed to produce the same oxygen saturation of haemoglobin. This is reflected in a DPG-dependent shift in the oxygen dissociation curve.

Measurement of the concentration of DPG in red cells may also be useful in identifying the probable site of an enzyme deficiency in the metabolic pathway. In general, enzyme defects cause an increase in the concentration of metabolic intermediates above the level of the block and a decrease in concentration below the block. Thus DPG is increased in PK deficiency and decreased in hexokinase deficiency. In most other disorders of the glycolytic pathway, however, the DPG concentration is normal, because increased activity through the pentose phosphate pathway allows a normal flux of metabolites through the triose part of the glycolytic pathway.

MEASUREMENT OF RED CELL DPG

Various methods have been used to assay DPG. Krimsky[29] used the catalytic properties of DPG in the conversion of 3-phosphoglycerate (3PG) to 2-phosphoglycerate (2PG) by phosphoglycerate mutase (PGM). At very low concentrations of DPG the rate of conversion is proportional to the concentration of DPG. This method is elegant and extremely sensitive but too cumbersome for routine use. A fluorimetric method was described by Lowry,[30] and this has been modified for spectrophotometry. Rose and Liebowitz[39] found that glycolate-2-phosphate increased the 2,3DPG phosphatase activity of phosphoglycerate mutase (PGM) and a quantitative assay of the substrate, DPG, was evolved on this basis.

Principle. DPG is hydrolysed to 3PG by the phosphatase activity of PGM stimulated by glycolate-2-phosphate. This reaction is linked to the conversion of NADH to NAD by glyceraldehyde-3-phosphate dehydrogenase (Ga3PD) and phosphoglycerate kinase (PGK):

$$2,3DPG \xrightarrow[\text{(glycolate-2-phosphate)}]{\text{2,3DPG phosphatase}} 3PG + Pi$$

$$3PG + ATP \xrightarrow{\text{PGK}} 1,3DPG + ADP$$

$$1,3DPG + NADH \xrightarrow{\text{Ga3PD}} Ga3P + Pi + NAD^+$$

The fall in absorbance at 340 nm, as NADH is oxidized, is measured.

Reagents

Triethanolamine buffer. 0.2 mol/l, pH 8.0.

Dissolve 9.3 g of triethanolamine hydrochloride in *c* 200 ml of water; then add 0.5 g of disodium EDTA and 0.25 g of $MgSO_4.7H_2O$. Adjust the pH to 8.0 with 2 mol/l KOH (*c* 15 ml) and make up the volume to 250 ml with water.

ATP, sodium salt. 20 mg/ml. Dissolved in buffer, this is stable for several months when frozen.

NADH, sodium salt. 10 mg/ml. When dissolved in buffer this is relatively unstable and should be made freshly each day.

Glyceraldehyde-3-phosphate dehydrogenase / Phosphoglycerate kinase. Mixed crystalline suspension in ammonium sulphate (Sigma, Code No. 366–2).

Phosphoglycerate mutase. Crystalline suspension from rabbit muscle in ammonium sulphate (*c* 2500 u/ml).

Glycolate-2-phosphate. 2-Phosphoglycolic acid (Sigma), 10 mg/ml. When dissolved in water this is stable for several months when frozen.

Method

Freshly drawn blood in EDTA or heparin may be used. If there is an unavoidable delay in starting the assay, blood (4 volumes) should be added to CPD anticoagulant (1 volume) and stored at 4°C. A control blood sample should be taken at the same time.

DPG levels are stable for 48 h if the blood is stored in this way. The haemoglobin, red cell count and PCV should be measured on part of the sample. It is not necessary to remove leucocytes or platelets.

Deproteinization. Add 1 ml of blood to 3 ml of ice-cold 80 g/l trichloracetic acid (TCA) in a 10 ml conical centrifuge tube.

Shake the tube vigorously, preferably on an automatic rotor mixer and then allow to stand for 5–10 min for complete deproteinization. The shaking is important; otherwise some of the precipitated protein will remain on the surface of the mixture.

Centrifuge at about 1200g for 5–10 min at 4°C to obtain a clear supernatant. The DPG in the supernatant is stable for 2–3 weeks when stored at 4°C, and indefinitely if frozen.

Reaction

Deliver the reagents into a silica or high quality glass cuvette, with a 1 cm light path. The following quantities are for a 4 ml cuvette:

	Test	*Blank*
Triethanolamine buffer	2.50 ml	2.50 ml
ATP	100 µl	100 µl
NADH	100 µl	100 µl
Deproteinized extract	250 µl	–
Ga-3-PD/PGK mixture	20 µl	20 µl
PGM	20 µl	20 µl
Water	–	250 µl
	3.00 ml	3.00 ml

Warm the mixtures at 30°C for 10 min and record the absorbance of both test and blank mixtures at 340 nm. Then start the reaction by the addition of 100 µl of glycolate-2-phosphate.

Remeasure the absorbance (in 35 min) of the test and blank mixtures on completion of the reaction.

Make further measurements after a further 5 min to make sure the reaction is complete.

Only one blank is required for each batch of test samples.

Calculation

DPG (µmol/ml blood)

$$= (\Delta A \text{ test} - \Delta A \text{ blank}) \times \frac{3.10}{6.22} \times 16$$

$$= (\Delta A \text{ test} - \Delta A \text{ blank}) \times 8 = D$$

where 3.10 = the volume of reaction mixture, 6.22 = mmolar extinction coefficient of NADH at 340 nm and 16 = dilution of original blood sample (1 ml in 3.0 ml of TCA, 0.25 ml added to cuvette).

The results of DPG assays are best expressed in terms of haemoglobin content or red cell volume. Thus, if the result of the above calculation is represented by D, then:

$$D \times \frac{1000}{(Hb)} = DPG \text{ in µmol/g Hb}$$

or

$$D \times \frac{1000}{(Hb)} \times \frac{64}{1000} = DPG \text{ in µmol/µmol Hb}$$

and

$$D \times \frac{1}{PCV}$$
$$= DPG \text{ in µmol/ml (packed) red cells,}$$

where Hb = haemoglobin in g/l of whole blood and 64 is the mol wt of haemoglobin $\times 10^{-3}$.

The molar ratio of DPG to haemoglobin in normal blood is about 0.75:1.

Normal range

4.5–5.1 µmol/ml packed red cells or 10.5–16.2 µmol/g haemoglobin.

Each laboratory should determine its own normal range.

Significance of DPG concentration

An increase in DPG concentration is found in most conditions in which the arterial blood is undersaturated with oxygen, as in congenital heart and chronic lung diseases; in most acquired anaemias; at high altitudes; in alkalosis, and in hyperphosphataemia. Decreased DPG levels occur in hypophosphataemic states and in acidosis.

Acidosis, which shifts the oxygen dissociation curve to the right, causes a fall in DPG, so that the oxygen dissociation curve of whole blood from patients with chronic acidosis (such as patients in diabetic coma or pre-coma) may have nearly normal dissociation curves. A rapid correction of the acidosis will lead to a major shift of the curve to the left, that is to a marked increase in the affinity of haemoglobin for oxygen, which may lead to tissue hypoxia. Caution should therefore be exercised in correcting acidosis.

From the diagnostic point of view, the main importance of DPG determination is (1) in haemolytic anaemias and (2) in the interpretation of changes in the oxygen affinity of blood.

1. As already mentioned, increased or decreased DPG may be associated with glycolytic enzyme defects, and increased DPG (up to 2–3 times normal) is particularly characteristic of most patients with PK deficiency. Although this finding certainly cannot be regarded as diagnostic, a normal or low DPG makes PK deficiency most unlikely.

2. Whenever a shift in the oxygen dissociation curve is observed, and an abnormal haemoglobin with altered oxygen affinity is suspected, determination of DPG is essential. Indeed, there is a simple correlation between DPG level and p_{50}, from which it is possible to work out whether any change in p_{50} is explained by an altered level of DPG.[18]

DPG levels are generally slightly lower than normal in HS and this probably accounts for the slight erythrocytosis which is sometimes seen after splenectomy.

THE OXYGEN DISSOCIATION CURVE

The oxygen dissociation curve is the expression of the relationship between the partial pressure of oxygen and the saturation of haemoglobin with oxygen. Details of this relationship and the physiological importance of changes in this relationship were worked out in detail at the beginning of this century by the great physiologists Hüfner, Bohr, Barcroft, Henderson and many others. Their work was summarized by Peters and Van Slyke in *Quantitative Clinical Chemistry, Volume 1*.[38] The relevant chapters of this book have been reprinted and it would be difficult to better their description of the importance of the oxygen dissociation curve:

The physiological value of haemoglobin as an oxygen carrier lies in the fact that its affinity for oxygen is so nicely balanced that in the lungs haemoglobin becomes 95–96% oxygenated, while in the tissues and capillaries it can give up as much of the gas as is demanded. If the affinity were much less, complete oxygenation in the lungs could not be approached: if it were greater, the tissues would have difficulty in removing from the blood the oxygen they need. Because the affinity is adjusted as it is, both oxyhaemoglobin and reduced haemoglobin exist in all

parts of the circulation but in greatly varied proportions.

MEASURING THE OXYGEN DISSOCIATION CURVE

Determination of the oxygen dissociation curve depends upon two measurements: the partial pressure of oxygen (pO_2) with which the blood is equilibrated, and the proportion of haemoglobin which is saturated with oxygen. Methods for determining the dissociation curve fall into three main groups:

1. The pO_2 is set by the experimental conditions and the percent saturation of haemoglobin is measured.

2. The percentage saturation is predetermined by mixing known proportions of oxygenated and deoxygenated blood and the pO_2 is measured.

3. The change in oxygen content of the blood is plotted continuously against pO_2 during oxygenation or deoxygenation and the percent saturation calculated.

The multiplicity of methods available for measuring the oxygen dissociation curve suggests that no method is ideal. The advantages and disadvantages of the various techniques have been reviewed.[3,43] The standard method with which new methods are compared is the gasometric method of Van Slyke and Neill.[46] This method is slow and demands considerable expertise and is not suitable for most haematological laboratories. The method described below[40] is based on similar principles to that of Van Slyke and Neill but employs spectrophotometric measurement of reduced oxyhaemoglobin rather than direct gasometric measurement. The method may be used for suspensions of red cells as well as dilute haemoglobin solutions.

Commercial instruments are now available for performing the test and drawing the complete oxygen dissociation curve. Such analysers are extremely quick and accurate and therefore ideal for laboratories performing multiple ' determinations.

Method

Principle. Oxygen at known pO_2 is added stepwise to a tonometer which contains a dilute suspension of red cells in which the haemoglobin is completely deoxygenated. The haemoglobin in the cells is equilibrated with the gas and the percent saturation is measured spectrophotometrically after each addition. Because the haemoglobin concentration is low there is a negligible shift in the pO_2 in the gas phase after equilibration.

Apparatus

Tonometer-cuvette. This is not available commercially but can be made in a glass-blowing workshop*.

A tonometer, 5 cm high by 5 cm maximum diameter, is made from Pyrex glass. To one end is fused a high vacuum stopcock† with a single side arm at right angles to the main axis of the

apparatus. Small scratches should be made around the entry hole so that air can be admitted slowly. To the other end of the tonometer is fused, via a graded seal, a silica cuvette, 1 cm in light path and 4 ml in volume. Silica cuvettes should be used since the fusion process will distort ordinary glass cuvettes. The joints should be made to withstand pressures of at least 100 kPa (1 atmosphere). The whole apparatus (Fig. 13.7) should be no more than 20 cm high. The total volume of the tonometer and additions is measured. The stopcock is greased with silicone grease, taking care that none gets into the apparatus.

Spectrophotometer. Double-beam spectrophotometer with modified cuvette housing (e.g. Pye-Unicam, S.P.8000).

High vacuum pump.

Gas burette. Made from a graduated 3 ml pipette.

Reagents

Stock phosphate buffer, pH 7.43. 80 ml of

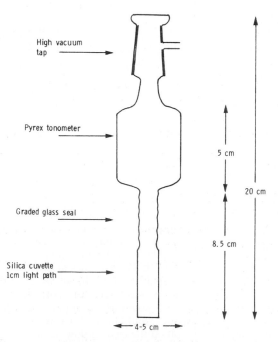

Fig. 13.7   Apparatus used in determination of oxygen dissociation curve.

---

*As designed by Professor E. R. Huehns and colleagues at University College Hospital, London.

†Quickfit, high vacuum stopcock TH6 (Baird and Tatlock (London) Ltd), suitably modified, is appropriate.

150 mmol/l Na_2HPO_4 and 20 ml of 150 mmol/l NaH_2PO_4.

Working buffer. Add 1 volume of stock buffer to 4 volumes of 154 mmol/l (9 g/l) NaCl. The pH must be 7.43 ± 0.01.

Other phosphate buffers of suitable pH may be prepared for studying the Bohr effect.

Method

Weigh the freshly greased tonometer. Dilute 2–4 drops of heparinized blood in about 10 ml of working buffer. This should give an absorbance of between 1.5 and 2.5 when measured at 576 nm. Connect with reinforced rubber tubing and evacuate via the side-arm of the stopcock using a high vacuum pump. Close the stopcock and disconnect the tonometer from the pump. Allow the cell suspension to run into the main body of the tonometer and then rotate it horizontally in a water-bath at 37°C for 3 min. This allows equilibration between the gases in the blood and buffer and the vacuum. Repeat the evacuation and equilibration twice more to ensure complete deoxygenation of the haemoglobin.

After a further equilibration, dry the cuvette, wipe it clean and place it in the appropriate part of the spectrophotometer.

After 30 s, to allow movement of red cells to stop, record the absorbance between 500 and 600 nm as a continuous spectrum. Then remove the tonometer from the spectrophotometer, dry the interior of the side arm, and attach the side arm to the gas burette.

Let a known volume of air (about 2 ml) into the tonometer through the side arm, the exact amount of air being measured by movement of the mercury bubble and recorded. Again equilibrate the Hb with the gas in the tonometer by rotating the apparatus at 37°C for 3 min.

Measure the absorbance over the same range once more after 30 s.

Add further volumes of air in the same way and repeat the process after each addition. In this way a family of curves is built up until finally the stopcock is opened to the air and the haemoglobin becomes fully saturated.

Read the absorbance at 540, 560 and 576 nm from the tracings.

Finally weigh the tonometer and its contents.

Notes

1. The pH of the buffer solution is critical and every care should be taken to ensure its accurate preparation.

2. Reinforced rubber tubing should be used for connections between the stopcock side arm and both the high vacuum pump and the gas burette, to ensure an air-tight seal.

3. It is vital that the position of the tonometer in the spectrophotometer is identical for all readings; a spring-loaded cuvette holder should be employed.

4. Always test a normal control blood in parallel.

Calculation

$$pO_2 \text{ (mmHg)} = \frac{\left(P - \dfrac{H \times SVP}{100}\right) \times 0.21}{V - v} \times A$$

where P = atmospheric pressure in mmHg[*]; H = relative humidity in percent; SVP = saturated vapour pressure at room temperature in mmHg; 0.21 = fraction of O_2 in air; V = volume of tonometer in ml; v = volume of contents in ml, and A = volume of air added in ml.

$$V = W_2 - W_1$$

where W_2 = weight of tonometer + contents and W_1 is weight of tonometer alone, assuming sp gr 1.0 for the blood/buffer suspension.

% saturation of Hb

$$= \frac{(A_{540} - A_{540}^{deoxy}) + (A_{560}^{deoxy} - A_{560})}{(A_{540}^{oxy} - A_{540}^{deoxy}) + (A_{560}^{deoxy}) - A_{560}^{oxy})} \times 100$$

or

% saturation of Hb

$$= \frac{(A_{576} - A_{576}^{deoxy} + (A_{560}^{deoxy} - A_{560})}{(A_{576}^{oxy} - A_{576}^{deoxy}) + (A_{560}^{deoxy}) - A_{560}^{oxy})} \times 100,$$

---

[*] $\times 0.133$ kPa.

where A_{540}, A_{560} and A_{576} are the absorbances of the partially saturated Hb at the appropriate wavelength and A^{deoxy} and A^{oxy} indicate the absorbance of the totally desaturated and totally oxygenated samples, respectively. The results are then plotted as a graph to obtain the full dissociation curve.

Assessment of the method

The method has the advantages that the curve can be determined on a small sample of blood and that it is relatively quick (about 45 min for a complete curve) and fairly simple. It is, too, a reasonably inexpensive method, providing the spectrophotometer can be used for other purposes. The method is particularly suitable for determining the 'n' value of a haemoglobin and calculating the Bohr effect. Its major disadvantage is that dilute suspensions of blood do not behave like whole blood and that the curve determined in this way gives no indication of what is happening in vivo to the $p_{50}O_2$. For these reasons it is useful for diagnostic work in identifying abnormal haemoglobins but it is not useful for research work which requires a knowledge of shifts in the oxygen affinity of blood in vivo.

Interpretation

Figure 13.8 shows the sigmoid nature of the oxygen dissociation curve of Hb A and the effect of hydrogen ions on the position of the curve. A shift of the curve to the right indicates decreased affinity of the haemoglobin for oxygen and hence an increased tendency to give up oxygen to the tissues: a shift to the left indicates increased affinity and so an increased tendency for haemoglobin to take up and retain oxygen. Hydrogen ions, DPG and some other organic phosphates such as ATP shift the curve to the right. The amount by which the curve is shifted may be expressed by the $p_{50}O_2$, i.e. the partial pressure of oxygen at which the haemoglobin is 50% saturated.

The oxygen affinity, as represented by the $p_{50}O_2$, is related to compensation in haemolytic anaemias.[2] 1 g of haemoglobin can carry about 1.34 ml of O_2. Fig. 13.9 shows the O_2 dis-

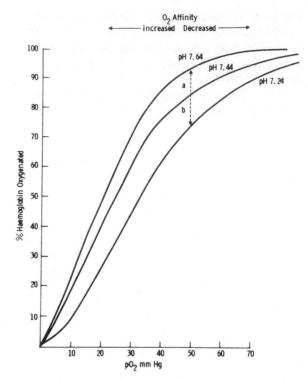

Fig. 13.8 The effect of pH upon the oxygen dissociation curve.

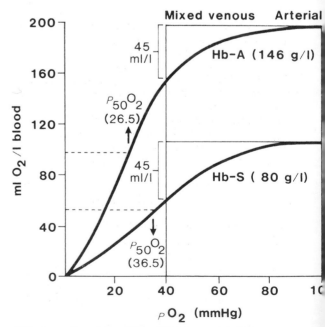

Fig. 13.9 The effect of O_2 affinity on O_2 delivery to tissues.

sociation curves of Hb A and Hb S plotted according to the volume of oxygen contained in 1 litre of blood when the haemoglobin concentrations are 146 g/l and 80 g/l, respectively. The $p_{50}O_2$ of Hb A is given as 26.5 mmHg (3.5 kPa) and Hb S as 36.5 mmHg (4.8 kPa). It will be seen that in the change from arterial to venous saturation the same volume of oxygen is given up despite the difference in haemoglobin concentration. Patients with a high $p_{50}O_2$ achieve a stable haemoglobin at a lower level than normal and this should be taken into account when planning transfusion for these patients.

The Bohr effect

Bohr et al described the effect of CO_2 on the oxygen dissociation curve.[12] An increase in CO_2 concentration produces a shift to the right, i.e. a decrease in oxygen affinity. It was soon realized that this effect was mainly due to changes in pH, although CO_2 itself has some direct effect. The Bohr effect is given a numerical value, $\Delta \log p_{50}O_2/\Delta pH$, where $\Delta \log p_{50}O_2$ is the change in $p_{50}O_2$ produced by a change in pH (ΔpH). The normal value of the Bohr effect at physiological pH and temperature is about 0.45.

Hill's constant

Hill thought that there was a constant ('n') which represented the number of molecules of oxygen which would combine with 1 molecule of haemoglobin.[24] Experiment showed that the value was 2.6 rather than the expected 4. The explanation for this lies in the effect of binding 1 molecule of oxygen by haemoglobin on the affinity for binding further oxygen molecules by haemoglobin, the so-called allosteric effect of haem-haem interaction: 'n' is a measure of this effect and the calculation of the 'n' value helps in identifying abnormal haemoglobins,[1] the molecular abnormality of which leads to abnormal haem-haem interaction.

Abbreviations used in this chapter

ADP, AMP, ATP	Adenosine di-, mono- or tri-phosphate
ALD	Aldolase
DHAP	Dihydroxyacetone phosphate
1,3DPG	1,3-Diphosphoglycerate
DPG	2,3-Diphosphoglycerate
DPGM	Diphosphoglycerate mutase
2,3DPGPase	2,3-Diphosphoglycerate phosphatase
DTNB	5,5'-Dithiobis(2-nitrobenzoic) acid) (Ellman's reagent)
En	Enolase
F1,6P	Fructose-1,6-diphosphate
F6P	Fructose-6-phosphate
Ga3P	Glyceraldehyde-3-phosphate
Ga3PD	Glyceraldehyde-3-phosphate dehydrogenase
G6P	Glucose-6-phosphate
2DG6P	2-Deoxyglucose-6-phosphate
G6PD	Glucose-6-phosphate dehydrogenase
GPI	Glucose phosphate isomerase
GPx	Glutathione peroxidase
GR	Glutathione reductase
GSH	Reduced glutathione
GSSG	Oxidized glutathione
Hx	Hexokinase
LAC	Lactate
LDH	Lactate dehydrogenase
NAD	Nicotine adenine dinucleotide
NADH	Reduced form of NAD
NADP	Nicotine adenine dinucleotide phosphate
NADPH	Reduced form of NADP
Pi	Inorganic phosphate
PEP	Phosphoenolpyruvate
PFK	Phosphofructokinase
6PG	6-Phosphogluconate
6PGD	6-Phosphogluconate dehydrogenase
3PG, 2PG	3- (or 2-) Phosphoglycerate
PGK	Phosphoglycerate kinase
PGM	Phosphoglyceromutase
P5N	Pyrimidine-5'-nucleotidase
PK	Pyruvate kinase
Ru5P	Ribulose-5-phosphate
TPI	Triose phosphate isomerase

REFERENCES

[1] BELLINGHAM, A. J. (1972). The physiological significance of the Hill parameter 'n'. *Scandinavian Journal of Haematology*, **9**, 552.

[2] BELLINGHAM, A. J. and HUEHNS, E. R. (1968). Compensation in haemolytic anaemias caused by abnormal haemoglobins. *Nature (London)*, **218**, 924.

[3] BELLINGHAM, A. J. and LENFANT, C. (1971). Hb affinity for O_2 determined by O_2-Hb dissociation analyser and mixing technique. *Journal of Applied Physiology*, **30**, 903.

[4] BENESCH, R. and BENESCH, R. E. (1967). The effect of organic phosphates from the human erythrocyte on the allosteric properties of haemoglobin. *Biochemical and Biophysical Research Communications*, **26**, 162.

[5] BEUTLER, E. (1984). *Red cell Metabolism. A Manual of Biochemical Methods*, 2nd edn. Grune & Stratton, Orlando, FL.

[6] BEUTLER, E. (1978). Why has the autohemolysis test not gone the way of the cephalin floculation test? *Blood*, **51**, 109.

[7] BEUTLER, E. (1989). Glucose-6-phosphate dehydrogenase: new perspectives. *Blood*, **73**, 1397.

[8] BEUTLER, E., BLUME, K. G., KAPLAN, J. C., LÖHR, G. W., RAMOT, B. and VALENTINE, W. N. (1977). International Committee for Standardization in Haematology. Recommended methods for red-cell enzyme analysis. *British Journal of Haematology*, **35**, 331.

[9] BEUTLER, E., BLUME, K. G., KAPLAN, J. C., LÖHR, G. W., RAMOT, B. and VALENTINE, W. N. (1979). International Committee for Standardization in Haematology. Recommended screening test for glucose-6-phosphate dehydrogenase (G-6-PD) deficiency. *British Journal of Haematology*, **43**, 465.

[10] BEUTLER, E., DURON, O. and KELLY, B. (1963). Improved method for the determination of blood glutathione. *Journal of Laboratory and Clinical Medicine*, **61**, 882.

[11] BEUTLER, E. and MITCHELL, M. (1968). Special modification of the fluorescent screening method for glucose-6-phosphate dehydrogenase deficiency. *Blood*, **32**, 816.

[12] BOHR, C., HASSELBACH, K. and KROGH, A. (1904). Ueber einen in biologischer Beziehung wichtigen Einfluss, den die Kohlensäurespannung des Blutes auf dessen Sauerstoffbindungübt. *Skandinavisches Archiv für Physiologie*, **16**, 402.

[13] BREWER, G. J., TARLOV, A. R. and ALVING, A. S. (1962). The methemoglobin reduction test for primaquine-type sensitivity of erythrocytes. A simplified procedure for detecting a specific hypersusceptibility to drug hemolysis. *Journal of the American Medical Association*, **180**, 386.

[14] CHANUTIN, A. and CURNISH, R. R. (1967). Effect of organic and inorganic phosphates on the oxygen equilibrium of human erythrocytes. *Archives of Biochemistry and Biophysics*, **121**, 96.

[15] COOPER, R. A. (1970). Lipids of human red cell membrane: normal composition and variability in disease. *Seminars in Hematology*, **7**, 296.

[16] DACIE, J. (1985). *The Haemolytic Anaemias, Vol. 1. The Hereditary Haemolytic Anaemias, Part 1*, (a) p. 146, (b) p. 352. Churchill Livingstone, Edinburgh.

[17] de GRUCHY, G. C, SANTAMARIA, J. N., PARSONS, I. C. and CRAWFORD, H. (1960). Nonspherocytic congenital hemolytic anemia. *Blood*, **16**, 1271.

[18] DUHM, J. (1971). Effects of 2,3-diphosphoglycerate and other organic phosphate compounds on oxygen affinity and intracellular pH of human erythrocytes. *Pflügers Archiv für die gesampte Physiologie des Menschen und der Tiere*, **326**, 341.

[19] GALL, J. C., BREWER, G. J. and DERN, R. J. (1965). Studies of glucose-6-phosphate dehydrogenase activity of individual erythrocytes: the methemoglobin-elution test for identification of females heterozygous for G6PD deficiency. *American Journal of Human Genetics*, **17**, 359.

[20] GOTTFRIED, E. L. and ROBERTSON, N. A. (1974). Glycerol lysis time of incubated erythrocytes in the diagnosis of hereditary spherocytosis. *Journal of Laboratory and Clinical Medicine*, **84**, 746.

[21] GOTTFRIED, E. L. and ROBERTSON, N. A. (1974). Glycerol lysis time as a screening test for erythrocyte disorders. *Journal of Laboratory and Clinical Medicine*, **83**, 323.

[22] GRIMES, A. J, LEETS, I. and DACIE, J. V. (1968). The autohaemolysis test: appraisal of the method for the diagnosis of pyruvate kinase deficiency and the effect of pH and additives. *British Journal of Haematology*, **14**, 309.

[23] GUNN, R. B., SILVERS, D. N. and ROSSE, W. F. (1972). Potassium permeability in β-thalassaemia minor red blood cells. *Journal of Clinical Investigation*, **51**, 1043.

[24] HILL, A. V. (1910). The possible effect of the aggregation of the molecules of haemoglobin on its dissociation curves. *Journal of Physiology*, **40**, 4.

[25] INTERNATIONAL COMMITTEE FOR STANDARDIZATION IN HAEMATOLOGY (1979). Recommended methods for the characterisation of red cell pyruvate kinase variants. *British Journal of Haematology*, **43**, 275.

[26] INTERNATIONAL COMMITTEE FOR STANDARDIZATION IN HAEMATOLOGY (1989). Recommended screening test for pyrimidine 5'-nucleotidase deficiency. *Clinical and Laboratory Haematology*, **11**, 55.

[27] JACOB, H. S. and JANDL, J. H. (1964). Increased cell membrane permeability in the pathogenesis of hereditary spherocytosis. *Journal of Clinical Investigation*, **43**, 1704.

[28] KONRAD, P. N., VALENTINE, W. N. and PAGLIA, D. E. (1972). Enzymatic activities and glutathione content of erythrocytes in the newborn. Comparison with red cells of older normal subjects and those with comparable reticulocytosis. *Acta Haematologica*, **48**, 193.

[29] KRIMSKY, I. (1965). D-2, 3-Diphosphoglycerate. In *Methods of Enzymatic Analysis*. Ed. H. U. Bergmeyer, p. 238. Academic Press, New York.

[30] LOWRY, O. H., PASSONNEAU, J. V., HASSELBERGER, F. X. and SCHULZ, D. W. (1964). Effect of ischemia on known substrates and cofactors of the glycolytic pathway in brain. *Journal of Biological Chemistry* **239**, 18.

[31] LUBIN, B. H. and OSKI, F. A. (1967). An evaluation of screening procedures for red cell glucose-6-phosphate dehydrogenase deficiency in the newborn infant. *Journal of Pediatrics*, **70**, 788.

[32] LUZZATTO, L. and MEHTA, A. (1989). Glucose-6-phosphate dehydrogenase deficiency. In *The Metabolic Basis of Inherited Disease*. Eds. C. R. Scriver, A. L. Beaudet, W. S. Sly and D. Valle, pp. 2237–2265. McGraw-Hill, New York.

[33] LYON, M. F. (1961). Gene action in the X-chromosomes of the mouse (*Mus musculus* L.). *Nature (London)*, **190**, 372.

[34] MIWA, S., FUJII, H., TAKEGAWA, S., NAKATSUJI, T., YAMOTO, K., ISHIDA, Y. and NINOMIYA, N. (1980). Seven

pyruvate kinase variants characterised by the ICSH recommended methods. *British Journal of Haematology*, **45**, 575.

[35] MIWA, S., NAKASHIMA, K., ARIYOSHI, K., SHINOHARA, K., ODA, E. and TANAKA, T. (1975). Four new pyruvate kinase (PK) variants and a classical PK deficiency. *British Journal of Haematology*, **29**, 157.

[36] MURPHY, J. R. (1967). The influence of pH and temperature on some physical properties of normal erythrocytes and erythrocytes from patients with hereditary spherocytosis. *Journal of Laboratory and Clinical Medicine*, **69**, 758.

[37] PARPART, A. K., LORENZ, P. B., PARPART, E. R., GREGG, J. R. and CHASE, A. M. (1947). The osmotic resistance (fragility) of human red cells. *Journal of Clinical Investigation*, **26**, 636.

[38] PETERS, J. P. and VAN SLYKE, D. D. (1931). Hemoglobin and oxygen. In *Quantitative Clinical Chemistry, Vol. 1, Interpretations*, p. 525. Williams & Wilkins, Baltimore.

[39] ROSE, Z. B. and LIEBOWITZ, J. (1970). Direct determination of 2,3-diphosphoglycerate. *Annals of Biochemistry and Experimental Medicine*, **35**, 177.

[40] ROSSI-FANELLI, A. and ANTONINI, E. (1958). Studies on the oxygen and carbon monoxide equilibria of human myoglobin. *Archives of Biochemistry and Biophysics*, **77**, 478.

[41] SELWYN, J. G. and DACIE, J. V. (1954). Autohemolysis and other changes resulting from the incubation in vitro of red cells from patients with congenital hemolytic anemia. *Blood*, **9**, 414.

[42] SUESS, J., LIMENTANI, D., DAMESHEK, W. and DOLLOFF, M. J. (1948). A quantitative method for the determination and charting of the erythrocyte hypotonic fragility. *Blood*, **3**, 1290.

[43] TORRANCE, J. D. and LENFANT, C., (1969–70). Methods for determination of O_2 dissociation curves, including Bohr effect. *Respiration Physiology*, **8**, 127.

[44] TORRANCE, J., WEST, C. and BEUTLER, E. (1977). A simple radiometric assay for pyrimidine 5'-nucleotidase. *Journal of Laboratory and Clinical Medicine*, **90**, 563.

[45] VALENTINE, W. N., FINK, K., PAGLIA, D. E., HARRIS, S. R. and ADAMS, W. S. (1974). Hereditary .haemolytic anaemia with human erythrocyte pyrimidine 5'-nucleotidase deficiency. *Journal of Clinical Investigation*, **54**, 866.

[46] VAN SLYKE, D. D. and NEILL, J. M. (1924). The determination of gases in blood and other solutions by vacuum extraction and manometric measurement. *Journal of Biological Chemistry*, **61**, 523.

[47] VULLIAMY, T. J., D'URSO, M., BATTISTUZZI, G., ESTRADA, M., FOULKES, N. S., MARTINI, G., CALABRO, V., POGGI, V., GIORDANO, R., TOWN, M., LUZZATO, L. and PERSICO, G. (1988). Diverse point mutations in the human glucose-6-phosphate dehydrogenase gene cause enzyme deficiency and mild or severe hemolytic anemia. *Proceedings of the National Academy of Sciences of the USA.*, **85**, 5171.

[48] WORLD HEALTH ORGANIZATION SCIENTIFIC GROUP (1967). Standardization of procedures for the study of glucose-6-phosphate dehydrogenase. *Technical Report Series, No. 366.* WHO, Geneva.

[49] WORLD HEALTH ORGANIZATION SCIENTIFIC GROUP ON GLUCOSE-6-PHOSPHATE DEHYDROGENASE (1990). *Bulletin of World Health Organization*, **67**, 601.

[50] YOSHIDA, A., BEUTLER, E. and MOTULSKY, A. G. (1971). Human glucose-6-phosphate dehydrogenase variants. *Bulletin of the World Health Organization*, **45**, 243.

[51] ZANELLA, A., IZZO, C., REBULLA, P., ZANUSO, F., PERRONI, L. and SIRCHIA, G. (1980). Acidified glycerol lysis test: a screening test for spherocytosis. *British Journal of Haematology*, **45**, 481.

[52] ZINKHAM, W. H. (1959). An in-vitro abnormality of glutathione metabolism in erythrocytes from normal newborns: mechanism and clinical significance. *Pediatrics*, **23**, 18.

14. Investigation of abnormal haemoglobins and thalassaemia

Revised by Milica Brozović and Joan Henthorn

The haemoglobin molecule   249
  Structural variants of haemoglobin   250
   Thalassaemia syndromes   252
   Increased Hb F in adult life   254
Investigation of patients suspected of suffering from a
  haemoglobinopathy   255
Investigation of structural variant   256
Collection of blood and preparation of haemolysates   257
  Control samples   258
  Quality assurance   258
Cellulose acetate electrophoresis at alkaline pH   258
Citrate agar electrophoresis, pH 6.0   261
Agar gel electrophoresis   262
Cellulose acetate electrophoresis, pH 6.5   262
Iso-electric focusing 262
Globin chain electrophoresis   264
Tests for Hb S   266
  Sickling in whole blood   266
  Hb S solubility test   267
  Hb S detection with monoclonal antibody   268
  Screening of newborn   268
Diagnosis of an unstable haemoglobin haemolytic
  anaemia   268

Heat instability test   268
Isopropanol stability test   269
n-Butanol stability test   269
Detection of haemoglobin M   270
Altered affinity haemoglobins   271
Suggested use of electrophoretic techniques in differential
  diagnosis of variants   271
Investigation of thalassaemia   272
Estimation of Hb A_2 274
  By elution from cellulose acetate   274
  By micro-column chromatography   275
Estimation of percentage of slow-moving haemoglobin
  variants in mixtures of haemoglobin   276
High performance liquid chromatography (HPLC)   278
Estimation of Hb F   279
  Modified Betke method   279
  Jonxis and Visser's method   280
  Radial immunodiffusion (RID)   280
Intracellular distribution of Hb F   281
Iron status in thalassaemia   282
Red cell inclusions   283
  Demonstration of Hb H   283
Fetal diagnosis of globin gene disorders   284

THE HAEMOGLOBIN MOLECULE

Human haemoglobin is formed of two pairs of globin chains to each of which is attached one molecule of haem. Six variants are normally formed: three are transient embryonic haemoglobins referred to as Hb Gower 1, Hb Gower 2 and Hb Portland; Hb F is the predominant haemoglobin of fetal life, and Hb A (more than 95%) and Hb A_2 (1–3.5%) are the characteristic haemoglobins of adults. Hb F, although present in large amounts at birth (65–95%), is normally formed subsequently only in traces.

The individual chains formed in post-natal life are designated α, β, γ and δ. Hb A is formed of two α chains and two β chains ($\alpha_2\beta_2$); Hb F is formed of two α chains and two γ chains ($\alpha_2\gamma_2$),

and Hb A_2 of two α chains and two δ chains ($a_2\delta_2$). The α chain is thus common to all three types of haemoglobin molecule.

The α chain is directed by two α genes, $\alpha 1$ and $\alpha 2$, on chromosome 16, and the β and δ chains by single genes on chromosome 11. The γ chain is directed by two genes, $^G\gamma$ and $^A\gamma$, also on chromosome 11. The globin genes are shown in Fig. 14.1.

The four chains are associated in the form of a tetramer: the $\alpha_1\beta_1$ contact is the strongest and involves many amino acids with many interlocking side chains; the $\alpha_1\beta_2$ contact is less extensive, while the contacts between like chains are relatively weak. The binding of a molecule of haem

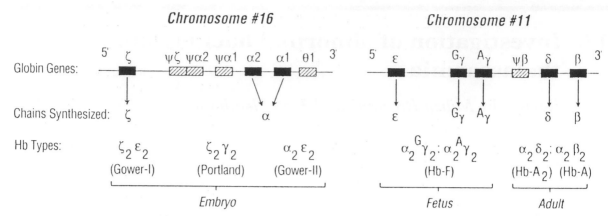

Fig. 14.1   Location of the α-globin gene cluster on chromosome 16 and that of the β-globin gene cluster on chromosome 11. The black boxes represent functional genes. The α- and γ-globin genes are duplicated; the two α-globin genes have the same product while the products of the two γ-globin genes are slightly different ($^{G}\gamma = \gamma136Gly$; $^{A}\gamma = \gamma136Ala$).

into a 'haem pocket' in each chain is vital for the oxygen-carrying capacity of the molecule and stabilizes the whole molecule. If the haem attachment is weakened, the globin chains dissociate into dimers and monomers.

It is now realized that many naturally occurring genetically determined (inherited) variants of human haemoglobin exist and that although many are harmless some have serious clinical effects. Collectively, the clinical syndromes resulting from disorders of haemoglobin are referred to as 'haemoglobinopathies'. They can be grouped into three main categories:

1. Those due to structural variants of haemoglobin, such as Hb S.
2. Those due to failure to synthesize haemoglobin normally, as in the thalassaemias.
3. Those due to failure to complete the normal neonatal switch from fetal haemoglobin (Hb F) to adult haemoglobin (Hb A). These comprise a group of disorders referred to as hereditary persistence of fetal haemoglobin (HPFH).

STRUCTURAL VARIANTS OF HAEMOGLOBIN

The alterations in the structure of haemoglobin are usually brought about by point mutations affecting one or, less often, a few bases coding for amino acids of the globin chain. An example of such a point mutation is Hb S caused by the substitution of valine for glutamic acid in position 6 of the β-globin chain ($\beta^{6Glu \rightarrow Val}$). Less commonly, structural change is caused by deletion or by extension of the globin chain. For example, five amino acids are deleted in the β chain of Hb Gun Hill; in Hb Constant Spring 31 amino acids are added to the α chain.

Many variant haemoglobins are haematologically and clinically silent, because the underlying mutation causes no alteration in the function, solubility or stability of the haemoglobin molecule. Some structural variants are associated with disease states in the homozygous or even heterozygous state; these mutations affect the physical or chemical properties of the haemoglobin molecule resulting in changes in haemoglobin solubility, stability or oxygen-binding properties.

HAEMOGLOBINS WITH ALTERED SOLUBILITY

The most common haemoglobin variant in this group is sickle haemoglobin or Hb S. Hb S differs from Hb A in a single amino acid: glutamic acid in position 6 of the β chain is replaced by valine.

Table 14.1   Clinical syndromes encountered with structural variants

Hb	Genotype	Name	Clinical problems
S	β^A/β^S	Sickle cell trait	None
	β^S/β^S	Sickle cell anaemia	Severe haemolytic anaemia, vaso-occlusive episodes
C	β^A/β^C	C trait	None
	β^C/β^C	C disease	Occasional mild anaemia
D^{Punjab}	β^A/β^D	D trait	None
	β^D/β^D	D disease	Occasional mild anaemia
O^{Arab}	β^A/β^{OArab}	O trait	None
	$\beta^{OArab}/\beta^{OArab}$	O disease	Haemolytic anaemia
Interactions	β^S/β^C	SC disease	Mild anaemia, vaso-occlusive problems
	$\beta^S/\beta^{DPunjab}$	SD disease	As for sickle cell anaemia
	β^S/β^{OArab}	SO disease	As for sickle cell anaemia
	β^{0thal}/β^S	Sickle-β^0thal	As for sickle cell anaemia
	β^{+thal}/β^S	Sickle-β^+thal	Mild sickle cell disease
	β^{thal}/β^C	C-βthal	Mild haemolytic anaemia
	β^{thal}/β^D	D-βthal	Mild haemolytic anaemia
	$\beta^{thal}/\beta^{OArab}$	O-βthal	Thalassaemia intermedia

As a result of this minute difference, Hb S has poor solubility and deformability in the de-oxygenated state and can polymerize within the red cell. The red cell shows a characteristic shape change due to polymer formation and becomes distorted and rigid, the so called sickle cell. In addition, intracellular polymers lead to red-cell membrane changes, generation of oxidant substances and abnormal adherence of red cells to vascular endothelium.

Clinical syndromes associated with common structural variants and those due to their interaction with β-thalassaemia are shown in Table 14.1.

Sickle cell disease[36]

Sickle cell disease or disorder is a collective name for a group of conditions characterized by the formation of sickle red cells and is common in people of African descent, but is also found in other ethnic groups.

The homozygous state, sickle cell anaemia or Hb SS causes moderate to severe haemolytic anaemia. The main clinical disability arises from repeated episodes of vascular occlusion by sickled red cells resulting in acute crises and eventually in end-organ damage. The severity of sickle cell anaemia is extremely variable. This is partly due to the effects of inherited modifying factors, such as interaction with α-thalassaemia or a mild allele of β⁺-thalassaemia, or increased synthesis of Hb F, and partly to socioeconomic conditions and other factors that influence general health.[36]

Sickle cell trait (Hb AS), the heterozygous state, is very common, affecting millions of people world-wide. There are no associated haematological abnormalities. In-vivo sickling occurs only at very high altitudes and at low oxygen pressures (such as encountered when deep sea diving); spontaneous haematuria, due to sickling in the kidneys, is found in about 1% of people with Hb AS.

Other forms of sickle cell disease

SC disease (Hb SC) is a compound heterozygous state for Hb S and Hb C. This results in a milder form of sickle cell disease with predominantly vascular problems. *Sickle β-thalassaemia* arises as a result of inheritance of one Hb S and one β-thalassaemia gene. Africans and West Indians with the condition are usually heterozygous for a mild β⁺-thalassaemia allele resulting in the production of about 20% of Hb A. This gives rise to a mild sickling disorder. Inheritance of Hb S and β^0-thalassaemia trait is associated with a severe sickle cell disease. Interaction of Hb S with Hb D^{Punjab} or with Hb O^{Arab} gives rise to a severe sickle cell disorder.

Haemoglobin C (Hb C) is the second most common structural haemoglobin variant. The substitution of glutamic acid in position 6 of the β chain by lysine results in a haemoglobin molecule with high positive charge, decreased solubility and 'paracrystal' formation. Heterozygotes are asymptomatic, but target cells are present in blood films. Homozygotes may have mild anaemia with numerous target cells. Interaction with β^0- and β^+-thalassaemia trait results in mild or moderate haemolytic anaemia.

UNSTABLE HAEMOGLOBINS[10,41]

Amino-acid substitutions close to the haem molecule, or at the points of contact between globin chains, affect protein stability and result in intracellular precipitation of globin chains. The precipitated globin chains attach to the red cell membrane giving rise to Heinz bodies. Changes in membrane properties may lead to severe haemolytic anaemia, often aggravated by oxidant drugs. Most variants are symptomatic in the heterozygous state. Hb Köln is the most common variant in this rare group of disorders.

HAEMOGLOBINS WITH ALTERED OXYGEN AFFINITY

Mutations which *increase O_2 affinity* are associated with benign life-long erythrocytosis. This may be confused with polycythaemia rubra vera and inappropriately treated with cytotoxic drugs.

Haemoglobin variants with *decreased O_2 affinity* are less common and are usually associated with mild anaemia and cyanosis.

Hb Ms are another rare group of variants. Such haemoglobins have a propensity to form methaemoglobin, generated by the oxidation of ferrous iron in haem to ferric iron, which is incapable of binding oxygen. Despite marked cyanosis, there are few clinical problems. Most are associated with substitutions which disrupt the normal six-ligand state of haem iron.

Methaemoglobinaemia is also found in congenital NADH methaemoglobin reductase deficiency, as well as after exposure to oxidant drugs and chemicals (nitrates, quinones, chlorates, phenacetin, dapsone and many others).

Carbon monoxide binds avidly to haem to form *carboxyhaemoglobin*. Carboxyhaemoglobin cannot bind oxygen and toxicity results from generalized tissue anoxia.

Sulphaemoglobin is a green pigmented derivative of haemoglobin. Sulphur is incorporated into the porphyrin ring giving the characteristic absorption spectrum at 620 nm. It forms through irreversible oxidation of haem by drugs and chemicals.

THALASSAEMIA SYNDROMES[40]

The thalassaemia syndromes are a heterogeneous group of inherited anaemias characterized by defects in the synthesis of one or more of the globin chains that form the haemoglobin tetramer. The clinical syndromes associated with thalassaemia arise from the combined consequences of inadequate haemoglobin production and of unbalanced accumulation of globin chains. The former causes anaemia with hypochromasia and microcytosis; the latter leads to ineffective erythropoiesis and haemolysis. Clinical manifestations range from completely asymptomatic microcytosis to profound anaemia incompatible with life and even death in utero (see Table 14.2). This clinical heterogeneity arises as a result of the variable severity of the primary genetic defect in haemoglobin synthesis and of co-inherited modulating factors, such as the capacity to synthesize increased amount of Hb F.

Thalassaemias are inherited as pathological alleles of one or more globin genes located on either chromosome 11 (for β, γ and δ chains) or

Table 14.2   Clinical syndromes of thalassaemia

Clinically asymptomatic
Silent carriers
  α^+-Thalassaemia trait
  Rare forms of β-thalassaemia trait
Thalassaemia minor (mild anaemia, low MCH and MCV)
  α^0-thalassaemia trait
  α^+/α^+-homozygotes
  β^0-thalassaemia trait
  β^+-thalassaemia trait
  δ/β-thalassaemia trait

Thalassaemia intermedia
Some β^+/β^+-thalassaemia homozygotes
Interaction of β^0/β^0 or β^+/β^+ with α-thalassaemia
Interaction of β^0/β^0 or β^+/β^+ with triple α-thalassaemia
Hb H disease
α^0/Hb Constant Spring thalassaemia
$\beta^0/\delta\beta$- or $\beta^+/\delta\beta$-thalassaemia compound heterozygotes
$\delta\beta/\delta\beta$-Thalassaemia
Some cases of Hb E/β thalassaemia and Hb Lepore/β thalassaemia
Rare cases of heterozygotes for β gene mutation involving exon 3

Thalassaemia major (transfusion dependent)
β^0/β^0-Thalassaemia
β^+/β^+-Thalassaemia
β^0/β^+-Thalassaemia
β^0/Hb Lepore, β^+/Hb Lepore thalassaemia
β^0/Hb E, β^+/Hb E thalassaemia

on chromosome 16 (for α chains). They are encountered in every population in the world but are most common in the Mediterranean littoral and near equatorial regions of Africa and Asia. Gene frequencies in the thalassaemia belt range from 2.5 to 15%.

β-THALASSAEMIA SYNDROMES[37]

Many different mutations cause β-thalassaemia and its related disorders. These mutations affect every step in the pathway of globin gene expression: transcription; processing of the mRNA precursor; translation of mature mRNA; and post-translational integrity of the β chain. Over 100 mutations have been described. Most types of β-thalassaemia are due to point mutations affecting one or a few bases that code for amino acids making up the globin chain, but some large deletions are also known. Certain mutations are particularly common in some communities. This helps to simplify pre-natal diagnosis which is carried out by detecting the exact mutation in fetal DNA.

The effect of different mutations varies greatly. At one end of the spectrum are a group of rare mutations involving exon 3 of the β globin gene which are so severe that they may produce the clinical syndrome of thalassaemia intermedia in the heterozygous state. At the other end are mild alleles which produce thalassaemia intermedia in homozygous state, and some which are so mild that they are completely haematologically 'silent', with normal MCV and Hb A_2 in the heterozygous state. In between are the great majority of β^+ and β^0 alleles which cause β-thalassaemia major in the homozygous or compound heterozygous state, and a mild anaemia with microcytosis and raised Hb A_2 in the heterozygous state.[6]

β-*Thalassaemia major* is a severe, transfusion-dependent inherited anaemia. There is a profound defect of β chain production. Excess of α chains accumulate and precipitate in the red cell precursors in the bone marrow causing cell death—the so-called ineffective erythropoiesis. The few cells which leave the marrow are laden with precipitated α chains and are rapidly removed by the RES. The constant erythropoietic drive causes massive expansion of bone marrow and extramedullary erythropoiesis. Eighty percent of untreated children with β thalassaemia major die in the first 5 yr of life.

Heterozygotes for β chain alleles usually have a mild microcytic hypochromic anaemia with elevated Hb A_2 and F. Laboratory features of various β-thalassaemic syndromes are shown in Table 14.3.

α-THALASSAEMIA SYNDROMES[18]

There are four syndromes of α-thalassaemia: α^+ trait where one of the four globin gene loci fails to function, α^0 trait where two loci are dysfunctional, Hb H disease with three loci affected and Hb Bart's hydrops fetalis where all four are defective. These syndromes are usually due to deletions of one or more loci, but non-deletional forms account for almost 20% of all cases. α^+-thalassaemia is particularly common in Africa, and α^0-thalassaemia in South-East Asia. Laboratory features are shown in Table 14.3.

Hb Bart's hydrops fetalis occurs almost exclusively in South-East Asia. Affected fetuses are stillborn prematurely or die shortly after birth.

Table 14.3   Laboratory findings in thalassaemia

Phenotype	Genotype	Usual MCV	MCH	Hb A$_2$	Heinz bodies
α-Thalassaemia					
α-Thalassaemia trait	$-α/αα$ $(α^+/α)$	N	N	N or ↓	–
α-Thalassaemia trait	$-α/-α$ or $--/αα$ $(α^+/α^+$ or $α^0/α^0)$	N or ↓	N or ↓	N or ↓	+
Hb H disease:					
mild	$--/-α$ $(α^0/α^+)$	↓	↓	N or ↓	+++
severe	$--/αα^T$ $(α^0/α^T)$	↓	↓	N or ↓	+++
Hb Bart's hydrops	$--/--$ $(α^0/α^0)$	↓	↓	–	–
(α-Thalassaemia major)					
β-Thalassaemia					
β-Thalassaemia trait	$β^0/β$ or $β^+/β$	↓	↓	↑	–
δβ-Thalassaemia trait	$δβ^0/β$	↓	↓	N or ↓	–
β-Thalassaemia trait	$β^+/β$	↓	↓	N	–
with normal Hb A$_2$					
Hb Lepore trait	Hb Lepore/β	↓	↓	N	–
β-Thalassaemia	Heterogeneous	↓	↓	↑, N or ↓	–
intermedia					
β-Thalassaemia major	$β^0/β^0$, $β^0/β^+$. $β^+/β^+$	↓	↓	↑, N or ↓	–

Severe anaemia and anasarca are the hallmarks of this condition. Women carrying a hydropic fetus have a high incidence of severe toxaemia. Prenatal diagnosis should be offered whenever possible.

Hb H disease gives rise to haemolytic anaemia of variable severity; patients rarely require transfusion or splenectomy.

The $α^0$ *trait* manifests itself as a persistent microcytosis. Haemoglobin may be normal or slightly reduced. The $α^+$ *trait* can be completely silent with only borderline microcytosis and slightly reduced or normal MCH. The α-thalassaemia trait is more difficult to diagnose than β-thalassaemia trait because there is no characteristic elevation in Hb A$_2$ and F, and Hb H bodies cannot always be demonstrated. Definitive diagnosis can only be made by molecular biology methods.

Thalassaemic structural variants

These are abnormal haemoglobins characterized by both a biosynthetic defect and an abnormal structure (see Table 14.4).

INCREASED HAEMOGLOBIN F IN ADULT LIFE[44]

Haemoglobin production in humans is characterized by two major 'switches' in the haemoglobin

Table 14.4   Thalassaemic structural variants*

Haemoglobin	Structure	When heterozygous	When homozygous	In combination with other haemoglobinopathies
Lepore	Combination of δ and β chains due to unequal crossover	Microcytosis, mild anaemia	Thalassaemia major	With β-thalassaemia gives thalassaemia major
E**	$β^{26Glu→Lys}$ resulting in abnormal mRNA	Microcytosis, mild anaemia	Microcytosis, mild anaemia	With β-thalassaemia gives thalassaemia major
Constant Spring	Elongated α chain due to incorporation of 31 extra amino acids	Microcytosis, mild anaemia	Microcytosis, mild anaemia	With $α^0$ gives Hb H disease

*Many other thalassaemic structural variants have been described but are much rarer than the three shown in this table.
**13–30% frequency in Cambodia, Thailand, Vietnam and some parts of China.

composition of the red cells. During the first 3 months of gestation, human red cells contain embryonic haemoglobins (see p. 249), whereas during the last 6 months of gestation red cells contain predominantly fetal haemoglobin. The major transition from fetal to adult haemoglobin occurs in the perinatal period and by the end of the first year red cells have a haemoglobin composition that subsequently remains stable. The major haemoglobin is Hb A, but there are small amounts of Hb A_2 and Hb F. Only 0.5–1% of total haemoglobin in human red cells is Hb F and it is restricted to a few cells called 'F' cells. Both the number of F cells and the amount of Hb F per cell can be increased in various conditions, particularly if there is rapid bone marrow regeneration.

The general organization of human globin gene clusters is shown in Fig. 14.1. The products of two γ genes differ in only one amino acid: $^G\gamma$ has glycine in position 136, whereas $^A\gamma$ has alanine. In fetal red cells the ratio of $^G\gamma$ to $^A\gamma$ is 3:1; in adult red cells it is 2:3.

In recent years much interest has been aroused by the attempts to manipulate the fetal switch pharmacologically. If it were possible to switch Hb F synthesis reliably beyond the perinatal period, both thalassaemia major and sickle cell anaemia would be ameliorated.

Inherited abnormalities which increase Hb F[44,45]

More than 50 mutations which increase Hb F synthesis have been described. They result in one of two phenotypes, hereditary persistence of Hb F (HPFH) or δβ-thalassaemia; the distinction between these two types is blurred. The most common, the African type of HPFH is associated with a high concentration of Hb F (15–45%), pancellular distribution of Hb F on Kleihauer staining (see p. 137) and normal red cell indices. Mutations causing increased synthesis of Hb F are mostly deletions, but some non-deletion variants have also been described. The major clinical significance of these variants is their interaction with β-thalassaemia and Hb S. Compound heterozygotes have much milder clinical syndromes than the homozygotes.

Increased Hb F is also found in many other haematological conditions, including congenital hypoplastic anaemias (Blackfan-Diamond and Fanconi's), in the juvenile form of chronic granulocytic leukaemia and in some myelodysplastic syndromes. A small but significant increase in Hb F occurs in the presence of erythropoietic stress (haemolysis, bleeding, recovery from acute hypoplasia) and in the third trimester of pregnancy.

INVESTIGATION OF PATIENTS SUSPECTED OF SUFFERING FROM A HAEMOGLOBINOPATHY

Investigation of persons considered to be possibly suffering from a haemoglobinopathy is usually carried out to establish, first, if an abnormal haemoglobin molecule is present and if so, to ensure that patients who have a haemoglobinopathy of clinical significance are correctly managed, and that, whether with or without clinical problems, they receive, if necessary, adequate genetic counselling. Genetic counselling implies discussions with both partners and, where appropriate, consideration of the possibility of prenatal diagnosis of an affected fetus (see p. 294).

In the majority of patients the presence of a haemoglobinopathy may be accurately diagnosed from knowledge of the patient's ethnic origin and clinical history (including family history) and the results of physical examination combined with relatively simple haematological tests. The peripheral blood picture should always be considered first and the quantitative data must include a red cell count, calculation of red cell indices and measurement of haemoglobin and haematocrit. In some instances a reticulocyte count and a search for red cell inclusions give valuable information. A detailed examination of a well stained blood film must always be carried out. Assessment of iron status by estimation of serum iron and total iron-binding capacity, ferritin or zinc protoporphyrin, or bone marrow iron stores is sometimes necessary. Other important basic tests are haemoglobin electrophoresis, haemoglobin solubility and measurement of Hb A_2 and Hb F percentage. If it is possible to carry out all these tests accurately, a reliable diagnosis can usually be made without the need for more sophisticated investigations. However, definitive diagnosis of some thalassaemic syndromes can only be obtained using DNA technology (see Chapter 28 and p. 294). Individuals or families who require such investigation must be carefully selected on the basis of family history and on the results of the basic investigations described below.

The problems of diagnosis in large-scale screening programmes when individual histories and results of laboratory investigations are not available, are discussed on p. 268.

The majority of errors occurring in the detection of and identification of a haemoglobinopathy are due to either failure to obtain correct laboratory data or failure to interpret data correctly. To avoid laboratory error, quality control guidelines must be observed, and participation in local or national quality assessment schemes should be mandatory. Controls must be set up with all procedures described in this Chapter and each laboratory must establish its own normal range for quantitative tests. Interpretation of laboratory findings is a skill only fully achieved after much practice.

In this chapter a sequence of investigations is suggested based on procedures which should be available in any hospital laboratory. Isoelectric focusing and high performance liquid chromatography are available in specialist laboratories and are only briefly described. Globin chain synthesis was described in the 6th edition of this book.

Laboratory investigation of a suspected haemoglobinopathy should follow a definite but flexible protocol. The data obtained from the clinical findings, blood picture and electrophoresis will usually indicate in which direction to proceed. The investigation for a structural variant is described in the first section and that for a suspected thalassaemic syndrome in the second section of this chapter.

INVESTIGATION FOR A STRUCTURAL VARIANT

A suggested scheme of investigation is shown in Fig. 14.2 and a list of methods and approaches are given below.

METHODS AND APPROACHES USEFUL IN INVESTIGATING A SUSPECTED STRUCTURAL VARIANT

1. Blood count and film examination (p. 256).
2. Preparation of samples and controls (p. 257).
3. Quality assurance (p. 258).
4. Cellulose acetate electrophoresis, Tris buffer, pH 8.5 (p. 258).
5. Citrate agar or acid gel electrophoresis, pH 6.0 (p. 261).
6. Cellulose acetate electrophoresis, phosphate buffer, pH 6.5 (p. 262).
7. Iso-electric focusing (p. 262).
8. Globin chain electrophoresis, pH 8.6 and 6.0 (p. 264)

9. Tests for Hb S (p. 266).
10. Screening of newborn babies for Hb S (p. 268).
11. Stability tests (p. 268).
12. Detection of Hb M (p. 270).
13. Testing for altered affinity haemoglobins (p. 271).
14. How to distinguish common structural variants (p. 271).

Blood count

The blood count, including red cell count, haemoglobin, haematocrit and red cell indices, provides valuable information useful in the diagnosis of both α- and β-thalassaemia interactions with structural variants (Chapter 5), whilst a film examination may reveal characteristic red cell changes such as target cells in Hb AC and sickle cells in Hb SS (Chapter 7).

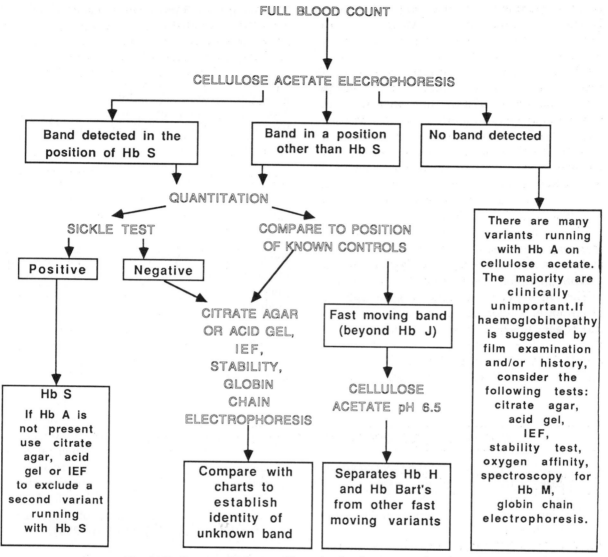

Fig. 14.2   Suggested scheme of investigation for structural variants.

Preparation of samples for investigation

Samples taken into any anticoagulant are satisfactory. Ethylenediaminetetra-acetic acid (EDTA) is the most convenient as this is used for the initial full blood count and film. Cells freed from clotted blood can also be used if necessary. The cells should be washed three times in isotonic saline (0.15 mol/l).

Preparation of a lysate for immediate use

Lyse 1 volume of washed packed cells in 4 volumes

of lysing reagent prepared as follows:

3.8 g EDTA, tetrasodium salt.
0.7 g potassium cyanide (KCN).
Water to 1 litre.

Such a lysate will not keep for more than 1–2 days at 4°C as it tends to gel. If necessary it can be frozen at –20°C for up to 1 month. Avoid repeated freezing and thawing.

Prepartion of a lysate for long-term storage

Lyse 2 volumes of washed packed cells in 1 volume of distilled water then add 1 volume of carbon tetrachloride (CCl$_4$). Alternatively, lyse by freezing and thawing, then add 2 volumes of CCl$_4$. After vigorous shaking, preferably using a mechanical agitator, centrifuge the mixture at 3000 rpm (1200g) for 30 min and transfer the clear solution to a clean tube and adjust the haemoglobin concentration to 100 g/l with water.

Samples can be stored frozen at $-20°C$ for up to 3 months. Avoid repeated freezing and thawing. In small aliquots in liquid nitrogen samples last almost indefinitely.

Preparation of control samples

The pattern shown by unknown samples must be compared with that shown by control lysates of known abnormal haemoglobins. A mixture of Hbs A, F, S and C must be included with each electrophoretic run alongside the samples under test. Such a mixture is prepared as follows.

1. Use fresh blood samples from a person with sickle trait (A+S), another with C trait (A+C), and a normal cord blood (A+F). (As an alternative, blood from a person with SC disease, and a cord blood may be used.)
2. Prepare lysates by the CCl$_4$ method given above.
3. Add a few drops of 0.3 mol/l KCN (20 g/l) to stabilize the haemoglobin as cyanmethaemoglobin (HiCN).
4. Mix equal volumes of the lysates and check by electrophoresis.

5. Dispense in 0.5 ml volumes and store at $-20°C$ for up to 3 months. Avoid repeated freezing and thawing. Samples stored in liquid nitrogen last almost indefinitely.

Controls may also be purchased in freeze-dried form; this is particularly useful for unusual variants. Most manufacturers of electrophoresis equipment have some controls in their catalogues.

Quality assurance[6]

All laboratories undertaking haemoglobin analysis should participate in an appropriate quality assurance programme. In the UK the National External Quality Assessment Scheme (NEQAS) provides samples for identification and quantitation of variant haemoglobins as well as for quantitation of Hb A$_2$ and F. Since these procedures are used to make or exclude the diagnosis of an inherited condition, it is essential to ensure adequate quality control of all methods. In-house protocols should be written with step-by-step instructions and any important points emphasized. In particular, in quantitative diagnostic analyses of Hb A$_2$ and Hb F, duplicates should agree to within 0.2% (SD<0.05%). All laboratories should check their normal range for the methods they use in order to ensure accuracy as well as precision. Particular attention should be given to the concentration of lysate for Hbs A$_2$ and F, and to the temperature of the reagents used for the estimation of Hb F (p. 279).

CELLULOSE ACETATE ELECTROPHORESIS AT ALKALINE pH[21,22]

For routine work, electrophoresis at pH 8.4–8.6 using a cellulose acetate membrane as a substrate is simple, rapid and sensitive. It is generally satisfactory in detecting most common haemoglobin variants.

Principle. At alkaline pH haemoglobin is a negatively charged protein and in an electric field will migrate towards the anode (+). Structural variants with surface charge differences will

separate from Hb A, those without a change in charge will not.

Equipment

Electrophoresis tank and power pack. Any horizontal electrophoresis tank which will allow a bridge gap of 7 cm. (Tanks with an adjustable bridge gap allow other electrophoretic procedures to be carried out.) A direct current power supply capable of delivering 350 V at 80 mA is suitable for both cellulose acetate and citrate agar electrophoresis.

Wicks of filter or chromatography paper.

Blotting paper.

Applicators. These are available from most manufacturers of electrophoresis equipment, but fine microcapillaries drawn from micro-haematocrit tubes are also satisfactory.

Cellulose acetate membranes. These are also available from most manufacturers of electrophoresis equipment. Plastic backed membranes (7.6 × 6.0 cm) are recommended.[13,29,33]

Staining equipment and drying oven.

pH meter. The pH meter must have an electrode suitable for use with Tris, as Tris interferes with the function of some electrodes. If an electrode can be calibrated with two standard buffers after soaking in Tris buffer for at least 15 min, it can be considered suitable.[6]

Reagents

Electrophoresis buffer. Tris/EDTA/borate (TEB) pH 8.5. Tris-(hydroxymethyl)aminomethane (Tris) 10.2 g, EDTA 0.6 g, boric acid 3.2 g, water to 1 litre. The buffer should be stored at 4°C and can be used repeatedly without deterioration.

Protein stain. Ponceau S 5 g, trichloracetic acid 7.5 g, water to 1 litre.

Destaining solution. 5% (v/v) acetic acid 50 ml, water to 1 litre.

Absolute methanol.

Clearing solution. Glacial acetic acid 125 ml, methanol 375 ml, polyethylene glycol 20 ml.

Method

The procedure described below may require modification to comply with instructions given by manufacturers of specific products.

1. Prepare a lysate according to one of the methods given on p. 257. Further dilute the sample 1:4 or 1:5 (to about 20 g/l) in water.

2. *With the power supply disconnected*, fill the compartments of the electrophoresis tank with TEB buffer. Soak and position the wicks.

3. In a separate dish soak the cellulose acetate membrane in TEB buffer for at least 5 min. It is important to immerse the membrane slowly, to avoid trapping air bubbles and ensuring even saturation of the membrane.

4. Blot the membrane between two pieces of absorbent paper, but do not let it dry out before sample application.

5. Place a small volume (10 µl) of each diluted sample into a sample well.

6. Dip the applicator into the sample wells.

7. Apply the samples to the cellulose acetate approximately 3 cm from one end of the membrane. Allow the applicator tips to remain in contact with the membrane for 3 s.

8. Place the membrane upside down across the bridge of the tank so that the cellulose acetate surface is in contact with the buffer, with the line of application at the cathode end.

9. Connect the power supply and run at 250–350 V for 20 min or until a visible separation is obtained. Do not be tempted to run for too long; it will not improve separation, and fast-moving fractions such as Hb H and Hb Bart's may be lost.

10. Disconnect the power supply, remove the membrane and stain in Ponceau S for 3–5 min.

11. Remove the membrane, drain, and elute the excess stain with three changes of destaining solution for 2 min each.

12. Dehydrate in absolute methanol for 2–3 min.

13. Immerse in clearing solution for 6–8 min.

14. Dry at 65°C for 4–6 min.

15. Label the membranes and store in a protective plastic envelope.

Interpretation and comments

The small volume of haemolysate applied by many commercially available applicators may lead to difficulty in detecting minor bands (such as those of Hb Constant Spring, Hb A_2 and A_2 variants, Hb Bart's and Hb H) unless the concentration of the lysate is carefully controlled.

It may be difficult to detect small amounts of Hb A in the presence of large amounts of Hb F; this is a particular problem when analysing neonatal samples. In this situation citrate agar electrophoresis should be used on all samples where Hb A is not detected. Alternatively, iso-electric focusing (IEF) may be used as the first-line method (see page 262).

Figure 14.3 shows the relative electrophoretic mobilities of some common Hb variants at pH 8.5 on cellulose acetate. Satisfactory separation of Hbs C, S, F, A, and J is obtained (Fig. 14.4), but it is not possible to differentiate between Hbs S, D and G nor between Hbs C, C^Harlem, E and O. Such differentiation can be obtained by using citrate agar electrophoresis or IEF.

When an abnormal Hb is found it is useful to measure the percentage of variant Hb; this can be done by the procedure for Hb A_2 estimation given on p. 274. The elution volume should be adjusted according to the amount of the variant under investigation. Alternatively, HPLC can be used if available. Quantitation of Hb S is particularly important where a transfusion regime aimed at suppressing the production of Hb S is being undertaken. In such patients maintaining the level of Hb S below 20% has been a factor in reducing morbidity and mortality. The quantitation of Hb S is also important in diagnosing the different interactions of Hb S with α- and β-thalassaemias as outlined in Table 14.5.

Of the fast-moving variants, Hb Bart's and Hb H can be distinguished by their movement on cellulose acetate using a phosphate buffer at pH 6.5 (p. 262). All samples showing a single band in the S or C position should be retested either by a citrate agar/acid gel method, or by IEF to exclude the possibility of a compound heterozygote such as Hb SD, SG, CE or CO^Arab.

Globin chain separation at both acid and alkaline pH is useful in identifying an abnormal globin chain (p. 264).

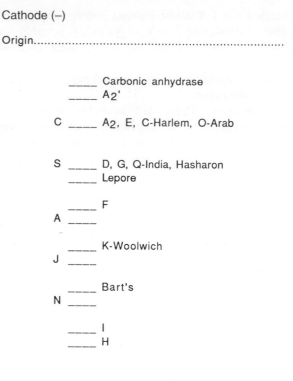

Fig. 14.3 Schematic representation of relative mobilities of some abnormal haemoglobins. Cellulose acetate pH 8.5.

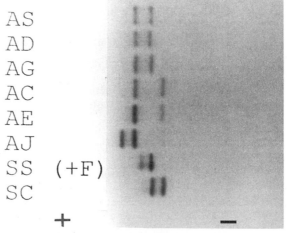

Fig. 14.4 Relative mobilities of some abnormal haemoglobins. Cellulose acetate pH 8.5.

Table 14.5   Results of laboratory investigations in interactions of Hb S and α- or β-thalassaemia in adults

	MCV	% S	% A	% A_2	% F
AS	N	35–48	52–65	<3.5	<1
SS	N	88–93	0	<3.5	5–10
S-β^0-Thalassaemia	L	88–93	0	>3.5	5–10
S-β^+-Thalassaemia	L	50–93	3–30	>3.5	1–10
S-HPFH	N	65–80	0	<3.5	20–35
AS-α^+-Thalassaemia	N/L	28–35	62–70	<3.5	<1
AS α^0 Thalassaemia	L	20–30	68–78	<3.5	<1
SS-α-Thalassaemia	N/L	88–93	0	<3.5	1–10

CITRATE AGAR ELECTROPHORESIS AT pH 6.0[28]

Reagents

Stock citrate buffer. Sodium citrate 147 g, water to 600 ml. Adjust the pH to 6.0 with 50% citric acid; then make up the volume to 1 litre with water. For the working buffer dilute the stock buffer 1:10 with water. Store at 4°C.

Agar gel plates. Agar powder 1 g added to 100 ml of working buffer. Heat the mixture in a boiling water-bath; when the solution is clear, dip a piece of firm plastic film (7.5 by 10 cm) in the hot agar and dry on a hotplate for 5 min. Place the pre-coated plate on a level surface and pipette on 9 ml of hot agar, ensuring an even spread and no air bubbles. Allow the agar to set before attempting to move the plate.

Staining solution. Bromophenol blue 100 mg, acetic acid 10 ml, water to 1 litre; or Ponceau S 5 g, trichloracetic acid 7.5 g, water to 1 litre.

Method

1. Dilute the lysates to be tested to 10–30 g of Hb/l, matching their Hb content closely to that of the controls. For the detection of minor Hb components, for instance in neonatal samples, a haemoglobin content of 100 g/l is recommended.

2. *With the power supply disconnected*, fill the compartments of the electrophoresis tank with cold working buffer. Soak and position the wicks.

3. Place a small volume (10 μl) of each diluted sample into a sample well.

4. Dip the applicator into the sample wells.

5. Apply the samples to the centre of the agar plate without cutting the surface of the gel. Allow the applicator tips to remain in contact with the plate for 15 s.

6. Place the plate upside down across the bridge of the tank so that the agar surface is in contact with the buffer, with the line of application in the centre.

7. Connect the power supply and run at a constant current of 50 mA for 60 min.

9. Disconnect the power supply, remove the plate and immerse in the staining solution for 3–5 min.

10. Remove the plate, drain and rinse in running water.

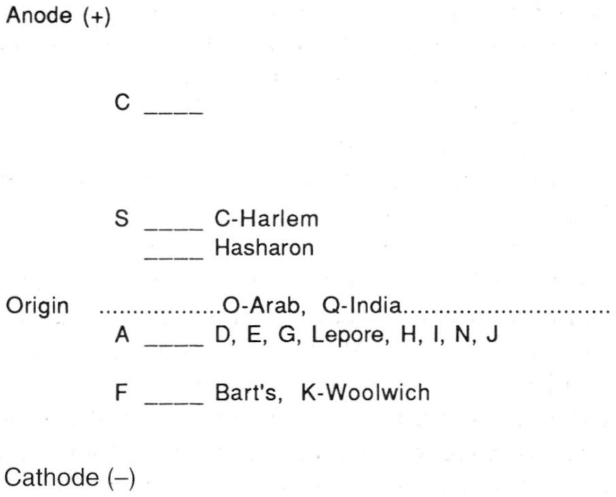

Anode (+)

C ____

S ____   C-Harlem
____   Hasharon

Origin   ....O-Arab, Q-India............
A ____   D, E, G, Lepore, H, I, N, J

F ____   Bart's, K-Woolwich

Cathode (−)

Fig. 14.5   Schematic representation of relative mobilities of some abnormal haemoglobins. Citrate agar pH 6.0.

11. Dehydrate in absolute methanol for 2–3 min.

12. Immerse in the clearing solution for 6–8 min.

13. Dry at 80°C for 2 h.

14. Label the membranes and store in a protective plastic envelope.

Interpretation and comments

Successful citrate agar electrophoresis presents more technical problems than cellulose acetate and controls are essential. The lysates must not have a haemoglobin content of more than 30 g/l (unless specific small bands are expected); lysates stronger than this give poor separation. Buffer at 4°C should be used and the tank kept cool during the run. Figure 14.5 shows the relative electrophoretic mobilities of some common Hb variants at pH 6.0 on citrate agar.

Agar gel electrophoresis

Commercial kits are now available using acid gel with a maleic acid buffer system. These are very easy to use and give good separation, but must be interpreted with caution as the migration of some variants is not identical to that seen in the traditional citrate agar pattern. Such kits can be obtained from various manufacturers[†]; charts are included showing the differing migrations.

CELLULOSE ACETATE ELECTROPHORESIS AT pH 6.5

Equipment

As described on p. 258.

Reagents

Electrophoresis buffer. KH_2PO_4 3.11 g, $Na_2HPO_4.2H_2O$ 1.87 g, water to 1 litre.

Protein stain. Ponceau S 5 g, trichloracetic acid 7.5 g, water to 1 litre.

Destaining solution. 5% (v/v) acetic acid 50 ml, water to 1 litre.

Absolute methanol.

Clearing solution. Glacial acetic acid 125 ml, methanol 375 ml, polyethylene glycol 20 ml.

Method

The procedure described is the same as that described on p. 259.

Interpretation and comments

Controls should include a cord blood sample containing Hb Bart's, a sample containing Hb H and one with another fast-moving variant such as Hb J. As Hbs H and Bart's are unstable and denature readily, the lysate should be made with fresh blood and stored lysates should not be used. Hb H migrates further towards the anode than Hb Bart's using this method. The amount of the variants can be measured by eluting the bands and using the method for Hb A_2 described on p. 274.

ISO-ELECTRIC FOCUSING (IEF)

Principle.[2,32]   Using IEF many more variants can be separated than by cellulose acetate. Pre-prepared plates of either polyacrylamide[*] or agarose gel[**] can be bought. The gels contain carrier ampholytes of low molecular weight and varying iso-electric points (pI). These molecules

[†]Beckman (UK), Progress Rd, Sands Industrial Estate, Bucks, HP12 4JL, UK; or Helena Laboratories, 1530 Lindbergh Drive, Beaumont, TX 77714, USA.
[*]LKB, Biotechnology, S-751 82, Uppsala, Sweden.
[**]Isolab Inc., Akron, OH, USA.

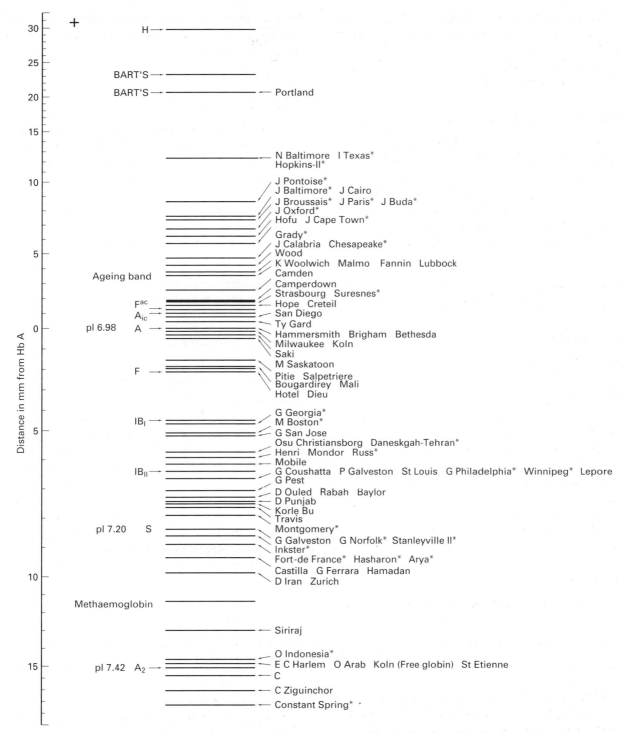

Fig. 14.6 Schematic representation of relative mobilities of some abnormal haemoglobins. Isoelectric focusing. Note the presence of two bands for Hb Bart's. *Indicates α-chain mutations. (Reproduced with permission from Basset et al.[2])

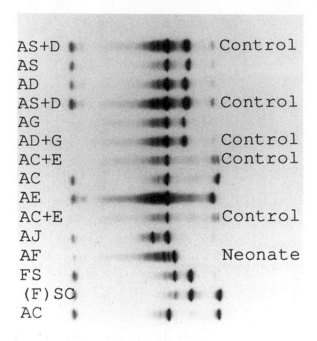

Fig. 14.7   Relative mobilities of some abnormal haemoglobins. Isoelectric focusing.

migrate to their respective pI when a current is applied, resulting in a stable pH gradient being formed; for Hb work a pH gradient of 6–8 is usually employed. On applying a lysate the Hb molecules are carried through the gel until they reach the area where their individual pI equal the corresponding pH on the gel. At this point the charge on the variant is zero, and migration ceases. The electric field counteracts diffusion, and the Hb variant forms a discrete thin band. In addition to lysates, unwashed blood samples can be used as can capillary samples collected on to filter paper and dried. The latter method is very suitable for samples which have to be transported long distances, and where only a few drops of blood can be obtained.

Method

For the exact method the manufacturer's instructions should be followed.

Interpretation and comments

IEF of old samples may produce irregular bands due to decomposition and/or oxidation of the haemoglobin molecule. Hb variants with pIs differing by 0.01 or greater can be separated. Figure 14.6 shows the relative iso-electric points of some common Hb variants and Fig. 14.7 shows the separation obtained.

GLOBIN CHAIN ELECTROPHORESIS[31,34]

Principle.   Electrophoresis of globin chains is useful in the investigation of unusual variants, as a means of determining whether the substitution is located in the α or β chain. Additionally, it can be used in the systematic identification of the suspected abnormal haemoglobin.

Whole blood lysates or prepared globin may be used; the haem groups and globin chains are dissociated with DL-dithiothreitol (DTT) and urea. This dissociated globin is then electrophoresed on cellulose acetate membranes using both alkaline and acid buffer systems.

ALKALINE GLOBIN CHAIN ELECTROPHORESIS

Reagents

Electrophoresis buffer. TRIS/EDTA/borate (TEB) buffer pH 8.5, Ponceau S stain, and acetic acid solution, as described on p. 259.
Urea.
DL-*dithiothreitol (DTT).*
Working buffer. Urea 108 g in 210 ml of TEB buffer. This should be freshly prepared for each run.

Method

1. Mix 0.5 ml of lysate, 0.5 ml of working buffer and 0.5 ml of DTT in a small tube. Allow to stand at room temperature for 30 min.

2. Add 2 ml of DTT to the remainder of the working buffer and mix thoroughly.

3. *With the power supply disconnected*, fill the compartments of the electrophoresis tank with working buffer. Soak and position the wicks.

4. In a separate dish soak the cellulose acetate membrane in working buffer for at least 5 min. It is important to immerse the membrane slowly, to avoid trapping air bubbles and ensuring even saturation of the membrane.

5. Blot the membrane between two pieces of absorbent paper, but do not let it dry out before sample application.

6. Place a small volume (10 µl) of each diluted sample into a sample well.

7. Dip the applicator into the sample wells.

8. Apply the samples to the cellulose acetate at the centre of the membrane. Allow the applicator tips to remain in contact with the membrane for 3 s.

9. Place the membrane upside down across the bridge of the tank so that the cellulose acetate surface is in contact with the buffer; mark the cathode end of the membrane.

10. Connect the power supply and run at 250 V, 1 mA per plate for 60 min.

11. Disconnect the power supply, remove the membrane and stain in Ponceau S for 3–5 min.

12. Remove the membrane, drain, and elute the excess stain with three changes of destaining solution for 2 min each until the background is clear.

13. Air dry.

14. Label the membranes and store in a protective plastic envelope.

ACID GLOBIN CHAIN ELECTROPHORESIS

Working buffer is prepared as described above, but the pH is adjusted to 6.0–6.2 with 300 g/l citric acid. The electrophoresis is carried out in the same way, substituting acid for alkaline working buffer, and observing the following differences: the application should be 1 cm from the anode and the power should be 150 V, 2 mA per plate for 90 min.

Pre-preparation of globin

If desired, globin may be pre-prepared but the whole procedure must be carried out in a well ventilated environment.

1. Add 500 µl of haemolysate (40 g/l) to 10 ml of acid/acetone mixture (98 volumes of acetone, 2 volumes of concentrated HCl) kept at –20°C. The globin will immediately form a white precipitate leaving the haem in solution.

2. Centrifuge at 100g for 5 min at –20°C.

3. Remove the supernatant and wash twice in acetone at –20°C, then once in ether at room temperature.

4. Remove the ether and allow the precipitate to dry at room temperature.

5. For use, dissolve 10 mg of globin in 0.5 ml of a solution prepared by dissolving 12.0 g of urea in water, adding 0.5 ml of DTT and diluting with water to 15 ml.

Interpretation and comments

The direction of migration of the globin chains is from anode to cathode, whilst in electrophoresis at alkaline pH on cellulose acetate whole haemoglobins migrate from the cathode to the anode. If the mobility of the Hb variant is known on alkaline cellulose acetate, then abnormal α and β chains can be differentiated. If the whole variant moves faster than Hb A on alkaline cellulose acetate, the abnormal chain will migrate on globin separation more slowly than its normal counterpart. The α chains move faster than the β chains and migrate nearer to the cathode. Thus, a haemoglobin which migrates rapidly on alkaline cellulose acetate due to an abnormal α chain will produce a *slow moving band* of α chains on globin separation, which will migrate between the normal α and β chains. Under the same circumstances, a *fast moving* haemoglobin due to an abnormal β chain will produce a *slow moving* band of β chains migrating behind the normal β chains.

The relative mobilities of some abnormal α and β chains are shown in Fig. 14.8.

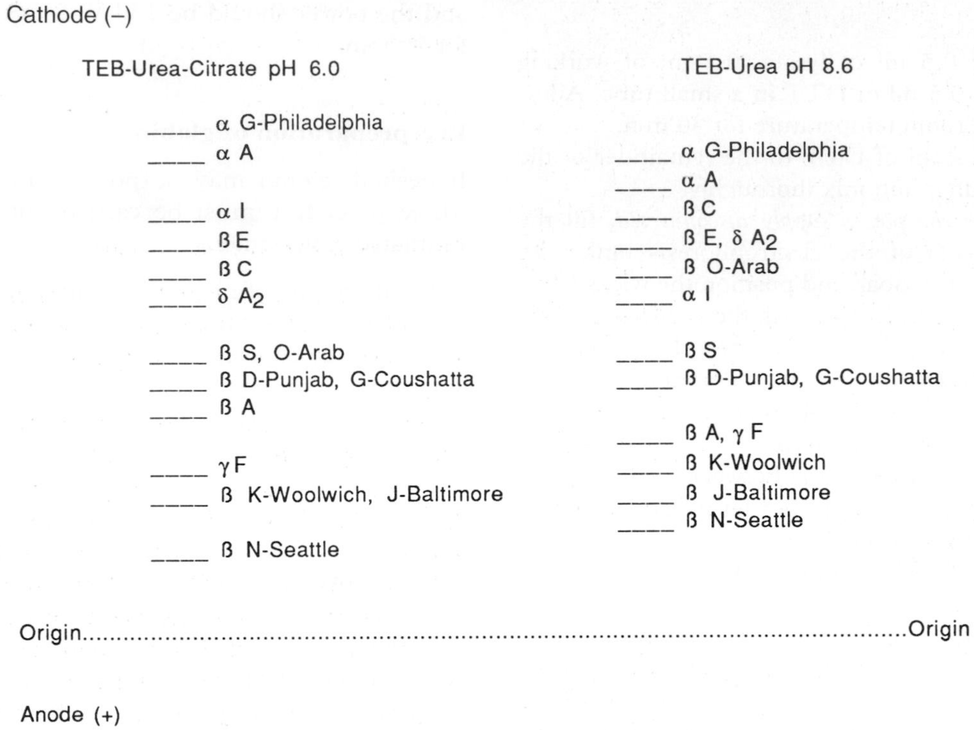

Cathode (−)

TEB-Urea-Citrate pH 6.0   TEB-Urea pH 8.6

_____ α G-Philadelphia   _____ α G-Philadelphia
_____ α A   _____ α A
                                                           _____ β C
_____ α I   _____ β E, δ A_2
_____ β E   _____ β O-Arab
_____ β C   _____ α I
_____ δ A_2

_____ β S, O-Arab   _____ β S
_____ β D-Punjab, G-Coushatta   _____ β D-Punjab, G-Coushatta
_____ β A

                                                           _____ β A, γ F
_____ γ F   _____ β K-Woolwich
_____ β K-Woolwich, J-Baltimore   _____ β J-Baltimore
                                                           _____ β N-Seattle
_____ β N-Seattle

Origin..Origin

Anode (+)

Fig. 14.8   Schematic representation of relative mobilities of some globin chains.

TESTS FOR Hb S

Tests to detect the presence of Hb S depend on the decreased solubility of the haemoglobin at low oxygen tensions.

SICKLING IN WHOLE BLOOD

The sickling phenomenon may be demonstrated in a thin wet film of blood (sealed with a petroleum jelly/paraffin wax mixture or with nail varnish). If Hb S is present, the red cells lose their smooth round shape and become sickled. This process may take up to 12 h in Hb S trait, whereas changes are apparent in homozygotes and compound heterozygotes after 1 h at 37°C. These changes can be hastened by the addition of a reducing agent such as sodium dithionate as follows.

Reagents

A. Disodium hydrogen phosphate (Na_2HPO_4). 0.114 mol/l (16.2 g/l).

B. Sodium dithionate ($Na_2S_2O_4$). 0.114 mol/l (19.85 g/l). Prepare freshly just before use.

Working solution. Mix 3 volumes of A with 2 volumes of B to obtain a pH of 6.8. Use immediately.

Method

Add 5 drops of the freshly prepared reagent to 1 drop of anticoagulated blood on a slide. Seal between slide and cover-glass with a petroleum jelly/paraffin wax mixture, or with nail varnish. Sickling takes place almost immediately in Hb S disease and should be obvious in Hb S trait within 1 h (Fig. 14.9). A positive control (AS not SS) must be included.

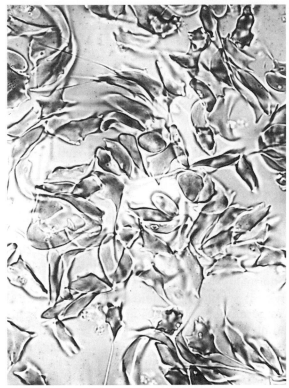

Fig. 14.9 Photomicrograph of sickled red cells. Hb SS. Sealed preparation of blood. Fully sickled filamentous forms predominate.

Hb S SOLUBILITY TEST[20]

Reagents

Phosphate buffer, pH 7.1. Potassium dihydrogen phosphate (KH_2PO_4) 33.78 g, dipotassium hydrogen phosphate ($K_2HPO_4.2H_2O$) 59.33 g, white saponin 2.5 g, water to 250 ml.

Working solution. Dissolve 0.1 g of sodium dithionate in 10 ml of buffer just before use.

Method

1. Place 1 ml of working buffer in a test tube and allow to warm to room temperature.

2. Add 0.05 ml of whole blood, mix well and leave to stand for 5 min.

3. Add 0.5 ml of diethyl ether, mix well and centrifuge at 1200*g* for 5 min.

4. A negative result shows a white band between the ether and the deep red subnatant, whilst a positive shows a red band above a pale pink or colourless subnatant.

5. A positive (Hb AS not SS) and a negative control must be run with every batch of solubility tests.

Interpretation and comments[4]

Positive results are given by the presence of Hb S and not by other haemoglobin variants with the same electrophoretic mobility such as Hb D and Hb G.

Positive results are also given by other haemoglobins with the valine for glutamic acid substitution at position 6 on the β chain such as Hb C^Harlem and Hb S^Travis but the electrophoretic mobility of these rare variants on cellulose acetate differs from that of Hb S. A positive solubility test merely indicates the presence of a sickling haemoglobin and does not differentiate between homozygotes and heterozygotes. In an emergency it may be necessary to decide if an individual suffers from sickle cell disease before the haemoglobin electrophoresis results are available. In these circumstances, if the solubility test is positive, a provisional diagnosis of sickle cell trait can be made if the blood count is normal and the blood film of normal appearance.[4] If the blood film shows any sickle or target cells, irrespective of the Hb concentration, a provisional diagnosis of sickle cell disease should be made. Always remember that the sickle test may be negative in infants with sickle cell disease (see below).

False-positive results can occur in blood with a low Hb concentration and have also been reported in severe leucocytosis, in hyperproteinaemia (such as myeloma), and in the presence of an unstable haemoglobin, especially after splenectomy.

False-negative results may be obtained if old or outdated reagents are used, and if the dithionite/buffer mixture is not freshly made. They may be given by the blood of infants under the age of 6 months, and in other situations when the Hb S is under 20%.

All sickle tests, whether positive or negative, must be checked by electrophoresis at the earliest opportunity.

DETECTION OF Hb S USING A MONOCLONAL ANTIBODY

Monoclonal antibodies have now been developed against several haemoglobin variants and can be used in ELISA assays; such a test for Hb S is marketed in kit form as Hemocard*. This kit contains both anti-Hb S and anti-Hb A. Thus with this test it is possible to differentiate homozygotes from heterozygotes. The antibodies are murine monoclonals that bind specifically to the amino acid at position 6 of the β chain. The antibodies are adsorbed onto suspended metal sol particles, which form a red complex with their specific haemoglobin molecule. This complex binds to the reaction vessel surface and remains whilst unbound antibody is washed away. This bound complex is indicative of a positive test.

The limit of detectability for Hb S is much lower than in the solubility test; the method is therefore suitable for infants. Very low (<7.5 g/dl) and very high (>22.5 g/dl) levels of Hb may give erroneous results; the samples under test should be adjusted accordingly. Samples containing Hb E with Hb S give a false-positive result for Hb A.

All tests, whether positive or negative, should be checked by electrophoresis at the earliest opportunity.

SCREENING OF THE NEWBORN FOR SICKLE CELL DISEASE[4]

Cord blood or a heel-prick sample from all babies at risk from sickle cell disease, i.e. babies of mothers with AS, SS, SC, SD, SE, Sβ+, Sβ0 and thalassaemia trait should be tested. In some areas, where haemoglobinopathies are common, all babies should be tested at birth.

If a cord blood specimen is used, it is important that it is collected by venepuncture of the umbilical vein to avoid contamination with maternal blood. Even a small amount of adult blood will make Hb F + Hb S (probable sickle cell anaemia) look like Hb F + Hb A + Hb S (sickle cell trait). Maternal contamination may also result in the Hb A band appearing stronger than the Hb F band. In such a case the test must be repeated on a heel-prick sample.

The baby's blood sample should be examined electrophoretically (see p. 258) using a technique which gives a good separation of Hb A and Hb F such as cellulose acetate at alkaline pH.[23] If any abnormality is detected, citrate agar gel electrophoresis at acid pH should also be undertaken. If a large number of babies are to be tested or the samples are sent to the laboratory as dried blood spots on filter paper, iso-electric focusing or HPLC may be the technique of choice.

Babies provisionally diagnosed as having SS, SC, SD, Sβ+ or Sβ0 thalassaemia should be retested within 6–8 weeks of birth. If the diagnosis is confirmed, they should be followed in a paediatric clinic, and immediately started on prophylactic penicillin to prevent pneumococcal infections and appropriately managed in the long term.[36] Babies with β-thalassaemia major will also be detected by the routine screening protocol; no Hb A will be detectable either at birth or when the babies are retested. The diagnosis of β-thalassaemia trait cannot be reliably made until 6 months of age.

TESTING FOR HAEMOGLOBIN INSTABILITY

Several methods are available for the demonstration of haemoglobin instability and three are given below.[7] Different haemoglobins may need different methods to demonstrate their unstable characteristics; if only one method can be performed, the n-butanol test is the simplest. The samples used should be as fresh as possible and no more than 1 week old. Choose samples for controls of the same age as the test sample; a normal cord blood sample can be used as a positive control.

HEAT INSTABILITY TEST[16,17]

Principle. When haemoglobin in solution is

---

*Isolab Inc., Akron, OH, USA.

heated the hydrophobic van der Waals bonds are weakened and the stability of the molecule is decreased. Under controlled conditions unstable haemoglobins precipitate while stable haemoglobin remains in solution.[8,16,17]

Reagent

Tris-HCl buffer, pH 7.4, 50 mmol/l. Tris 6.05 g, water to 1 litre. Adjust the pH to 7.4 with concentrated HCl.

Method

1. Add 0.2 ml of lysate, freshly prepared by the CCl_4 method given on p. 257, to a tube containing 1.8 ml of buffer. Include a positive (Hb F) and a negative (Hb A) control of the same age as the test sample.

2. Place the tubes in a water-bath at 50°C for 120 min. Examine the tubes at 60, 90 and 120 min for turbidity and fine flocculation.

Interpretation and comments

The normal control may give minimal cloudiness at 60 min but a major unstable haemoglobin will have undergone marked precipitation at 60 min and gross floccuation at 120 min.

ISOPROPANOL STABILITY TEST[8]

Principle

When haemoglobin is dissolved in a solvent such as isopropanol, which is more non-polar than water, the hydrophobic van der Waal's bonds are weakened and the stability of the molecule is decreased. Under controlled conditions unstable haemoglobins precipitate while stable haemoglobin remains in solution.

Reagents

Tris-HCl buffer, pH 7.4, 100 mmol/l. Tris 12.11 g, water to 1 litre. Adjust the pH to 7.4 with concentrated HCl.

Isopropanol, 17%. 17 volumes of isopropanol are made up to 100 volumes with buffer. The resultant 17% isopropanol solution may be stored in a tightly stoppered glass bottle for 3 months at 4°C.

Method

1. Add 0.2 ml of lysate, freshly prepared by the CCl_4 method given on p. 257, to a tube containing 2.0 ml of 17% isopropanol. Include a positive (Hb F) and a negative (Hb A) control of the same age as the test sample. Stopper each tube and mix by inversion.

2. Place the tubes in a water-bath at 37°C for 30 min. Examine the tubes at 5, 20 and 30 min for turbidity and fine flocculation.

Interpretation and comments

The normal control will remain clear at 20 min. At 30 min minimal cloudiness should be apparent, but significant precipitation will not occur until 40 min. A major unstable haemoglobin will have undergone marked precipitation at 5 min and gross flocculation at 20 min. A slightly unstable haemoglobin such as Hb E will show diffuse precipitation at 20 min.

Positive results may be given by samples containing as little as 10% Hb F or by samples containing increased methaemoglobin as a result of prolonged storage. If the normal sample undergoes premature precipitation, check the temperature of the water-bath, as it is likely to be over 37°C.

False-negative results should be avoided by continuing the incubation until the normal control undergoes precipitation.

n-BUTANOL STABILITY TEST[30]

Principle. When haemoglobin is dissolved in a solvent such as n-butanol, which is more non-polar than water, the hydrophobic van der Waals bonds are weakened and the stability of the molecule is decreased. Under controlled conditions unstable haemoglobins precipitate while stable haemoglobin remains in solution.

Reagents

Stock sodium phosphate buffer, 0.1 mol/l. $NaPO_4$

15.6 g, EDTA 3.7 g, water to 1 litre, adjust the pH to 7.4 with concentrated HCl. The buffer may be stored at room temperature.

n-Butanol.

Working solution. The working buffer is temperature-dependent; prepare as follows:

18–20°C n-butanol 6.5 ml, stock buffer to 1 litre.
21–23°C n-butanol 6.0 ml, stock buffer to 1 litre.
24–26°C n-butanol 5.5 ml, stock buffer to 1 litre.

Method

1. Add 0.2 ml of washed packed cells to a plastic tube containing 2.0 ml of working solution. Include a positive (Hb F) and a negative (Hb A) control of the same age as the test sample. Stopper each tube and mix by inversion; then remove the stopper. The RBCs should lyse giving a clear solution.

2. Place the tubes at room temperature and examine at 30, 60, 90 and 120 min for turbidity and fine flocculation.

Interpretation and comments

The normal control will remain clear at 120 min. A major unstable haemoglobin will have undergone marked precipitation at 90 min and gross flocculation at 120 min. A slightly unstable haemoglobin such as Hb E will show diffuse precipitation at 120 min. The test should be continued until the positive control shows precipitation.

Positive results may be given by samples containing as little as 10% Hb F or by samples containing increased methaemoglobin as a result of prolonged storage.

False-negative results should be avoided by continuing the incubation overnight.

DETECTION OF Hb M

Methaemoglobin (Hi) has iron present in the ferric form. Inherited variants of haemoglobin which undergo oxidation to metHb more readily than does Hb A are referred to as Hb Ms. They are the cause of one variety of a very rare condition, congenital methaemoglobinaemia. Methaemoglobin levels vary, but may be as high as 40% of the total haemoglobin.

Methaemoglobin variants may be detected electrophoretically, but almost all can be distinguished from metHb A (Hi A) by their absorption spectra. Each methaemoglobin has its own distinct absorption spectrum. Hi A has two absorption peaks at 502 nm and 632 nm, whilst the peaks for the varant Hb M methaemoglobins are shifted to shorter wavelengths (Fig. 14.10).

Reagent

Potassium ferricyanide, 0.1 mol/l.

Method

1. Lyse washed red cells from a blood sample

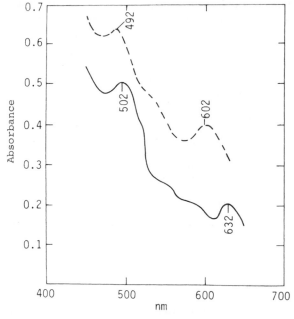

Fig. 14.10 Absorption maxima of methaemoglobins in the range 450–650 nm. —— Normal methaemoglobin; – – – Hb M Saskatoon. (Reproduced with permission from H. Lehmann and R. G. Huntsman, (1974). *Man's Haemoglobins,* 2nd edn, p. 214. North-Holland, Amsterdam.)

of known Hb A and of the test sample with water to give a concentration of about 1 g/l.

2. Convert the haemoglobin to Hi by the addition of 5 μl of potassium ferricyanide solution to each ml of haemolysate.

3. Leave for 10 min at room temperature.

4. Record the spectrum of Hi A on an automatic scanning spectrophotometer.

5. Now record the spectrum of Hi in the test sample.

ALTERED AFFINITY HAEMOGLOBINS

Electrophoretic techniques may or may not be helpful, depending on whether the amino-acid substitution involves a change in charge.

The most important investigation is the measurement of the oxygen dissociation curve (p. 241). The most significant finding is a decreased Hill's constant ('n' value), since this can only come about by a change in the structure of the haemoglobin. The p_{50} may be either increased or decreased. It must be borne in mind that the p_{50} alone may be modified by other factors such as the high concentration of 2,3-DPG in pyruvate kinase deficiency.

SUGGESTED METHODS HELPFUL IN THE DIFFERENTIAL DIAGNOSIS OF COMMON STRUCTURAL VARIANTS

Suggested methods are given in Table 14.6. Figure 14.11 gives a comparison of some common variants using different techniques.

Table 14.6 Methods helpful in the differential diagnosis of common structural variants

Initial finding on cellulose acetate electrophoresis	Most likely variant	Differentiation
Band in position of Hb S	Hb S, D, G-Phil, Lepore	Blood count, quantitation, solubility test, citrate agar/acid gel electrophoresis, IEF
Band in position of Hb C	Hb C, E, O-Arab	Quantitation, citrate agar/acid gel electrophoresis, IEF
Very fast band	Hb I, H	H bodies, cellulose acetate electrophoresis at pH 7.0

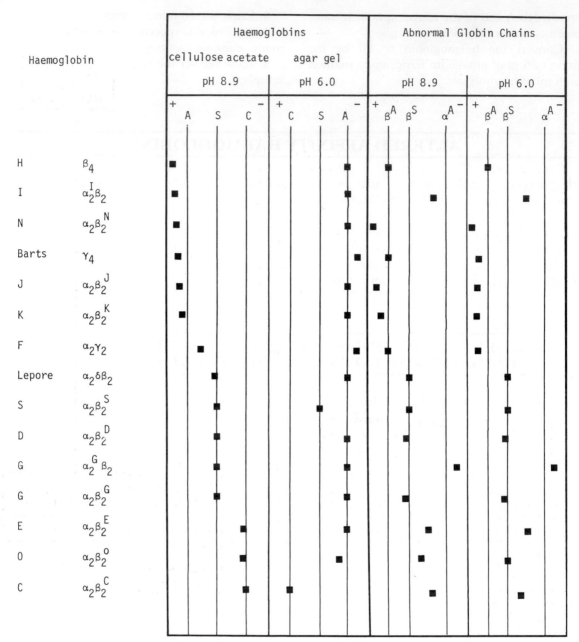

Fig. 14.11 Comparison of the relative mobilities of some abnormal haemoglobins by different methods. The position of Hb A, Hb S and Hb C and their corresponding chains are indicated by the vertical lines. (Adapted from ICSH.[21])

INVESTIGATION OF THALASSAEMIA

A suggested scheme of investigations is shown in Fig. 14.12 and the methods used are listed below.

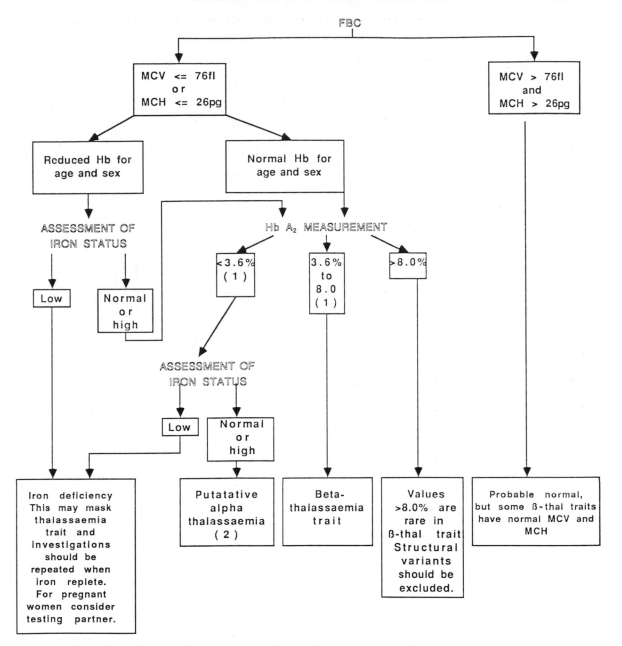

1. Values between 3.3% and 3.8% need careful assessment and should be repeated using a second method.
2. A$_2$ values in alpha thalassaemia are usually below 2.5%.
   Some types of beta thalassaemia trait have normal Hb A$_2$ values.

Fig. 14.12   Suggested scheme of investigation for thalassaemia.

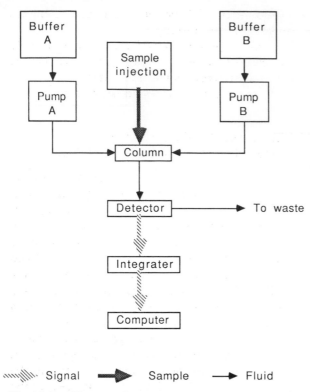

∿∿∿〟 Signal   ➡   Sample   ⟶   Fluid

Fig. 14.13 Diagramatic representation of HPLC showing the flow of sample and buffers.

METHODS FOR INVESTIGATION OF THALASSAEMIA

1. Blood count.
2. Hb A_2 measurement by cellulose acetate elution (p. 274).
3. Hb A_2 measurement by microcolumn chromatography (p. 275).
4. High performance liquid chromatography (HPLC) (p. 278).
5. Estimation of Hb F (p. 279).
6. Assessment of the distribution of Hb F (p. 281).
7. Assessment of iron status (p. 282).
8. Demonstration of red cell inclusion bodies (p. 283).
9. DNA analysis (p. 284).

Blood count

The blood count, including red cell count, haemoglobin, haematocrit and red cell indices,

provides valuable information useful in the diagnosis of both α- and β-thalassaemia.

ESTIMATION OF Hb A_2

A raised Hb A_2 level is characteristic of heterozygous β-thalassaemia, and its accurate measurement is required for the diagnosis or exclusion of β-thalassaemia trait. Estimations may be made by elution after cellulose acetate electrophoresis, or by chromatography, either microcolumn or high performance liquid chromatography (HPLC).

MEASUREMENT OF Hb A_2 BY ELUTION FROM CELLULOSE ACETATE

***Principle**. Hb A_2 is separated from Hb A on cellulose acetate electrophoresis at pH 8.9, eluted into buffer and the percentage calculated by measuring and comparing the absorbance of the Hb A_2 eluate and an eluate prepared from the remaining haemoglobin.

Equipment

Electrophoresis tank and power pack. See p. 258.
Wicks of double filter paper.
10 μl microcapillary pipette.
Cellulose acetate membranes. 10 by 5 cm is a suitable size.
pH meter. See p. 259.

Reagents

1. *Electrophoresis buffer.* Tris/EDTA/Borate (TEB) pH 8.9. Tris 14.4 g, EDTA 1.5 g, boric acid 0.9 g, water to 1 litre. The buffer should be stored at 4°C and the pH checked before use.

2. *Working buffer.* KCN 200 mg, stock buffer 100 ml; water to 2 litres. Adjust to pH 8.5 with concentrated HCl.

Method[29,43]

The procedure described below may require modification to comply with instructions given by manufacturers of specific products.

1. Prepare haemolysate according to the CCl_4 method given on p. 257.

2. *With the power supply disconnected*, fill the compartments of the electrophoresis tank with TEB buffer. Soak and position the wicks.

3. In a separate disk soak the cellulose acetate membrane in TEB buffer for at least 5 min. It is important to immerse the membrane slowly, to avoid trapping air bubbles and ensuring even saturation of the membrane.

4. Blot the membrane between two pieces of absorbent paper, but do not let it dry out before sample application.

5. Stretch the strips across the bridges of the tank so that they are connected to the buffer chambers by a double layered wick of filter paper.

6. Apply 10 μl of haemolysate (100 g/l) to the cathode end of the membrane by micropipette. The application should stretch to within 0.5 cm of the edge of the strip.

7. Connect the power supply and run at 3 mA for 30–40 min or until a good separation is obtained.

8. Disconnect the power supply, remove the membrane and cut the Hb A_2 and Hb A zones into small pieces and elute into 1.5 ml and 15 ml of buffer respectively.

9. Allow to elute with occasional mixing for 20–30 min.

10. Remove the eluted pieces and centrifuge the eluates at 1200*g* for 5 min to sediment the debris.

11. Measure the absorbance of each eluate at 413 nm using a spectrophotometer, and using TEB buffer as the blank.

12. Calculate as follows:

$$\% \text{ Hb } A_2 = \frac{A^{413} \text{ Hb } A_2}{(10 \times A^{413} \text{ Hb A}) + A^{413} \text{ Hb } A_2} \times 100$$

Interpretation and comments

If a haemoglobin variant is present, the eluate used to calculate the major Hb fraction must include this variant. Particular care must be taken when cutting strips on which Hb S is present, as the separation between Hb S and Hb A_2 is diminished. This method is unsuitable in the presence of Hbs C, Hb C^{Harlem}, Hb E and Hb

O^{Arab} as they all have electrophoretic mobilities similar to that of Hb A_2.

Methaemoglobin formation in a stored sample may cause less clear separation between bands, thus making estimations less reliable.

For interpretation of results see p. 279.

MEASUREMENT OF Hb A_2 BY MICROCOLUMN CHROMATOGRAPHY

Principle. Microcolumn chromatography depends on the interchange of charged groups on the ion exchange resin with charged groups on the haemoglobin molecule. When a mixture of haemoglobins is adsorbed onto the resin a particular haemoglobin component may be eluted from the column using a buffer (developer) with a specific pH and/or ionic strength, while a second component (either a single haemoglobin or a mixture of haemoglobins) may be eluted by changing the pH or ionic strength of the developer. The separation of haemoglobin components in such a system will depend on such factors as the pH or ionic strength of the developers used for the equilibration of the column; and for the elution, the type of resin, the volume of the sample added, the size of the column, the gradient and the flow rates.

The methods described below use the anion exchange resin diethylaminoethyl (DEAE) cellulose (Whatman DE-52 microgranular pre-swollen), with Tris-HCl developers[12] or glycine-KCN developers.[19]

MEASUREMENT OF Hb A_2 BY MICROCOLUMN CHROMATOGRAPHY WITH TRIS-HCl DEVELOPERS[12]

Buffers

Stock buffer 1.0 mol/l Tris. Tris 121.1 g; water to 1 litre.

Working buffer 1. KCN 200 mg; stock buffer 100 ml; water to 2 litres; adjust to pH 8.5 with concentrated HCl.

Working buffer 2. KCN 200 mg; stock buffer 100 ml; water to 2 litres; adjust to pH 8.3 with concentrated HCl.

Working buffer 3. KCN 200 mg; stock buffer

100 ml; water to 2 litres; adjust to pH 7.0 with concentrated HCl.

Important: If the developers are stored at 4°C they must be allowed to come to room temperature before use.

Method

1. Prepare the slurry by adding 10 g of DE-52 to 200 ml of buffer 1. Mix gently, then adjust the pH of the thoroughly suspended resin to 8.5 with concentrated HCl. Allow the resin to settle, remove the supernatant and resuspend the resin in a further 200 ml of Buffer 1. Check that the pH is steady at 8.5; this normally takes about 10 min. Allow the resin to settle and remove enough buffer so that the settled resin constitutes about half the total volume.

2. Set up disposable pipettes with short stems vertically in a stand. Place either a 3 mm glass bead or a small piece of cotton wool in the tapered part of the pipette to act as a support for the slurry. If cotton wool is used it should be first moistened with buffer 1 and only loosely packed into the pipette tip.

3. Fill the pipette with thoroughly suspended resin slurry and allow the column to pack under gravity to a height of about 6 cm.

4. Dilute 1 drop of lysate (100 g/l) with 5 drops of Buffer 1.

5. When all the excess buffer has drained from the column, but before it starts to dry out, gently apply the diluted lysate to the top of the column and allow it to be adsorbed onto the resin. Do not allow the surface of the column to dry out.

6. Apply Buffer 2 gently to the column with a piece of polythene tubing attached to the top of the pipette acting as a reservoir. About 9 ml of Buffer 2 should be used to elute the Hb A$_2$ band, the greater part of which should elute between 4 and 6 ml. Collect the eluate in a 10 ml flask and make the volume up to 10 ml with the remaining Buffer 2.

7. Elute the remaining Hb A, using 10 ml of Buffer 3; collect the eluate and make the volume up to 25 ml with the remaining Buffer 3. If, at any stage, the flow through the column stops, it should be discarded.

8. Read the absorbance of the eluted haemoglobins at 413 nm in a spectrophotometer, using water as a blank. Calculate the Hb A$_2$ as follows:

$$\% \text{ Hb A}_2 = \frac{\text{A}^{413} \text{ Hb A}_2}{\text{A}^{413} \text{ Hb A}_2 + (2.5 \times \text{A}^{413} \text{ Hb A})} \times 100$$

Interpretation and comments

The amount of haemoglobin applied to the column must be carefully controlled. Overloading the column with more than 7–8 mg of haemoglobin will cause contamination of the Hb A$_2$ fraction with Hb A. Less than 2 mg of haemoglobin will result in an eluate with an absorbance too low for accurate measurement.

The flow-rate of the column may be adjusted by altering the height of the reservoir above the column. A flow-rate of 10–20 ml/h is satisfactory. Raising the reservoir increases the flow-rate and broadens the A$_2$ band on the column but does not affect its elution or quantity.

Modified procedure for samples containing slow-moving variants

The above procedure may be modified to make it suitable for samples containing slow-moving variants such as Hb S; a longer column is required.[11] The column is packed with the prepared slurry to the height of 16 cm, and the Hb A$_2$ is eluted using pH 8.3 buffer as above. The slow moving Hb is eluted with Tris-HCl buffer at pH 8.2, and if the proportion of the variant is to be estimated the eluate is collected in a 10 ml volumetric flask. The remaining Hb A is eluted with pH 7.0 buffer and collected as above. The Hb S and Hb A$_2$ can be calculated as follows:

$$\% \text{ Hb S} = \frac{2.5 \times \text{A}^{413} \text{ Hb S}}{\text{A}^{413} \text{ HbA}_2 + (2.5 \times \text{A}^{413} \text{ Hb S}) + (2.5 \times \text{A}^{413} \text{ Hb A})} \times 100$$

$$\% \text{ Hb A}_2 = \frac{2.5 \times \text{A}^{413} \text{ Hb A}_2}{\text{A}^{413} \text{ HbA}_2 + (2.5 \times \text{A}^{413} \text{ Hb S}) + (2.5 \times \text{A}^{413} \text{ Hb A})} \times 100$$

Interpretation and comments

A normal and a high Hb A$_2$ control should be tested with every batch of samples. Each laboratory must establish its own normal range and this should not differ significantly from that determined by elution from cellulose acetate. Efremov[11] quotes a normal range of 1.5–3.5%, mean 2.5 ± 0.15%.

For interpretation of results see p. 279.

MEASUREMENT OF Hb A$_2$ BY MICROCOLUMN CHROMATOGRAPHY WITH GLYCINE-POTASSIUM CYANIDE DEVELOPERS[19]

The method described below is suitable for samples containing slow-moving variants such as Hb S. The elution of Hb A$_2$ is dependent on the pH of the ion exchanger and is relatively less sensitive to the pH of the developer.

Reagents

Developer A. Glycine 15.0 g, KCN 0.1 g, water to 1 litre.
Developer B. NaCl 9.0 g, water to 1 litre.

Method

1. Prepare the slurry by adding 50 g of DE-52 to 250 ml of buffer 1. Mix gently, then allow to settle and remove the supernatant. Repeat this process at least twice, then adjust the pH of the thoroughly suspended resin to 7.6 with 0.1 mol/l HCl. This adjustment should be made very slowly since the molarity of the developer is an important factor in the elution of haemoglobin fractions. If the slurry is made too acidic it should be discarded since any attempt to readjust it would increase the total ionic concentration and therefore alter the elution pattern. The slurry may be stored for up to 3–4 weeks but the pH should be checked and if necessary readjusted before use.

2. Set up disposable pipettes with short stems vertically in a stand. Place either a 3 mm glass bead or a small piece of cotton wool in the tapered part of the pipette to act as a support for the slurry. If cotton wool is used it should be first moistened with developer A and only loosely packed into the pipette tip. Prepared columns may be stored after topping up with Developer A and closing both ends. Remove excess buffer before use.

3. Fill the pipette with thoroughly suspended resin slurry and allow the column to pack under gravity to a height of about 6 cm.

4. Check each batch of columns with a Hb AS lysate. The Hb A$_2$ should elute in the first 3–4 ml and the Hb S in the next 15–20 ml of the developer.

5. Dilute 1 drop of lysate (100 g/l) with 6 drops of water.

6. When all the excess buffer has drained from the column, but before it starts to dry out, gently apply the diluted lysate to the top of the column, and allow it to be adsorbed onto the resin. Do not allow the surface of the column to dry out.

7. Apply Developer A gently to the column with a piece of polythene tubing attached to the top of the pipette acting as a reservoir. About 3–4 ml of developer should be used to elute the Hb A$_2$ band. Collect the eluate in a 5 ml flask and make the volume up to 5 ml with Developer A.

8. Elute the remaining Hb A, or Hb S + Hb A, using 15–20 ml of Developer B; collect the eluate and make the volume up to 25 ml with Developer B. If, at any stage, the flow through the column stops, it should be discarded.

9. Read the absorbance of the eluted haemoglobins at 413 nm in a spectrophotometer, using water as a blank. Calculate the Hb A$_2$ as follows:

$$\% \text{ Hb A}_2 = \frac{A^{413} \text{ Hb A}_2}{A^{413} \text{ Hb A}_2 + (5 \times A^{413} \text{ Hb A})} \times 100.$$

Interpretation and comments

In general, similar comments apply to both the Tris and the glycine methods. Hb A$_2$ percentages tend to be slightly lower with the former, but with either procedure there should be no overlap between normal and β-thalassaemia trait subjects.[12] An advantage of the glycine KCN method is a reduced sensitivity to minor changes in the pH of the developer; an added advantage is that it may be used for samples containing Hb S.

To estimate the percentage of Hb S and the remaining haemoglobin as well as that of Hb A$_2$, Hb A$_2$ is eluted in the first 3–4 ml with developer A; Hb S is eluted in the next 15–20 ml of the

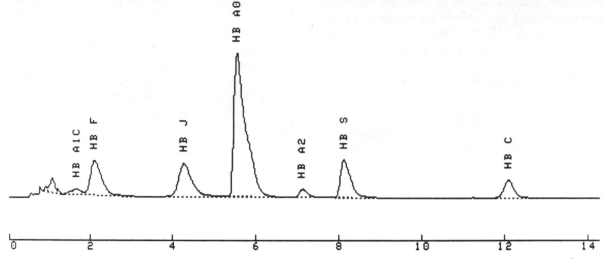

Fig. 14.14   A mixture of haemoglobins separated by HPLC.

same developer A, and the remaining haemoglobin with Developer B. The eluate containing Hb A_2 is diluted to 5 ml and the eluates containing Hb S and the remaining haemoglobin diluted to 25 ml. To ensure elution of all the Hb A_2 in the first 3–4 ml, and all the Hb S in the next 15–20 ml, the pH of the ion exchanger may need adjustment following a test chromatogram.[19]

HIGH PERFORMANCE LIQUID CHROMOTOGRAPHY (HPLC)[35]

Principle. HPLC for haemoglobin work uses the same principle as microcolumn chromatography which is given on p. 275. A typical column filler is 5 μm spherical silica gel. The surface of the support is modified by carboxyl groups to have a weakly cationic charge, which allows the separation of haemoglobin molecules with different charges by ion exchange. Elution of the charged molecules is achieved by a continually changing salt gradient; fractions are detected as they pass through an ultraviolet/visible light detector, and recorded on an integrating computer system. Analysis of the area under these absorption peaks gives the percentage of the fraction detected.

Many systems are available from various manufacturers*; the best systems allow variable alteration of the salt gradient in order to provide optimum conditions for the elution of different haemoglobin fractions, and should support some preparatory analysis work such as reverse phase HPLC if desired. Fig. 14.13 (p. 274) shows a schematic representation of an HPLC system and Fig. 14.14 shows a chromatogram of a mixture of different haemoglobins.

Results from such systems can be obtained in a few minutes and are accurate and reproducible, but as with every method of haemoglobin analysis, each laboratory must establish its own normal range and controls should be run with every batch. If the system is being used for the identification of Hb variants, elution times can be compared with those of known controls; actual times however are affected by the age of the column. A better comparision can be obtained using the relative elution time (RET), which is calculated by dividing the elution time of the variant with that of the main Hb A fraction.

To prolong the life of the column it is important to follow the manufacturers' instructions with regard to the strength of haemoglobin

---

*Bio-rad Laboratories; Shimadzu; LKB Biotechnology.

in the sample to be injected, and to centrifuge the sample before injection in order to remove any debris.

Interpretation of Hb A$_2$ values[1,6,11,25,38]

Hb A$_2$	>8.0%	A$_2$ values of >8.0% are rare. Exclude a structural variant; repeat Hb A$_2$ estimation.
Hb A$_2$	3.8–8.0%	β-thalassaemia trait, unstable Hbs.
Hb A$_2$	3.4–3.7%	Iron deficiency in β-thalassaemia trait. Additional δ-chain variant in a β-thalassaemia trait. (Total A$_2$ must be measured.) Interaction of α- and β-thalassaemia.
Hb A$_2$ (contd.)	3.4–3.7%	Presence of Hb S, making precise measurement difficult. Interaction of α-thalassaemia and Hb S. Analytical error. Repeat analysis by another method if possible.
Hb A$_2$	1.6–3.5%	Normal result. δβ-Thalassaemia. Rare cases of β-thalassaemia trait. α$^+$-Thalassaemia.
Hb A$_2$	<1.6%	α^0-Thalassaemia. Hb H disease. Additional δ-chain variant present. (Total Hb A$_2$ must be measured.)

ESTIMATION OF Hb F[14]

Hb F may be estimated by several methods based on its resistance to denaturation at alkaline pH or by HPLC. Of the alkaline denaturation methods that of Betke et al[3] is reliable for small amounts (below 10–15%) of Hb F, whilst for levels over 50%, and in cord blood, the method of Jonxis and Visser[24] is preferable; it is, however, not reliable at levels below 10%.

Recently, immunological methods have been devised to measure Hb F by immunodiffusion[9]— there are commercially available kits*—and by enzyme linked immuno-assay (ELISA).[27]

MODIFIED BETKE METHOD FOR THE ESTIMATION OF Hb F[3]

Principle. To measure the percentage of Hb F in a mixture of haemoglobins, sodium hydroxide is added to a lysate and after a set time denaturation is stopped by adding saturated ammonium sulphate. The ammonium sulphate lowers the pH and precipitates the denatured haemoglobin. After filtration, the quantity of undenatured (unprecipitated) haemoglobin is measured. The proportion of alkali-resistant (fetal) haemoglobin is then calculated as a percentage of the total amount of haemoglobin present.

Reagents

Cyanide solution. Potassium cyanide 0.2 g, potassium ferricyanide 0.2 g, water to 1 litre.

Sodium hydroxide solution 1.2 mol/l. Sodium hydroxide 48.0 g, water to 1 litre.

Saturated ammonium sulphate.

Method

1. All reagents should be allowed to reach room temperature before use. Add 0.6 ml of lysate (100 g/l) to 10 ml of cyanide solution to make a cyanmethaemoglobin (HiCN) solution.

2. Add 0.2 ml of sodium hydroxide solution to 2.8 ml of the HiCN solution. Mix thoroughly and leave for exactly 2 min at room temperature.

3. Add 2.0 ml of saturated ammonium sulphate, mix thoroughly and allow to stand for 10 min.

---

*Helena Laboratories.

4. Filter through a Whatman No. 42 filter paper and collect the filtrate.

5. Using the remaining HiCN solution as the standard, read the absorbance of the filtrate and the standard in a spectrophotometer at either 413 nm or 520 nm.

6. Calculate the percentage of Hb F as follows:

$$\% \, Hb \, F = \frac{A^{413} \, filtrate \times 100}{A^{413} \, standard \times 20}$$

Interpretation and comments

A normal and a raised Hb F control should be tested with every batch of samples. The raised Hb F control should not contain more than 10% Hb F, and can be prepared from a mixture of cord and adult blood. Each laboratory must establish its own normal range and this should not differ significantly from published values; for adults the range is 0.2–1.0%.

Zago et al[46] reported variability in the capacity of different batches of filter paper to absorb haemoglobin from the filtrate which in some instances may be responsible for a distinct drop in the normal range.

For interpretation of results see p. 282.

METHOD OF JONXIS AND VISSER[24]

Principle. The increased resistance of Hb F to denaturation by alkali is detected by recording the change in absorption at 576 nm each min caused by the addition of ammonium hydroxide. At this wavelength the absorption of oxyhaemoglobin differs from that of the alkali haemochromogen which is formed on denaturation.

When the logarithm of the percentage of haemoglobin remaining undenatured is plotted against time a straight line is obtained. By extrapolation to time zero the percentage of Hb F in the original sample can be calculated.

Reagents

Ammonium hydroxide solution. NH$_4$OH 100 g, distilled water to 1 litre.

Sodium hydroxide solution 0.06 mol/l. Sodium hydroxide 2.4 g, water to 1 litre.

Method

1. All reagents should be allowed to reach room temperature before use. Add 0.1 ml of blood or lysate (100 g/l) to 10 ml of water and mix.

2. Add 2 drops of ammonium hydroxide solution and mix.

3. Measure the absorbance in a spectrophotometer at 576 nm (A_B).

4. Add 0.1 ml of the same blood or lysate to 10 ml of sodium hydroxide solution; then add 2 drops of ammonium hydroxide solution and mix thoroughly.

5. Measure the absorbance in a spectrophotometer at 576 nm every min for 15 min (A_T); then incubate the solution at 37°C for 15 min, cool to room temperature and measure the absorbance (A_E). The ratio A_B:A_E should be constant.

6. Calculate the percentage of undenatured haemoglobin at each min as follows:

$$\frac{A_T^{576} - A_E^{576}}{A_B^{576} - A_E^{576}} \times 100.$$

7. Plot the percentage on the logarithmic scale of semi-logarithmic paper against time. This should produce a straight line from which the original amount of Hb F at time zero can be found by extrapolation.

Interpretation and comments

The comments about control samples and normal ranges made for the Betke method also apply here. In addition, the Jonxis and Visser method requires an accurate spectrophotometer, as the maximum absorption peak at 576 nm is very narrow and the difference in extinction between oxyhaemoglobin and alkali haemochromogen is relatively small.

For interpretation of results see p. 282.

RADIAL IMMUNODIFFUSION (RID)[9]

The RID procedure can be used for the quantitation of Hb F. The principle is based on an antibody-antigen reaction; the anti-Hb F is incorporated into the gel support medium resulting in the formation of a visible opaque precipitin ring.

The square of the diameter of this ring is directly proportional to the concentration of Hb F. A standard curve must be prepared from samples containing known levels of Hb F plotted against their haemoglobin concentrations. Helena Laboratories market a kit providing prepared plates, a microdispenser and a measuring device.

The RID method is simple but the formation of the precipitin rings requires at least 18 hours incubation at room temperature. For this reason, rapid diagnostic work is not possible. Care must be taken with sample application as damage to the plate wells results in asymetrical precipitin rings and erroneous measurements.

ASSESSMENT OF THE INTRACELLULAR DISTRIBUTION OF Hb F

Differences in the intracellular distribution of Hb F are used to differentiate between heterozygotes for δβ-thalassaemia and the African type of hereditary persistence of fetal haemoglobin (HPFH). In the former it can be shown that not all red cells contain Hb F (heterocellular distribution), whilst in the latter every cell contains Hb F (pancellular distribution), although there is some variability in content from cell to cell. It has been suggested that a heterocellular distribution may be more apparent than real and merely reflects the threshold for detection of Hb F by the particular technique used. Higher levels of Hb F tend to give a more pancellular distribution than lower levels. For this reason results should be treated with caution and not used to make a diagnosis in isolation.

Two techniques have been widely used for demonstrating intracellular Hb F distribution. The most frequently used is the acid elution test of Kleihauer[26] which was originally developed for the detection of fetal red cells in the maternal circulation following transplacental haemorrhage. This method is described on p. 137. Less frequently used is the more sensitive immunofluorescent technique described below.

IMMUNOFLUORESCENT METHOD[46]

Principle. Anti-Hb F antibody binds specifically and quantitatively to Hb F in fixed red cells. These cells can be identified after treatment with a second fluorescent labelled antibody directed against the anti-Hb F.

Equipment

Glass slides.
Coplin jars.
Microscope. Equipped with accessories for UV fluorescence.
Moist chamber. Made from a Petri dish with moistened filter paper in the bottom.

Reagents

Phosphate buffered saline (PBS), pH 7.1. See p. 578.
Rabbit anti-human Hb F serum. Dilute the antiserum 1 in 64 in PBS; store in small aliquots at −20°C. Stable for several months.
Sheep (or goat) anti-rabbit immunoglobulin labelled with fluorescein isothiocyanate. Dilute 1 in 32 in PBS; store in small aliquots at −20°C. Stable for several months.
Fixative. Acetone 90 ml, methanol 10 ml.

Method

1. Prepare thin blood films and allow to dry overnight.
2. Fix for 5 min at room temperature, shake off excess fixative and rinse immediately in PBS. If the films are too thick they will peel off at this stage.
3. Rinse the slides in water and allow to dry.
4. Layer 5 μl of the anti-Hb F antisera onto the slide.
5. Incubate in the moist chamber at 37°C for 30 min or at room temperature for 60 min.
6. Rinse the slides thoroughly in PBS to remove any unbound antiserum.

7. Rinse the slides in water and allow to dry.

8. Layer 5 μl of the anti-rabbit antisera onto the slide.

9. Incubate in the moist chamber at 37°C for 30 min or at room temperature for 60 min.

10. Rinse the slides thoroughly in PBS to remove any unbound antiserum.

11. Rinse the slides in water and allow to dry.

12. Examine microscopically using a ×40 objective and filters suitable for use with fluorescein *iso*thiocyanate. To quantitate the number of Hb F-containing cells, count the total number of cells in a field under white light using an eyepiece grid, then the number of stained cells under the UV light. If the level of Hb F is less than 10% at least 2000 cells should be counted.

Comments

In normal adults, from 0.1–7.0% of cells show detectable fluorescence. The proportion of positive cells correlates well with the percentage of Hb F as measured by alkali denaturation at levels between 0.5 and 5.0%. As little as 1 pg of Hb F per cell can be detected, giving much greater sensitivity than the acid elution method. This increased sensitivity however, may make a heterocellular distribution appear pancellular if the proportion of Hb F if greater than 10%.[14]

Interpretation of Hb F values[6,45]

| Hb F | 0.2–1.0% | Normal result. |
| Hb F | 1.0–5.0% | In 30–50% of β-thalassaemia traits. |

Hb F (contd.)	1.0–5.0%	Some heterozygotes for a Hb variant. Some homozygotes for a Hb variant. Some compound heterozygotes for a Hb variant and β-thalassaemia trait. Some individuals with haematological disorders (aplastic anaemia, myelodysplastic syndromes, etc). Some pregnant women (third trimester). Sporadically in the general population, particularly in Afro-Carribeans.
Hb F	5.0–20.0%	Occasional β-thalassaemia trait. Some homozygotes for a Hb variant. Some compound heterozygotes for a Hb variant and β-thalassaemia trait. Some types of heterozygous HPFH. δβ-thalassaemia.
Hb F	15.0–45.0%	Heterozygous HPFH—African type. (Usually above 20%.) Some cases of β-thalassaemia intermedia.
Hb F	>45.0%	β-thalassaemia major. Some cases of β-thalassaemia intermedia. Homozygous African type HPFH. Neonates.

ASSESSMENT OF IRON STATUS IN THALASSAEMIA

Concurrent iron deficiency makes the diagnosis of thalassaemia trait more difficult as it masks the typical blood picture and causes reduced Hb A_2 synthesis.[1,25,38] In a β-thalassaemia trait, dependent on the severity of the anaemia, the Hb A_2 value may be reduced to borderline, or even to normal levels. In α-thalassaemia trait Hb A_2 levels may be below 1.0%.

Whenever possible, individuals should not be investigated for the presence of thalassaemia trait if they are iron deficient. Iron stores are usually replete after 3–4 months of treatment with iron. If a pregnant woman is suspected of having a thalassaemia trait, it is not possible to wait for the correction of iron deficiency to establish the diagnosis. The woman and her partner should be tested without delay and globin chain synthesis or preferably DNA analysis of globin chains carried out if both are suspected of having a thalassaemia trait (see Chapter 28).

In addition to traditional methods for iron assessment such as serum iron and TIBC and ferritin measurement, estimation of zinc protoporphyrin (ZPP) is of potential value in haematology. It can be carried out on an EDTA sample and is a measure of iron incorporation at the cellular level.

MEASUREMENT OF ZINC PROTOPORPHYRIN (ZPP) IN RED CELLS

Principle. Haem is formed in the developing red cell by insertion of iron into a preformed porphyrin ring. In the event of an insufficient supply of iron, or impaired iron utilization, zinc is substituted for iron into protoporphyrin IX. The ZPP formed in the chelation process is stable and remains in the red cell throughout its life-span. Thus the level of ZPP in the red cell is a functional indicator of iron utilization at the time of cell maturation. ZPP can be measured in whole blood using a front face fluorometer*.

Method

The manufacturer's instructions as to the exact method of use should be followed.

Interpretation and comments

Samples should be washed before testing to remove interfering substances such as bilirubin. Grossly haemolysed samples are not suitable for testing.

A normal and iron-deficient control should be tested with every batch of samples and each laboratory must establish its own normal range. This method does not measure iron overload. High values are found in iron deficiency, lead poisoning and in the anaemias of chronic disorders in which iron release from the reticuloendothelial system is blocked.

---

*Helena Laboratories.

RED CELL INCLUSIONS

The most important red cell inclusions found in the haemoglobinopathies are Hb H inclusion bodies (precipitated β-chain tetramers) found in α-thalassaemia,[39] α-chain inclusions found in β-thalassaemia major[15,40] and Heinz bodies found in unstable haemoglobin diseases.[17,42]

Precipitated α-chains are found in the cytoplasm of nucleated red cell precursors of patients with β-thalassaemia major; they can be demonstrated by supravital staining with methyl violet (as can Heinz bodies) and appear as irregularly shaped bodies close to the nucleus of normoblasts. After splenectomy they may also be found in the peripheral blood normoblasts and reticulocytes. Heinz bodies (insoluble denatured globin chains) form as a result of chemical poisoning and drug intoxication, and develop spontaneously in G-6PD deficiency and in the unstable haemoglobin diseases. They are usually only seen in the peripheral blood after splenectomy. When due to the presence of an unstable haemoglobin they may be demonstrated in the peripheral blood of patients with an intact spleen if their blood is kept at 37°C for 24–48 h. The use of methyl violet and of brilliant cresyl blue in the demonstration of precipitated α-chains and Heinz bodies is described in Chapter 8.

DEMONSTRATION OF Hb H INCLUSION BODIES

Reagent

Staining solution. 1.0% brilliant cresyl blue or new methylene blue. New batches of stain must be tested with a known positive control, as the redox action of the dyes may vary from batch to batch.

Method

1. Mix 2 volumes of fresh blood (within 24 h of collection) with 1 volume of staining solution.
2. Incubate at 37°C for 2 h, or at room temperature for 4 h.
3. Resuspend the cells and spread a thin blood film.
4. Examine the film as for a reticulocyte count. The inclusion bodies appear as multiple greenish-blue dots like the pitted pattern on a golf ball.

They can be readily distinguished from the precipitated dots and filaments of a reticulocyte.

Interpretation and comments

In α^+-thalassaemia trait only a very occasional H body (1:1000 to 1:10 000) is usually seen; they are more numerous in α^0-thalassaemia but the number of cells developing inclusions does not help in differentiating the various gene deletion patterns seen in α-thalassaemia, and the absence of demonstrable inclusions does not preclude a diagnosis of α-thalassaemia trait. In Hb H disease inclusions are found in more than 30% of red cells.

FETAL DIAGNOSIS OF GLOBIN GENE DISORDERS[5]

Prenatal diagnosis is carried out if the fetus is at risk of thalassaemia major or a severe form of sickle cell disease such as sickle cell anaemia. Two approaches to fetal diagnosis are available: globin chain synthesis (used if the putative father is not available) and DNA analysis. DNA can be obtained from a chorionic villus sample or from amniotic fluid. Methods used for DNA analysis are described in Chapter 28.

When a potentially at risk couple is detected they will require counselling and if a fetal diagnosis is requested, it is necessary to confirm the parental haemoglobin phenotype. The family or parental blood samples are sent to the diagnostic centre and the timing of fetal sampling is arranged.

Sample requirements

Blood samples for globin chain synthesis have to be fresh (received within a few hours of collection) and transported at 4°C. Blood samples for DNA analysis can be sent by overnight delivery without refrigeration but must be processed within 3 days of collection at the latest. 10 ml of blood in EDTA or heparin are required

from each parent. If restriction fragment length polymorphism (RFLP) linkage analysis is required, the following additional samples are needed: blood from either a homozygous normal or affected child, or from a heterozygous child and one set of grandparents, or if no child is available, blood from both sets of grandparents. The samples must be carefully and clearly labelled and the family tree drawn. Particulars of all haematological tests must be given.

Chorionic villus samples must be dissected free of any maternal tissue and sent by overnight delivery in tissue culture medium or preferably, in a special buffer obtainable from the DNA diagnosis laboratory. Amniotic fluid samples (15–20 ml are needed) must be received within 24 h of collection. If a longer transit time is unavoidable, the amniocytes should be resuspended in tissue culture medium.

It is essential that follow-up data are obtained on all cases that have undergone fetal diagnosis. This should include tests on cord blood or heel prick sample at birth and a test at 6 months to confirm the carrier state. Whenever possible DNA analysis of the child's globin genes should be carried out.

REFERENCES

1   ALPERIN, J. B., DOW, P. A. and PETEWAY, M. B. (1977). Haemoglobin A_2 levels in health and various hematological disorders. *American Journal of Clinical Pathology*, **67**, 219.

2   BASSET, P., BEUZARD, Y., GAREL, M. C. and ROSA, J. (1978). Isoelectric focusing of human hemoglobins: its application to screening, to characterization of 70 variants and to study of modified fractions of normal hemoglobins. *Blood*, **51**, 971.

3   BETKE, K., MARTI, H. R. and SCHLICHT, L. (1959). Estimation of small percentage of foetal haemoglobin. *Nature*, **184**, 1877.

4   BRITISH COMMITTEE FOR STANDARDIZATION IN HAEMATOLOGY (1991). Haemoglobinopathy screening. In *Standard Haematology Practice*. Ed. B. Roberts, p. 43. Blackwell Scientific Publications, Oxford.

5   BRITISH COMMITTEE FOR STANDARDIZATION IN HAEMATOLOGY (1994). Guidelines for fetal diagnosis of globin gene disorders. *Journal of Clinical Pathology*, **47**, 199.

6   BRITISH COMMITTEE FOR STANDARDIZATION IN HAEMATOLOGY (1994). Guidelines for the investigation of the α and β thalassaemia traits. *Journal of Clinical Pathology*, **47**, 289.

7   CARRELL, R. W. (1986). The hemoglobinopathies: methods of determining hemoglobin instability (unstable hemoglobins). *Methods in Haematology*, **15**, 109.

8   CARRELL, R. W. and KAY, R. (1972). A simple method for the detection of unstable haemoglobins. *British Journal of Haematology*, **23**, 615.

9   CHUDWIN, D. S. and RUCKNAGEL, D. L. (1974). Immunological quantification of hemoglobins F and A_2. *Clinica Chimica Acta*, **50**, 413.

10   DACIE, J. V. (1988). *The Haemolytic Anaemias, Vol. 2: The Hereditary Haemolytic Anaemias*, 3rd edn, Part 2, p. 322. Churchill Livingstone, Edinburgh.

11   EFREMOV, G. D. (1986). The hemoglobinopathies: quantitation of hemoglobins by microchromatography. *Methods in Hematology*, **15**, 72.

12   EFREMOV, G. D., HUISMAN, T. H. J., BOWMAN, K., WRIGHTSTONE, R. and SCHROEDER, W. A. (1974). Microchromatography of hemoglobins: II A rapid method for the determination of Hb A_2. *Journal of Laboratory and Clinical Medicine*, **83**, 657.

13   FAIRBANKS, V. F. (1980). *Hemoglobinopathies and Thalassaemias. Laboratory methods and case studies*. B. C. Decker, New York.

14   FELICE, A. E. (1986). The hemoglobinopathies: quantitation of fetal hemoglobin. *Methods in Hematology*, **15**, 91.

15   FESSAS, P. (1963). Inclusions of hemoglobin in erythroblasts and erythrocytes of thalassaemia. *Blood*, **21**, 21.

16   GRIMES, A. J. and MEISLER, A. (1962). Possible cause of Heinz bodies in congenital Heinz body anaemia. *Nature (London)*, **194**, 190.

17   GRIMES, A. J., MEISLER, A. and DACIE, J. V. (1964). Congenital Heinz-body anaemia: further evidence on the cause of Heinz-body production in red cells. *British Journal of Haematology*, **10**, 21.

18   HIGGS, D. R. (1993). α-Thalassaemia. In *The Haemoglobinopathies. Bailliere's Clinical Haematology*. Eds. D. R. Higgs, and D. J. Weatherall, Vol. 6, p. 117. Baillière Tindall, London.

19   HUISMAN, T. H. J., SCHROEDER, W. A., BRODIE, A. R.,

MAYSON, S. M. and JAKURAY, J. (1975). Microchromatography of hemoglobins III. A simplified procedure for the determination of hemoglobin A_2. *Journal of Laboratory and Clinical Medicine*, **86**, 700.

20   HUNTSMAN, R. G., BARCLAY, G. P. T., CANNING, D. M. and YAWSON, G. I. (1970). A rapid whole blood solubility test to differentiate the sickle cell trait from sickle cell anaemia. *Journal of Clinical Pathology*, **23**, 781.

21   INTERNATIONAL COMMITTEE FOR STANDARDIZATION IN HEMATOLOGY (1978). Simple electrophoretic system for presumptive identification of abnormal hemoglobins. *Blood*, **52**, 1058.

22   INTERNATIONAL COMMITTEE FOR STANDARDIZATION IN HEMATOLOGY (1978). Recommendations for a system for identifying abnormal hemoglobins. *Blood*, **52**, 1065.

23   INTERNATIONAL COMMITTEE FOR STANDARDIZATION IN HEMATOLOGY (1988). Recommendations for neonatal screening for haemoglobinopathies. *Journal of Clinical and Laboratory Haematology*, **10**, 335.

24   JONXIS, J. H. P. and VISSER, H. K. A. (1956). Determination of low percentages of fetal hemoglobin in blood of normal children. *American Journal of Diseases of Children*, **92**, 588.

25   KATAMIS, C., PANAYOTIS, L., METAXOTOU-MAVROMATI, A. and MATSANIATIS, N. J. (1972). Serum iron and unsaturated iron binding capacity in β-thalassaemia trait: their relation to the levels of Hb A, A_2 and F. *Medical Genetics*, **9**, 154.

26   KLEIHAUER, E. (1974). Determination of fetal hemoglobin: elution technique. In *The Detection of Hemoglobinopathies*. Eds. R. M. Schmidt, T. H. J. Huisman and H. Lehmann, p. 20. CRC Press, Cleveland, OH.

27   MAKLER, M. T. and PESCE, A. J. (1980). ELISA assay for measurement of hemoglobin A and hemoglobin F. *American Journal of Clinical Pathology*, **74**, 673.

28   MARDER, V. J. and CONLEY, C. L. (1959). Electrophoresis of hemoglobin on agar gel. Frequency of hemoglobin D in a Negro population. *Bulletin of the Johns Hopkins Hospital*, **105**, 77.

29   MARENGO-ROWE, A. J. (1965). Rapid electrophoresis and quantitation of haemoglobins on cellulose acetate. *Journal of Clinical Pathology*, **18**, 790.

30   MOLCHANOVA, T. P. (1993). A new screening test for unstable hemoglobins using n-butanol and red blood cells. *Hemoglobin*, **17**, 81.

31   NEDA, S. and SCHNEIDER, R. G. (1969). Rapid identification of polypeptide chains of hemoglobin by cellulose acetate electrophoresis of hemolysates. *Blood*, **34**, 230.

32   RIGHETTI, P. G., GIANAZZA, E., BIANCHI-BOSISIO, A. and COSSU, G. (1986). The hemoglobinopathies: conventional isoelectric focusing and immobilized pH gradients for hemoglobin separation and identification. *Methods in Hematology*, **15**, 47.

33   SCHNEIDER, R. G. (1974). Identification of hemoglobin by electrophoresis. In *The Detection of Hemoglobinopathies*. Eds. R. M. Schmidt, T. H. J. Huisman, and H. Lehmann, p. 11. CRC Press, Cleveland, OH.

34   SCHNEIDER, R. G. (1974). Differentiation of electrophoretically similar hemoglobins—such as S, D, G, and P or A_2, C, E and O—by electrophoresis of the globin chains. *Clinical Chemistry*, **20**, 1111.

35   SCHROEDER, W. A., SKELTON, J. B. and SKELTON, J. R.

(1980). Separation of hemoglobin peptides by high performance liquid chromatography (HPLC). *Hemoglobin*, **4,** 551.

[36] SERJEANT, G. R. (1992). *Sickle Cell Disease*, 2nd edn. Oxford University Press, Oxford.

[37] THEIN, S. W. (1993). β-thalassaemia. In *The Haemoglobinopathies. Bailliere's Clinical Haematology*, Eds. D. R. Higgs and D. J. Weatherall, Vol. 6, p. 151. Baillière Tindall, London.

[38] WASI, P., NA-NAKORN, S., POOTRAKUL, S., SOOKANEK, M., DISTHASONGCHAN, P., PORNPATKUL, M. and PANICH, V. (1969). Alpha-and beta-thalassemia in Thailand. *Annals of New York Academy of Sciences*, **165,** 60.

[39] WEATHERALL, D. J. (1983). The thalassemias: hematologic methods. *Methods in Hematology*, **6,** 27.

[40] WEATHERALL, D. J. and CLEGG, J. B. (1981). *The Thalassaemia syndromes*, 3rd edn. Blackwell Scientific Publications, Oxford.

[41] WHITE, J. M. (1974). The unstable haemoglobin disorders. *Clinics in Haematology*, **3,** 333.

[42] WHITE, J. M. and DACIE, J. V. (1971). The unstable hemoglobins—molecular and clinical features. *Progress in Hematology*, **7,** 69.

[43] WOOD, W. G. (1983). The thalassemias: hemoglobin analysis. *Methods in Hematology*, **6,** 31.

[44] WOOD, W. G. (1993). Increased Hb F in adult life. In *The Haemoglobinopathies. Bailliere's Clinical Haematology*. Eds. D. R. Higgs and D. J. Weatherall, Vol 6, p. 177. Baillière Tindall, London.

[45] WOOD, W. G., STAMATOYANNOPOULOS, G., LIM, G. and NUTE, P. E. (1975). F cells in the adult: normal values and levels in individuals with hereditary and acquired elevations of Hb F. *Blood*, **46,** 671.

[46] ZAGO, M. A., WOOD, W. G., CLEGG, J. B., WEATHERALL, D. J., O'SULLIVAN, M. and GUNSON, H. (1979). Genetic control of F-cells in human adults. *Blood*, **53,** 977.

15. Laboratory methods used in the investigation of paroxysmal nocturnal haemoglobinuria (PNH)

Revised by L. Luzzatto and P. Hillmen

Acidified-serum test (Ham Test)   289
  with magnesium   290
Significance of acidified-serum test   290
Sucrose lysis test   291
'Cold antibody lysis' test   291

Flow cytometry   292
  GPI-linked proteins   292
Other PNH tests   293
PNH-like cells   293
Preparation of AET cells   293
Summary   293

Paroxysmal nocturnal haemoglobinuria is an acquired disorder in which the patient's red cells are abnormally sensitive to lysis by normal constituents of plasma. In its classical form it is characterized by haemoglobinuria during sleep (nocturnal haemoglobinuria), jaundice and haemosiderinuria. Not uncommonly, however, PNH presents as an obscure anaemia without obvious evidence of intravascular haemolysis or develops in a patient suffering apparently from aplastic anaemia or more rarely from myelosclerosis or leukaemia.[8,16,48]

PNH red cells are unusually susceptible to lysis by complement.[14,43] This can be demonstrated in vitro by a variety of tests, e.g. the acidified-serum (Ham),[14,24] sucrose,[19,24] thrombin,[7] cold-antibody lysis,[9] inulin[3] and cobra-venom[25] tests. In the acidified-serum, inulin and cobra-venom tests complement is activated via the alternative (Pillemer) pathway, while in the cold-antibody test, and probably in the thrombin test, complement is activated by the classical sequence initiated through antigen-antibody interaction. In the sucrose lysis test a low ionic strength is thought to lead to the binding of IgG molecules non-specifically to the cell membrane and to the subsequent activation of complement via the classical sequence. In addition, the alternative pathway appears to be activated.[29] In each test PNH cells undergo lysis because of their greatly increased sensitivity to lysis by complement.

Minor degrees of lysis may be observed in the cold-antibody lysis and sucrose tests with the red cells from a variety of dyserythropoietic anaemias, e.g. aplastic anaemia, megaloblastic anaemia and myelosclerosis.[4,28] Weak positive results in these tests have thus to be interpreted with care. PNH red cells, however, almost always undergo major amounts of lysis in these tests.

A characteristic feature of a positive test for PNH is that not all the patient's cells undergo

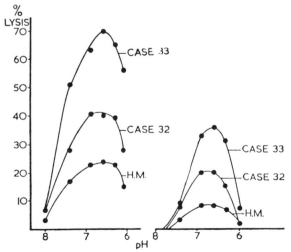

Fig. 15.1 Effect of pH on lysis in vitro of PNH red cells by human sera. The red cells of three patients (Cases 32, 33 and H.M. of different sensitivity) were used, and two fresh normal sera, one serum being more potent than the other.

lysis, even if the conditions of the test are made optimal for lysis (Fig. 15.1). This is because only a proportion of any patient's PNH red cell population is hypersensitive to lysis by complement. This population varies from patient to patient, and there is a direct relationship between the proportion of red cells that can be lysed (in any of the diagnostic tests) and the severity of in-vivo haemolysis.

The phenomenon of some red cells being sensitive to complement lysis and some insensitive was studied quantitatively by Rosse and Dacie who obtained two-component complement sensitivity curves in a series of PNH patients.[43] Later, Rosse and his coworkers reported that in some cases three populations of red cells could be demonstrated.[40–42]

1. Very sensitive (Type III) cells, 10–15 times as sensitive as normal cells.
2. Cells of medium sensitivity (Type II), 3–5 times as sensitive as normal cells.
3. Cells of normal sensitivity (Type I).

In vivo, the proportion of Type-III cells parallels the severity of the patient's haemolysis.

PNH is an acquired clonal disorder[36] arising due to a somatic mutation occurring in a haemopoietic stem cell. It has been demonstrated that a proportion of granulocytes, platelets and lymphocytes are part of the PNH clone as well as a proportion of the red cells.[26,35] The characteristic feature of cells belonging to the PNH clone is that they are deficient in several cell-membrane bound proteins including red cell acetylcholinesterase,[1,5,11,12] neutrophil alkaline phosphatase,[2,17,27] decay accelerating factor (DAF or CD55),[34,38] homologous restriction factor (HRF)[15,55] and membrane inhibitor of reactive lysis (MIRL or CD59),[10,22,23] amongst others. DAF, HRF and CD59 all have roles in the protection of the cell against complement mediated attack. CD59 inhibits the formation of the terminal complex of complement, and it has been established that the deficiency of CD59 is largely responsible for the complement sensitivity of PNH red cells. PNH type III erythrocytes have a complete deficiency of CD59 whereas PNH Type-II erythrocytes have only a partial deficiency and it is this difference which accounts for their variable sensitivities to complement.[44,45] The

analysis of these deficient proteins on PNH cells by flow cytometry, particularly of the red cells and neutrophils, has recently become a useful research and diagnostic tool. By comparing the proportion of cells with deficient CD59 to the percentage lysis in the Ham test it has been possible to assess the sensitivity of the Ham test. The standard Ham test is reasonably good at estimating the proportion of PNH red cells as long as they are PNH Type-III cells and that they comprise less than 20% of the total. In cases in which the PNH cells are Type II and more than 20% are present, the standard Ham test significantly underestimates the proportion of PNH red cells. The standard Ham test can be negative when there are less than 5% PNH Type-III cells or less than 20% PNH Type-II cells. When the Ham test is supplemented with magnesium, to optimize the activation of complement, the percentage lysis gives a more accurate estimation of the proportion of PNH cells (Fig. 15.2).[30]

Certain chemicals, in particular sulphydryl compounds, can act on normal red cells in vitro

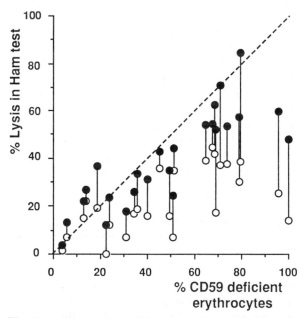

Fig. 15.2 Comparison of the proportion of CD59 deficient red cells with the lysis in the Ham test. The percentage lysis in the Ham test with added magnesium (●) and without added magnesium (○) is plotted against the proportion of CD59 deficient red cells in the same samples from 25 patients with PNH (P. Hillmen, M. Bessler, D. Roper and L. Luzzatto, unpublished observation).

so as to increase their complement sensitivity. In this way PNH-like red cells can be created in the laboratory and can be used as useful reagents (p. 293).

ACIDIFIED-SERUM TEST (HAM TEST)

Principle. The patient's red cells are exposed at 37°C to the action of normal or the patient's own serum suitably acidified to the optimum pH for lysis (pH 6.5–7.0) (Fig. 15.1).

The patient's red cells can be obtained from defibrinated, heparinized, oxalated, citrated or EDTA blood, and the test can be satisfactorily carried out even on cells which have been stored at 4°C for up to 2–3 weeks in ACD or Alsever's solution, if kept sterile. The patient's serum is best obtained by defibrination, for if in PNH it is obtained from blood allowed to clot in the ordinary way at 37°C or at room temperature it will almost certainly be found to be markedly lysed. Normal serum should similarly be obtained by defibrination, but serum derived from blood allowed to clot spontaneously at room temperature or at 37°C can be used. Normal serum known to be strongly lytic to PNH red cells is to be preferred to patient's serum, the lytic potentiality of which is unknown. However, if the test is positive using normal serum it is important, particularly if the patient appears not to be suffering from overt intravascular haemolysis, to obtain a positive result using the patient's serum, in order to exclude HEMPAS (see p. 290). The variability between the sera of individuals in their capacity to lyse PNH red cells is shown in Fig. 15.1. The activity of a single individual's serum also varies from time to time[37] and it is always important to include in any test, as a positive control, a sample of known PNH cells or artificially created 'PNH-like' cells (see p. 293).

The sera should be fresh, i.e. used within a few hours of collection. Their lytic potency is retained for several months at –70°C, but at 4°C, and even at –20°C, this deteriorates within a few days.

Method

Deliver 0.5 ml samples of fresh normal serum, group AB- or ABO-compatible with the patient's blood, into six (three pairs) of 75 × 12 mm glass tubes. Place two tubes at 56°C for 10–30 min in order to inactivate complement. Keep the other two pairs of tubes at room temperature and add to the serum in two of the tubes one-tenth volumes (0.05 ml) of 0.2 mol/l HCl. Add similar volumes of acid subsequently to the inactivated serum samples. Then place all the tubes in a 37°C water-bath.

While the serum samples are being dealt with, wash samples of the patient's red cells and of control normal red cells (compatible with the normal serum) twice in 9.0 g/l NaCl and prepare 50% suspensions in the saline. Then add one-tenth volumes of each of these cell suspensions (0.05 ml) to single tubes containing unacidified fresh serum, acidified fresh serum and acidified inactivated serum, respectively. Mix the contents carefully and leave the tubes at 37°C. Centrifuge them after about 1 h.

Table 15.1 The acidified-serum test with added magnesium

Reagent	Test (ml)			Controls (ml)		
	1	2	3	4	5	6
Fresh normal serum	0.5	0.5	0	0.5	0.5	0
Heat-inactivated normal serum	0	0	0.5	0	0	0.5
0.2 mol/l HCl	0	0.05	0.05	0	0.05	0.05
50% patient's red cells	0.05	0.05	0.05	0	0	0
50% normal red cells	0	0	0	0.05	0.05	0.05
Magnesium chloride (250 mmol/l; 23.7 g/l)	0.01	0.01	0.01	0.01	0.01	0.01
Lysis (in a positive test)	Trace (2%)	+++ (30%)	–	–	–	–

Add 0.05 ml of each cell suspension to 0.55 ml of water so as to prepare a standard for subsequent quantitative measurement of lysis and retain 0.5 ml of serum for use as a blank. For the measurement of lysis, deliver 0.3 ml volumes of the supernatants of the test and control series of cell-serum suspensions, and of the blank serum and of the lysed cell suspension equivalent to 0% and 100% lysis, respectively, into 5 ml of 0.4 ml/l ammonia or Drabkin's reagent. Measure the lysis in a photoelectric colorimeter using a yellow-green (e.g. Ilford 625) filter or in a spectrophotometer at a wave-length of 540 nm.

If the test cells are from a patient with PNH, they will undergo definite, although, as already mentioned, incomplete lysis in the acidified serum. Very much less lysis, or even no lysis at all, will be visible in the unacidified serum. No lysis will be brought about by the acidified inactivated serum. The normal control sample of cells should not undergo lysis in any of the three tubes.

In PNH 10–50% lysis is usually obtained, when lysis is measured as liberated haemoglobin. Exceptionally, there may be as much as 80% lysis or as little as 5%.

The red cells of a patient who has been transfused will undergo less lysis than before the transfusion, because the normal transfused cells, despite circulation in the patient, behave normally. In PNH, it is characteristic that a young cell (reticulocyte-rich) population, such as the upper red cell layer obtained by centrifugation, undergoes more lysis than the red cells derived from mixed whole blood.

ACIDIFIED-SERUM TEST WITH ADDITIONAL MAGNESIUM (MODIFIED HAM TEST)

Principle. The sensitivity of the Ham test can be improved by the addition of magnesium to the test to enhance the activation of complement.

Method

The method is identical to that for the standard Ham test (see above) with the addition of 10 μl of 250 mM magnesium chloride (final concentration = 4 mM) to each tube prior to the incubation (Table 15.1).

SIGNIFICANCE OF THE ACIDIFIED-SERUM TEST

A positive acidified-serum test, carried out with proper controls, denotes the PNH abnormality, and PNH cannot be diagnosed unless the acidified-serum test is positive. The addition of magnesium chloride increases the sensitivity of the acidified-serum test, and it remains specific for PNH*.

The only disorder other than PNH that may appear to give a clear-cut positive test is a rare congenital dyserythropoietic anaemia, CDA Type II or HEMPAS.[6,53] In contrast to PNH, however, HEMPAS red cells undergo lysis in only a proportion (about 30%) of normal sera; moreover, they do not undergo lysis in the patient's own acidified serum and the sucrose lysis test is negative. The expression of GPI-linked proteins in HEMPAS is normal. In HEMPAS, lysis appears to be due to the presence on the red cells of an unusual antigen which reacts with a complement-fixing IgM antibody ('anti-HEMPAS') present in many, but not in all, normal sera.[53]

Heating at 56°C inactivates the lytic system and, if there is lysis in inactivated serum, the test cannot be considered positive. Markedly spherocytic red cells or effete normal red cells may lyse in acidified serum, probably due to the lowered pH, and such cells may lyse, too, in acidified inactivated serum.

It must be stressed that PNH red cells are not unduly sensitive to lysis by a lowered pH per se. The addition of the acid adjusts the pH of the serum-cell mixture to the optimum for the activity of the lytic system. As is shown in Fig. 15.1, it is possible to construct pH-lysis curves, if different concentrations of acid are used. The optimum pH for lysis is between pH 6.5 and 7.0 (measurements made after the addition of the red cells to the serum).

---

*Whenever the acidified-serum test is positive it is recommended that a direct antiglobulin test (p. 457) should also be carried out. If this is positive, it could be due to a lytic antibody which has given a false positive acidified-serum test. This can be confirmed by appropriate serological studies (see Chapter 24). In addition, in such complex cases a more definitive test for PNH, which is now available, is flow cytometry after reaction of the red cells with anti-CD59 (p. 292).

SUCROSE LYSIS TEST[18,19,24]

An iso-osmotic solution of sucrose (92.4 g/l) is required. This can be stored at 4°C for up to 2–3 weeks.

For the test, set up two tubes, one containing 0.05 ml of fresh normal group AB or ABO-compatible serum diluted in 0.85 ml of sucrose solution and the other containing 0.05 ml of serum diluted in 0.85 ml of saline. Add to each tube 0.1 ml of a 50% suspension of washed red cells. After incubation at 37°C for 30 min, centrifuge the tubes and examine for lysis. If lysis is visible in the sucrose-containing tube, measure this in a photoelectric colorimeter or a spectrophotometer (see above), using the tube containing serum diluted in saline as a blank and a tube containing 0.1 ml of the red cell suspension in 0.9 ml of 0.4 ml/l ammonia in place of the sucrose-serum mixture as a standard for 100% lysis.

Interpretation

The sucrose lysis test is based on the fact that red cells absorb complement components from serum at low ionic concentrations.[30,33] PNH cells, because of their great sensitivity will undergo lysis but normal red cells do not. The red cells from some cases of leukaemia[4] or myelosclerosis[50] may undergo a small amount of lysis, almost always <10%; in such cases the acidified-serum test is usually negative and PNH should not be diagnosed. In PNH, lysis varies from 10% to 80%, but exceptionally may be as little as 5%. Sucrose lysis and acidified-serum lysis of PNH red cells are fairly closely correlated. The sucrose lysis test is typically negative in HEMPAS (see p. 290).

'COLD-ANTIBODY LYSIS' TEST

The greatly increased sensitivity of PNH red cells to complement can be dramatically demonstrated if the cells are suspended in dilutions of a high-titre cold agglutinin (anti-I) in the presence of fresh human serum complement.[9] Using suitable dilutions of the reagents, PNH red cells undergo marked lysis whereas normal red cells undergo little or no lysis. This reaction, the basis of the cold-antibody lysis test, is, however, not quite specific for PNH as the red cells from some patients with various types of dyserythropoietic anaemia may undergo minor, or rarely moderate, amounts of lysis.[28]

An anti-I serum is required (titre at 4°C, >8000), which when used unacidified fails to lyse at room temperature most normal human red cells, i.e. a typical anti-I serum from a patient suffering from the cold haemagglutinin disease. Such sera keep their properties for years if frozen at −20°C. The serum should be distributed in 0.5–1.0 ml volumes in a number of tubes to avoid repeated thawing and freezing.

Method

Make a 1 in 50 or 1 in 100 dilution of the anti-I serum in fresh normal group AB or ABO-compatible serum. Deliver two 0.5 ml volumes of the serum into 75 × 12 mm tubes and add 0.5 ml volumes of a 5% suspension of washed normal and test (? PNH) red cells, respectively, to the serum samples. Add a further 0.5 ml volume of the washed test cells to a tube containing 0.5 ml of saline to serve as a standard for the quantitative measurement of lysis. Retain 0.5 ml of the diluted serum as a blank. After 1 h at room temperature centrifuge the two tubes containing the serum-cell suspensions, and add 0.3 ml volumes of their supernatants to 5 ml of 0.4 ml/l ammonia or Drabkin's reagent. Measure lysis in a photoelectric colorimeter using a yellow-green (e.g. Ilford 625) filter or in a spectrophotometer at a wavelength of 540 nm. Add 0.3 ml of the diluted red cell suspension to a further 5 ml of the diluent to give a standard for 100% lysis.

If a potent complement-fixing (i.e. lytic) anti-I antiserum is available, a very sensitive anti-I lysis test can be carried out using diluted human AB serum as complement. This is the basis of the complement lysis sensitivity test and the less elaborate 'four-tube complement lysis sensitivity' test.[43] These tests are probably more specific for PNH than is the original and very simple cold-antibody lysis test.

Significance of the 'cold-antibody lysis' test

The cold antibody lysis test is a sensitive test for the diagnosis of PNH. The complement lysis sensitivity test has the advantage that it differentiates PNH Type-III red cells from PNH Type-II red cells. A more convenient method to differentiate these is by the analysis of CD59 on red cells by flow cytometry. This, however, requires a flow cytometer. Hence the inclusion of the cold-antibody lysis test in this chapter.

FLOW CYTOMETRY—ANALYSIS OF THE GPI-LINKED* PROTEINS ON RED CELLS

Principle. The patient's red cells are stained with a fluorescein-labelled antibody which is specific for one of several GPI-linked proteins, e.g. CD59, DAF and LFA-3, which are deficient in PNH red cells. The stained cells are then analysed with a flow cytometer.

The patient's red cells can be obtained in any of the anticoagulants described for the Ham test. The cells, if taken into ACD, can be stored for 2–3 weeks prior to analysis. Fluorescein-conjugated anti-CD59 (MEM 43, Cymbus Bioscience Ltd, Southampton, UK) gives excellent results when used for red-cell analysis. It is important to use the conjugated antibody, as staining with unconjugated anti-CD59 followed by a fluorescein-conjugated second layer antibody may result in artefact, probably due to red-cell agglutination. There is no suitable anti-DAF antibody commercially available at present. Anti-LFA-3 (BRIC5, Bioproducts Laboratories, UK, used at 20 µg/ml) gives reproducible results for red cell analysis, but the level of LFA-3 expression on PNH Type-II cells is higher than that of many other GPI-linked proteins and thus studying LFA-3 expression is useful but not ideal.[21]

Method

Chill 1×10^6 cells in 50 µl of PBS on ice with 50 µl of monoclonal antibody (MoAb) for 30 min. Wash twice in PBS + azide (200 mg/l), and then chill with fluorescein-labelled goat anti-mouse antibody on ice in the dark for 30 min. Wash twice in PBS + azide, and then fix with approximately 0.5 ml of 1% formaldehyde in Isoton II (Coulter). Analysis is performed using a flow cytometer. A negative control antibody should always be used to assess the fluorescence of cells lacking the antigen. The cells from a normal subject should be stained as an additional control to verify that negative cells in the test sample are true PNH cells and not artefactual.

FLOW CYTOMETRY—ANALYSIS OF THE GPI-LINKED PROTEINS ON NEUTROPHILS

Principle. A proportion of the patient's neutrophils have been demonstrated to be part of the PNH clone in all patients with PNH. GPI-linked proteins which are suitable for analysis include CD16, CD59, DAF, CD67 and CD24.[39,52] There are available numerous fluorescein-conjugated antibodies to CD16 which are suitable for analysis, for example fluorescein-conjugated anti-Leu-11a (Becton Dickinson) or fluorescein-conjugated anti-CD59 (Cymbus Biosciences).

Method

The patient's neutrophils are obtained by collecting blood, anticoagulating with preservative-free heparin (10 units/ml) and obtaining a buffy coat. The formation of a buffy coat can be accelerated

---

*Glycosylphosphatidylinositol-linked.

by adding 1ml of 6% hetastarch in 0.9% sodium chloride (Hespan, DuPont) to 10 ml of blood. 1–2 $\times 10^6$ cells are analysed. It is important that all the subsequent staining and washing is performed at 4°C to minimize non-specific staining. Chill the cells in 50 μl of PBS on ice with 50 μl of monoclonal antibody (MoAb) for 30 min. Wash twice in PBS + 0.1% bovine serum albumin (PBS + BSA), and then chill with fluorescein-labelled goat anti-mouse antibody on ice in the dark for 30 min. Wash twice in PBS + BSA, and then fix with approximately 0.5 ml of 1% formaldehyde in Isoton II. For conjugated antibodies a single incubation step only is required followed by a wash and then fixing prior to analysis. Analysis is performed using a flow cytometer. Appropriate normal controls and negative controls should always be tested in parallel to the patient's samples.

A negative control antibody should always be used to assess the fluorescence of cells lacking the antigen. The cells from a normal subject should be stained as an additional control to verify that negative cells in the test sample are true PNH cells and not an artefact.

Significance of flow cytometric analysis

The presence of a population of cells with a deficiency of more than one GPI-linked protein is diagnostic of PNH (Fig. 15.3). It is important to analyse more than one protein because there are extremely rare cases in which an inherited deficiency of one protein has been described (i.e. the Inab-phenotype[31,32,51]—a deficiency of DAF due to a defect of the structural gene for DAF; inherited deficiency of CD59[54] due to a defect of the CD59 structural gene). Analysis of the expression of CD59 on erythrocytes allows the identification of PNH type II as well as PNH Type-III red cells. This is important because although patients with only PNH Type-II red cells do not usually suffer from significant haemolysis they may suffer some of the complications of PNH, such as thrombosis. The analysis of neutrophils for GPI-linked proteins is more difficult than red cell analysis. It is, however, probably more sensitive as the proportion of abnormal neutrophils is usually higher than the proportion

of PNH red cells because of the reduced survival of PNH red cells compared to normal and because of the effect of transfusions. Thus flow cytometry applied to neutrophils is a more sensitive method for the diagnosis of PNH than methods relying on the complement sensitivity of PNH red cells.

OTHER TESTS FOR PNH

Various other tests which depend upon the complement sensitivity have been used for the diagnosis of PNH. These include the thrombin test,[7] the cobra venom test,[25] the heat resistance test[20] and the inulin test.[3] None of these tests is superior to the Ham test and most are inferior. These tests will not be described in detail but readers are referred to the 7th edition of this book should a detailed account be required.

PNH-LIKE RED CELLS

By treating normal red cells with certain chemicals it is possible to increase their complement sensitivity so that they take on many of the characteristics of PNH cells.[46] The chemicals include sulphydryl compounds such as L-cysteine, reduced gluthathione (GSH), 2-aminoethyl-*iso*-thiouronium bromide (AET) and 2-mercaptobenzoic acid (MBA).[13] AET and MBA cells can be used conveniently as a positive control for in-vitro lysis tests for PNH.[49]

Preparation of AET cells[47]

Prepare an 8 g/l solution of AET and adjust its pH to 8.0 with 5 mol/l NaOH. Collect normal blood into ACD and wash it twice in 9 g/l NaCl (saline). Add 1 volume of the packed cells to 4 volumes of the AET solution in a 75 × 12 mm glass tube which is then stoppered. Mix the contents gently and place the tube at 37°C for 10–20 min. (According to Jenkins, the optimal time of incubation varies from red cell sample to red cell sample.[24]) Then wash the cells repeatedly with large volumes of saline until the supernatant is colourless. The red cells are now ready to use.

SUMMARY

The Ham test remains the main diagnostic test

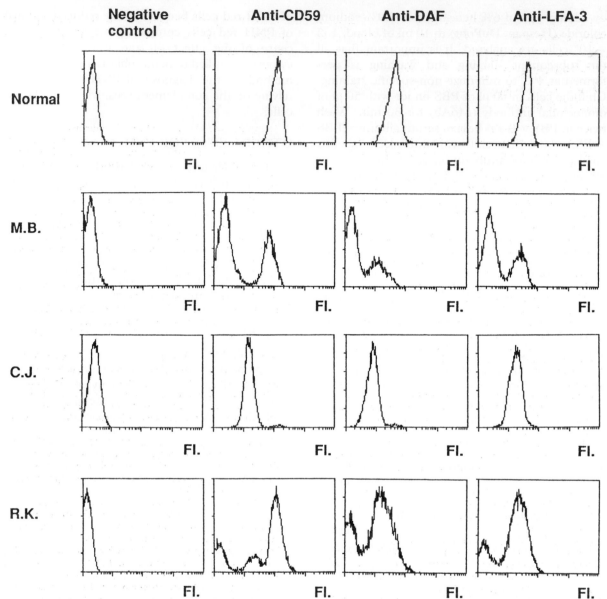

Fig. 15.3   Expression of GPI-linked proteins on the red cells in PNH. Flow cytometry of the erythrocytes from a normal control and 3 patients with PNH stained with a negative control antibody and antibodies to several GPI-linked proteins.
M.B: 2 populations; normal and absent GPI-linked proteins.
C.J: Mainly reduced GPI-linked proteins, but there is also a very small normal component present.
R.K: 3 populations; normal, reduced and absent GPI-linked proteins.
Fl.: fluorescence intensity.

for PNH. If carried out with additional magnesium chloride, and performed with the necessary controls, it is even more sensitive and it remains specific for the diagnosis of PNH. The inclusion of a further test, such as the sucrose lysis test, is optional. The use of flow cytometry gives a better estimate of the size of the PNH clone and identifies the type of red cell abnormality. However, more experience and expensive equipment is required to perform flow cytometry reliably than to perform a Ham test. Flow cytometry is a useful diagnostic test in certain circumstances, especially when the patient is heavily transfused, and therefore neutrophils must be analysed; or when following a patient after bone marrow transplantaion. Flow cytometry may also be useful in the follow-up of groups of patients with aplastic anaemia as clonal evolution into PNH may be detected at an earlier stage.

REFERENCES

[1] AUDITORE, J. V. and HARTMANN, R. C. (1959). Paroxysmal nocturnal hemoglobinuria: II. Erythrocyte acetylcholinesterase defect. *American Journal of Medicine*, **27**, 401.

[2] BECK, W. S. and VALENTINE, W. N. (1965). Biochemical studies on leucocytes. II. Phosphatase activity in chronic lymphatic leucemia, acute leucemia and miscellaneous hematologic conditions. *Journal of Laboratory and Clinical Medicine*, **38**, 245.

[3] BRUBAKER, L. H., SCHABERG, D. R., JEFFERSON, D. H. and MENGEL, C. E. (1973). A potential rapid screening test for paroxysmal nocturnal hemoglobinuria. *New England Journal of Medicine*, **288**, 1059.

[4] CATOVSKY, D., LEWIS, S. M. and SHERMAN, D. (1971). Erythrocyte sensitivity to in-vitro lysis in leukaemia. *British Journal of Haematology*, **21**, 541.

[5] CHOW, F.-L., TELEN, M. J. and ROSSE, W. F. (1985). The acetylcholinesterase defect in paroxysmal nocturnal hemoglobinuria: evidence that the enzyme is absent from the cell membrane. *Blood*, **66**, 940.

[6] CROOKSTON, J. H., CROOKSTON, M. C., BURNIE, K. L., FRANCOMBE, W. H., DACIE, J. V., DAVIS J. A. and LEWIS, S. M. (1969). Hereditary erythroblastic multinuclearity associated with a positive acidified-serum test: a type of congenital dyserythropoietic anaemia. *British Journal of Haematology*, **17**, 11.

[7] CROSBY, W. H. (1950). Paroxysmal nocturnal hemoglobinuria. A specific test for the disease based on the ability of thrombin to activate the hemolytic factor. *Blood*, **5**, 843.

[8] DACIE, J. V. and LEWIS, S. M. (1972). Paroxysmal nocturnal haemoglobinuria: clinical manifestations, haematology and nature of the disease. *Series Haematologica*, **5**, 3.

[9] DACIE, J. V., LEWIS, S. M. and TILLS, D. (1960). Comparative sensitivity of the erythrocytes in paroxysmal nocturnal haemoglobinuria to haemolysis by acidified normal serum and by a high-titre cold antibody. *British Journal of Haematology*, **6**, 362.

[10] DAVIES, A., SIMMONS, D. L., HALE, G., HARRISON, R. A., TIGHE, H., LACHMANN, P. J. and WALDMANN, H. (1989). CD59, an LY-6-like protein expressed in human lymphoid cells, regulates the action of the complement membrane attack complex on homologous cells. *Journal of Experimental Medicine*, **170**, 637.

[11] DE SANDRE, G., GHIOTTO, G. and MASTELLA, G. (1956). L'acetilcolinesterasi eritrocitaria. II. Rapporti con le malattie emolitiche. *Acta Medica Patavina*, **16**, 310.

[12] DE SANDRE, G. AND GHIOTTO, G. (1960). An enzymic disorder in the erythrocytes of paroxysmal nocturnal haemoglobinuria: a deficiency in acetylcholinesterase activity. *British Journal of Haematology*, **6**, 39.

[13] FRANCIS, D. A. (1983). Production of PNH-like red cells using 2-mercaptobenzoic acid. *Medical Laboratory Sciences*, **40**, 33.

[14] HAM, T. H. and DINGLE, J. H. (1939). Studies on destruction of red blood cells. II. Chronic hemolytic anemia with paroxysmal nocturnal hemoglobinuria: certain immunological aspects of the hemolytic mechanism with special reference to serum complement. *Journal of Clinical Investigation*, **18**, 657.

[15] HANSCH, G. M., SCHONERMARK, S. and ROEICKE, D. (1987). Paroxysmal nocturnal hemoglobinuria type III: lack of an erythrocyte membrane protein restricting the lysis by C5b-9. *Journal of Clinical Investigation*, **80**, 7.

[16] HANSEN, N. E. and KILLMAN, S.-A. (1969). Paroxysmal nocturnal haemoglobinuria. A clinical study. *Acta Medica Scandinavica*, **184**, 525.

[17] HARTMANN, R. C. and AUDITORE, J. V. (1959). Paroxysmal nocturnal hemoglobinuria I. Clinical studies. *American Journal of Medicine*, **27**, 389.

[18] HARTMANN, R. C. and JENKINS, D. E. Jr (1966). The 'sugar water' test for paroxysmal nocturnal hemoglobinuria. *New England Journal of Medicine*, **275**, 155.

[19] HARTMANN, R. C., JENKINS, D. E. Jr and ARNOLD, A. B. (1970). Diagnostic specificity of sucrose hemolysis test for paroxysmal nocturnal hemoglobinuria. *Blood*, **35**, 462.

[20] HEGGLIN, R. and MAIER, C. (1944). The 'heat resistance' of erythrocytes. A specific test for the recognition of Marchiafava's anemia. *American Journal of Medical Sciences*, **207**, 624.

[21] HILLMEN, P., HOWS, J. M. and LUZZATTO, L. (1992). Two distinct patterns of glycosylphosphatidylinositol (GPI) linked protein deficiency in the red cells of patients with paroxysmal nocturnal haemoglobinuria. *British Journal of Haematology*, **80**, 399.

[22] HOLGUIN, M. H., WILCOX, L. A., BERNSHAW, N. J., ROSSE, W. F. and PARKER, C. J. (1989). Relationship between the membrane inhibitor of reactive lysis and the erythrocyte phenotypes of paroxysmal nocturnal hemoglobinuria. *Journal of Clinical Investigation*, **84**, 1387.

[23] HOLGUIN, M. H., FREDRICK, N. J., BERNSHAW, L. A., WILCOX, L. A., and PARKER, C. J. (1989). Isolation and characterization of a membrane protein from normal human erythrocytes that inhibits reactive lysis of the erythrocytes of paroxysmal nocturnal hemoglobinuria. *Journal of Clinical Investigation*, **84**, 7.

[24] JENKINS, D. E. Jr (1979). Paroxysmal nocturnal hemoglobinuria hemolytic systems. In *A Seminar on Laboratory Management of Hemolysis*, pp. 45–49. American Association of Blood Banks, Washington.

[25] KABAKÇI, T., ROSSE, W. F. and LOGUE, G. L. (1972). The lysis of paroxysmal nocturnal haemoglobinuria red cells by serum and cobra factor. *British Journal of Haematology*, **23**, 693.

[26] KINOSHITA, T., MEDOF, M. E., SILBER, R., and NUSSENZWEIG, V. (1985). Distribution of decay-accelerating factor in the peripheral blood of normal individuals and patients with paroxysmal nocturnal hemoglobinuria. *Journal of Experimental Medicine*, **162**, 75.

[27] LEWIS, S. M. and DACIE, J. V. (1965). Neutrophil

(leucocyte) alkaline phosphatase in paroxysmal nocturnal haemoglobinuria. *British Journal of Haematology*, **11**, 549.

[28] LEWIS, S. M., DACIE, J. V. and TILLS, D. (1961). Comparison of the sensitivity to agglutination and haemolysis by a high-titre cold antibody of the erythrocytes of normal subjects and of patients with a variety of blood diseases including paroxysmal nocturnal haemoglobinuria. *British Journal of Haematology*, **7**, 64.

[29] LOGUE, G. L., ROSSI, W. F. and ADAMS, J. P. (1973). Mechanisms of immune lysis of red blood cells in vitro. I. Paroxysmal nocturnal hemoglobinuria cells. *Journal of Clinical Investigation*, **52**, 1129.

[30] MAY, J. E., ROSSE, W. F., and FRANK, M. M. (1973). Paroxysmal nocturnal hemoglobinuria: alternative-complement-pathway-mediated lysis induced by magnesium. *New England Journal of Medicine*, **289**, 705.

[31] MERRY, A. H., RAWLINSON, V. I., UCHIKAWA, M., DAHA, M. R. and SIM, R. B. (1989). Studies on the sensitivity to complement-mediated lysis of erythrocytes (Inab phenotype) with a deficiency of DAF (decay accelerating factor). *British Journal of Haematology*, **73**, 248.

[32] MERRY, A. H., RAWLINSON, V. I., UCHIKAWA, M., WATTS, M. J. and SIM, R. B. (1989). Lack of abnormal sensitivity to complement-mediated lysis in erythrocytes deficient only in decay accelerating factor. *Biochemical Society Transactions*, **17**, 514.

[33] MOLLISON, P. L. and POLLEY, M. J. (1964). Uptake of γ-globulin and complement by red cells exposed to serum at low ionic strength. *Nature (London)*, **203**, 535.

[34] NICHOLSON-WEBBER, A., MARCH, J. P., ROSENFIELD, S. I. and AUSTEN, K. F. (1983). Affected erythrocytes of patients with paroxysmal nocturnal hemoglobinuria are deficient in the complement regulatory protein, decay accelerating factor. *Proceedings of the National Academy of Sciences of the U.S.A.*, **80**, 5066.

[35] NICHOLSON-WELLER, A., SPICIER, D. B. and AUSTEN, K. F. (1985). Deficiency of the complement regulating protein 'decay accelerating factor' on membranes of granulocytes, monocytes, and platelets in paroxysmal nocturnal hemoglobinuria. *New England Journal of Medicine*, **312**, 1091.

[36] ONI, S. B., OSUNKOYA, B. O. and LUZZATTO, L. (1970). Paroxysmal nocturnal hemoglobinuria: evidence for monoclonal origin of abnormal red cells. *Blood*, **36**, 145.

[37] PACKMAN, C. H., ROSENFELD, S. I., JENKINS, D. E. Jr, THIEM, P. A. and LEDDY, J. P. (1979). Complement lysis of human erythrocytes. Differing susceptibility of two types of paroxysmal nocturnal hemoglobinuria cells to C5b-9. *Journal of Clinical Investigation*, **64**, 428.

[38] PANGBURN, M. K., SCHREIBER, R. D. and MÜLLER-EBERHARD, H. F. (1983). Deficiency of an erythrocyte membrane protein with complement regulatory activity in paroxysmal nocturnal hemoglobinuria. *Proceedings of the National Academy of Sciences U.S.A.*, **80**, 5430.

[39] PLESNER, T., HANSEN, N. E. and CARLSEN, K. (1990). Estimation of PI-bound proteins on blood cells from PNH patients by quantitative flow cytometry. *British Journal of Haematology*, **75**, 585.

[40] ROSSE, W. F. (1972). The complement sensitivity of PNH cells. *Series Haematologica*, **5**, 101.

[41] Rosse, W. F. (1973). Variations in the red cells in paroxysmal nocturnal haemoglobinuria. *British Journal of Haematology*, **24**, 327.

[42] ROSSE, W. F., ADAMS, J. P. and THORPE, A. M. (1974).

The population of cells in paroxysmal nocturnal haemoglobinuria of intermediate sensitivity to complement lysis: significance and mechanism of increased immune lysis. *British Journal of Haematology*, **28**, 281.

[43] ROSSE, W. F. and DACIE, J. V. (1966). Immune lysis of normal human and paroxysmal nocturnal hemoglobinuria (PNH) red blood cells. 1. The sensitivity of PNH red cells to lysis by complement and specific antibody. *Journal of Clinical Investigation*, **45**, 736.

[44] ROSSE, W. F., HOFFMAN, S., CAMPBELL, M., BOROWITZ, M., MOORE, J. O. and PARKER, C. J. (1991). The erythrocytes in paroxysmal nocturnal haemoglobinuria of intermediate sensitivity to complement lysis. *British Journal of Haematology*, **79**, 99.

[45] SHICHISHIMA, T., TERASAWA, T., HASHIMOTO, C., OHTO, H., UCHIDA, T. and MARUYAMA, Y. (1991). Heterogenous expression of decay accelerating factor and CD59/membrane attack complex inhibition factor on paroxysmal nocturnal haemoglobinuria (PNH) erythrocytes. *British Journal of Haematology*, **78**, 545.

[46] SIRCHIA, G. and FERRONE, S. (1972). The laboratory substitutes of the red cell of paroxysmal nocturnal haemoglobinuria (PNH): PNH-like red cells. *Series Haematologica*, **5**, 137.

[47] SIRCHIA, G., FERRONE, S. and MERCURIALI, F. (1965). The action of two sulfhydryl compounds on normal human red cells. Relationship to red cells of paroxysmal nocturnal hemoglobinuria. *Blood*, **25**, 502.

[48] SIRCHIA, G. and LEWIS, S. M. (1975). Paroxysmal nocturnal haemoglobinuria. *Clinics in Haematology*, **4**, 199.

[49] SIRCHIA, G., MARUBINI, E., MERCURIALI, F. and FERRONE, S. (1973). Study of two *in vitro* diagnostic tests for paroxysmal nocturnal haemoglobinuria. *British Journal of Haematology*, **24**, 751.

[50] STRATTON, F. and EVANS, D. I. K. (1967). Lysis of P.N.H. cells in solutions of low ionic strength. *British Journal of Haematology*, **13**, 862.

[51] TELEN, M. J. and GREEN, A. M. (1989). The Inab phenotype: characterization of the membrane protein and complement regulatory defect. *Blood*, **74**, 437.

[52] VAN DER SCHOOT, C. E., HUIZINGA, T. W. J., VAN'T VEER-KORTHOF, E. T., WIJMANS, R., PINKSTER, J. and VON DEM BORNE, A. E. G. K. (1990). Deficiency of glycosyl-phosphatidylinositol-linked membrane glycoproteins of leukocytes in paroxysmal nocturnal hemoglobinuria, description of a new diagnostic cytofluorometric assay. *Blood*, **76**, 1853.

[53] VERWILGHEN, R. L., LEWIS, S. M., DACIE, J. V., CROOKSTON, J. H. and CROOKSTON, M. C. (1973). HEMPAS: congenital dyserythropoietic anaemia (type II). *Quarterly Journal of Medicine*, **42**, 257.

[54] YAMASHINA, M., UEDA, E., KINOSHITA, T., TAKAMI, T., OJIMA, A., ONO, H., TANAKA, H., KONDO, N., ORIL, T., OKADA, N., OKADA, H., INOUE, K. and KITANI, T. (1990). Inherited complete deficiency of 20-kilodalton homologous restriction factor (CD59) as a cause of paroxysmal nocturnal hemoglobinuria. *New England Journal of Medicine*, **323**, 1184.

[55] ZALMAN, L. S., WOOD, L. M., FRANK, M. M. and MULLER-EBERHARD, H. J. (1987). Deficiency of the homologous restriction factor in paroxysmal nocturnal hemoglobinuria. *Journal of Experimental Medicine*, **165**, 572.

16. Investigation of haemostasis

Revised by M. A. Laffan and A. E. Bradshaw

The blood vessel 297
Platelets 298
Blood coagulation 300
The coagulation limiting mechanism 302
The fibrinolytic system 303
General approach to investigation of haemostasis 303
Notes on equipment and collection of samples 305

Prothrombin time (PT) 307
Activated partial thromboplastin time (APTT) 308
Thrombin time (TT) 309
Second line investigations 310
Mixing experiments using the APPT 312
Mixing experiments using the PT 313
Correction tests using the TT 314
Reptilase time 314

The haemostatic mechanisms have several important functions. First to maintain blood in a fluid state whilst it remains circulating within the vascular system. Second to arrest bleeding at the site of injury or blood loss by formation of a haemostatic plug. Third, they must ensure the eventual removal of the plug when healing is complete. Normal physiology thus constitutes a delicate balance between these conflicting tendencies and a deficiency or exaggeration of any one may lead to either thrombosis or haemorrhage. There are at least five different components involved; blood vessels, platelets, plasma coagulation factors, their inhibitors and the fibrinolytic system. In this chapter a brief review of normal haemostasis is presented followed by a discussion on the general principles of basic tests used to investigate haemostasis. More detailed tests to identify specific abnormalities are discussed in Chapters 17 and 18.

THE BLOOD VESSEL

General structure of the blood vessel

The blood vessel wall has three layers: intima, media and adventitia. The intima consists of endothelium and subendothelial connective tissue and is separated from the media by the elastic lamina interna. Endothelial cells form a continuous monolayer lining all blood vessels. The structure and the function of the endothelial cells vary according to their location in the vascular tree, but they all share three important characteristics: they are 'non-thrombogenic', that is, they do not react with plasma or the cellular elements of the blood; they play an active role in supplying nutrients to the subendothelial structures, and they act as a barrier to macromolecules and particulate matter circulating in the blood stream. The permeability of the endothelium may vary under different conditions to allow various molecules and cells to pass.

Endothelial cell function[2,16,17]

The luminal surface of the endothelial cell is covered by the glycocalyx, a proteoglycan coat. It contains heparin sulphate and other glycosaminoglycans which are capable of activating antithrombin III, an important inhibitor of coagulation enzymes. Beneath the glycocalyx, there is a lipid bilayer membrane containing ADPase, an enzyme which degrades ADP which is a potent platelet agonist (see p 323). There are also various membrane-lined structures, such as vesicles and 'pits', which participate in transport across the membrane.

The endothelial cell also participates in vasoregulation: on one hand it metabolizes and inactivates vasoactive peptides; on the other hand, the endothelial cell can produce prostacyclin and thus inhibit platelet aggregation (see below). It can also generate angiotensin II, a local vasoconstrictor. Thrombin generated at the site of injury is rapidly bound to a specific product of the endothelial cell, thrombomodulin. When bound to this protein, thrombin can activate the protein C system to degrade and inhibit factors Va and VIIIa. Thrombin also stimulates the endothelial cell to produce plasminogen activator. The endothelium can also synthesize protein S, the cofactor for protein C. Finally endothelium produces von Willebrand factor (vWF) essential for platelet adhesion to the subendothelium. This is stored in specific granules called Weibel Palade bodies and is secreted partly into the circulation and partly towards the subendothelium.

The subendothelium[11,24]

The subendothelium consists of connective tissues composed of collagen, elastic tissues, proteoglycans and non-collagenous glycoproteins, including fibronectin and vWF. After vessel wall damage has occurred these components are exposed and are then responsible for platelet adherence. This appears to be mediated by vWF binding to collagen, particularly under high shear rate, but also to the microfibrils which have a greater affinity for vWF under some conditions. vWF then undergoes a conformational change. Platelets then bind to altered vWF and thence to the subendothelium via their surface membrane glycoprotein Ib.

Vasoconstriction[24]

Vessels with muscular coats contract following injury thus helping to arrest blood loss. Although not all coagulation reactions are enhanced by reduced flow, this probably assists in the formation of a stable fibrin plug. Vasoconstriction also occurs in the microcirculation in vessels without smooth muscle cells. Endothelial cells themselves can produce vasoconstrictors such as angiotensin II. In addition, activated platelets produce thromboxane (TXA_2) which is a potent vasoconstrictor.

PLATELETS

Platelets are small fragments of cytoplasm derived from megakaryocytes. On average they are 1.5–3.5 μm in diameter but may be larger in some disease states. They do not contain a nucleus and are bounded by a typical lipid bilayer membrane. Beneath the outer membrane lies the marginal band of microtubules which maintain the shape of the platelet and depolymerize when aggregation begins. The central cytoplasm is dominated by the three types of platelet granules: the dense granules, α granules, and lysosomal granules. The contents of these various granules are detailed in Table 16.1. Finally there exists the dense tubular system and the canalicular membrane system; the latter of which communicates with the exterior. It is not clear how all these elements act together to perform such functions as contraction and secretion, characteristic of platelet activation.

The platelet membrane. This is the site of interaction with the plasma environment and with damaged vessel wall. It consists of phospholipids, cholesterol, glycolipids and at least nine glycoproteins, named GpI–GpIX. The membrane phospholipids are asymmetrically distributed, with sphingomyelin and phosphatidylcholine predominating in the outer leaflet, and phosphatidylethanolamine, -inositol and -serine in the inner leaflet.

The contractile system of the platelet. This consists of the dense microtubular system and

Table 16.1   Contents of platelet granules

Dense (δ) granules	α Granules	Lysosomal vesicles
ATP	PF4	Galactosidases
ADP	β-Thromboglobulin	Fucosidases
GDP	Fibrinogen	Hexosaminidase
GTP	FVIII	Glucuronidase
Calcium	vWF	+ others
Serotonin	Thrombospondin	
Pyrophosphate	Fibronectin	
	PDGF	
	PAI-1	

the circumferential microfilaments which maintain the disc shape. Actin is the main constituent of the contractile system, but myosin and a regulatory calcium binding protein, calmodulin, are also present.

Platelet function in the haemostatic process[27]

When the vessel wall is damaged, the subendothelial structures, including basement membrane, collagen and microfibrils, are exposed. Surface bound vWF binds to GpIb on circulating platelets resulting in an initial monolayer of adhering platelets. Once activated, platelets immediately change shape from a disc to a tiny sphere with numerous projecting pseudopods. After adhesion of a single layer of platelets to the exposed subendothelium, platelets stick to one another to form aggregates. Fibrinogen, fibronectin and the glycoprotein Ib–IX complex are essential at this stage to increase the cell to cell contact and facilitate aggregation. Certain substances (agonists) react with specific platelet membrane receptors and initiate platelet aggregation and further activation. The agonists include: exposed collagen fibres, ADP, adrenaline, serotonin and certain arachidonic acid metabolites including thromboxane $A_2(TXA_2)$. In areas of non-linear blood flow such as may occur at the site of an injury, locally damaged red cells release ADP which further activates platelets.

Platelet aggregation

Platelet aggregation may occur by at least two independent but closely linked pathways.[28] The first pathway involves arachidonic acid metabolism. Activation of phospholipase enzymes releases free arachidonic acid from the membrane phospholipids. About 50% of free arachidonic acid is converted by a lipo-oxygenase enzyme to a series of products including leucotrienes which are important chemoattractants of white cells. The remaining 50% of arachidonic acid is converted by the enzyme cyclo-oxygenase into labile cyclic endoperoxides, most of which are in turn converted by thromboxane synthetase into TXA_2. TXA_2 has profound biological effects, causing platelet granule release and local vasoconstriction, as well as further local platelet aggregation. It exerts these effects by raising intracellular cytoplasmic free calcium concentration and binding to specify granule receptors. TXA_2 is very labile with a half-life of less than 1 min before being degraded into the inactive thromboxane B_2 (TXB_2) and malonyldialdehyde.

The second pathway of activation and aggregation can proceed completely independently from the first one: various platelet agonists, including thrombin and collagen, produce a brisk increase in the free cytoplasmic calcium to cause the release reaction. Calcium is released from the dense tubular system to form complexes with calmodulin; this complex and the free calcium act as co-enzymes for the release reaction, for the activation of different regulatory proteins, as well as of actin and myosin and the contractile system, and also for the liberation of arachidonic acid from membrane phospholipids and the generation of TXA_2.

The aggregating platelets align together into loose reversible aggregates, but after the release reaction of the platelet granules, a larger, firmer aggregate forms. Changes in the platelet membrane configuration now occur: 'flip-flop' arrangement of the surface brings the negatively charged phosphatidylserine and inositol on to the outer leaflet, thus generating platelet factor 3 (procoagulant) activity. At the same time specific receptors for various coagulation factors are exposed on the platelet surface and help coordinate the assembly of the enzymatic complexes. Local generation of thrombin will then further activate platelets.

Platelets are not activated if in contact with healthy endothelial cells. The 'non-thrombogenicity' of the endothelium is due to a combination of control mechanisms exerted by the endothelial cell: synthesis of prostacyclin, capacity to bind thrombin and activate the protein C system and ability to inactivate vasoactive substances, etc. (see p. 302). Prostacyclin released locally binds to specific platelet membrane receptors and then activates the membrane-bound adenylate cyclase (producing c-AMP). c-AMP inhibits platelet aggregation by inhibiting arachidonic acid metabolism and the release of free cytoplasmic calcium ions.

BLOOD COAGULATION[19]

The central event in the coagulation pathways is the production of thrombin which acts upon fibrinogen to produce fibrin and thus the fibrin clot. This clot is further strengthened by the crosslinking action of factor XIII which itself is activated by thrombin. The two commonly used coagulation tests, the activated partial thromboplastin time (APTT) and the prothrombin time (PT) have been used historically to define two pathways of coagulation activation; the intrinsic and extrinsic paths, respectively. However, it is clear that this bears only a limited relationship to the way coagulation is activated in vivo. For example, deficiencies of the contact factors or of factor VIII both produce marked prolongation of the APTT but only the deficiency of the latter is associated with a haemorrhagic tendency. Moreover, there is considerable evidence that activation of factor IX (intrinsic pathway) by factor VIIa (extrinsic pathway) is crucial to establishing coagulation after an initial stimulus has been provided by factor VII-tissue factor (TF) activation of FX.[5] See Fig 16.1.

Investigation of the coagulation system centres on the coagulation factors but the activity of these proteins is also greatly dependent on specific surface receptors and phospholipids largely presented on the surface of platelets but also by activated endothelium. The necessity for calcium in many of these reactions is frequently utilized to control their activity in vitro. The various factors are described below, as far as possible in their functional groups and their properties detailed in Table 16.2.

The contact activation system

This system comprises factor XII (Hageman factor), high molecular weight kininogen (HMWK) (Fitzgerald factor) and prekallikrein/kallikrein (Fletcher factor). As mentioned above these factors do not appear to be essential for haemostasis in vivo. There is some evidence that their ability to activate the fibrinolytic system may be functionally more important.

The contact activation system results in the generation of factor XIIa which is able to activate factor XI thus initiating the coagulation cascade of the intrinsic pathway. When bound to a

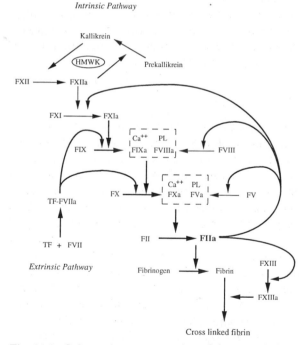

Fig. 16.1 Schematic representation of the coagulation cascade. The major interactions are shown by the bold arrows. Inhibitory factors and clot-limiting mechanisms are not shown. PL, phospholipid; HMWK, high molecular weight kininogen.

Table 16.2   The coagulation factors

No.	Factor	RMM*	Half-life	Concentration in plasma (mg/dl)
I	Fibrinogen	340 000	90 h	150.0–400.0
II	Prothrombin	72 000	60 h	10.0–15.0
V	–	330 000	12–36 h	0.5–1.0
VII	–	48 000	6 h	1.0
VIII	–	200 000	12 h	<0.01
vWF	–	800 000–140 000 000	24 h	0.5–1.0
IX	–	57 000	12 h	0.01
X	–	58 000	24 h	0.75
XI	–	160 000	40 h	1.2
XII	–	80 000	48–52 h	0.4
Pre-kallikrein	–	85 000	48–52 h	0.3
HMWK	–	110 000	6.5 days	2.5
XIII	–	32 000	3–5 days	2.5

*Relative molecular mass (molecular weight).

negatively charged surface, factor XII and prekallikrein are able to reciprocally activate one another by limited proteolysis but the initiating event is not clear. Possibly a conformational change in factor XII on binding results in limited auto-activation which triggers the process. HMWK acts as a co-factor by facilitating the attachment of prekallikrein and factor XI, with which it circulates in a complex, to the negatively charged surface.[23] It has been shown in in-vitro studies that platelets can provide the necessary negatively charged surface for this mechanism and also possess specific receptors for factor XI.

Tissue factor

Tissue factor is the co-factor for the extrinsic pathway. It is a lipoprotein which is membrane bound and present in many tissues and on the surface of stimulated inflammatory cells such as macrophages. It is likely in most situations where damage to vessel walls has occurred that TF is responsible for the activation of coagulation. TF combines with factor VII in the presence of calcium ions and this complex is then capable of activating factor X to factor Xa. Factor Xa in turn converts factor VII to its active two-chain form thus increasing its coagulant activity. The factor VII-TF complex can activate both factor X and factor IX and therefore two routes to thrombin production are stimulated. Factor Xa may subsequently bind to tissue factor pathway inhibitor (TFPI) and then to factor VIIa to form a quaternary complex. This mechanism therefore functions to shut off the extrinsic pathway after the initial stimulus to coagulation has been provided.

The vitamin K dependent factors

This group comprises factors II, VII, IX and X. However, it is important to remember that the anticoagulant proteins S and C are also vitamin K dependent. Each of these proteins contains a number of glutamic acid residues at its amino terminus that are γ-carboxylated by a vitamin K dependent mechanism. This results in a novel amino acid, γ-carboxyglutamic acid, which appears to be important in binding the factor to phospholipid.[22] Because this binding is crucial for coordinating the interaction of the various factors, the proteins produced in the absence of vitamin K (PIVKAs) which are not γ-carboxylated are essentially functionless. The vitamin K dependent factors are pro-enzymes or zymogens which require cleavage of a small peptide (activation peptide) in order to become functional. Measurement of these activation peptides has become a useful test for measuring coagulation activation.

Labile factors

Factors VIII and V are the two most labile of the coagulation factors and are rapidly lost from stored blood or heated plasma. They share considerable structural homology and are co-factors for the serine proteases FIX and FX, respectively.

Finally, they both require proteolytic activation by factor IIa or Xa in order to function. Factor VIII circulates in combination with von Willebrand factor (vWF) which is present in the form of large multimers of a basic 200 000 kD monomer.[29] Von Willebrand factor serves to stabilize factor VIII and protect it from degradation. In the absence of vWF the survival of factor VIII in the circulation is extremely short, i.e. a few minutes instead of the normal 8–12 h. vWF may also serve to deliver factor VIII to platelets adherent to a site of vascular injury. Once factor VIII has been cleaved and activated by thrombin it no longer binds to vWF.

Fibrinogen

Fibrinogen is a large dimeric protein, each half consisting of three polypeptides named $A\alpha$, $B\beta$ and $G\gamma$ held together by 12 disulphide bonds. The two monomers are joined together by a further three disulphide bonds. Fibrin is formed from fibrinogen by thrombin cleavage of the A and B peptides from fibrinogen. This results in fibrin monomers that associate to form a polymer that is the visible clot. The central E domain exposed by thrombin cleavage then binds with a complementary region on the outer or D domain of another monomer. The monomers thus assemble into a staggered overlapping two-stranded fibril. More complex interactions subsequently lead to branched and thickened fibre formation.[10,14]

Factor XIII

The initial fibrin clot is held together by non-covalent interactions and can be deformed and resolubilized. Factor XIII which is also activated by thrombin is able to covalently cross-link these fibrin monomers. Factor XIII is a transglutaminase which joins a glutamine residue on one chain to a lysine on an adjacent chain. This loss of resolubility is the basis of the screening test for factor XIII deficiency.

THE COAGULATION LIMITING MECHANISM[13]

Clearly, the production of the fibrin clot must be limited to the site of injury and not allowed to propagate indefinitely. A number of mechanisms exist to ensure that this is so. Firstly there are a number of proteins which bind to and inactivate the enzymes of the coagulation cascade. Probably the first of these to become active is tissue factor pathway inhibitor (TFPI) which rapidly quenches the factor VII-TF complex that initiates coagulation. It does this in combination with factor Xa so that coagulation is thereafter dependent on the small amount of thrombin that has been generated.

The principal physiological inactivator of thrombin is antithrombin ATIII which belongs to the serpine group of proteins. This binds to factor IIa forming an inactive thrombin-antithrombin complex (TAT) which is subsequently cleared from the circulation by the liver. This process is greatly enhanced by the presence of heparin. ATIII is responsible for approximately 60% of thrombin inactivating capacity in the plasma, the remainder is provided by heparin cofactor II and less specific inhibitors such as $\alpha2$ macroglobulin. ATIII is also capable of inactivating factors X, IX, XI and XII but to lesser degrees than thrombin.

As thrombin spreads away from the area of damage it is also bound by thrombomodulin on the surface of endothelial cells. In doing so it is changed from a primarily procoagulant protein to an anticoagulant one. Whilst remaining available for binding to ATIII, thrombin bound to thrombomodulin no longer cleaves fibrinogen. It now has a greatly enhanced preference for Protein C (PC) as a substrate. Protein C activated by thrombin cleavage acts to limit and arrest coagulation by inactivating factors Va and VIIIa. This action is further enhanced by its co-factor protein S which does not require prior activation. There is some evidence that a second as yet uncharacterized co-factor for protein C exists.[4] Protein C is subsequently inactivated by its own specific inhibitor.

THE FIBRINOLYTIC SYSTEM[3]

The deposition of fibrin and its removal are regulated by the fibrinolytic system. Although this is a complex multicomponent system with many activators and inhibitors it centres around the fibrinogen- and fibrin-cleaving enzyme plasmin.[26] Plasmin circulates in its inactive precursor form, plasminogen, which is activated by proteolytic cleavage. The principal plasminogen activator (PA) in man is tissue plasminogen activator (t-PA) which is another serine protease. t-PA and plasminogen are both able to bind to fibrin via the amino acid lysine. When they are both bound the rate of plasminogen activation is markedly increased and thus plasmin is generated preferentially at its site of action and not free in plasma. The principal other physiological PA in humans is called urokinase (u-PA). This single chain molecule (scu-PA) is activated by plasmin or kallikrein to a two-chain derivative (tcu-PA) which is not fibrin-specific in its action. However, the extent to which this is important in vivo is not clear and the identification of cell surface receptors for u-PA suggests that its primary role may be extravascular. The contact activation system also appears to generate some plasminogen activation via FXIIa. The degradation products released by the action of plasmin on fibrin are of diagnostic use and are discussed below.

PAI-1 (plasminogen activator inhibitor-1) is a potent inhibitor of t-PA, produced primarily by endothelial cells but also found in hepatocytes, platelets and placenta. Levels in plasma are highly variable. It is a member of the serpin family and is active against t-PA and tcu-PA but not scu-PA. A second inhibitor PAI-2 has also been identified, originally from human placenta, but its role and importance are not yet established.

The main physiological inhibitor of plasmin in plasma is α2-antiplasmin which inhibits plasmin function by forming a 1:1 complex (plasmin-anti plasmin complex; PAP). This reaction in free solution is extremely rapid but depends on the availability of free lysine-binding sites on the plasmin. Thus, fibrin-bound plasmin in the clot is not accessible to the inhibitor. Deficiencies of the fibrinolytic system are rare but have sometimes been associated with a tendency to thrombosis.

GENERAL APPROACH TO INVESTIGATION OF HAEMOSTASIS

This section begins with some general points regarding the collection of samples for investigation and the general principles underlying the analyses. Following this the basic or first-line screening tests of haemostasis are described. These tests are generally used as the first step in investigation of an acutely bleeding patient, a person with a suspected bleeding tendency or as a precaution before an invasive procedure is carried out. They have the virtue that they are easily performed and the patterns of abnormalities obtained point clearly to the appropriate next set of investigations. If should be remembered, however, that these tests may be normal in the presence of a mild but significant bleeding diathesis such as vWD. These questions are dealt with further in Chapter 17.

Despite their simplicity it is clearly important that the results obtained from the first-line tests are reproducible and accurate. This requires attention to blood sample collection and processing, selection, preparation and storage of reagents and the use of appropriate controls and standards. Laboratories should participate in local or national quality assessment schemes.

Principles of laboratory analysis

It is worth remembering that the tests of coagulation performed in the laboratory are attempts to mimic in vitro processes that normally occur in vivo. Not surprisingly this may give rise to misleading results. One of the most striking is the gross prolongation of the APTT in complete factor XII deficiency in the absence of any bleeding tendency. Similarly, the amount of factor VII required to produce a normal PT is greatly in excess of the amount required for normal haemostasis. Conversely, as previously mentioned, normal screening tests do not necessarily imply that the patient has entirely normal haemostasis. The only in-vivo test of coagulation that is commonly performed is the bleeding time and even with this test there are notable discrepancies between the results and the clinical bleeding propensity.

The more detailed investigations of coagulation proteins also require caution in their interpretation — depending on the type of assay performed. These can be divided into three principal categories.

Immunological[7]

These include immuno-diffusion, immuno-electrophoresis, radioimmunometric assays, latex agglutination tests and tests using enzyme-linked antibodies. Fundamentally, all these tests rely on the recognition of the protein in question by a polyclonal or monoclonal antibody. They are often easy to perform, particularly convenient for large batches, and can be bought as kits with standardized controls. The obvious drawback of these assays is that they may tell you nothing about the functional capacity of the antigen detected. It is preferable therefore that they are always carried out in parallel with a functional assay.

Assays using chromogenic peptide substrates (amidolytic assays)

The serine proteases of the coagulation cascade have narrow substrate specificities. It is possible to synthesize a short peptide specific for each enzyme that has a dye (p-nitroaniline; p-NA) attached to the terminal amino acid. When the synthetic peptide reacts with the specific enzyme the dye is released and the rate of its release or the total amount released can be measured photometrically. This gives a measure of the enzyme activity present.[1,8]

Chromogenic substrate assays can be classified into direct and indirect assays. Direct assays can be further sub-classified into primary assays in which a substrate specific for the enzyme to be measured is used and secondary assays in which the enzyme or pro-enzyme measured is used to activate a second protease for which a specific substrate is available. Specific substrates are available for kallikrein, factor Xa, thrombin, activated protein C, plasmin and urokinase. Indirect assays are used to measure naturally occurring inhibitors and some platelet factors.

It should be remembered that the measurement of amidolytic activity is not the same as the measurement of biological activity in a coagulation assay. This is particularly important when dealing with the molecular variants of various coagulation factors. Nevertheless, the continuing development of more specific substrates with good solubility and high affinity for individual enzymes, together with rapid advances in automation, make chromogenic substrate assays increasingly popular. The assays can be carried out in a tube when a spectrophotometer is used to measure the intensity of the colour development, or in a microtitre plate when the colour is noted by eye.

Coagulation assays

These assays are functional bioassays and rely on comparison with a control or standard preparation with a known level of activity. The assay can be performed using either a one-stage or two-stage system. In the one-stage system optimal amounts of all the clotting factors are present except the one to be determined, which should be as near to nil as possible. The best one-stage system is provided by a substrate plasma either obtained from a severely congenitally deficient patient or artificially depleted by immuno-adsorption. In the two-stage assay, the coagulation enzyme is generated in a two-step system and there is no requirement for a factor-deficient substrate plasma. The principles of bioassay, its standardization and limitations are considered in detail in Chapter 17.

Coagulation techniques are also used in mixing tests to identify a missing factor in an emergency, or to identify and estimate quantitatively an inhibitor or anticoagulant. The advantage of this type of assay is clearly that it most closely approximates to the activity in vivo of the factor in question. However, they can be technically more difficult to perform than the other types described above.

Other assays

These include measurement of coagulation factors using snake venoms, assay of ristocetin cofactor and the clot solubility test for factor XIII.

Technical errors

Some common 'technical' errors

An artifactual abnormality of the clotting time occurs in the following situations:

1. Faulty collection of the sample, resulting in it

undergoing partial clotting, can lead to a shortening of the APTT.

2. Excess citrate or insufficient blood so that the volume of citrate in relation to the blood is incorrect.
3. An unsuitable anticoagulant, such as EDTA, used in collecting the sample.
4. Collection of blood through a line that has at some stage been in contact with heparin. This leads to a marked prolongation of the APTT.
5. Contamination of the kaolin/platelet substitute reagent with a trace of thromboplastin. This can shorten the APTT.
6. Incorrect water-bath temperature.

NOTES ON EQUIPMENT AND COLLECTION OF SAMPLES

Collection of venous blood

Venous blood samples should be obtained whenever possible, even from the neonate. Peripheral blood tests require modification of techniques, experienced operators and locally established normal ranges; they are not an easy alternative to tests on venous blood.[25] Blood is withdrawn without undue venous stasis and without frothing into a plastic syringe or an evacuated system. The venepuncture must be 'clean'; blood from indwelling catheters should never be used for tests of haemostasis, as they are prone to dilution or heparin contamination. For investigation of acute haemostatic failure, 10 ml of citrated blood (9 volumes of blood to 1 volume of 31.3 g/l aqueous trisodium citrate dihydrate or 38 g/l aqueous trisodium citrate pentahydrate) are required as well as an appropriate amount of blood taken into a screw-cap container containing dried EDTA so that a full blood count and platelet count can be carried out and a blood film made. The blood is thoroughly mixed with the anticoagulant by inverting the container several times. The samples should be brought to the laboratory as soon as possible. If urgent fibrinolysis tests are contemplated, the blood samples

should be kept on crushed ice until delivered to the laboratory.

Preparation of platelet-poor plasma

Platelet-poor plasma (PPP) is prepared by centrifugation at 2000g for 15 min at 4°C (approximately 4000 rev/min in a standard bench centrifuge). It should be kept at room temperature if it is to be used for prothrombin time tests, factor VII assays or platelet function testing, and at 4°C for other assays; the testing should preferably be completed within 2 h of collection. The samples may be frozen at −40°C for several weeks without a significant loss of activity in the case of most of the haemostatic components to be assayed.

Control blood samples

Control blood samples, obtained from a healthy subject, are treated as described above. Care should be taken when handling all plasma samples, whether test or control, because of the risk of transmission of hepatitis and HIV. Alternatively, commercial freeze-dried control plasma samples tested for viral contamination can be used.

Equipment

Water-baths set at 37°C should have a tolerance of no more than ± 0.5°C as temperature markedly affects the speed of clotting reactions. A water-bath with plastic or glass sides is preferable and some type of cross-illumination helps to determine the exact time of appearance of fibrin. At least four stop-watches are needed unless the laboratory is equipped with an automatic coagulometer. Automatic pipettes are also required.

If coagulometers are used, it is important to ensure that their temperature control and the mechanism for detecting the end-point are functioning properly. Although such instruments reduce observer error when a large number of samples are tested, it is important to apply stringent control to the instrument at all times to ensure accuracy and precision.

Reagents

Some reagents are common to most if not all first-line tests. They are described here, whereas the reagents specific for one test or assay only are described with the details of the relevant test.

$CaCl_2$. The working solution is best prepared from a commercial molar solution. Small volumes of 0.025 mol/l concentration should be frequently prepared and stored for short periods of time to avoid proliferation of microorganisms. Prewarmed $CaCl_2$ should always be discarded at the end of the working day.

Barbitone buffered saline pH 7.3–7.4 is recommended for most clotting tests. See p. 577 for preparation of barbitone buffered saline, pH 7.4.

Glyoxaline buffer. Dissolve 2.72 g of glyoxaline (imidazole) and 4.68 g of NaCl in 650 ml of water. Add 148.8 ml of 0.1 mol/l HCl and adjust the pH to 7.4. Adjust the volume to 1 litre with water.

Owren's veronal buffer

Sodium acetate	3.89 g.
Barbitone sodium	5.89 g.
Sodium chloride	6.8 g.

Dissolve the salts in 800 ml of water.
Add 21.5 ml of 1mol/l HCl, then make up to 1 litre with water, mix and check that the pH is 7.35.

Handling of samples and reagents

All plasma samples should be kept in plastic or siliconized glass tubes and placed on melting ice or at 4°C until used, except when cold activation of factor VII and platelets is to be avoided, in which case the plasma is then kept at room temperature. All pipetting should be performed using disposable plastic pipettes or automatic pipette tips. The actual clotting tests are performed at 37°C in new round-bottom glass tubes of standard size (10 or 12 mm external diameter). Ideally, all glassware should be disposable. If the tubes have to be re-used, scrupulous cleaning using chromic acid and a detergent such as 2% Decon 90 is essential.

Eliminating a time trend

The potential instability of biological reagents used in tests of haemostasis makes it desirable to arrange results so as to reduce bias related to time. Thus, if there is a significant length of time between the results with the patient's plasma and the results with the control sample, the difference may be due to the deterioration of one or more of the reagents or of the plasma itself rather than to a true defect or deficiency. In the simplest case, if there are two samples A and B, the readings should be carried out in the order A_1, B_1, B_2, A_2. Additional specimens are allowed for by inserting further letters into the design.[9]

The end-point

The visual properties of a clot depend to some extent on the rate of its formation: the shorter the clotting time the more opaque is the clot and the easier it is to detect. A slowly forming clot may appear as mere fibrin wisps. In manual work, the observer must try to adopt a uniform convention in selecting the moment in clot formation which will be accepted as the end-point. It is also important to ensure that the tube can be watched with its lower part under the water or while quickly dipped in and out so as to avoid cooling and a slowing down of the clot formation. Bubbles also make the determination of the end-point difficult. In instrumental work the coagulometer must be shown to detect long clotting times reliably and reproducibly. The various coagulometers available have different means of detecting the end-point which may make comparison of results difficult.

PROTHROMBIN TIME

Principle. The test measures the clotting time of plasma in the presence of an optimal concentration of tissue extract (thromboplastin) and indicates the overall efficiency of the extrinsic clotting system.[21] Although originally thought to measure prothrombin, the test is now known to depend also on reactions with factors V, VII and X, and on the fibrinogen concentration of the plasma.

Reagents

Patient's and control plasma samples. Platelet-poor plasma from the patient and control (see below) is obtained as described on p. 305. Note that plasma stored at 4°C may have a shortened prothrombin time as a result of factor VII activation in the cold.[15]

Thromboplastin. Thromboplastins are tissue extracts obtained from different species and different organs. Because of the potential hazard of slow viral and other infections from handling human brain, its use as a source of thromboplastin is no longer recommended. The majority of thromboplastins now in use are extracts of rabbit brain or lung. Each preparation has a different sensitivity to clotting factor deficiencies and defects, in particular to the defect induced by oral anticoagulants (see Chapter 19, p. 368). In addition, even the same type of thromboplastin may show variation between batches. Whenever possible, a preparation calibrated against the International Reference Thromboplastin should be used; a calibrated commercially available thromboplastin will have its International Sensitivity Index (ISI) determined and clearly labelled. For further details, see p. 369. It is also important to remember that some thromboplastins are not sensitive to an isolated factor VII deficiency. If the manufacturer does not state in the accompanying literature that the reagent is sensitive to factor VII, it is advisable to check whether it is capable of detecting this deficiency by performing a prothrombin time on a known factor-VII-deficient plasma.

CaCl$_2$. 0.025 mol/l.

Method

Deliver 0.1 ml of plasma into a glass tube placed in a water-bath and add 0.1 ml of thromboplastin. Wait 1–3 min to allow the mixture to warm. Then add 0.1 ml of warmed CaCl$_2$ and mix the contents of the tube. Start the stop-watch and record the end-point. Carry out the test in duplicate on the patient's and the control plasma. When a number of samples are to be tested as a batch, the samples and controls must be suitably staggered to eliminate the time bias.

Expression of results

The results are expressed as the mean of the duplicate readings in seconds or as the ratio of the mean patient's time to the mean normal control time. The control plasma is obtained from 20 normal men and women (non-pregnant and not on oral contraceptives) and the logarithmic mean normal PT (LMNPT) calculated. For further details and a discussion of the importance of the one-stage prothrombin time test in oral anticoagulant control, when results may be reported as an International Normalized Ratio (INR), see also Chapter 19.

Normal values

Normal values depend on the thromboplastin used, the exact technique and whether visual or instrumental end-point reading is used. With most rabbit thromboplastins the normal range of the prothrombin time is between 11 and 16 s. Each laboratory should establish its own normal range.

Interpretation

The common causes of prolonged one-stage prothrombin times are:

1. The administration of oral anticoagulant drugs (vitamin K antagonists).
2. Liver disease, particularly obstructive.
3. Vitamin K deficiency.

4. Disseminated intravascular coagulation.
5. Rarely, a previously undiagnosed factor VII, X, V or prothrombin deficiency or defect (see

pp. 328 and 341). *Note*: With factor X or factor V deficiency the APTT will also be prolonged.

ACTIVATED PARTIAL THROMBOPLASTIN TIME (APTT)[12,20]

This test is also known as the partial thromboplastin time with kaolin (PTTK) and the kaolin cephalin clotting time (KCCT).

Principle The test measures the clotting time of plasma after the activation of contact factors but without added tissue thromboplastin, and so indicates the overall efficiency of the intrinsic pathway. To standardize the activation of contact factors, the plasma is first pre-incubated with kaolin. A standardized phospholipid is provided to allow the test to be performed on platelet-poor plasma. The test depends not only on the contact factors and on factors VIII and IX, but also on the reactions with factors X, V, prothrombin and fibrinogen. It is also sensitive to the presence of circulating anticoagulants (inhibitors) and heparin.

Reagents

Platelet-poor plasma. From the patient and a control, stored as described previously.

Kaolin. 5 g/l (laboratory grade) in barbitone buffered saline, pH 7.4 (p. 577). Add a few glass beads to aid resuspension. The suspension is stable at room temperature. Other insoluble surface active substances such as celite or elagic acid can also be used.

Phospholipid. Many reagents are available; these contain different phospholipids. Each laboratory should use the reagent it is familiar with. When choosing a phospholipid reagent for the APTT, it is important to establish that the reagent is sensitive to deficiencies of factors VIII:C, IX and XI at concentrations of 20 to 25 IU/dl.[18] Reagents which fail to detect this reduction in factor VIII:C are too insensitive for routine use.

$CaCl_2$. 0.025 mol/l.

Method

Mix equal volumes of the phospholipid reagent and the kaolin suspension and leave in a glass tube in the water-bath at 37°C. Place 0.1 ml of plasma into a new glass tube. Add 0.2 ml of the kaolin-phospholipid solution, mix the contents and start the stop-watch simultaneously. Leave at 37°C for 10 min with occasional shaking. At exactly 10 min add 0.1 ml of pre-warmed $CaCl_2$ and start a second stop-watch. Record the time taken for the mixture to clot. Repeat the test at least once on both the patient's and the control plasma. It is possible to do four tests at 2-min intervals if sufficient stop-watches are available.

Expression of results

Express the results as the mean of the paired clotting times.

Normal range

30–40 s. The actual times depend on the reagents used and the duration of the pre-incubation period. These variables also greatly alter the sensitivity of the test to minor or moderate deficiencies of the contact activation system. Laboratories can choose appropriate conditions to achieve the sensitivity they require. Each laboratory should calculate its own normal range.

Interpretation

The common causes of a prolonged APTT are:

1. Disseminated intravascular coagulation.
2. Liver disease.
3. Massive transfusion with stored blood.
4. Administration of heparin or contamination with heparin.
5. A circulating anticoagulant.
6. Deficiency of a coagulation factor other than factor VII.

The APTT is also moderately prolonged in patients on oral anticoagulant drugs and in the presence of vitamin K deficiency. Occasionally, a patient with previously undiagnosed haemophilia or another congenital coagulation disorder presents with a prolonged APTT (see Chapter 17). If the patient's APTT is abnormally long, the equal mixture test must be set up (see below).

Deficiency or circulating anticoagulant?

In cases with a long APTT, a 50:50 mixture of normal and test plasma should be tested. If the APTT of the mixture is reduced by more than 50% of the difference between the two individual clotting times; i.e. the normal plasma corrects the prolonged times, the patient probably has a deficiency of one or more clotting factors. This mixture should be incubated at 37°C for 2 h before testing because factor VIII inhibitors are time-dependent in their action. Controls should be incubated for the same length of time as this results in a lengthening of the APTT of normal plasma. If the normal plasma fails to correct, an inhibitor or anticoagulant may be present. For details of testing for inhibitors, see p. 339.

THROMBIN TIME (TT)

Principle. Thrombin is added to plasma and the clotting time measured. The thrombin time is affected by the concentration and reaction of fibrinogen, and by the presence of inhibitory substances, including fibrinogen/fibrin degradation products (FDP) and heparin. The clotting time and the appearance of the clot are equally informative.

Reagents

Platelet-poor plasma. From the patient and a control.

Thrombin solution. A commercial bovine thrombin is used. It is stored frozen as a 50 NIH unit solution, and freshly diluted in barbitone buffered saline in a plastic tube so as to give a clotting time of normal plasma of 17 s (usually c7–8 NIH thrombin units per ml). Shorter times with normal plasma may fail to detect mild abnormalities.

Method

Place 0.1 ml of barbitone buffered saline, pH 7.4 (p. 577) and 0.1 ml of control plasma in a glass tube at 37°C. Add 0.1 ml of thrombin and start the stop-watch. Measure the clotting time and observe the nature of the clot, e.g. whether transparent or opaque, firm or wispy, etc. Repeat the procedure with two tubes containing patient's plasma in duplicate, and then with a second sample of control plasma.

Expression of results

The results are expressed as the mean of the duplicate clotting times in seconds for the control and the test plasma.

Normal range

A patient's thrombin time should be within 2 s of the control (i.e. 15–19 s). Times of 20 s and over are definitely abnormal.

Interpretation of results

The common causes of prolonged thrombin time are:

1. Hypofibrinogenaemia as found in disseminated intravascular coagulation (DIC) and, more rarely, in a congenital defect or deficiency.

2. Raised concentrations of FDP, as encountered in DIC or liver disease.

3. Extreme prolongation of the TT is nearly always due to the presence of heparin which interferes with the thrombin-fibrinogen reaction. If the presence of heparin is suspected a Reptilase time test should be carried out (see p. 314).

4. Dysfibrinogenaemia, found either congenitally or acquired in liver disease, or in neonates.

A transparent bulky clot is found if fibrin polymerization is abnormal, as is the case in liver disease and some congenital dysfibrinogenaemias.

A gross elevation of the plasma fibrinogen concentration may also prolong the thrombin time. Correction can be obtained by diluting the patient's plasma with saline (see p. 313).

first-line tests described above often gives a reasonably clear indication of the underlying defect and determines the appropriate further tests required to define it. The patterns are outlined in Table 16.3 and discussed in detail below. The further tests which include specific factor assays and tests for DIC are found in Chapter 17.

Interpretation of first-line tests

The pattern of abnormalities obtained using the

Table 16.3   First-line tests used in investigating acute haemostatic failure

Test			Platelet count	Condition
PT	APTT	TT		
1. N	N	N	N	Disorder of platelet function. Factor XIII deficiency. Disorder of vascular haemostasis. Normal haemostasis
2. Long	N	N	N	Factor VII deficiency. Early oral anticoagulation
3. N	Long	N	N	Factors VIII:C, IX, XI, XII, prekallikrein, HMWK deficiency. von Willebrand's disease. Circulating anticoagulant
4. Long	Long	N	N	Vitamin K deficiency. Oral anticoagulants. Factors V, VII, X and II deficiency
5. Long	Long	Long	N	Heparin. Liver disease. Fibrinogen deficiency. Hyperfibrinolysis
6. N	N	N	Low	Thrombocytopenia
7. Long	Long	N	Low	Massive transfusion. Liver disease
8. Long	Long	Long	Low	DIC. Acute liver disease

N, Normal.

SECOND-LINE INVESTIGATIONS

Relevant second-line investigations are discussed with each of the possible patterns of abnormalities detected by the first-line tests.

1. PT: normal
   APTT: normal
   Thrombin time: normal
   Platelet count: normal

If all the first-line investigations are normal in a patient who continues to bleed from the site of an injury or after surgery, there are five possible diagnoses:

1. A disorder of platelet function, either congenital or acquired.
2. Factor XIII deficiency.
3. A vascular disorder of haemostasis.
4. Bleeding from a severely damaged vessel or vessels with normal haemostasis.
5. A mild coagulation disorder that is below the sensitivity of the routine tests to detect or which has been masked by the administration of blood products. This will include mild factor VIII deficiency (e.g. around 30% of normal) and some cases of von Willebrand's disease.

The second-line investigations required in this situation are the bleeding time, the clot solubility test and specific factor assays for the common deficiencies such as factor VIII or factor IX deficiency. These are described in Chapter 17.

2. PT: long
APTT: normal
Thrombin time: normal
Platelet count: normal

This combination of results is only found in:

1. The rare congenital factor VII deficiency.
2. At the start of oral anticoagulant therapy.

Factor VII assay is described in Chapter 17 (p. 328). It is usually possible to establish from the history whether the patient has received oral anticoagulant drugs within the preceding 12–36 h.

3. PT: normal
APTT: long
Thrombin time: normal
Platelet count: normal

An isolated prolonged APTT is found in:

1. Congenital deficiencies or defects of the intrinsic pathway, i.e. haemophilia A, haemophilia B, factor XI and factor XII deficiency, as well as in prekallikrein and high molecular weight kininogen deficiencies.
2. von Willebrand's disease, when it is usually associated with a prolonged bleeding time.
3. In the presence of circulating anticoagulants (inhibitors).
4. A common cause of a prolonged APTT is heparin, either because the patient is on treatment or because of sample contamination. However, the thrombin time is extremely sensitive to heparin and will also be prolonged. A Reptilase time should then be performed.

The next diagnostic step is to establish whether the patient has a deficiency or an inhibitor by performing the 50:50 mixture test described on p. 339. Mixing tests should be done immediately, followed by the specific assay, as described in Chapter 17, p. 340.

4. PT: long
APTT: long
Thrombin time: normal
Platelet count: normal

The main causes of a prolonged prothrombin and partial thromboplastin time in a patient who is bleeding either from a single site or has a generalized bleeding tendency are:

1. Lack of vitamin K. In this case the prothrombin time is usually relatively more prolonged than is the APTT.
2. The administration of oral anticoagulant drugs. The prothrombin time is usually more prolonged than is the APTT.
3. Liver disease.
4. Rare congenital defects of factors V, X, prothrombin, and combined V and VIII:C deficiency.

Mixing experiments using the prothrombin time may be useful if there is no history of anticoagulant therapy and no obvious reason for failure of vitamin K absorption, e.g. parenteral feeding, long-term antibiotic treatment, etc.

5. PT: long
APTT: long
Thrombin time: long
Platelet count: normal

Abnormalities in all three screening coagulation tests are found:

1. In the presence of heparin.
2. In hypo- and dys-fibrinogenaemias.
3. In some cases of liver disease.
4. In systemic hyperfibrinolysis.

To distinguish between these conditions, carry out thrombin time correction tests, the Reptilase or ancrod time, and measure the FDP concentration in plasma.

6. PT: normal
APTT: normal
Thrombin time: normal
Platelet count: low

If the only abnormality is a low platelet count its possible causes must be investigated. The usual approach is to perform a bone-marrow aspirate to exclude marrow failure and establish whether megakaryocytes are present. If the number of megakaryocytes in the marrow is normal, further investigations are undertaken to establish the cause of the presumed peripheral destruction of platelets.

7. PT: long
APTT: long
Thrombin time: normal
Platelet count: low

This pattern of abnormalities of the screening tests is found:

1. After massive transfusion with stored blood which contains adequate amounts of fibrinogen but does not contain factors VIII or V or platelets.
2. In some cases of chronic liver disease, especially cirrhosis.

8. PT: long
APTT: long
Thrombin time: long
Platelet count: low

All the first-line tests are abnormal in:

1. Acute disseminated intravascular coagulation (DIC).
2. Some cases of acute liver necrosis with DIC.

It is only exceptionally necessary to confirm the diagnosis of DIC with additional tests, e.g. by estimating FDP concentration and by carrying out a screening test for the presence of fibrin monomers.

MIXING EXPERIMENTS USING THE APTT

Principle

Plasma samples found to have a prolonged APTT are further investigated to define the abnormality by performing mixing or correction tests. Correction of the abnormality by the additive indicates that the reagent must contain the substance deficient in the test sample. An abnormal APTT is repeated on 50:50 mixtures of a known congenitally deficient plasma and the test plasma, or on 50:50 mixtures of aged/absorbed plasma and test plasma until correction is obtained and the missing factor identified.

Reagents

Platelet-poor plasma. From the patient and a control.

Plasma deficient in factors VIII, IX and XI. Note that individuals deficient in factor XII, pre-kallikrein or high molecular weight kininogen rarely if ever bleed despite a prolonged APTT.

Aged plasma. Platelet-poor plasma from a healthy donor is collected into a one-ninth volume of potassium oxalate (14 g of potassium oxalate per litre), and separated under sterile conditions and incubated at 37°C for 2–3 days. The prothrombin time at the end of this time should not exceed 90 s. Volumes of plasma are then delivered into plastic tubes and stored at –40°C. Aged plasma is deficient in factors V and VIII.

Absorbed plasma. Aluminium hydroxide gel (aluminia) is prepared by mixing 1 g of moist gel* with 4 ml of water to a smooth suspension. A one-tenth volume of aluminium hydroxide suspension is added to platelet-poor plasma prepared from a healthy subject, mixed and incubated for 2 min at 37°C. The mixture is then centrifuged to sediment the gel. The supernatant plasma is deficient in factors II (prothrombin), VII, IX and X.

---

*e.g. BDH Merck Ltd.

Other reagents. As described under partial thromboplastin time with kaolin (p. 308).

Method

Perform APTT on control, patient's and a known deficient plasma, followed by APTT on 50:50 (0.05 ml of each) mixtures of the control and a known deficient plasma and of patient's and a known deficient plasma. Perform all the tests in duplicate using a balanced order to avoid time bias; or perform APTT on mixtures of control, test, aged and absorbed plasma. Note that mixing experiments to detect factor VIII inhibitors require incubation for 2 h (see p. 340).

Interpretation

The failure to correct by a plasma with a known congenital defect indicates that the factor missing in the patient is the same as that missing in the known deficient plasma. Correction indicates that the factor missing in the known plasma and that missing in the patient's plasma are not identical. In many instances only a partial correction is possible because the congenitally deficient plasma samples may have been stored for long periods of time or are freeze-dried commercially-obtained preparations. It is therefore essential always to include a control normal plasma and mixtures with a control normal plasma in every experiment.

The interpretation of mixing tests with aged and absorbed plasma is shown in Table 16.4.

Table 16.4   Interpretation of mixing experiments with the APTT

APTT of test plasma corrected with		Interpretation
Aged plasma	Al(OH)$_3$ plasma	
No	Yes	Factor VIII deficiency
Yes	No	Factor IX deficiency
Yes	Yes	Factor XI or XII deficiency

MIXING EXPERIMENTS USING THE PROTHROMBIN TIME

Principle. The test plasma is mixed with aged and absorbed plasma to establish which factor is lacking.

Reagents

Platelet-poor plasma. From the patient and a control.
Absorbed plasma. See above.
Aged plasma. See p. 311.
Other reagents. As for prothrombin time.

Method

Measure the prothrombin time of 50:50 mixtures of test plasma and control with aged and absorbed plasma in a balanced order.

Interpretation

The results can be interpreted using Table 16.5.

Table 16.5   Interpretation of mixing experiments using the prothrombin time

PT of test plasma corrected with		Interpretation
Aged plasma	Al(OH)$_3$ plasma	
No	Yes	Factor V: deficiency
Yes	No	Factor X deficiency
Yes	Partial	Prothrombin deficiency

CORRECTION TESTS USING THE THROMBIN TIME

Principle. The tests utilize certain physico-chemical properties of reagents to bind to inhibitors or abnormal molecules and normalize the prolonged thrombin time. Protamine sulphate has a net electropositive charge and interacts with heparin, as well as binding to FDP, neutralizing the inhibitory effects of both. Toluidine blue is also a charged reagent which will neutralize heparin but has no effect on FDP. Interestingly, toluidine blue normalizes the thrombin time in some dysfibrinogenaemias, probably by interacting with the excess of sialic acid attached to the fibrinogen molecules. See Table 16.6.

Reagents

Patients and control plasma.
Protamine sulphate. 1% and 10% in 9 g/l NaCl.
Toluidine blue. 0.05 g in 100 ml of 9 g/l NaCl.

Table 16.6   Interpretation of correction tests using the thrombin time (TT)

Saline	TT of test plasma corrected with		Toluidine blue	Interpretation
	Normal plasma	Protamine sulphate		
No	Yes	No	No	Deficiency
No	Var	No	Yes	Dysfibrinogenaemia of liver disease
No	Var	Yes	Yes	High concentration of FDP

Var, variable.

Bovine thrombin. As described under thrombin time (p. 309).

Method

Perform the test as described for thrombin time, replacing 0.1 ml of saline in the test with protamine sulphate or toluidine blue solution. Also perform a thrombin time on a 50:50 mixture of control and test plasma.

Interpretation

See Table 16.6.

Comment

The end-point may be difficult to see in samples with a low fibrinogen content in the presence of toluidine blue owing to the dark colour of the reagent. Grossly elevated fibrinogen concentrations or the presence of a paraprotein can cause a prolonged time not corrected by either protamine or toluidine blue. Diluting the test plasma in saline will shorten the thrombin time.

REPTILASE OR ANCROD TIME[6]

Reptilase, a purified enzyme from the snake *Bothrops atrox*, and ancrod (Arvin), a similar enzyme from the snake *Agkistrodon rhodostoma*, may be used to replace thrombin in the thrombin time test.

The venoms are reconstituted as directed by the manufacturers, and the test is performed exactly as described for the thrombin time. The snake venoms are not inhibited by heparin and will give normal times for the clotting of normal plasma in the presence of heparin. The clotting times will, however, remain prolonged in the presence of raised FDP or abnormal or reduced fibrinogen.

REFERENCES

[1]BLOMBACK, M. and EGBERG, M. (1987). Chromogenic peptide substrates in the laboratory diagnosis of clotting disorders. In *Haemostasis and Thrombosis*. Eds. A. L. Bloom and D. P. Thomas, p. 967. Churchill Livingstone, Edinburgh.

[2]CHESTERMAN, C. N. and BERNDT, M. C. (1986). Platelet and vessel wall interaction and the genesis of atherosclerosis. *Clinics in Haematology*, **15**, 323.

[3]COLLEN, D. and LINJEN, H. R. (1991). Basic and clinical aspects of fibrinolysis and thrombolysis. *Blood*, **78**, 3114.

[4]DAHLBACK, B., CARLSSON, M. and SVENSSON, P. J. (1993). Familial thrombophilia due to a previously unrecognised mechanism characterised by poor anticoagulant response to activated protein C: Prediction of a cofactor to activated protein C. *Proceedings of the National Academy of Sciences USA*, **90**, 1004.

[5]DAVIE, E. W., FUJIKAWA, K. and KISIEL, W. (1991). The coagulation cascade: initiation, maintenance and regulation. *Biochemistry*, **30**, 10363.

[6]FUNK, C., GMUR, J., HEROLD, R. and STRAUB, P. W. (1971). Reptilase[R] — a new reagent in blood coagulation. *British Journal of Haematology*, **21**, 43.

[7]GIDDINGS, J. C. (1987). Immunoanalysis of haemostatic components. In *Haemostasis and Thrombosis*. Eds. A. L. Bloom and D. P. Thomas, p. 982. Churchill Livingstone, Edinburgh.

[8]HUTTON, R. A. (1987). Chromogenic substrates in haemostasis. *Blood Reviews*, **1**, 201.

[9]INGRAM, G. I. C., BROZOVIC, M. and SLATER, N. (1982). *Bleeding Disorders*. p. 243. Blackwell Scientific Publications, Oxford.

[10]LAMMLE, B. and GRIFFIN, J. H. (1985). Formation of fibrin clot: the balance of procoagulant and inhibitory factors. *Clinics in Haematology*, **14**, 281.

[11]LEGRANGE, Y. J. and FAUVEL-LAFEVE, F. (1992). Molecular mechanism of the interaction of subendothelial microfibrils with blood platelets. *Nouvelle Revue Française d'Hématologie*, **34**, 17.

[12]MACPHERSON, J. C. and HARDISTY, R. M. (1961). A modified thromboplastin screening test. *Thrombosis et Diathesis Haemorrhagica*, **6**, 492.

[13]MANNUCCI, P. M. and OWEN, W. G. (1987). Basic and clinical aspects of proteins C and S. In *Haemostasis and Thrombosis*. Eds. A. L. Bloom and D. P. Thomas, p. 452. Churchill Livingstone, Edinburgh.

[14]MARDER, V. J., FRANCIS, C. W. and DOOLITTLE, R. F., (1982). Fibrinogen. Structure and physiology. In *Haemostasis and Thrombosis*. Eds. R. W. COLEMAN, J. HIRSH, V. J. MARDER and E. W. SALZMAN, p. 145. J. B. Lippincott Co., Philadelphia.

[15]MILLER, G., SEGATCHIAN, M. J., WALTER, S. J., HOWARTH, D. J., THOMPSON, S. G., ESNOUF, M. P. (1986). An association between the factor VII coagulant activity and thrombin activity induced by surface/cold exposure of normal human plasma. *British Journal of Haematology*, **62**, 379.

[16]NAWROTH, P. P., HANDLEY, D. A. and STERN, D. M. (1986). The multiple levels of endothelial cell-coagulation factor interactions. *Clinics in Haematology*, **15**, 293.

[17]NAWROTH, P. P., KISIEL, W. and STERN, D. M. (1985). The role of endothelium in the homeostatic balance of haemostasis. *Clinics in Haematology*, **14**, 531.

[18]O'BRIEN, P. F., NORTH, W. R. S. and INGRAM, G. I. C. (1981). The diagnosis of mild haemophilia by the partial thromboplastin time. WFH/ICTH study of the Manchester method. *Thrombosis and Haemostasis*, **45**, 162.

[19]OGSTON, D. and BENNET, B. (1991). Blood coagulation mechanism. In *Recent Advances in Blood Coagulation*. Ed. L. Poller, Vol. 6, p. 1. Churchill Livingstone, Edinburgh.

[20]PROCTOR, R. R. and RAPAPORT, S. I. (1961). The partial thromboplastin time with kaolin. A simple screening test for first stage plasma clotting factor deficiencies. *American Journal of Clinical Pathology*, **36**, 212.

[21]QUICK, A. J. (1942). *The Hemorrhagic Diseases and the Physiology of Hemostasis*. Thomas, Illinois.

[22]SADOWSKI, J. A., BOVILL, E. G. and MANN, K. G. (1991). Warfarin and the metabolism of vitamin K. In *Recent Advances in Blood Coagulation*. Ed. L. Poller, Vol. 6, p. 93. Churchill Livingstone, Edinburgh.

[23]SCHMAIER, A. H. and COLEMAN, R. W. (1985). The contact phase of coagulation: a review and specific techniques to study its components. In *Blood Coagulation and Haemostasis. A Practical Guide*. Ed. J. M. Thomson, p. 22. Churchill Livingstone, Edinburgh.

[24]SIXMA, J. J. (1987). Role of platelets, plasma proteins and vessel wall in haemostasis. In *Haemostasis and Thrombosis*. Eds. A. L. Bloom and D. P. Thomas, p. 283. Churchill Livingstone, Edinburgh.

[25]STUART, J., PICKEN, A. M., BREEZE, G. R. and WOOD, B. S. B. (1973). Capillary blood coagulation profile in the newborn. *Lancet*, **ii**, 1467.

[26]WALKER, I. D. and DAVIDSON, I. F. (1985). Fibrinolysis. In *Blood Coagulation and Haemostasis. A Practical Guide*. Ed. J. M. Thomson, p. 208. Churchill Livingstone, Edinburgh.

[27]WARE, J. A. and HEISTAD, D. D. (1993). Platelet endothelium interactions. *New England Journal of Medicine*, **328**, 628.

[28]YARDUMIAN, D. A., MACKIE, I. J. and MACHIN, S. J. (1986). Laboratory investigation of platelet function: a review of methodology. *Journal of Clinical Pathology*, **39**, 701.

[29]ZIMMERMAN, T. S. and MEYER, D. (1987). Structure and function of factor VIII and von Willebrand factor. In *Haemostasis and Thrombosis*. Eds. A. L. Bloom and D. P. Thomas, p. 131. Churchill Livingstone, Edinburgh.

17. Investigation of a bleeding tendency

Revised by M.A. Laffan and A. E. Bradshaw

Vascular disorders   318
Bleeding time   318
Investigation of platelet function   319
   Platelet aggregation   320
Investigation of a coagulation factor deficiency or defect   325
   Parallel line bioassays   326
   Normal standard plasma pool   327
Factor VII assay   328
Investigation of intrinsic pathway   329
Investigation of von Willebrand's disease   331
   vW:Ag ELISA assay   333
   Multimeric analysis   334
   Ristocetin cofactor   336
Investigation of a circulating anticoagulant   339

Factor VIII:C inhibitor assay   340
Investigation of a prolonged PT and APTT   341
Taipan venom assay   342
Factor X assay   342
Factor V assay   343
Investigation of a-, hypo- or dysfibrinogenaemia   344
Clot solubility test   344
Disseminated intravascular coagulation   345
   Fibrinogen assay   345
   Detection of FDP   346
   Fibrin monomers   346
Investigation of carriers of coagulation defects   347
Monitoring factor replacement therapy   348
Cross-linked fibrin D-dimers   349

The investigation of a suspected bleeding tendency may begin from three different points:

1. Investigating a clinically suspected bleeding tendency. In this case the investigation properly begins with the bleeding history which may suggest an acquired or congenital disorder of primary or secondary haemostasis. If the bleeding history or family history is significant, then appropriate specific tests should be performed, notwithstanding the results of screening tests such as the PT, APTT, etc.

2. Following up an abnormal first-line test. In this case the abnormalities already detected will determine the appropriate further investigations (see Chapter 16).

3. Investigation of acute haemostatic failure. This is often in the context of an acutely ill or post-operative patient. Investigations are therefore directed towards detecting disseminated intravascular coagulation (DIC) or a previously undetected coagulation defect. The availability of a normal pre-morbid coagulation screen and further questioning to determine a bleeding history can be extremely useful in this respect.

Table 17.1   Substances which commonly affect platelet function

Agents which affect prostanoid synthesis
Aspirin
Non-steroidal anti-inflammatory drugs
Corticosteroids
Membrane stabilizing agents
α Antagonists
β Blockers
Antihistamines
Tricyclic antidepressants
Local anaesthetics
Antibiotics
Penicillin
Cephalosporins
Agents which increase c-AMP activity
Dipyridamole
Aminophylline
Prostanoids
Others
Heparin
Dextran
Ethanol
Clofibrate
Phenothiazine
Garlic

Comprehensive clinical evaluation, including the patient's history, the family history and the family tree, as well as the details of the site, frequency and the character of haemorrhagic manifestations (purpura, bruising, large haematomata, haemarthroses, etc.), is required to establish a definitive diagnosis. It is also desirable to undertake a series of screening tests before proceeding to more specific tests. The results of the screening investigations, taken in conjunction with clinical information, usually point to the additional appropriate method of analysis.

The common patterns of results obtained on screening investigations are shown in Table 16.3 (p. 310).

INVESTIGATION OF THE VASCULAR DISORDERS OF HAEMOSTASIS

Vascular disorders of haemostasis are those which arise due to defect or deficiency of the vessel wall. This may be due to one of the inherited disorders of collagen or to an acquired disorder such as amyloid or scurvy.

In general the tests of coagulation available in the laboratory will be of little help in elucidating such defects. The only test of any use is the bleeding time. Tests of capillary resistance are of little value. A careful clinical history and physical examination are most likely to provide the basis for diagnosis. Particular attention should be paid to previous scars, associated signs of the inherited syndromes and evidence of systemic disease. In some cases a tissue biopsy may be useful.

THE BLEEDING TIME

Principle. A standard incision is made on the volar surface of the forearm and the time the incision bleeds is measured. Cessation of bleeding indicates the formation of haemostatic plugs which are in turn dependent on an adequate number of platelets and on the ability of the platelets to adhere to the subendothelium and to form aggregates.[9]

STANDARDIZED TEMPLATE METHOD[23]

Materials

Sphygmomanometer.
Cleansing swabs.
Template bleeding time device. Such as 'Simplate' (General Diagnostics).
Filter paper. 1 mm thick.
Stop-watch.

Method

Place a sphygmomanometer cuff around the patient's arm above the elbow, inflate to 40 mmHg and keep it at this pressure throughout the test. Clean the volar surface of the forearm with 70% ethanol and choose an area of skin which is devoid of visible superficial veins. Press a sterile metal template with a linear slit 7–8 mm long firmly against the skin aligned along the long axis of the arm and use a scalpel blade with a guard so arranged that the tip of the blade protrudes 1 mm through the template slit. In this way make an incision 6 mm long and 1 mm deep. Modifications of the template and blade making two simultaneous cuts with a spring mechanism are commercially available.

Blot off gently but completely with filter paper at 15-s intervals the blood exuding from the cut. Avoid contact with the wound during this procedure. When bleeding has ceased, carefully oppose the edges of the incision and apply an adhesive strip to lessen the risk of keloid formation and an unsightly scar.

Normal range

2.5–9.5 min.

IVY'S METHOD[18]

The test is similar to the template method, but instead of a standardized incision two separate punctures, 5–10 cm apart, are made in quick succession using a disposable lancet. Any microlance with a cutting depth of 2.5 mm and width of just over 1 mm is suitable; it can be inserted to its maximum depth without fear of penetrating too deeply. A source of inaccuracy with Ivy's method is the tendency for the puncture wound to close before bleeding has ceased.

Normal range

2–7 min. Ideally, each laboratory should determine its own normal range.

Interpretation of results

A prolonged bleeding time may be due to:

1. *Thrombocytopenia*. It is advisable to check the platelet count before carrying out the bleeding time test. Patients with a platelet count below $50 \times 10^9/l$ may have a very long bleeding time and the bleeding may be difficult to arrest.

2. *Disorders of platelet function*. They may be congenital; such as thrombasthenia, storage pool defect, etc. (see below), or acquired; due to drugs, the presence of a paraprotein, or platelet abnormalities per se as in myelodysplastic syndromes.

3. von Willebrand's disease, due to defective platelet adherence to the subendothelium in the absence of a normal amount or of normally functioning von Willebrand factor (vWF) (see p. 331).

4. Vascular abnormalities, as found in Ehler-Danlos's syndrome, or in pseudoxanthoma elasticum.

5. Occasionally, severe deficiency of factor V or XI, or afibrinogenaemia.

INVESTIGATION OF A SUSPECTED DISORDER OF PLATELET FUNCTION, INHERITED OR ACQUIRED

(For investigation assays of von Willebrand's disease, see p. 331; for diagnosis of thrombocytopenia, see p. 63 and 77.)

Abnormalities of platelet function all lead to signs and symptoms characteristic of defects of primary haemostasis: bleeding into the mucous membranes and small skin ecchymoses. The patient may also suffer from abnormal intraoperative bleeding and oozing from small cuts or wounds.

LABORATORY INVESTIGATION OF PLATELETS AND PLATELET FUNCTION

The peripheral blood platelet count and the skin bleeding time are the first-line tests of platelet function. If the results of these two tests are within the normal limits, it is unlikely that a clinically important platelet defect is responsible for the bleeding tendency. Additional information may be obtained by inspecting a fresh blood film which may show abnormalities of platelet size or morphology which may be of diagnostic importance.

If the screening procedures suggest a disorder of platelet function, further tests should be organized. Drugs and certain foods (Table 17.1) may affect platelet function tests, and the patient must be asked to refrain from taking such substances for at least 7 days before the test.

The usual sequence of investigation is shown in Fig. 17.1 in the form of a flow chart. Platelet function tests can be divided into five main groups (Table 17.2): adhesion tests, aggregation tests, assessment of the granular content and the release reaction, investigation of the prostaglandin pathways and tests of platelet coagulant activity.

Tests of *platelet retention or adhesion* by a glass bead column are rarely used today because of the lack of specificity. More sophisticated tests based on the Baumgartner technique of passing whole blood over everted rabbit aorta denuded of endothelial cells are very useful research tools, but unsuitable for the routine laboratory.

In contrast, studies of *platelet aggregation* are mandatory in investigating platelet function, particularly in patients with a normal platelet count and a prolonged bleeding time. A turbidometric technique using patient's own platelet-rich plasma is commonly used; numerous platelet

Table 17.2   Platelet function tests

Adhesion tests	
Retention in a glass-bead column	
Baumgartner's technique	
Aggregation tests	
Turbidometric technique using	
ADP	
Collagen	
Ristocetin	
Adrenalin	Endoperoxide
Thrombin	analogues U44069,
Arachidonic acid.	U46619.
	Calcium ionophore
	A21387
Investigation of granular content and release	
Dense bodies	Electron microscopy.
	ADP and ATP content
	(bioluminescence).
	Serotonin release
Granules	β-Thromboglobulin.
	Platelet factor 4.
	vWF
Prostaglandin pathways	
TXB_2 radio-immune assay	
MDA assay using thiobarbituric acid	
Studies with radioactive arachidonic acid	
Platelet coagulant activity	
Prothrombin consumption index	

activating agents or agonists can be applied. Details of the technique and the agonists, as well as the diagnostic patterns encountered, are discussed in detail below.

The *granular content* of the platelets can be assessed by electron microscopy or by measuring the substances released (Table 17.2). Adenine nucleotide and serotonin release from the dense granules are probably best measured by a specialist laboratory. The release of β-thromboglobulin and platelet factor 4 can be measured using commercial radio-immunoassay kits, but there are problems with reproducibility and interpretation of the results. The release from the α granules is mostly investigated as a marker of in-vivo platelet activation and thrombotic tendency. Platelet vWF is measured to diagnose variants of von Willebrand disease. Platelet-derived growth factor can also be measured by some specialized laboratories.

If the initial aggregation studies suggest a defect in the prostaglandin pathways, TXB_2 can

be estimated quantitatively by radio-immune assay. Highly specific assays of various steps in arachidonic acid metabolism are also available but are outside the scope of a routine laboratory.

Platelet coagulant activity—the completion of the membrane 'flip-flop'—can be indirectly measured using the prothrombin consumption index. However, this test is rarely performed now; it was described in the previous edition.

PLATELET AGGREGATION[5,6,8,30]

Principle. The absorbance of platelet-rich plasma falls as platelets aggregate. The amount and the rate of fall are dependent on platelet reactivity to the added agonist if other variables, such as temperature, platelet count and mixing speed are controlled. The absorbance changes are monitored on a chart recorder, using a technique originally developed by Born.[5,6]

Reagents

Test and control platelet-rich plasma. The patient and control should be off all drugs, beverages and foods which may affect aggregation for at least 10 days (see p. 317) and preferably should have fasted overnight as the presence of chylomicra may also disturb the aggregation patterns. Twenty ml of venous blood are collected with minimal venous occlusion and added to a one-tenth volume of trisodium citrate (see p. 576) contained in a plastic or siliconized container. The blood should not be chilled because cold activates the platelets. Platelet-rich plasma (PRP) is obtained by centrifuging at room temperature (*c* 20°C) for 10–15 min at 150–200*g*. The PRP is carefully removed, avoiding contamination with red cells or buffy coat, and placed in a stoppered plastic tube. PRP should be stored at room temperature until tested and is stable for about 3 h. It is important to test all samples after a similar interval of time (say 1 h) and to store them at the same temperature in order to minimize variation.

Test and control platelet-poor plasma (PPP). The remaining blood is centrifuged at 2000*g* for 20 min to obtain platelet-poor plasma (PPP).

Standardization of PRP. A platelet count is performed on the PRP. The number of platelets

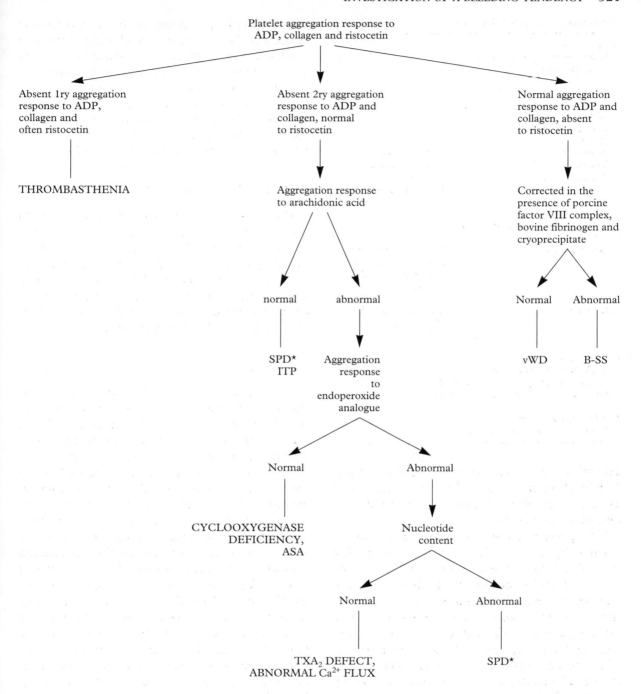

Fig. 17.1 Flow chart for investigation of suspected platelet dysfunction. SPD, storage pool defect; ITP, coating of platelets by auto-antibodies in idiopathic thrombocytopenic purpura; vWD, von Willebrand's disease; B-SS, Bernard-Soulier syndrome; ASA, effect of aspirin ingestion. *Some cases.

will influence aggregation responses if the count falls outside 200–400 × 10^9/l. For very high PRP counts, the count should be adjusted by diluting the PRP in the patient's PPP. Platelet counts below 200 × 10^9/l give rise to diminished aggregation responses. Further centrifugation of PRP is not recommended because it induces platelet activation. The control PRP should be diluted to the same count and tested as a comparison.

PRP should always be stored in tightly stoppered tubes which are filled nearly to the top, to avoid changes in pH which also affect platelet aggregation and tests of nucleotide release.

Aggregating agents

The five aggregating agents listed below should be sufficient for the diagnosis of most functional disorders. For research purposes and when investigating unusual kindreds, other agonists listed in Table 17.2 may also be used.

ADP. The anhydrous sodium salt of adenosine 5-diphosphate is used. A stock solution is prepared by dissolving 4.93 mg of the trisodium salt or 4.71 mg of the disodium salt in 10 ml of 9 g/l NaCl, pH 6.8. This makes a 1 mmol/l solution. It is stored in 0.5 ml volumes at −40°C until use and remains stable for up to 3 months at this temperature. Once thawed, the solution must be used within 3 h and then discarded. For aggregation testing, prepare 100, 50, 25, 10 and 5 μmol/l solutions.

Collagen (Hormon-Chemie, Munich). This is a 1 mg/ml stock solution. For use it is diluted in the buffer supplied with the collagen or in 5% dextrose to obtain concentrations of 10 and 40 μg/l. When diluted 1:10 in PRP (see below), the final concentrations will be 1 and 4 μg/ml.

Ristocetin sulphate (H. Lundbeck, Copenhagen). Each vial contains 100 mg of ristocetin and should be stored at 4°C until dissolved; 8 ml of 9 g/l NaCl are added to each vial so as to obtain a 12.5 mg/ml solution. This is then stored at −40°C in 0.5 ml volumes until used. Ristocetin may be refrozen after use. It should never be used in concentrations of greater than 1.4 mg/ml as protein precipitation may occur in plasma and give rise to false results.

Arachidonic acid. Na-salt, 99% pure. The con-

tents of a 10 mg vial are dissolved in 1.5 ml of sterile water by gentle mixing to give a 20 mmol/l stock solution. This may be frozen in 0.5 ml volumes at −20°C for later use. A working solution is prepared by making doubling dilutions of the stock in saline to give 5 and 10 mmol/l solutions.

Adrenaline. 1-Epinephrine bitartarate. 3.33 mg are dissolved in 10 ml of water to prepare a 1 mmol/l stock solution. It is stored in 0.5 ml volumes at −40°C. 20 and 200 μmol/l solutions are prepared for use in barbitone buffered saline, pH 7.4.

Note: All aggregation reagents should be kept on ice until used.

Method

Centrifugation may cause cellular release of ADP and platelet refractoriness to aggregation, and the actual aggregation test should not be started within 30 min of preparing the PRP. However, the tests should be completed within 3 h and whenever possible within 2 h of preparing the PRP. Platelets left standing at room temperature (*c*20°C) become increasingly reactive to adrenaline and in some cases to collagen; the rate of change increases after 3 h.

Switch the aggregometer on about 30 min before the tests are to be performed to allow the heating block to warm up to 37°C. Set the stirring speed to 900 rpm. Pipette the appropriate volume of PRP (this varies depending on the make of the aggregometer used) into a plastic tube or cuvette. Place the tube in the heating block. After 1 min insert the stirrer into the plasma. Set the transmission to 0 on the chart recorder. Replace with a cuvette containing PPP and set the transmission to 100%. Repeat this procedure until no further adjustments are needed and the pen traverses most of the width of the chart paper in response to the difference in absorbance between the PRP and PPP.

Allow the PRP to warm up to 37°C for 2 min and then add 1:10 vol of the agonist. Record the change in absorbance until the response reaches a plateau or for 3 min (whichever is sooner). Repeat this procedure for each agonist. The starting amount for each agonist is the lowest concentration prepared as described above. (See Fig.

17.2). If no release is obtained, increase the concentration until a satisfactory response is obtained.

Interpretation

Normal platelet aggregation curves are shown in Fig. 17.2.

ADP. Low concentrations of ADP (<0.5 to 2.5 μmol/l) cause primary or reversible aggregation. First, ADP binds to a membrane receptor and releases Ca^{2+} ions. A reversible complex with extracellular fibrinogen forms and the platelets undergo a shape change reflected by a slight increase in absorbance. After this, the bound fibrinogen adds to the cell-to-cell contact and reversible aggregation occurs. At very low concentrations of ADP, platelets may disaggregate after the first phase. In the presence of higher concentrations of ADP an irreversible secondary wave aggregation is associated with the release of dense and α-granules due to activation of the arachidonic acid pathway. If only high doses of

ADP are used, defects in the primary wave (measuring the second pathway as described on p. 299) will be missed.

Collagen. The aggregation response to collagen is preceded by a short 'lag' phase lasting between 10 and 60 s. The duration of the lag phase is inversely proportional to the concentration of collagen used and to the responsiveness of the platelets tested. This phase is succeeded by a single wave of aggregation due to the activation of the arachidonic acid pathway and the release of the granules. Higher doses of collagen (>2 μg/ml) cause a sudden increase in intra-platelet calcium concentration and this may bring about the release reaction without activating the prostaglandin pathway. Collagen responses should therefore always be measured using 1 and 4 μg/ml concentrations.

Ristocetin. Ristocetin reacts with vWF and the membrane receptor to induce platelets to clump together ('agglutination'). It does not activate any of the three aggregation pathways and does not initially cause granule release. The response is

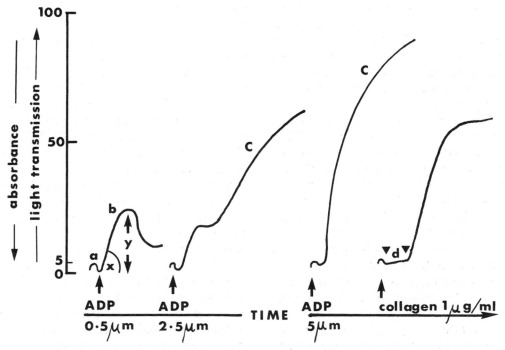

Fig. 17.2   Traces obtained during the aggregation of platelet-rich plasma. (a) Shape change. (b) Primary wave aggregation. (c) secondary wave aggregation. x°, Angle of the initial aggregation slope. y, Height of the aggregation trace. d, Lag phase. μm = μmol/l. (Reproduced with the permission of authors and publisher from Yardumian et al.[30])

assessed on the basis of the angle of the initial slope. The platelet response to 1.2 mg/ml is initially studied. Concentrations above 1.4 mg/ml may cause nonspecific platelet 'agglutination' due to an interaction between ristocetin and fibrinogen and protein precipitation. For a detailed discussion on ristocetin 'agglutination' in von Willebrand's disease, see p. 336.

Arachidonic acid. Arachidonic acid induces thromboxane A_2 generation and granule release even if there is a defect of agonist binding to the surface membrane or of the phospholipase-induced release of endogenous arachidonate. If steps further along the pathway are impaired, such as absence or inhibition of cyclo-oxygenase, arachidonic acid will not produce normal aggregation.

Adrenaline. No shape change precedes aggregation, but the response thereafter resembles the ADP response. Such a response is usually obtained with concentrations of 2–10 μmol/ml. Some clinically normal people have severely reduced responses to adrenaline.[27]

The pattern of responses in various disorders of platelet function is shown in Table 17.3. For a discussion of hyperaggregability, see p. 360.

Calculation of results[8,30]

Results can be expressed in one of three ways:

1. As a percentage fall in absorbance measured at 3 min after the addition of an agonist (see Fig. 17.2; y). This does not provide any information on the shape of the curve.

2. By the initial slope of the aggregation tracing (see Fig. 17.2; x°). This indicates the rate of aggregation but does not show whether or not secondary aggregation has occurred.

3. By the minimum amount of agonist required to induce a secondary response.

Normal range

The platelets of normal subjects usually produce a single reversible primary wave with 1 μmol/l ADP or less, biphasic aggregation with ADP at 2.5 μmol/l, and a single irreversible wave at 5 or 10 μmol/l. A single phase response is observed after a lag phase lasting not more than 1 min with 1 and 4 μg/ml of collagen. A single phase or biphasic response is seen with 1.2 mg/ml of ristocetin and after 50 and 100 μmol/l of arachidonic acid. Biphasic aggregation is observed with 2–10 μmol/l of adrenaline. A response to a low concentration of ristocetin (0.5 mg/ml) is abnormal and is a feature of type IIb vWD (see below).

Some common technical problems associated with platelet aggregation are shown in Table 17.4.

FURTHER INVESTIGATION OF PLATELET FUNCTION

If an abnormal aggregation pattern is observed it is advisable to check the assessment on at least one further occasion. If the aggregation tests are persistently abnormal, and the patient is not

Table 17.3 Differential diagnosis of disorders of platelet function

Condition	Platelet		Aggregation with:				
	Count	Size	ADP	Col	Ri	AA	FVIII
Thrombasthenia	N	N	0	0	Ab	0	Ab
Bernard-Soulier syndrome	Large	Large	N	N	0	N	0
Storage pool defect	N	N	1	Ab	1/0	1/0	1/0
Cyclo-oxygenase deficiency	N	N	1/N	Ab	N	Ab	–
Thromboxane synthetase deficiency	N	N	1/N	Ab	N	Ab	–
Aspirin ingestion	N	N	1	Ab	N/Ab	Ab	N/Ab
Ehler-Danlos syndrome	N	N	N	Ab	N	N	–
von Willebrand disease	N	N	N	N	0	N	N

N, normal; 0, absent; 1, primary wave only; Ab, abnormal; Col, collagen; Ri, ristocetin; AA, arachidonic acid; FVIII, porcine factor VIII complex/bovine fibrinogen.
Note that many other defects, such as found in oculo-cutaneous albinism, Chediak-Higashi syndrome, grey platelet syndrome, etc., have also been described.

Table 17.4 Technical factors which may influence platelet aggregation tests

Centrifugation. At room temperature, *not* at 4°C. Should be sufficient to remove red cells and white cells but not the largest platelets. Residual red cells in the PRP may cause apparently incomplete aggregation.

Time. For 30 min after the preparation of PRP, platelets are refractory to the effect of agonists. Progressive increase in reactiveness occurs thereafter, more marked from 2 h onward.

Platelet count. Slow and weak aggregation observed with platelet counts below 150 or over $400 \times 10^9/l$.

pH. <7.7 inhibits aggregation; pH >8.0 enhances aggregation.

Mixing speed. <800 rpm or >1200 rpm slows aggregation.

Haematocrit. >0.55 is associated with less aggregation, especially in the 2ry phase due to the increased concentration of citrate in PRP. It may also be difficult to obtain enough PPP. Centrifuging twice may help.

Temperature. <35°C causes decreased aggregation except to low dose ADP which may be enhanced.

Dirty cuvette. May cause spontaneous platelet aggregation or interfere with the optics of the system.

Air bubbles in the cuvette. Cause large irregular oscillations even before the addition of agonists.

No stir bar. No response to any agonist obtained.

taking any drugs or substances known to interfere with platelet function, the following tests should be done (see also Fig. 17.1 and Table 17.3):

1. If thrombasthenia or the Bernard-Soulier syndrome is suspected, an analysis of membrane glycoproteins is necessary.

2. If a release abnormality is suspected, additional agonists including synthetic endoperoxide analogues and calcium ionophores should be used in testing for aggregation. In addition, the total adenine nucleotide content of the platelets and the amount released after maximal stimulation should be measured using a firefly bioluminescence technique.[8,11]

3. Whenever possible electron microscopic studies of platelet ultrastructure should be carried out.

4. Factor VIII:C, vWF:Ag and ristocetin cofactor assay should be carried out on all patients investigated for an abnormality of platelet function who show abnormal ristocetin 'agglutination', or in whom all platelet function tests are normal.

5. Plasma assays of β-thromboglobulin and platelet factor 4 are described in Chapter 18 (p. 360) as tests of hypercoagulability. They are also used to detect α-granule deficiency states, such as the grey platelet syndrome.

INVESTIGATION OF A BLEEDING DISORDER DUE TO A COAGULATION FACTOR DEFICIENCY OR DEFECT

When the screening tests indicate that an individual has a coagulation defect, the plasma concentration of the coagulation factors should be assayed. Such assays not only establish the diagnosis of the deficiency or defect, they also assess its severity, and can be used to monitor replacement therapy and to detect the carrier state in families in which one or more members are affected by a congenital bleeding disorder.

An individual may have a deficiency of a coagulation factor because of impaired synthesis or because a variant of the molecule is synthesized which is deficient in clotting activity. In both instances the results of assays based on coagulation tests will be subnormal, but when a variant molecule is being produced, the result of an immunological assay may be normal or near normal. In many congenital bleeding disorders, immunological assays form an important part of the diagnostic procedure and of management.

GENERAL PRINCIPLES OF PARALLEL LINE BIOASSAYS OF COAGULATION FACTORS.[1,17]

If two materials containing the same coagulation factor are assayed in a specific assay system in a range of dilutions, and the clotting times are plotted against the plasma concentration on linear graph paper, curved dose response lines are obtained. If the plot is redrawn on double-log paper, a sigmoid curve with a straight middle section is obtained (Fig. 17.3). If the dilutions of the test and standard materials are chosen carefully, it should be possible to draw two straight parallel lines. The horizontal distance between the two lines represents the difference in potency ('strength' or concentration) of the factor assayed. If the test line is to the right of the standard it contains less of the factor than the standard; if to the left, it contains more.

When setting up and performing a parallel line assay, a number of measures must be taken to ensure that the assay is valid and reliable.

1. *Dilution range.* This should be chosen so that the coagulation times lie on the linear portion of the sigmoid curve. For example, when assaying factor VIII:C by one-stage assay, dilutions giving times between 60 and 100 s are chosen if the blank clotting time is over 120 s. (The blank consists of a mixture of buffer and substrate or deficient plasma which provides all factors except the one to be measured.)

2. *Number of dilutions.* At least three dilutions of the standard and the test are assayed to give the best graphical or mathematical solution.

3. *Responses.* Dilutions of the test sample should be chosen so that the clotting times fall within the range obtained for the standard. The standard curve should not be extrapolated beyond this range.

4. *Duplicates and replicates.* Duplicates are obtained from the same dilution of the sample and sometimes by sub-sampling from the same incubation mixture. Replicates are true repeats involving a fresh dilution and fresh reagents. Normally, coagulation times are measured on duplicates. Replicates are sometimes used for particularly difficult assays.

5. *Temporal drift.* This has already been dis-

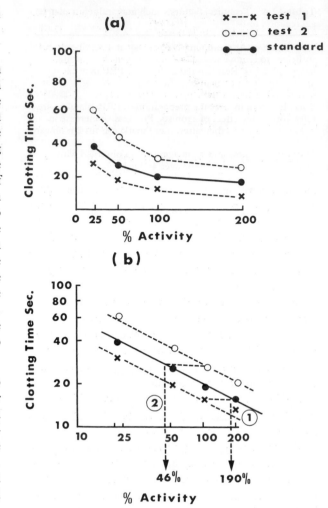

Fig. 17.3   Parallel line bioassay of factor VII.
(a) Clotting times with 1 in 5, 1 in 10, 1 in 20 and 1 in 40 dilutions of test and standard plasma plotted on linear graph paper. (b) The same data plotted on double log paper. Three parallel straight lines are obtained. The horizontal shift of the test line represents the difference in potency. In this case test 1 has a potency of 190% and test 2 a potency of 46%.
The 1 in 10 dilution of the standard plasma is assigned a potency of 100%.

cussed in Chapter 16 (p. 306). Duplicates in a coagulation assay should always be tested in a balanced order, e.g. ABCCBA.

Standard plasma

The use of a suitable standard is crucial for an accurate assay. The concentration of some coagulation factors may vary as much as fourfold in different normal plasma samples and it is therefore inadvisable to use plasma from any one person as representing 100% clotting activity. A normal plasma pool is the only satisfactory standard for coagulation factor assays. The larger the number of donors in the pool, the more likely the pool clotting activity will be c 100% or 100 units/dl.

Collection of blood samples and preparation of the pool. Add 9 volumes of venous blood to 1 volume of citrate (see p. 305). Prepare platelet-poor plasma by centrifuging at 2000g for 15 min. Remove the supernatant carefully without disturbing the buffy-coat or red cells. Pool the plasma samples in a plastic container and store in 1.0 ml volumes frozen, preferably at −40°C or below.

Most pools are made from between 6 and 40 donors. Larger pools are preferable and it is best to include individuals of both sexes, aged between 20 and 60. Women taking oestrogen-containing oral contraceptives should not contribute to the standard pool.

Calibration of standard pools. Whenever possible, the normal pool should be calibrated against a freeze-dried reference material already calibrated against the international standard. The reference material may be a national standard or a commercial standard. The international standards and reference preparations for factor VIII:C, vWF:Ag and factor IX are available from the National Institute of Biological Standards and Control, which holds them on behalf of the WHO (see p. 590).

In the absence of reference materials the laboratory should follow the procedure set out below to calibrate its own normal pool and assign it a value of 100 u/dl.

Suggested calibration procedure. The most important principle of calibration is repetition needed to minimize possible errors at each stage of calibration. It is necessary to carry out at least four independent assays, and preferably six. An independent assay is an assay for which a new ampoule of standard is opened, or if a freeze-dried standard is not availabe, for which a new set of dilutions are prepared from frozen or fresh previous reference plasma. Each plasma must be tested in duplicate; two replicate assays should be carried out each day, and the procedure repeated on at least 4 days (four independent assays). Whenever possible more than one operator should be involved.

Comparison should always be made with the previous normal pool. The potency of the new normal pool is calculated for each replicate assay on each day and an overall mean value calculated. The calibration also enables an assessment of the precision of the method used.

Calculation of results

The results can be worked out graphically or mathematically. For a graphical solution, mean values for duplicate clotting times are plotted against the dilutions on double-log paper. The dilutions are converted to decimals; the lowest dilution of the standard is assigned a value of 100% or 1.0 (see Fig. 17.3). Best-fit lines are drawn through each set of points. Non-parallel or grossly curved lines indicate an invalid assay and should be discarded (see p. 330). To obtain the actual potency of the test sample in terms of the standard, a horizontal line is drawn through both dose response lines to cut the test sample line where it crosses 1.0 or 100%. A vertical line is then dropped on to the concentration axis and the relative potency of the test sample read directly off the concentration scale.

Mathematical solutions are better than graphical ones, as they provide exact criteria for parallelism and curvature. Computer or calculator programs can be used to calculate the results.

Variability of coagulation assays

Within one laboratory, variability is most commonly due to a dilution error, differences in the composition of reagents, failure to take the time-trend into account, and because of differences in experience and technique between operators. A coefficient of variation of 15–20% is not uncommon for factor VIII:C assay. Furthermore, the variability increases if like is not compared with like; e.g. if concentrate preparations are assayed against plasma.

Variability between laboratories is much higher. Apart from the factors described for the within-laboratory variability, there is the major effect of differences in methods and in the composition of reagents. Comparability between laboratories improves if standardized reagents are used.

The unavoidable variability associated with coagulation assays makes the use of reliable reference materials imperative.

INVESTIGATION OF A SUSPECTED FACTOR VII DEFICIENCY OR DEFECT

The investigation of an isolated prolonged one-stage prothrombin time in an individual with a life-long history of bleeding includes a one-stage factor VII assay. If a reduced concentration of factor VII is found, further tests should include immunoassays of factor VII and whenever possible a family study.

ONE-STAGE ASSAY OF FACTOR VII

Principle. The assay of factor VII is based on the prothrombin time. The assay compares the ability of dilutions of the patient's plasma and of a standard plasma to correct the prothrombin time of a substrate plasma.

Reagents

Platelet-poor plasma from the patient.
Standard plasma. For details see p. 327.
Factor VII deficient plasma. Commercial or from a patient with known severe deficiency. Plasma from dogs with severe congenital deficiency can also be used.
Barbitone buffered saline. See p. 306.
Thromboplastin. Rabbit brain thromboplastin known to be sensitive to factor VII deficiency (see p. 307). The thromboplastin should be diluted 1 in 20 in buffered saline.
$CaCl_2$. 0.025 mol/l.

Method

Prepare 1 in 5, 1 in 10, 1 in 20 and 1 in 40 dilutions of the standard and test plasma in buffered saline. Transfer 0.1 ml of each dilution to a glass tube and add to it 0.1 ml of deficient (substrate) plasma, and 0.1 ml of dilute thromboplastin. Mix and allow to warm to 37°C. Add 0.1 ml of $CaCl_2$ and start the stop-watch. Record the clotting time. A blank must be included with every assay and all tests carried out in duplicate, and in balanced order.

Calculation of results

Plot the clotting times of the test and standard against the concentration of factor VII on 3 cycle × 2 cycle log paper. Read the concentration as shown in Fig. 17.3. (Some automated coagulometers produce computed values using mathematical formulae.)

Normal range

50–200 u/dl (for discussion of units see p. 327).

Interpretation

Patients with a congenital deficiency have factor VII levels of 30 u/dl and less. The concentration measured varies according to the thromboplastin used in the assay. A small proportion of patients have normal factor VII antigen despite abnormal functional activity.

INVESTIGATION OF A PATIENT WITH A SUSPECTED INTRINSIC PATHWAY DEFICIENCY OR DEFECT

An isolated prolongation of the APTT in a patient with a life-long bleeding disorder may be due to a deficiency or defect of one of the following factors: factor VIII:C or vWF, factor IX or factor XI. Individuals with factor XII, prekallikrein and HMWK deficiencies do not usually bleed and the prolonged APTT is most often an incidental finding. The first step would be to carry out mixing experiments in order to discover which factor is lacking (see p. 309) and whether an inhibitor is present (see Fig. 17.4). The missing factor should then be estimated quantitatively using a coagulation assay. Further tests may become necessary to elucidate the nature of the disorder.

ONE-STAGE ASSAY OF FACTOR VIII:C[16,17]

Principle. The one-stage assay for factor VIII:C is based on the APTT. It consists of comparing the ability of dilutions of the patient's plasma and of a standard plasma to correct the

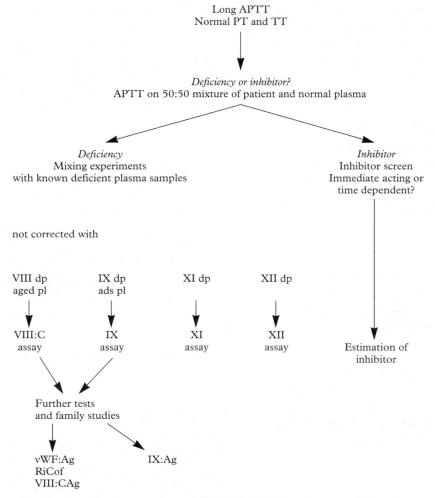

Fig. 17.4 Flow chart for investigating a prolonged APTT. dp, Deficient plasma; aged pl, aged plasma; ads pl, adsorbed plasma; vWF:Ag, von Willebrand factor antigen; IX:Ag, factor IX antigen; VIII:CAg, factor VIII:C antigen, RiCof: Ristocetin cofactor.

APTT of a plasma known to lack factor VIII:C, but containing all other factors required for normal coagulation. An identical principle applies to the assays of factors IX, XI and XII. Assays of von Willebrand factor are described separately.

Reagents

Platelet-poor plasma. From the patient.

Standard plasma. See p. 327.

Factor VIII deficient plasma (substrate plasma). If using a commercial plasma, the reagent should be reconstituted according to the manufacturer's instructions. If a haemophiliac donor is used, his factor VIII:C concentration should be less than 1% and his plasma should be free of inhibitors. The plasma should be stored in suitable volumes, e.g. 2 ml, at –40°C until used. All samples obtained from patients must be considered potentially infective. Patient samples should be tested for antibodies to HIV and hepatitis C virus and for HBs antigen. Alternatively, plasma depleted of factor VIII:C by immuno-adsorption can be used.

Kaolin. 5 mg/ml in barbitone buffered saline.

Barbitone buffered saline. See p. 306.

Phospholipid solution (platelet substitute). As described on p. 589.

CaCl$_2$. 0.025 mol/l.

Ice-bath.

Method

Place the kaolin, phospholipid and CaCl$_2$ at 37°C, and the patient's, standard and substrate plasma in the ice-bath until used.

Make 1 in 10 dilutions of the test and standard plasma in buffered saline in plastic tubes in the ice-bath. If the test plasma is suspected of having a very low factor VIII:C content, make a 1 in 5 dilution instead. Using 0.2 ml volumes, make doubling dilutions in buffered saline to obtain 1 in 20 and 1 in 40 dilutions. Place 0.1 ml of the three dilutions (1 in 10, 1 in 20 and 1 in 40) in glass tubes.

Add to each dilution 0.1 ml of freshly reconstituted or thawed substrate plasma and warm up at 37°C. Add 0.2 ml of the phospholipid/kaolin mixture, mix the contents of the tube and start a master stop-watch. At 10 min exactly add the CaCl$_2$ and start a second stop-watch. Record the clotting time.

The dilutions should be tested at 2-min intervals on the master watch. The assay must end with a blank consisting of 0.1 ml of buffered saline and 0.1 ml of substrate plasma. A balanced order of testing should be followed.

Calculation of results

Plot the clotting times of the test and standard against the concentration of factor VIII:C on 4 cycle × 3 cycle log paper. Read the concentration as shown in Fig. 17.3. It is important to obtain straight and parallel lines if the result is to be accurate. The reasons for non-parallelism and curvature are:

1. Technical error. Repeat the assay with new dilutions.

2. Activation of the plasma by poor collection. A new sample should be collected.

3. A low concentration of factor VIII:C in the test plasma gives rise to non-parallel lines. Stronger concentrations of plasma should be prepared and tested.

4. The presence of an inhibitor. The tests described on p. 339 should be carried out.

Some automated coagulometers produce computed values using mathematical formulae. If the standard plasma is calibrated in terms of international units, the result can be expressed in IU. For example, if the standard plasma has a factor VIII:C concentration of 65 IU/dl and the test is shown to have 20% of the activity of the standard, the test plasma will have a factor VIII concentration of 13 IU/dl (20% of 65 IU).

Normal range

50–200 IU/dl.

Interpretation

Some clinically normal people have factor VIII:C concentrations of 35–50 IU/dl. Values below 30 IU/dl are unequivocally abnormal; values below 50 IU/dl are significant in carriers (see p. 347).

A reduced factor VIII:C concentration is found in:

1. Haemophilia A.
2. Some carriers of haemophilia A.
3. von Willebrand disease, types I and III, and some cases of type II.
4. Rare congenital combined deficiency of factors VIII:C and V.
5. Disseminated intravascular coagulation.
6. Circulating anticoagulant (inhibitor).

Further tests in haemophilia A

Factor VIII:CAg (IRMA) and vWF:Ag (RiCoF) (described below) should be measured and the patient's family investigated.

Other one-stage assays based on the APTT

Factors IX, XI and XII can be measured in an identical manner using an appropriate substrate plasma. The normal values for these factors are given in Table 17.5. If low values are detected in

Table 17.5 Normal range and some causes of increased plasma concentration for factors of the intrinsic pathway

Factor	Normal range (IU/dl)	Increased
VIII:C	50–200	In acute phase reaction, stress, exercise, pregnancy, chronic liver disease, vasculitic diseases
IX	40–160	In pregnancy, in women taking oestrogen-containing contraceptives
XI	40–160	
XII	30–150	

a patient with a history of bleeding, immunoassays should be undertaken to establish whether there is any cross-reacting material, and family studies should be carried out.

Isolated factor IX or XII deficiency may be acquired as a result of a selective urinary loss in the nephrotic syndrome. An acquired low factor IX concentration has also been described in Sheehan's syndrome and Gaucher's disease.

INVESTIGATION OF A SUSPECTED VON WILLEBRAND'S DISEASE[3,8,17]

A diagnosis of von Willebrand's disease should be considered in individuals with a history of bleeding who show a prolonged bleeding time and APTT in screening tests. All factor VIII activities, that is VIII:C concentration, vWF:Ag concentration and ristocetin cofactor activity

(RiCoF), should be measured. If an abnormality is detected, further investigations, such as crossed immuno-electrophoresis (CIE) of vWF:Ag and the multimer analysis of the plasma should be performed. In normal plasma, each multimer of vWF (a large molecule consisting of four to over

Table 17.6 Classification of von Willebrand's disease

Type	Inheritance	VIII:C	vWF:Ag	RiCoF	CIE	Multimer analysis
I	Autos. dominant	L	L	L	N	Normal pattern
IIa*	Autos. dominant	L or N	L or N	L	Abn	Large and intermediate multimers absent from plasma and platelets, abnormal triplets
IIb	Autos. dominant	L or N	L or N	L or N	Abn	Large multimers absent from plasma only, normal triplets
IIc	Autos. recessive	N	N	L	Abn	Large multimers absent from plasma and platelets, abnormal triplets
III	Autos. recessive	L	L	0	ND	None detected

L, low; N, normal; 0, absent; ND, none detected; autos, autosomal; CIE, crossed immuno-electrophoresis.
*Types IId, e, and f are also described with different abormalities of the multimeric structure.
Some forms of vW disease Type II may show normal or even enhanced ristocetin 'agglutination' in platelet-rich plasma (see Fig. 17.5).

20 subunits of vWF) is seen to be composed of a 'triplet', a dark central band sandwiched between two lighter bands; high molecular weight multimers predominate. In von Willebrand's disease, there may be either no vWF:Ag detectable, or the high molecular weight forms necessary for normal platelet adhesion may be lacking, or the triplet pattern may be abnormal. On the basis of these results von Willebrand's disease can be classified as shown in Table 17.6.

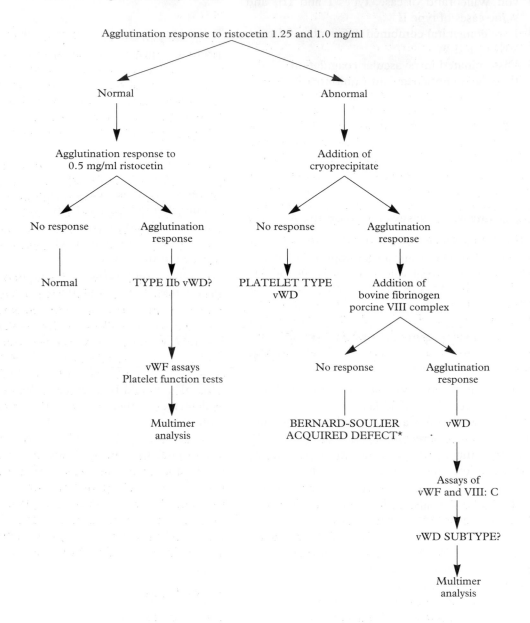

Fig. 17.5 Flow chart for investigating von Willebrand's disease.
*Acquired defect of platelet 'agglutination' response to ristocetin, most commonly found in myelodysplastic syndromes.

ENZYME-LINKED IMMUNOSORBENT ASSAY (ELISA) FOR VON WILLEBRAND FACTOR ANTIGEN[2]

Principle. ELISA involves coating a special microtitre plate with a primary antibody to vWF:Ag. A suitable dilution of the test plasma is added to the wells allowing the vWF:Ag to bind to the primary antibody. After removal of excess antigen by washing the plate, a second antibody, conjugated to an enzyme, usually peroxidase, and called the 'tag' antibody, is added and this binds to the vWF:Ag already bound to the plate. On addition of a specific substrate, a colour change occurs. After the reaction has been stopped with acid the optical density (OD) of each well can be measured using an electronic plate reader and the OD is directly proportional to the amount of vWF:Ag present in the test plasma. The primary antibody can be substituted by a monoclonal antibody specifically raised against the glycoprotein Ib binding site on the von Willebrand factor (available from Porton, Cambridge), and the method is then found to closely correlate with the functional activity of the von Willebrand factor measured as ristocetin cofactor activity (RiCoF).

Reagents

0.05M Carbonate buffer. 1.59g Na_2CO_3, 2.93 g $NaHCO_3$, 0.2 g NaN_3 in 1 litre of distilled water (pH 9.6).

0.01M Phosphate buffered saline. 0.39 g $NaH_2PO_4.2H_2O$, 2.68 g $Na_2HPO_4.12H_2O$, 8.47 g NaCl in 1 litre distilled water (pH 7.2).

0.1 M Citrate phosphate buffer. 8.8 g citric acid, 24.0 g $Na_2HPO_4.12H_2O$ in 1 litre distilled water (pH 5.0).

Anti vWF:Ag antiserum.
Anti vWF:Ag conjugated with peroxidase.
Platelet-poor (100%) calibration plasma.
Platelet-poor plasma (tests and control).
1,2-o-Phenylenediamine dihydrochloride (OPD).
1 M Sulphuric acid.
Hydrogen peroxide 20 vol.
Tween 20.

Method

Dilute the anti-human vWF:Ag 1:500 in 0.05 M carbonate buffer (i.e. 40 µl antibody in 20 ml buffer) and add 100 µl to each well of the microtitre plate. Incubate for 1 h at room temperature in a moist chamber. Discard antibody and wash 3 times by immersion in a trough of PBS with 0.5 ml/l Tween for 2 min, followed by inversion onto absorbent paper.

Prepare dilutions of the 100% standard 1:10, 1:20, 1:40 and 1:60 in PBS with 1 ml/l Tween. Dilute patients' and control plasmas 1:10, 1:20 and 1:40 in the same way and add 100 µl of each dilution in duplicate to the wells of the microtitre plate. Incubate for 1 h as before and repeat washing.

Dilute the anti-human vWF:Ag-peroxidase conjugate 1:500 in 1 ml/l PBS-Tween (i.e. 40 µl antibody in 20 ml buffer) and add 100 µl to each well. Incubate for 1 h. Wash twice in 0.5 ml/l PBS Tween and once in 0.1 M citrate phosphate buffer.

Dissolve 40 mg of substrate (OPD) in 15 ml citrate phosphate buffer. Add 10 µl of 20 volume hydrogen peroxide to the substrate solution immediately before use, and then add 100 µl to each well.

When the yellow colour has reached an intensity where a mid-yellow ring is clearly visible in the bottom of the wells, stop the reaction by the addition of 150 µl of 1 M sulphuric acid. Read the optical density across the plate at 492 nm using a microtitre plate reader. Plot the standard curve on log-linear graph paper. vWF:Ag levels are obtained by reading from the reference curve.

Normal range

50–200 IU/dl.

Interpretation

The results must be interpreted in conjunction with the results of factor VIII:C assay and the ristocetin cofactor assay (Table 17.6). VWF:Ag can also be measured by an immunoelectro-phoretic assay. The Laurell rocket method for this is described in the 7th edition of this book.

MULTIMERIC ANALYSIS OF VON WILLEBRAND FACTOR ANTIGEN IN PLASMA SAMPLES[13]

Principle. Plasma samples are diluted in a buffer containing 8 M urea and SDS to ensure mobility of protein is related to size and not molecular charge. Samples are electrophoresed through an agarose stacking gel at pH 8.8. After running overnight on a cooling platten, the protein is fixed in the gel, washed, and incubated with radiolabelled antibody to vWF followed by extensive washing. An X-ray film is exposed to the dried gel and an autoradiograph produced.

Reagents

Rabbit anti-human vWF:Ag. DAKO Laboratories.
^{125}Iodine. Amersham International.
Chloramine T.
Sodium metabisulphite.
PD-10 Sephadex G-25M Columns. Pharmacia.
Bovine serum albumin.
Bio-Rad DNA grade ultrapure agarose.
Sodium dodecyl sulphate (SDS).
Glycine.
Sodium EDTA.
Hydrochloric acid.
Propan-2-ol.
Acetic acid.
Trisma base.
Bromophenol blue.
Bovine IgG fraction.
Rabbit plasma. Wellcome reagents.
Deionized water.
Sodium phosphate.

Preparation of ^{125}I labelled antibody

Mix 50 µl of antiserum with *c* 2 mCi (20 µl) ^{125}I. Add 10 µl of freshly prepared chloramine T (50 mg in 10 ml 0.5 M sodium phosphate buffer) and mix for 30 s. Add 100 µl sodium metabisulphite (12 mg in 10 ml sodium phosphate buffer). Pass the mixture down a Sephadex column. The column is equilibrated in PBS and the eluant is PBS containing 1% bovine serum albumin. Collect approximately 1 ml fractions; the radioactivity counts begin to occur after about three fractions. Pool the radioactive fractions and dispose of the column containing free iodine. Aliquot the labelled antibody and store in working aliquots (approximately 10 aliquots) at −40°C for up to a maximum of 3 months. Usual precautions for working with radioactive material should be observed.

Stock solutions

2 M Tris.
3 M HCl.
0.01 M Na$_2$ EDTA.
The above three reagents may be stored at 4°C for up to 3 months.

Preparation of buffers and reagents

Running buffer

37.5 ml–2 M Tris.
4.45 ml–3 M HCl.
Make up to 50 ml with water, check pH is 8.8.
May be stored at 4°C for up to 2 weeks.

Sample buffer stock

500 ml 2 M Tris.
10 ml stock EDTA.
Make up to 100 ml with water.
May be stored at 4°C for up to 4 weeks.

For use

9.61 g urea.
0.4 g SDS.

Dissolve in sample buffer and make up to 20 ml.
May need warming to dissolve.
Carefully adjust the pH to 8.0 with 1M HCl —
use within 1 day of preparation.
10% SDS. 1 g SDS dissolved in deionized water
to a final volume of 10 ml. Store at 4°C to
prevent bacterial growth, warm to room
temperature just before use. Discard after 4
weeks of storage.

Electrophoresis buffer

57.6 g glycine.
12.0 g Tris base.
2.0 g SDS.
Dissolve and make up to 2 litres with water; make
up fresh on day of use.

Fixative

100 ml propan-2-ol.
40 ml acetic acid.
Make up to 400 ml with water.

Preparation of gels

Running gel (1.6% agarose, 0.1% SDS)

0.8 g agarose.
12.5 ml running buffer.
37.0 ml water.
0.5 ml 10% SDS.
Dissolve by boiling — SDS may be added to the
molten agarose to prevent frothing. The
hydrophilic side of standard gel-bond is stuck to
a clean glass slide (110 × 205 mm) by a few
drops of water. Gels are cast between the
hydrophobic side and a clean glass plate
separated by a 1 mm spacer. Bulldog clips are
used to clamp the mould together which is
warmed at 37°C prior to the addition of molten
agarose. The resultant gel is allowed to set at
4°C.

Preparation of samples

Plasma samples are diluted in the sample buffer:
50 µl sample.
700 µl sample buffer.
15µl 1% bromophenol blue dye.

Electrophoresis

The LKB cooling system used should be set at
8°C to achieve a gel temperature of 13°C. Wicks
are prepared from J cloths and Whatman No. 1
24 cm filter papers, cut to the length of the agarose
gel. 500 ml of electrophoresis buffer is placed in
each reservoir of the Shandon tank. The mould is
carefully disassembled by sliding the gel-bond off,
leaving the gel on the glass plate. Using a
template, cut 10 wells (10 × 2 mm) in the gel. The
gel is placed on the cooling platten and the moist
filter paper wicks are overlaid the gel by 2 mm at
both ends. Moist cloth wicks are then placed over
the paper wicks by all but the 2 mm which
overlays the stacking gel, and allowed to dip into
the buffer in each reservoir.

20 ml of diluted sample are pipetted into each
well and the gels electrophoresed at a constant
current of 5 mA per gel (approx. 65 V). After
approximately 90 min when the blue dye has

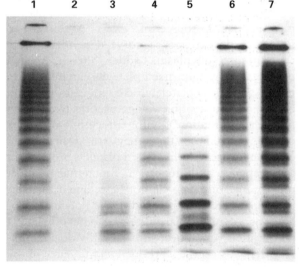

**Fig. 17.6 Autoradiograph of the electrophoretic
analysis of vWF multimer patterns.** The largest
multimers appear at the top of the gel. The normal pattern
with numerous large multimers and a triplet pattern visible in
the smaller multimers is shown in lane 7. Lanes 1 and 6 are
compatible with Type-I vWD in which there is a generalized
decrease in multimer numbers but retaining the normal triplet
pattern. In lane 2 there is virtually no vWF detected
indicating Type-III vWD. Lanes 3 and 5 show both
abnormality of vWF amount and multimer pattern indicating
Types IIa and IId, respectively. In lane 4 there is selective loss
of the large multimers typical of Type-IIb vWD. For more
detailed discussion, see ref. 26.

migrated 1 cm any liquid in the well is removed and the wells are refilled with molten gel. Electrophoresis is restarted at the same current. After a total of 18–20 h the dye will have run off the gel and into the wick. Gels are then fixed for 1 h and the gel gently removed from the glass plate.

After washing in 3 changes of distilled water for a total of 3 h gels are transferred to a small plastic tray and washed with 100 ml 1% bovine IgG in PBS, then in PBS followed by 10% rabbit plasma in PBS, each wash being about 20 min. Gels are then washed in PBS for the remainder of the day, when 100 ml of the labelled rabbit antibody, diluted in PBS, are added to the gel and the tray left to mix overnight behind a lead shield.

The labelled antibody is carefully removed and poured to waste down the radioactive sink. Extensive washing of the gel in 3% saline for 24 h is followed by washing in 0.9% saline and distilled water throughout the 4th day. After mounting the gel on the hydrophilic side of the gel bond it may be dried in a hot-air oven.

Dried gels are placed against Kodak X Omat X-ray film in between intensifying screens in a cassette. They are left overnight in a deep-freeze refrigerator, preferably at −70°C, warmed for 30 min, then developed.

Interpretation[26]

See Fig 17.6.

RISTOCETIN COFACTOR ASSAY[22]

Principle. Washed platelets do not 'agglutinate' in the presence of ristocetin unless normal plasma is added as a source of vWF. 'Agglutination' follows a dose response curve dependent upon the amount of plasma added. Fresh washed platelets or formalin-fixed platelets can be used in the assay. Fixed platelets take longer to prepare, but are not susceptible to aggregation (as distinct from 'agglutination') with ristocetin, and they can be stored so that they are available for emergency use. Fresh washed platelets are quicker to prepare, and retain a functional platelet membrane, but they cannot be retained for later use. Commercial lyophilized washed platelet preparations are also available. The type of platelet preparation which best suits an individual laboratory depends on the work-load and urgency of the test. Where there are large batches of non-urgent assays, there may be no advantage in using fixed platelets. Commercial preparations may not be economical.

ASSAY USING FRESH PLATELETS

Reagents

K_2EDTA. 0.134 mol/l.
Citrate-saline. One volume of 31.1 g/l trisodium citrate + 9 volumes of 9 g/l NaCl.

EDTA-citrate-saline. One volume of 0.134 mol/l K_2EDTA + 9 volumes of citrate-saline.

Method

Collect 40–60 ml of normal blood into a one-tenth volume of EDTA-saline in flat-bottom plastic universal containers. Do not use conical bottom containers. Centrifuge at 150–200**g** at room temperature (c 20°C) for 15 min.

Pipette, using a plastic pipette, the platelet-rich plasma into a plastic container. Mark the level of plasma on the tube. Centrifuge at 1500–2000**g** to obtain a platelet button.

Discard the platelet-poor plasma. Resuspend the platelet button in a 2 ml volume pipetteful of EDTA-citrate-saline by gently squeezing the liquid up and down a pipette until a smooth suspension is formed. Add EDTA-citrate-saline to the 20 ml mark.

Centrifuge at 1500–2000**g** for 15 min. Discard the supernatant. Resuspend in EDTA-citrate-saline and leave at room temperature for 20 min to elute the ristocetin cofactor off the platelets.

Centrifuge again, discard the supernatant, resuspend in EDTA-citrate-saline two more times to a total of four washes.

Centrifuge at 1500–2000g for 15 min. Discard the supernatant and resuspend in citrate-saline using a volume slightly under the original plasma volume (marked on the container). Centrifuge at 800g for 5 min to remove platelet clumps, white cells and red cells.

Remove the platelet-rich supernatant carefully. Perform a platelet count and dilute the platelet-rich suspension with citrate-saline until the platelet count is about 200×10^9/l.

Leave the platelets at room temperature for 30–45 min to allow the platelets to recover from the trauma of washing and centrifugation.

Reagents for assay

Citrate-saline.
Ristocetin. 100 mg/ml. Stored frozen in 1 ml volumes.
Plasma standard.
Platelet-poor plasma. From the patient or patients.

Assay method

Confirm that the washed platelets do not 'agglutinate' with ristocetin in the absence of added plasma. Deliver 0.5 ml of citrate-saline into an aggregometer cuvette and 0.4 ml of the platelet suspension + 0.1 ml of citrate-saline into another cuvette. Place in the warming block and allow to warm. Add 5 µl of ristocetin and record at 1 cm/min for 2 min. The absorbance due to citrate-saline alone is taken to represent 100% agglutination, and that due to platelets alone represents zero (%) agglutination (blank). The absorbance due to the platelet suspension must not exceed 5 divisions on the chart paper. If it is greater, the platelets must be washed again and the procedure repeated. The reading of this blank must be repeated every hour.

All plasma samples and ristocetin should be kept in an ice-bath.

Standard curve. A standard curve is obtained by making doubling dilutions, 1 in 2 to 1 in 32 in citrate-saline, of the standard plasma (donor pool, commercial reference plasma or other reference materials). The absorbance due to a mixture of 0.4 ml of citrate-saline and 0.1 ml of plasma dilution is taken to represent 100% agglutination and that due to the mixture of 0.4 ml of platelet suspension and 0.1 ml of plasma dilution zero (0%) agglutination.

Add 5 µl of ristocetin to the cuvette containing the mixture giving zero agglutination and record the agglutination for 2 min. Test each dilution of the standard plasma in a similar way.

The patient's plasma is tested at two dilutions, depending on the expected concentration of vWF in the plasma. Both dilutions should give agglutination within the range of that of the standard curve.

Reset 100% and zero aggregation for each patient.

A reading of the platelet blank should be repeated at hourly intervals. If the reading differs from the original, the difference must be subtracted from the results of subsequent tests.

Results

Measure 'agglutination' at 1 or 2 min depending on the strength of 'agglutination'. All responses must be compared on the same time scale and not read at maximum 'agglutination'.

Plot the standard curve on semi-log paper with 'agglutination' on the linear scale and the concentration of vWF in u/dl on the log scale (see Fig. 17.7). For assay purposes, assign the 1 in 2 dilution of standard plasma a value of 50 u/dl. (Each batch of standard is precalibrated as described on p. 327 and may not necessarily be 100 u/dl.)

Read the patient's vWF concentration directly off the standard curve, correct for the dilution factor and average the two results from the different dilutions.

Normal

50–200 u/dl.

Interpretation

The vWF concentration measured by ristocetin cofactor assay can only be interpreted in conjunction with other factor VIII:C and vWF:Ag assays, as shown in Table 17.6, p. 331.

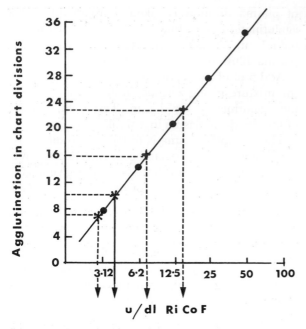

Fig 17.7   Ristocetin cofactor assay. The standard curve is plotted on semi-log paper. Each test plasma is assayed in two dilutions. Plasma 1 (+) produced the following readings: 1 in 4 dilution: 16 divisions of the chart paper = 7 u (× 4 (dilution factor) = 28 u/dl); 1 in 2 dilution: 22 divisions = 13 u/dl (× 2 (dilution factor) = 26 u/dl). The mean of the two readings is 27 u/dl. Plasma 2 (⋆) gave the following results. 1 in 2 dilution: 7 divisions = 2.5 u (× 2 (dilution factor) = 5 u/dl). 1 in 4 dilution: 5 divisions (not shown). This result was similar to the blank and the plasma was next tested undiluted, giving a reading of 10 divisions = 4 u/dl. The mean is 4.5 u/dl (very low).

ASSAY USING FORMALIN-FIXED PLATELETS

Reagents

Sodium citrate solution. 32 g/l trisodium sodium citrate ($Na_3C_6H_5O_7.2H_2O$).
   K_2EDTA. 0.134 mol/l.
   2% formalin (40% formaldehyde). In 9 g/l NaCl.
   0.05% sodium azide. In 9 g/l NaCl.

Method

Citrated blood in a blood donation bag, obtained from a normal individual or from a therapeutic venesection carried out on a patient with a normal platelet count can be used. ACD or CPD solution from the donor bag is ejected through the taking needle and replaced by the equivalent volume of sodium citrate. Collect *c* 500 ml of blood.

Centrifuge the blood at 300*g* for 15 min at room temperature. Separate the platelet-rich plasma (PRP) and add 9 volumes of PRP to 1 volume of EDTA solution. Incubate for 1 h at 37°C to reverse the effect of ADP released during the preparation. Add an equal volume of 2% formalin and leave at 4°C for 1 h. Centrifuge at 200*g* for 10 min at 4°C. Decant the supernatant and recentrifuge it at 250*g* for 20 min at 4°C. Discard the supernatant and resuspend the platelet sediment in chilled (4°C) 9 g/l NaCl. Wash the platelets twice more. After the final wash resuspend the platelets in the sodium azide solution. Adjust the platelet count to 300–500 × 10⁹/l. The suspension is stable for 1 month at 4°C.

Reagents for assay

Buffer for plasma dilutions. Barbitone buffer, pH 7.4, containing 40 mg/ml of bovine serum albumin (p. 577).
   Ristocetin, plasma standard and patient's platelet-poor plasma. As described in the previous assay.

Assay method

Follow the method described for washed fresh platelets. Prepare all plasma dilutions in the albumin-containing buffer.

Results, interpretation and normal range

As described for the washed platelet assay.

INVESTIGATION OF A PATIENT WITH A CIRCULATING ANTICOAGULANT (INHIBITOR)[4,19]

Circulating anticoagulants or acquired inhibitors of coagulation factors are immunoglobulins arising either in congenitally deficient individuals as a result of the administration of the missing factor or in previously haemostatically normal subjects as a part of an auto-immune process.

Of the anticoagulants which cause a bleeding tendency, antibodies to factor VIII:C are most common. They develop in 15% or more of haemophiliacs. Inhibitors directed against vWF and factors IX, V, XI, XII, etc., are very rare. The commonest anticoagulant in haemostatically normal people is the lupus anticoagulant, but despite the prolongation of clotting tests in vitro, this anticoagulant predisposes to thrombosis and its diagnosis and investigation is therefore considered on p. 351. Only the factor VIII:C inhibitor assays are described in detail in this section. Inhibitors against factors VIII:C fall into two general categories: those with simple kinetics, and those with complex kinetics. Patients with haemophilia usually develop antibodies with simple kinetics; this inhibitor reacts with factor VIII:C in a linear fashion and the antigen/antibody complex has no factor VIII:C activity. Complex inhibitors usually arise in non-haemophilic individuals. Inactivation of factor VIII:C is at first rapid, but it then slows as the antigen/antibody complex either dissociates or displays some factor VIII:C activity. In some patients diluted plasma can neutralize more factor VIII:C than an undiluted sample.

INHIBITOR (ANTICOAGULANT) SCREEN BASED ON THE APTT[19]

Principle. Circulating anticoagulants or inhibitors affecting the APTT may act immediately or be time-dependent. Normal plasma mixed with a plasma containing an immediately acting inhibitor will have little or no effect on the prolonged clotting time. In contrast, if normal plasma is added to a plasma containing a time-dependent inhibitor, the clotting time of the latter will be substantially shortened. However, after 1–2 h, correction will be abolished, and the clotting time will become long again. In order to detect both types of inhibition, normal plasma and test plasma samples are mixed and tested immediately and then after incubation at 37°C for 120 min.

Reagents

Normal plasma. A pool of 20 donors as described on p. 327

Platelet-poor plasma. From the patient.

Reagents for the APTT (see p. 308).

Method

Prepare three plastic tubes as follows: place 0.5 ml of normal plasma in a first tube, 0.5 ml of the patient's plasma in a second tube, and a mixture of 0.25 ml of normal and 0.25 ml of patient's plasma in a third tube. Incubate the tubes for 120 min at 37°C and then place all three tubes in an ice-bath or on crushed ice.

Make a 50:50 mixture of the contents of tubes 1 and 2: this tube serves to check for the presence of an immediate inhibitor. Perform APTTs in duplicate on all four tubes.

Results and interpretation

See Table 17.7.

Confusion may arise in the presence of inhibitor if different clotting factors are assayed.

Table 17.7 Interpretation of the inhibitor screen based on the APTT

Tube	Content	Clotting time		
1	Normal plasma	Normal	Normal	Normal
2	Patient's plasma	Long	Long	Long
3	50:50 mixture, patient:normal, incubated 2 h	Normal	Long	Long
4	50:50 mixture, patient:normal, no incubation	Normal	Long	Normal
Interpretation:		Deficiency	Immediately acting inhibitor	Time-dependent inhibitor

For instance, if a patient's plasma contains an inhibitor directed against factor VIII and the factor IX level in that plasma is assayed using factor IX deficient plasma, then the clotting times in the factor IX assay will be prolonged. This may lead to the mistaken conclusion that the patient has factor IX deficiency. Clotting factors should always be assayed at multiple dilutions. If the inhibitor is specifically directed against one clotting factor, that factor will appear to be equally deficient at all dilutions of patient's plasma. The assayed level of other clotting factors will increase with increasing dilution as the inhibitor is diluted out.

QUANTITATIVE MEASUREMENT OF FACTOR VIII:C INHIBITORS[19]

Principle. Factor VIII inhibitors are time-dependent. Thus if factor VIII:C is added to plasma containing an inhibitor and the mixture is incubated, factor VIII:C will be progressively neutralized. If the amount of factor VIII:C added and the duration of incubation are standardized, the strength of the inhibitor may be measured in units according to how much of the added factor VIII:C is destroyed.

In the Bethesda method described below, the unit is defined as the amount of inhibitor which will neutralize 50% of 1 unit of factor VIII:C in 2 h at 37°C.

Dilutions of test plasma are incubated with an equal volume of the normal plasma pool at 37°C. The normal plasma pool is taken to represent 1 unit of factor VIII:C. Dilutions of a control normal plasma containing no inhibitor are treated in the same way. An equal volume of normal plasma mixed with buffer is taken to represent the 100% value.

At the end of the incubation period the residual factor VIII:C is assayed and the inhibitor strength calculated from a graph of residual factor VIII:C activity versus inhibitor units.

Reagents

Glyoxaline buffer. See p. 306.
Kaolin. 5 mg/ml.
Factor VIII:C deficient plasma.
Standard plasma. Normal plasma pool.
Platelet substitute. Phospholipid (see p. 589); also available commercially.

Method

Pipette into each of a series of plastic tubes 0.2 ml of normal pool plasma. Add 0.2 ml of glyoxaline buffer to the first tube (this tube serves as the 100% value); add 0.2 ml of test plasma dilutions in glyoxaline buffer to each of the other tubes. If the patient's inhibitor has been assayed previously, this can be used as a guide to the dilutions that should be used. If the patient has not been tested before, a range of dilutions should be set up ranging from undiluted plasma to a 1 in 50 dilution.

Cap, mix and incubate all the tubes for 2 h at 37°C. Then immerse all the tubes in an ice-bath. Perform factor VIII:C assays on all the incubation mixtures.

Calculation of results

Record the residual factor VIII:C percentage for each mixture assuming the assay value of the control to be 100%. The dilution of test plasma that gives the residual factor VIII:C percentage nearest to 50% (between 30 and 60%) is chosen for calculating the strength of inhibitor. How the results are calculated is shown in Table 17.8 and Fig. 17.8 for three different patients: one had a mild inhibitor only detected in undiluted plasma, one a stronger inhibitor with simple kinetics and one an inhibitor with complex kinetics.

Interpretation

If the residual factor VIII:C activity is between 80% and 100%, the plasma sample does not contain an inhibitor. If the residual activity is less than 60% the plasma unequivocally contains an inhibitor. Values between 60% and 80% are borderline and repeated testing on additional samples is needed before the diagnosis can be established.

Tests for other inhibitors

Factor IX inhibitors can be measured in a system identical to that described above. Because factor IX inhibitors act immediately, there is no need for prolonged incubation: the mixtures can be assayed after 5 min at 37°C.

The activity of the inhibitor against porcine factor VIII can be measured by substituting Hyate C (porcine factor VIII, concentrate, appropriately diluted) for normal plasma.

Table 17.8 Example of the calculation of Bethesda units in three plasma samples

Patient	Plasma dilution	% residual VIII:C	Calculation u × dilution	Inhibitor in Bethesda u
A	Undiluted	61	0.70×1	= 0.07
B	1 in 5	33	1.60×5	= 8.0
	1 in 10	55	0.85×10	= 8.5
	1 in 15	68	0.55×15	= 8.3
C	1 in 5	40	1.30×5	= 6.5
	1 in 10	55	0.85×10	= 8.5
	1 in 15	61	0.70×15	= 10.5
	1 in 20	65	0.60×20	= 12

Patient A has a mild inhibitor, patient B an inhibitor with simple kinetics and patient C an inhibitor with complex kinetics. All values are chosen for the percent residual factor VIII:C activity close to 50%. The units are calculated from Fig. 17.8. (Modified from Kasper & Ewing.[19])
Note that in patients B and C the results should be reported as 8.5 Bethesda units; In C the calculated level of inhibitor may continue to rise with increasing dilution.

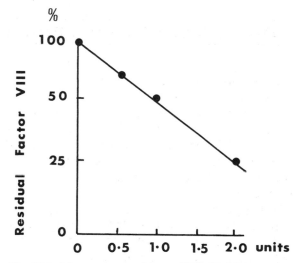

Fig. 17.8 Measurement of factor VIII:C inhibitors.
Relationship between the residual factor VIII:C activity in a standard plasma and the inhibitor activity of a test plasma can be read off this plot. At 50% inhibition the test plasma contains 1 Bethesda inhibitor unit per ml. See also Table 17.8.

INVESTIGATION OF A PATIENT WHOSE APTT AND PT ARE PROLONGED

A prolonged APTT and PT but a normal TT in a patient with a bleeding disorder may be due to a defect or deficiency of one of the factors of the common pathway: factor X, factor V or prothrombin. In addition, the patient could be suffering from the much rarer combined deficiency of factors V and VIII:C. Liver disease and vitamin K deficiency should always be excluded, even in the presence of a family history of bleeding. Mixing tests illustrated on p. 329 may help to pinpoint the defect; the missing factor or factors should be estimated quantitatively. Further tests (including chromogenic and immunoassays as well as immuno-electrophoresis) may be necessary to elucidate the nature of the defect.

TAIPAN VENOM ASSAY FOR PROTHROMBIN.

Principle. The venom of the snake *Oxyuranus scutellatus*, or Taipan venom, converts prothrombin into thrombin in the presence of calcium and phospholipid. This action is not dependent on factors V or X. If a source of fibrinogen is included in the system, the resultant clotting times are proportional to the concentration of prothrombin in the plasma tested.

The best source of fibrinogen is adsorbed oxalated bovine plasma: it provides antithrombin in excess and eliminates the effect of antithrombins in the test plasma.

Reagents

Taipan venom. Commercially available.
Adsorbed oxalated bovine plasma.
Platelet substitute. See p. 589; also available commercially.
Barbitone buffered saline (see p. 306).
Platelet-poor plasma. From the patient.
Standard plasma.
$CaCl_2$. 0.025 mol/l.

Method

Prepare 1 in 5, 1 in 10, 1 in 20, 1 in 40 and 1 in 80 dilutions of the test and standard plasma in buffered saline in plastic tubes. Place 0.1 ml of each dilution in a glass tube, add 0.1 ml of platelet substitute and 0.1 ml of bovine plasma. Warm at 37°C; then add 0.2 ml of a mixture of equal volumes of $CaCl_2$ and Taipan venom, start a stop-watch and record the clotting time. Repeat for each dilution of the standard and test plasma.

Calculation

Plot the clotting times against the reciprocal of the dilutions on *linear* graph paper. Straight but not necessarily parallel lines should be obtained. To calculate the result, express the result with each dilution of the test sample in relation to the standard and calculate the mean of all the readings.

Normal range

50–200 u/dl.

Interpretation

Congenital prothrombin deficiency is very uncommon. Its basis is the presence of an abnormal prothrombin molecule. The condition has been described as dysprothrombinaemia. Before making this diagnosis it has, however, to be differentiated from various acquired disorders and the presence of the lupus anticoagulant (see p. 351).

A two-stage assay for prothrombin was described in the 6th edition of this book.

FACTOR X ASSAY[12]

Principle. Factor X is assayed by a one-stage procedure using Russell Viper venom (RVV). RVV is insensitive to factor VII deficiency and if the venom is used instead of thromboplastin, prolongation of the prothrombin time reflects a deficiency of factors X, V and prothrombin. By incorporating an excess of factor V and prothrombin in the system, the concentration of factor X can be sensitively measured.

Reagents

Platelet-poor plasma. From the patient.
Standard plasma
$CaCl_2$. 0.025 mol/l.
Barbitone buffered saline. See p. 306.
Factor-X-deficient plasma. Commercially available.
Platelet substitute. See p. 589; also commercially available.
Russell viper venom (Burroughs Wellcome). Add 2 ml of buffered saline to the vial: this

results in a 1 in 10 000 dilution of the venom. To provide the working reagent the venom is combined with platelet substitute. Dilute the platelet substitute 1 in 5 with buffered saline. Add 0.1 ml of the solution of the venom to 2.9 ml of platelet substitute so as to achieve a final dilution of 1 in 300 000. This mixture must be prepared fresh before every assay.

Method

Prepare in plastic tubes 1 in 5, 1 in 10, 1 in 20 and 1 in 40 dilutions of both the test and the standard plasma in buffered saline. Transfer 0.1 ml of each dilution into a glass tube and add 0.1 ml of factor X deficient plasma. Warm to 37°C. Then add 0.1 ml of the RVV/platelet substitute mixture, start the stop-watch and mix. At exactly 30 sec add 0.1 ml of $CaCl_2$. Record the clotting time. Repeat for each dilution of the test and standard plasma. Always include a blank containing buffered saline instead of a plasma dilution. Test in balanced order to avoid time-trend.

Results

Plot the clotting times against factor X concentration using 2 cycle × 3 cycle log paper. The lines should be straight and parallel. Read the factor X concentration of the test from the intercept with the standard curve, as shown previously.

Normal range

50–200 u/dl.

Interpretation

Factor X deficiency is a rare disorder and affected families have abnormal, variant proteins. Immunoassays and tests of factor X activation are necessary to confirm the diagnosis. Isolated acquired factor X deficiency has also been described in association with amyloidosis and investigations to exclude amyloidosis and paraproteinaemia may be required.

FACTOR V ASSAY

Principle. Factor V assay is a one-stage procedure based on the prothrombin time. It is carried out in the same way as the assay of factor VII. Factor V deficient plasma is, however, used as substrate.

Reagents

Factor V deficient plasma. This is prepared by ageing normal plasma. Blood from a healthy individual is collected into a one-ninth volume of 14 g/l potassium oxalate. Plasma is separated by centrifuging at 2000*g* for 15 min. The plasma is kept at 37°C under sterile conditions for 3 days, then stored in 2 ml volumes at –30°C until used.

Other reagents are described on p. 328.

Normal range

50–200 u/dl.

Interpretation

It is important to ensure that the test sample is fresh and that a low result is not due to ageing of the patient's plasma. Factor V deficiency is very rare, combined deficiency of factors V and VIII:C even rarer. Factor VIII:C assays should be carried out in all individuals found to have a deficiency of factor V. Acquired factor V deficiency is also uncommon; it has been found as part of the consumption coagulopathy resulting from DIC and very rarely in untreated chronic granulocytic leukaemia (personal observation).

Factor V assays are now often used as part of the assessment of hepatocellular damage.

INVESTIGATION OF A PATIENT SUSPECTED OF AFIBRINOGENAEMIA, HYPOFIBRINOGENAEMIA OR DYSFIBRINOGENAEMIA

The patient usually has a prolonged APTT, PT and thrombin time. The prolongation of the PT is usually less marked than that of the APTT and thrombin time. There may be either a history of bleeding or of recurrent thrombotic events. Fibrinogen should be measured quantitatively using a clot weight method as described below or a thrombin-based estimation (see p. 345).

FIBRINOGEN ESTIMATION (DRY CLOT WEIGHT)

Principle. Fibrinogen in plasma is converted into fibrin by clotting with thrombin and calcium. The resulting clot is weighed.

Reagents

Citrated platelet-poor plasma.
$CaCl_2$. 0.025 mol/l.
Bovine thrombin. 50 NIH u/ml.

Method

Pipette 1 ml of plasma into a 12 × 75 mm glass tube and warm to 37°C. Place a wooden applicator or swab stick in the tube, add 0.1 ml of $CaCl_2$ and 0.9 ml of thrombin and mix. Incubate for 15 min at 37°C.

Gently wind the fibrin clot onto the stick, squeezing out the serum. Wash the clot in a tube containing at first 9 g/l NaCl, then water. Blot the clot carefully with filter paper, remove the fibrin from the stick and put into acetone for 5–10 min. Dry the clot in a hot air oven or over a hot lamp for 30 min. Allow it to cool and weigh.

Results

The fibrinogen level is expressed as g/l, i.e. the weight of fibrin obtained from 1 ml of plasma × 1000.

Normal range

1.5–4.0 g/l.

Further investigations

Whenever a congenital fibrinogen abnormality is suspected, DIC and hyperfibrinolysis must be excluded: FDP should not be in excess and there should be no evidence of the consumption of other coagulation factors and platelets (see p. 345).

Immunological or chemical determination of fibrinogen is the next step in investigation. In dysfibrinogenaemias there is often a normal or even raised plasma fibrinogen concentration using these methods although the functional assays indicate a deficiency. Other tests which may be helpful are the Reptilase time, fibrinopeptide release, factor XIII cross-linking, tests of polymerization, binding to thrombin and lysis by plasmin. In some cases genomic DNA analysis can be performed.[20]

CLOT SOLUBILITY TEST FOR FXIII

Principle. Clots formed in the presence of factor XIII and Ca^{2+} are stable (due to cross-linking) for at least 1 h in 1% monochloracetic acid solution and in 5 mol/l urea, whereas clots formed in the absence of factor XIII dissolve rapidly.

Reagents

Platelet-poor plasma. From the patient and a control.
$CaCl_2$. 0.025 mol/l.
Monochloracetic acid. 10 g/l.
Urea. 5 mol/l in 9 g/l NaCl.

Method

Place 0.5 ml of the two plasma samples in glass tubes, add an equal volume of $CaCl_2$ solution to each and incubate for 30 min. Tap each tube gently to loosen the clot from the sides of the tube and add 3 ml of monochloracetic acid solution or 5 mol/l urea so that the clot is suspended. Leave at room temperature (c 20°C). Inspect the clot at 4 h if monochloracetic acid is used, and at 24 h if urea is used.

Interpretation

The control clot, if normal, shows no sign of dissolving. If the patient's factor XIII concentration is subnormal, the clot will completely dissolve. The presence of deficiency or defect must be confirmed by a combination of immunological and functional techniques, such as the incorporation of synthetic radioactive or fluorescein-labelled ester.[28,29] Kits are now available for direct assays of factor XIII functional activity.

DISSEMINATED INTRAVASCULAR COAGULATION (DIC)

The term DIC encompasses a wide range of clinical phenomena of varying degrees of severity. It is also sometimes referred to as consumptive coagulopathy because its characteristic feature is excessive and widespread activation of the coagulation mechanism with consequent consumption of clotting factors and inhibitors with loss of the normal regulatory mechanisms. In acutely ill patients this typically results in defibrination and a haemorrhagic diathesis. In some situations, however, the activation may be less marked resulting in a tendency to thrombosis. This latter phenomenon is typical of the coagulation activation seen in association with malignancy and may be associated with slightly shortened clotting times.

The diagnosis of acute DIC can generally be made from the basic first-line screening tests described in Chapter 16. Characteristically, the PT, APTT and TT are all prolonged and the fibrinogen level is markedly reduced. In association with the consumption of clotting factors responsible for these abnormalities there is also a fall in platelet count also due to consumption. Concomitantly there is activation of the fibrinolytic system and an increase in circulating fibrin(ogen) degradation products. These abnormalities form the basis for the diagnosis of DIC. More elaborate tests are not usually performed but can demonstrate reductions in individual clotting factors, ATIII and antiplasmin and increased levels of thrombin-antithrombin and plasmin-antiplasmin complexes and of activation peptides such as prothrombin F1+2. The first-line tests are described in the previous chapter; the assays for fibrinogen and its degradation products are described below.

FIBRINOGEN ASSAY (CLAUSS TECHNIQUE)[10]

Principle. Diluted plasma is clotted with a strong thrombin solution; the plasma must be diluted to give a low level of any inhibitors, i.e. FDPs and heparin. A strong thrombin solution must be used so that the clotting time over a wide range is independent of the thrombin concentration.

Reagents

Calibration plasma. With a known level of fibrinogen.
Platelet-poor plasma. From the patient and a control.
Thrombin solution. Freshly reconstituted to 100 NIH per ml in 9 g/l NaCl.
Owren's veronal buffer, pH 7.35. See p. 306.

Method

A calibration curve is prepared each time the batch of thrombin reagent is changed and this is used to calculate the results of unknown plasma samples.

Make dilutions of the calibration plasma in veronal buffer to give a range of fibrinogen concentrations, i.e. 1 in 5, 1 in 10, 1 in 20 and 1 in 40. 0.2 ml of each dilution is warmed to 37°C, 0.1 ml of thrombin solution is added and the clotting time is measured. Each test should be performed in duplicate. Plot the clotting time in seconds against the fibrinogen concentration in g/l on log/log graph paper. The 1 in 10 concentration is considered to be 100% and there should be a straight line correlation between 5–50 s. Make a 1 in 10 dilution of each patient's sample and clot 0.2 ml of the dilution with 0.1 ml of thrombin. Read the fibrinogen result off the calibration curve. The clot formed in this method may be 'wispy' due to the plasma being diluted, and end-point detection may be easier with automated equipment.

Normal range

2–4 g/l.

DETECTION OF FIBRINOGEN/FIBRIN DEGRADATION PRODUCTS (FDP) USING A LATEX AGGLUTINATION METHOD[14]

Principle. A suspension of latex particles is sensitized with specific antibodies to the purified FDP fragments D and E. The suspension is mixed on a glass slide with a dilution of the serum to be tested. Aggregation indicates the presence of FDP in the sample. By testing different dilutions of the unknown sample, a semi-quantitative assay can be performed.

Reagents

Venous blood. Collected into a special tube (provided with the kit) containing the anti-fibrinolytic agent and thrombin.
Thrombo-Wellcotest kit.
Positive and negative controls. Provided by the manufacturer.
Glycine buffer. Part of the kit.

Method

Allow the tube with blood to stand at 37°C until clot retraction commences. Then centrifuge the tube and withdraw the serum for testing.

Make 1 in 5 and 1 in 20 dilutions of serum in glycine buffer. Mix one drop of each serum dilution with one drop of latex suspension on a glass slide. Rock the slide gently for 2 min while looking for macroscopic agglutination. If a positive reaction is observed in the higher dilution, make doubling dilutions from the 1 in 20 dilution until macroscopic agglutination can no longer be seen.

Interpretation

Agglutination with a 1 in 5 dilution of serum indicates a concentration of FDP in excess of 10 μg/ml; agglutination in a 1 in 20 dilution indicates FDP in excess of 40 μg/ml.

Normal range

Healthy subjects have an FDP concentration less than 10 μg/ml. Concentrations between 10 and 40 μg/ml are found in a variety of conditions including acute venous thromboembolism, acute myocardial infarction, severe pneumonia and after major surgery. High levels are seen in systemic fibrinolysis associated with DIC and thrombolytic therapy with streptokinase.

SCREENING TESTS FOR FIBRIN MONOMERS[7,21]

Principle. When thrombin acts on fibrinogen some of the monomers do not polymerize but give rise to soluble complexes with plasma fibrinogen and FDP. These complexes can be associated in vitro by ethanol or protamine sulphate.

Reagents

Platelet-poor plasma. From the patient and a control.
Positive control. This is prepared by adding 0.1 ml of thrombin (0.2 NIH units/ml) to 0.9 ml of control plasma and incubating at 37°C for 30 min. Fibrin threads formed during the incubation are removed by centrifugation.
Protamine sulphate. 1% (10 g/l).

Ethanol. 50% (v/v) in water.

Method

1. *Protamine sulphate test.* Add 0.05 ml of protamine sulphate to 0.5 ml of patient's plasma and to 0.5 ml of positive control plasma. Incubate undisturbed at 37°C for 30 min. A positive result is indicated by the formation of a fine fibrin network or fibrin strands. The presence of amorphous material only is a negative result.

2. *Ethanol gelation test.* Add 0.15 ml of ethanol to 0.5 ml of patient's plasma and to 0.5 ml of the positive control plasma at room temperature (*c* 20°C). After gentle agitation inspect the tubes at 1 min intervals. A positive result is the formation of a definite gel within 3 min.

Interpretation

Positive gelation tests are found in:

1. The early stages of acute disseminated intravascular coagulation.
2. After major surgery.
3. Severe inflammatory illness, in particular lobar pneumonia.
4. Liver disease.

INVESTIGATION OF CARRIERS OF A CONGENITAL COAGULATION DEFICIENCY OR DEFECT[3,15,25]

Carrier detection is important in genetic counselling, and antenatal diagnosis may enable heterozygotes to consider abortion of a severely affected fetus. The information of value in carrier detection is derived from family studies, phenotype investigations and the determination of genotype.

FAMILY STUDIES

Haemophilia A and B (factor VIII:C and factor IX deficiency) are inherited by X-linked genes. This means that all the sons of a haemophiliac will be normal and all his daughters carriers. The children of a carrier have a 0.5 chance of being affected if they are sons, and a 0.5 chance of being carriers if they are daughters. The other coagulation factor defects are inherited as autosomal traits. Heterozygotes possess approximately half the normal concentration of the coagulation factor and are generally not affected clinically; only homozygotes have a significant bleeding tendency.

A detailed family study is important in all coagulation factor defects in order to establish the true nature of the defect and its severity. Patients often describe any familial bleeding tendency as haemophilia, and it is therefore essential to prove the exact defect in every new patient and family. In inbred kindreds the likelihood of homozygotes emerging is increased.

When a detailed family study has been carried out it may be possible to establish the statistical chance of inheriting a coagulation defect. For a review, see Graham et al.[15]

Phenotype investigation

Theoretically one might expect the concentration of the affected coagulation factor in the heterozygote or carrier to be roughly half that of normal. However, in the case of factor VIII and factor IX this is complicated by the phenomenon of X chromosome inactivation (XCI). Women possess two X chromosomes but in each cell only one of these two is utilized and the other is largely inactivated. The choice of which X is active is essentially random and varies over a normal distribution. Thus, in carriers of haemophilia A or B, the level of factor VIII or IX also varies over roughly a normal distribution depending on the proportions of the normal and haemophiliac containing Xs that are utilized. As a result, some carriers may have an entirely normal level of factor VIII or factor IX and others may be significantly deficient. This chromosome inactivation is sometimes referred to as Lyonization after Mary Lyon by whom it was first described.

In the case of factor VIII the level of vWF has sometimes been found to be useful. The ratio of VIII:C to vWF:Ag is reduced in most carriers and can be used in conjunction with the family history to determine a probability that the subject is a carrier. These estimations are further complicated by the fact that factor VIII levels behave as an acute phase reactant and may be elevated by a number of intercurrent factors including stress and exercise.

Genotype assignment

The advent of molecular biology and the cloning of many of the genes for coagulation factors, especially factor VIII and factor IX, has revolu-

tionized the approach to carrier determination. The discovery of genetic polymorphisms, some of which are multi-allelic, within the coagulation factor genes has meant that in most families the affected gene can be tracked and the carrier state determined with a high degree of probability. Increasingly, and particularly for factor IX, the genetic defect itself can be identified resulting in unequivocal genotypic assignment in every member of a family.

The techniques required for these analyses are described in Chapter 28. The whole problem of carrier determination and antenatal diagnosis has recently been dealt with in a comprehensive review by a WHO/WFH group.[24]

TESTS REQUIRED FOR MONITORING REPLACEMENT THERAPY IN COAGULATION FACTOR DEFECTS AND DEFICIENCIES

Replacement therapy requires the following:

1. Calculation of the dose of the material to be administered and its frequency.
2. Assessment of the response to the dose.
3. Monitoring of any untoward effects.

The *dose* to be administered is calculated from the patient's body weight and the rise in the plasma concentration of the defective coagulation factor that is desired. Thus, the patient's plasma concentration of the factor and the potency or strength of the therapeutic material must be known. For the vast majority of patients whose defect is known and its plasma concentration has been measured, and for whom a commercial freeze-dried factor concentrate is used, this means a calculation based on the following formulae:

For factor VIII:C the dose in IU per kg body weight = rise required in IU per dl divided by 2.

For factor XI, the dose in IU per kg body weight = rise required in IU per dl.

The rise required depends on the type of bleeding, the half-life and stability of the clotting factor used, and on the concentration of the

defective factor in the patient's plasma prior to treatment. For details, see Rizza and Jones.[25]

Assessment of the response to the therapy requires regular measurements of the plasma concentration of the coagulation factor infused by means of a functional assay. The response can be assessed from the formula:

Rise in IU per dl divided by dose in IU per kg body weight = K, which is approximately 2 for haemophilia A, and approximately 1 for haemophilia B (if concentrates are used).

The response is usually measured immediately after the administration of the therapeutic material. If the response is inadequate, this may have been due to an error in calculating the dose, or because the potency of the therapeutic material is less than expected, or because the patient is developing an inhibitor.

The main *untoward effects* are transmission of infection and the development of inhibitors. If the presence of an inhibitor is suspected, it must be confirmed using the tests described on p. 339 and later assessed quantitatively. For monitoring replacement and other types of therapy in patients with inhibitors, see Bloom.[4]

DETECTION OF CROSS-LINKED FIBRIN D-DIMERS USING A LATEX AGGLUTINATION METHOD

Principle. This is identical to the test previously described for fibrinogen/fibrin degradation products, but in this case the latex beads are coated with a monoclonal antibody directed specifically against fibrin D-dimer in human plasma or serum.

Reagents

Several manufacturers market kits for the measurement of D-dimers. These usually contain the latex suspension, dilution buffer and positive and negative controls.

As there is no reaction with fibrinogen, the need for serum is eliminated and measurements can be performed on plasma samples.

Method

The manufacturer's protocol should be followed.

Undiluted plasma is mixed with one drop of latex suspension on a glass slide and the slide is gently rocked for the length of time recommended in the kit. If macroscopic agglutination is observed, dilutions of the plasma are made until agglutination can no longer be seen.

Interpretation

Agglutination with the undiluted plasma indicates a concentration of D-dimers in excess of 200 mg/l. The D-dimer level can be quantified by multiplying the reciprocal of the highest dilution showing a positive result by 200 to give a value in mg/l.

Normal range

Plasma levels in normal subjects are <200 mg/l.

REFERENCES

[1] BARROWCLIFFE, T. W. and CURTISS, A. D. (1987). Principles of bioassay. In *Haemostasis and Thrombosis*. Eds. Bloom, A. L. and Thomas, D. P., 2nd edn, p. 996. Churchill Livingstone, Edinburgh.

[2] BARTLETT, A., DORMANDY, K. M., HAWKEY, C. M., STABLEFORTH, P. and VOLLER, A. (1976) Factor VIII related antigen: measurement by enzyme immunoassay. *British Medical Journal*, **1**, 994.

[3] BLOOM, A. L. (1987). Inherited disorders of blood coagulation. In *Haemostasis and Thrombosis*. Eds. Bloom, A. L. and Thomas, D. P., 2nd edn, p. 393. Churchill Livingstone, Edinburgh.

[4] BLOOM, A. L. (1987). The treatment of factor VIII inhibitors. In *Thrombosis and Hemostasis*. Eds. Verstraete, M., Vermylen, J., Lijnen, H. R. and Arnout, J., p. 108. International Society on Thrombosis and Haemostasis and Leuven University Press, Leuven.

[5] BORN, G. V. R. (1962). Aggregation of blood platelets by adenosine diphosphate and its reversal. *Nature*, **194**, 927.

[6] BORN, G. V. R. (1962). Quantitative investigations into the aggregation of blood platelets. *Journal of Physiology*, **162**, 67.

[7] BREEN, F. A. Jr. and TULLIS, J. L. (1986). Ethanol gelation: a rapid screening test for intravascular coagulation. *Annals of Internal Medicine*, **69**, 1197.

[8] BRITISH SOCIETY FOR HAEMATOLOGY (1988). Guidelines on platelet function testing. *Journal of Clinical Pathology*, **41**, 1322.

[9] CHANNING RODGERS, R. P. and LEVIN, J. (1990). A critical reappraisal of the bleeding time. *Seminars in Thrombosis and Hemostasis*, **16**, 1.

[10] CLAUSS, A. (1957). Rapid physiological coagulation method in determination of fibrinogen. *Acta Haematologica (Basel)*, **17**, 237.

[11] DAVID, J. L. and HERION, F. (1972). Assay of platelet ADP and ATP by the luciferase method. *Advances in Experimental Medicine and Biology*, **34**, 341.

[12] DENSON, K. W. E. (1961). The specific assay of Prower-Stuart Factor and Factor VII. *Acta Haematologica (Basel)*, **25**, 105.

[13] ENAYAT, M. S. and HILL, F. G. (1983). Analysis of the complexity of the multimeric structure of Factor VIII related antigen/vonWillebrand protein using a modified electrophoretic technique. *Journal of Clinical Pathology*, **36**, 915.

[14] GARVEY, M. B. and BLACK J. M. (1972). The detection of fibrinogen/fibrin degradation products by means of a new antibody coated latex particle. *Journal of Clinical Pathology*, **25**, 680.

[15] GRAHAM, J. B., ELSTON, R. C., BARROW, E. S., REISNER, H. M. and NAMBOODIRI, K. K. (1982). The hemophilias: statistical methods for carrier detection in hemophilias. *Methods in Hematology*, **5**, 156.

[16] HARDISTY, R. M. and MACPHERSON, J. C. (1962). A one stage factor VIII (antihaemophilic globulin) assay and its use on venous and capillary plasma. *Thrombosis et Diathesis Haemorrhagica*, **7**, 215.

[17] INGRAM, G. I. C., BROZOVIC, M. and SLATER, N. (1982).

Bleeding Disorders. Blackwell Scientific Publication, Oxford.

[18] IVY, A. C., NELSON, D. and BUCHER, G. (1940). The standardization of certain factors in the cutaneous 'venostasis' bleeding time technique. *Journal of Laboratory and Clinical Medicine,* **26,** 1812.

[19] KASPAR, C. K. and EWING, N. P. (1982). The Hemophilias: Measurement of inhibitor to factor VIII C (and IX C). *Methods in Hematology,* **5,** 39.

[20] LANE, D. A. and SOUTHAN, C. (1987). Inherited abnormalities of fibrinogen synthesis and structure. In *Haemostasis and Thrombosis.* Eds. Bloom, A. L. and Thomas, D. P., 2nd edn, p. 442. Churchill Livingstone, Edinburgh.

[21] LIPINSKI, B. and WOROWSKI, K. (1969). Detection of soluble fibrin monomer complexes in blood by means of protamine sulphate test. *Thrombosis et Diathesis Haemorrhagica,* **20,** 44.

[22] MACFARLANE, D. E., STIBBE, D. E., KIRBY, J., ZUCKER, M. B., GRANT, R. A. and MCPHERSON, J. (1975). A method for assaying Willebrand Factor (ristocetin cofactor). *Thrombosis et Diathesis Haemorrhagica,* **34,** 306.

[23] MIELKE, C. H., KENESHIRO, M. M., MAHER, I. A., WIENER, J. M. and RAPAPORT, S. I. (1969). The standardised normal Ivy bleeding time and its prolongation by aspirin. *Blood,* **34,** 204.

[24] PEAKE, I., LILLICRAP, D. P., BOULYJENKOV, E. et al (1993).

Report of a joint WHO/WFH meeting on the control of haemophlia: carrier detection and prenatal diagnosis. *Blood Coagulation and Fibrinolysis,* **43,** 313.

[25] RIZZA, C. R. and JONES, P. (1987). Management of patients with inherited blood coagulation defects. In *Haemostasis and Thrombosis.* Eds. Bloom, A. L. and Thomas, D. P., 2nd edn, p. 465. Churchill Livingstone, Edinburgh.

[26] RUGGERI, Z. M. (1991). Structure and function of von Willebrand's factor: relationship to von Willebrand's disease. *Mayo Clinic Proceedings,* **66,** 847.

[27] SCRUTTON, M. C., CLARE, K. A., HUTTON, R. A. and BRUCKDORFEN, K. R. (1981). Depressed responsiveness to adrenaline in platelets from apparently normal human donors. A familial trait. *British Journal of Haematology,* **49,** 303.

[28] STEINBERG, P. and STENFLO, J. (1979). A rapid and specific fluorescent activity staining procedure for transamidating enzymes. *Analytical Biochemistry,* **93,** 445.

[29] TYLER, H. M. (1966). A comparative study of the solvents commonly used to detect fibrin stabilization. *Thrombosis et Diathesis Haemorrhagica,* **16,** 61.

[30] YARDUMIAN, D. A., MACKIE, I. J. and MACHIN, S. J. (1986). Laboratory investigation of platelet functions: a review of methodology. *Journal of Clinical Pathology,* **39,** 701.

18. Investigation of a thrombotic tendency

Revised by M. A. Laffan and A. E. Bradshaw

Investigation of suspected acquired thrombotic tendency   351
  Lupus anticoagulant   351
  Kaolin clotting time   352
  Russell's viper venom time   354
  Platelet neutralization test   355
  Anti-cardiolipin assay   356
Investigation of fibrinolytic system   356
  Investigation of suspected dysfibrinogenaemia   356
  Investigation of plasminogen defect or deficiency   356
  Investigation of 'fibrinolytic potential'   357
  Euglobulin lysis time   357
  Fibrin plate lysis   358
  Venous occlusion test   358

t-PA amidolytic assay   359
  Plasminogen activator inhibitory assay   359
  α_2-Antiplasmin amidolytic assay   359
Platelet hyperreactivity   360
  β-thromboglobulin and platelet factor 4 assays   360
Investigation of inherited thrombotic syndromes   361
  Antithrombin III assay   361
  Protein C deficiency   362
  Protein S deficiency   363
ELISA of free and total protein S   364
Heparin cofactor II deficiency   365
Markers of coagulation activation   366

Investigations to exclude an acquired or inherited thrombotic tendency are carried out in neonates, children and young adults who develop venous thrombosis, those who have a strong family history of such events or have thrombosis at an unusual site, and in individuals of all ages with recurrent episodes of thrombo-embolism. These investigations are commonly instituted in venous thrombosis, but some unexplained arterial events, especially in young people, are also studied. In this chapter the investigations to diagnose or exclude an acquired thrombotic tendency are presented first, followed by a simplified battery of tests needed to establish the diagnosis of the more common inherited 'thrombophilias'. The British Committee for Standards in Haematology has published guidelines on the investigation and management of thrombophilia.[4]

INVESTIGATION OF A SUSPECTED ACQUIRED THROMBOTIC TENDENCY

An acquired thrombotic tendency is common and occurs in many conditions. An outline of appropriate investigations is described below and also shown in Table 18.1. A list of causes and probable mechanisms is outlined in Table 18.2

INVESTIGATION FOR THE PRESENCE OF LUPUS ANTICOAGULANT (LAC)

The lupus anticoagulant is an acquired auto-antibody found in a variety of auto-immune disorders and sometimes even in otherwise healthy

Table 18.1　Flow chart for investigating a suspected thrombotic tendency

First-line tests (APTT, PT, TT, and platelet count)	
1. Clotting times shorter than normal, platelet count raised	*?Acquired thrombotic tendency* To confirm or elucidate, measure: fibrinogen, VIII:C and vWF, fibrinolytic potential; inhibitors;* platelet hyperreactivity
2. Clotting times normal, platelet count normal	Either: *Acquired thrombotic tendency* Investigate as under 1. Or: *Congenital thrombophilia* Measure: plasma inhibitors and inactivators, plasminogen
3. APTT prolonged, PT normal or long, with an inhibitor pattern of behaviour	Investigate for: *Lupus anticoagulant*
4. TT prolonged	Investigate for: *Dysfibrinogenaemia*
5. All clotting tests slightly prolonged, platelets low, normal or high	*?Chronic DIC:* Measure: FDP and D-dimer; platelet hyperreactivity; inhibitors

*In some clinical situations such as nephrotic syndrome, in women taking oestrogen-containing contraceptive pills, etc.

individuals.[19] Lupus anticoagulants are immuno-globulins which bind to phospholipids active in coagulation and thus prolong the clotting times of phospholipid-dependent tests such as the PT or APTT. The name 'anticoagulant' is a misnomer since patients do not have a bleeding tendency. Instead, there is a clear association with recurrent venous thrombo-embolism, cerebrovascular accidents and other arterial events and, in women, with recurrent abortions in the second trimester.

Tests for the presence of the lupus anticoagulant should be carried out in all young individuals with unexplained thrombosis, and also in women with recurrent second trimester fetal loss. The detection of lupus anticoagulant should not preclude further investigation for other prethrombotic defects, such as co-existent ATIII, protein C and protein S deficiency. When lupus anticoagulant is present, the first-line tests usually show a normal TT and a prolonged APTT which is not corrected by mixing with normal plasma. The PT may be normal or prolonged. The results obtained in the APTT will depend on the reagent and method used as well as on the potency and avidity of the antibody. Even the most sensitive APTT method may fail to detect the lupus anticoagulant in a small number of patients. It is advisable to confirm or exclude its presence with one or more of the tests described below.

Tests for the lupus anticoagulant involving tissue thromboplastin are not recommended because many samples give false negative results. Some one-stage coagulation assays which utilize phospholipid reagents are also sensitive to the lupus anticoagulant.

It is essential that all the samples of plasma tested for the lupus anticoagulant should be as free of platelets as possible. This is achieved by further centrifugation of plasma at 2000g or by passing the test plasma through a 0.2 μm microfilter under pressure using a syringe.

Patients with the lupus anticoagulant may show other abnormalities, including thrombocytopenia, a positive direct antiglobulin test and a positive antinuclear factor test. In some rare cases, specific antibodies against coagulation factors are also found. Such patients may have a bleeding tendency. The tests used are: the kaolin clotting time, the dilute Russell's viper venom time, and the platelet neutralization test. At least two of these tests must be performed when investigating a patient with a suspected lupus anticoagulant.

The modification of the APTT using aluminium hydroxide and heating has been found to be unreliable and should not be used.

A recommended approach to the diagnosis of lupus anticoagulants has been published.[12]

KAOLIN CLOTTING TIME (KCT)[5,8]

Principle. When the APTT is performed in the absence of platelet substitute reagent, it is particularly sensitive to the lupus anticoagulant. If the test is performed on a range of mixtures of

Table 18.2 Acquired thrombotic tendency: aetiology, mechanisms of hypercoagulability and effects on haemostasis

Aetiology	Mechanisms of hypercoagulability	Effect on first-line tests	Other haemostatic effects
Acute phase reaction	Increase in VIII:C, vWF, fibrinogen and PAI	APTT and PT often short	Increased plasma concentration of acute reactants
Malignancy	Acute phase reaction and/or DIC due to release of tumour products	APTT, PT and TT may be long	Increased FDP, signs of activation of coagulation and of consumption
Myeloproliferative diseases	Increased blood viscosity and high platelet count with activation of haemostasis	APTT and PT may be short	Increased β-TG and PF4; increased acute reactants
Oestrogen-containing pill	Increased levels of vitamin-K-dependent factors, reduced ATIII; dose related	PT may be short	Increased plasma conc. of VII, IX, and XI; reduced ATIII concentration
Lupus anticoagulant	Anti-phospholipid antibodies interfering with coagulation	APTT long, PT variable	Tests for lupus anticoagulant positive; ATIII and PC conc. may be low
Nephrotic syndrome	Loss of ATIII in urine	Normal	Reduced plasma ATIII
Vasculitic diseases and angiopathies, including Behçet's syndrome	Stimulation of endothelium with acute phase reaction, fibrinolytic shut-down and platelet activation	Variable	Very high plasma vWF, VIII:C and fibrinogen; increased PAI, FDP, βTG and PF4
ARDS*	Low grade DIC	Variable	Reduced ATIII, PC, increased FDP, variable levels and acute reactants
Paroxysmal nocturnal haemoglobinuria	Not known; possibly platelet mediated	Normal	Platelet activation may be detected

*ARDS, adult respiratory distress syndrome.
vWF, von Willebrand factor; β-TG, β-thromboglobulin; PF4, platelet factor 4;
ATIII, antithrombin III; PC, protein C; PAI, plasminogen activator inhibitor.

normal and patient's plasma, different patterns of response are obtained indicating the presence of lupus anticoagulant, deficiency of one or more of the coagulation factors or the 'lupus cofactor' effect. This cofactor is now thought to be β-2-glycoprotein-1.

Reagents

Kaolin. 20 mg/l in Tris buffer, pH 7.4. (see p. 308.)
Normal platelet-poor plasma. Depleted of platelets by second centrifugation or microfiltration.
Patient's plasma. Also platelet-depleted.
$CaCl_2$. 0.025 mol/l.

Method

Mix normal and patient's plasma in plastic tubes in the following ratios of normal to patient's plasma: 10:0, 9:1, 8:2, 5:5, 2:8, 1:9 and 0:10. Pipette 0.2 ml of each mixture into a glass tube at 37°C. Add 0.1 ml of kaolin and incubate for 3 min, then add 0.2 ml of $CaCl_2$ and record the clotting time.

Results

Plot the clotting times against the proportion of normal : patient's plasma on linear graph paper as shown in Fig.18.1.

Interpretation

If pattern 1 is obtained, the patient has a classical lupus anticoagulant. Pattern 2 indicates a coagulation factor deficiency as well as lupus anticoagulant.

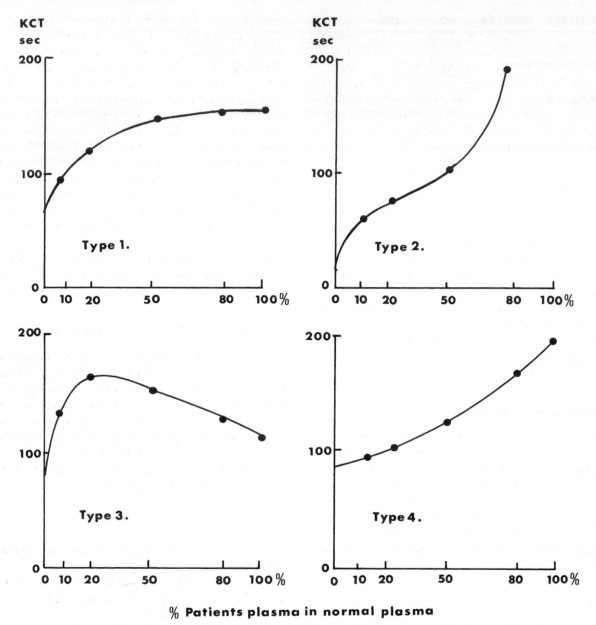

Fig. 18.1 Curves obtained using the kaolin clotting time (KCT) to test for the presence of the lupus anticoagulant. For explanation see text.

Pattern 3 is found in plasma containing the anticoagulant but also deficient in a cofactor necessary for the full inhibitory effect. Pattern 4 is seen in the absence of the lupus anticoagulant.

The crucial feature of these patterns which allows diagnosis to be made is a ratio of KCT at 20% test plasma to KCT at 100% normal control plasma of $\geqslant 1.2$; i.e.

$$\frac{\text{KCT (80\% N:20\% test)}}{\text{KCT 100\% N}} \geqslant 1.2.$$

DILUTE RUSSELL'S VIPER VENOM TIME[20,21]

Principle. Russell's viper venom (RVV) activates factor X in the presence of phospholipid and calcium ions. The lupus anticoagulant prolongs the clotting time by binding to the phospholipid and preventing the action of RVV. In the test described below, dilution of the venom and phospholipid makes it particularly sensitive for detecting the lupus anticoagulant.[21] Since RVV activates factor X directly, defects of the contact system, and factor VIII:C and IX deficiencies will not influence the test.

Reagents

Platelet-poor plasma. From the patient and a control.

Pooled normal plasma.

Glyoxaline buffer. 0.05 mol/l, pH 7.4 (p 306).

Russell's viper venom. Stock solution: 1 mg/ml in saline. For working solution dilute approximately 1 in 200 in buffer. The working solution is stable at 4°C for several hours.

Phospholipid. Platelet substitute (p. 589); also available commercially.

$CaCl_2$. 0.025 mol/l.

Reagent preparation

The RVV concentration is adjusted to give a clotting time of 30–35 s when 0.1 ml of RVV is added to the mixture of 0.1 ml of normal plasma and 0.1 ml of undiluted phospholipid. The test is then repeated using doubling dilutions of phospholipid reagent. The last dilution of phospholipid before the clotting time is prolonged by 2 s or more is selected for the test (thus giving a clotting time of 35–40 s).

Method

Place 0.1 ml of pooled normal plasma and 0.1 ml of dilute phospholipid reagent in a glass tube at 37°C. Add 0.1 ml of dilute RVV and, after warming for 30 s, add 0.1 ml of $CaCl_2$. Record the clotting time. Repeat the sequence using the test plasma. Calculate the ratio of the clotting times of the test and control (normal pool) plasma.

Interpretation

The normal ratio should be determined in each laboratory: it is usually between 0.9 and 1.05. Ratios greater than 1.05 suggest the presence of the lupus anticoagulant, or an abnormality of factors II, V or X. The presence of the lupus anticoagulant should be confirmed by testing a mixture of equal volumes of patient's and control plasma, and/or using the platelet neutralization test described below. The addition of normal plasma will correct an abnormal dilute RVV test result due to factor deficiency or defect, but will not do so in the presence of the lupus anticoagulant. The platelet neutralization procedure will shorten the clotting time in the dilute RVV test of plasma containing the lupus anticoagulant (see next test).

False-positive results may be obtained in patients on intravenous heparin, and the interpretation is difficult in patients receiving oral anticoagulants.

PLATELET NEUTRALIZATION TEST[21]

Principle. When platelets are used instead of phospholipid reagents in clotting tests, the tests become insensitive to the lupus anticoagulant. This appears to be due to the ability of the platelets to adsorb the lupus anticoagulant. To utilize this property of platelets, they must be washed to remove contaminating plasma proteins, and activated or 'fractured' to expose their coagulation factor binding sites.

Reagents

Commercial platelet extract reagent or washed normal platelets.

ACD anticoagulant solution, pH 5.4 (see p. 575). For use, 6 parts of blood are added to one part of this anticoagulant.

Na_2EDTA. 0.1 mol/l in saline.

Calcium-free Tyrode's buffer. To prepare, dissolve 8 g NaCl, 0.2 g KCl, 0.625 g Na_2HPO_4, 0.415 g $MgCl_2$ and 1.0g $NaHCO_2$ in 1 litre of water. Adjust pH if necessary to 6.5 with 1 mol/1 HCl.

Method

Collect normal blood into ACD and centrifuge at 270g for 10 min. Pipette the supernatant platelet-rich plasma (PRP) into a plastic container, and centrifuge for a second time to obtain more PRP, which is added to the first lot. Dilute the PRP with an equal volume of the calcium-free buffer, and add 1/10th volume of EDTA to give a final concentration of 0.01 mol/l. Centrifuge the mixture in a conical or round-bottom tube at 2000*g* for 10 min, and discard the supernatant. Gently re-suspend the platelet pellet in buffer and 0.01 mol/l EDTA, and centrifuge again. Again discard the supernatant, and resuspend the pellet in buffer alone. Then centrifuge the platelets a third time, and finally resuspend the pellet in buffer without EDTA to give a platelet count of at least 400 × 10⁹/l. The washed platelets may be stored below –20°C in volumes of 1–2 ml. Before use, they must be activated by repeatedly thawing and refreezing 3–4 times./

Use the washed platelets or the commercial reagent in the dilute RVV test or in the APTT in place of the usual phospholipid reagent. First, determine a suitable dilution by testing a range of doubling dilutions in the test system with control plasma. A suitable dilution will give a similar clotting time to that obtained using control plasma and the phospholipid reagent.

Interpretation

The addition of platelets to the dilute APTT system will shorten the clotting time when the lupus anticoagulant is present. It will not shorten the time when the prolongation is due to a factor deficiency or an inhibitor directed against a specific coagulation factor. However, the ability of different batches of platelets to perform this correction is variable and may vary further with storage. Accordingly, each time the test is performed a plasma sample known to contain a LAC should be tested in parallel to establish the efficacy of the platelets.

ANTI-CARDIOLIPIN ASSAY[9]

Individuals with the lupus anticoagulant almost always have other abnormalities due to the anti-phospholipid antibodies. The most frequent finding is the presence of anti-cardiolipin antibodies. These antibodies are detected using an immunoassay on microtitre plates or in coated polystyrene tubes. Commercial kits for the assay are available.

Care must be taken in the selection of control sera and in setting the cut-off point for normal values. It is also important to remember that anti-cardiolipin antibodies may be found after viral infections, including glandular fever, and after myocardial infarction.

INVESTIGATION OF THE FIBRINOLYTIC SYSTEM

Investigation of the fibrinolytic system consists of the measurement of fibrinogen and plasminogen concentration and their functional integrity, and the assessment of the fibrinolytic potential.

INVESTIGATION OF A SUSPECTED DYSFIBRINOGENAEMIA

Congenital dysfibrinogenaemia associated with thrombosis should be suspected in individuals with a prolonged thrombin time and a slightly or moderately reduced fibrinogen concentration in plasma (see Table 18.1). For details of investigation see p. 344.

INVESTIGATION OF A SUSPECTED PLASMINOGEN DEFECT OR DEFICIENCY

Inherited plasminogen deficiency or defect may account for about 2–3% of unexplained thromboses in young people.[14] However, the relationship between the deficiency and thrombosis is not clear. The laboratory screening should be carried out using a functional assay based on full transformation of plasminogen into plasmin by activators. Such assays can be caseinolytic, fibrin substrate or chromogenic.

CHROMOGENIC ASSAY FOR PLASMINOGEN[5]

Principle. In this two-step amidolytic assay plasminogen is first complexed with excess streptokinase. In the second step, the plasmin-like activity of the streptokinase-plasminogen complex is measured by its effect on a plasmin-specific peptide. The amount of the dye released is proportional to the amount of plasminogen available in the sample for complexing with streptokinase.

Reagents and method

Details can be found in the manufacturer's instructions. They vary with manufacturer and even from batch to batch of the same kit.

Normal range

80–120 u/dl.

Interpretation

Plasminogen concentration is reduced in the newborn, in patients with cirrhosis, with DIC and during and after thrombolytic therapy. Plasminogen is an acute phase reactant and an increased concentration is found in infection, trauma, myocardial infarction and malignant disease. The diagnosis of inherited plasminogen deficiency must be confirmed by functional tests using other activators, immunological assays and family studies.

INVESTIGATION OF 'FIBRINOLYTIC POTENTIAL'

The 'fibronolytic potential' is measured as the combined effect of plasminogen activators and inhibitors. The concentration of activators may be increased by venous occlusion or by the administration of DDAVP. The tests used are, firstly, the assays of plasminogen activators, using a fibrin substrate (euglobulin lysis time, fibrin plate lysis and many others) or a chromogenic substrate or ELISA techniques; and secondly, assays of inhibitors. The commonly used tests for inhibitors are the chromogenic assays of plasminogen activator inhibitor (PAI) and of α_2 antiplasmin (AP).[17,23]

EUGLOBULIN LYSIS TIME[5,22]

Principle. When plasma is diluted and acidified, the precipitate (euglobulin) which forms contains plasminogen activator (mostly t-PA), plasminogen and fibrinogen. Most of the inhibitors are left in the solution. The precipitate is redissolved, the fibrinogen clotted with thrombin and the time for clot lysis measured.

Reagents

Acetic acid. 0.01%
Bovine thrombin. 10 NIH u/ml.
Fresh platelet-poor plasma from the patient and control. As t-PA is very labile, blood must be collected into cooled sample tubes, placed on ice and processed immediately.
Glyoxaline buffer, pH 7.4. (See p. 306).

Method

Place venous blood in a plastic tube containing citrate; after mixing, keep the tube in an ice-bath. Centrifuge the sample as soon as possible (never later than 30 min after collection) at 4°C at 1200–1500g. Pipette 1.0 ml of plasma into 9 ml of acetic acid. Mix well and keep on ice for 15 min. Centrifuge at 4°C for 15 min, at 1500g, to deposit the white euglobulin precipitate. Discard the supernatant, invert the tubes, then wipe the walls with cotton wool on an applicator stick until completely dry inside. Add 0.5 ml of glyoxaline buffer and dissolve the precipitate. Place duplicate 0.3 ml volumes of patient's and control plasma dissolved euglobulin fraction in glass tubes and clot with 0.1 ml of thrombin. Leave undisturbed at 37°C and inspect for clot lysis at 15-min intervals.

Normal range

90–240 min.

Interpretation

The major cause of a long lysis time is the failure to maintain a low temperature throughout all the stages of the test. Exercise and prolonged venous stasis shorten the lysis times. There is also a significant diurnal variation: lysis time is longer in the morning than at noon or in the afternoon. Prolonged fibrinolysis (as found during fibrinolytic therapy) may result in plasminogen depletion and give rise to a falsely long time. In DIC, a low fibrinogen concentration in the patient's plasma gives a wispy clot which dissolves rapidly and results in a falsely short lysis time.

Long lysis times are found in the last trimester of pregnancy, in the post-operative period, after myocardial infarction, in obese individuals and in many cases of recurrent venous thrombosis. Very short lysis times are seen in some haematological or disseminated malignancies, and in cirrhosis.

LYSIS OF FIBRIN PLATES,[5,16]

Principle. Most commercially available fibrinogen preparations are contaminated with plasminogen. If a standard fibrinogen solution is poured into a Petri dish and clotted with $CaCl_2$ and thrombin, a solid fibrin plate is obtained. If the euglobulin fraction under test is placed on the plate, the plasminogen in the plate will be converted into plasmin and a zone of lysis will appear around the sample. The area of lysis will be proportionate to the concentration of plasminogen activator in the euglobulin fraction.

Reagents

Bovine fibrinogen.
Bovine thrombin. 50 NIH u/ml.
Calcium. 0.025 mol/l.
Barbitone buffered saline (see p. 306).
Platelet-poor plasma. From the patient and a control collected as described for euglobulin lysis time.

Equipment

Plastic Petri dishes.

Method

To prepare the fibrin plate, dilute the fibrinogen in buffered saline to obtain a final concentration of 1.5 g/l. Pipette 10 ml of diluted fibrinogen into a Petri dish. Place it on a level tray. Add 0.5 ml of $CaCl_2$ and 0.2 ml of thrombin solution. Mix the contents by swirling quickly. The plate clots within 10 to 20 s; it must clot evenly to be suitable for the test. Leave the plate undisturbed for 20 min. The prepared plates can then be kept for 3–4 days at 4°C.

Carefully apply 30 μl of the euglobulin fraction, prepared as described in the previous test, to the surface of the plate. There is no need to cut a well. Place in an incubator at 37°C for 24 h.

Perform all tests (patient and control) in duplicate.

Results

Calculate the zone of lysis by measuring two diameters in mm at right angles to each other. Multiply the two values to obtain the approximate area of lysis in mm^2.

Normal range

Variable, but usually between 40 and 60 mm^2.

Interpretation

The area of lysis may be difficult to define because of incomplete lysis. Only areas of complete, clear lysis should be measured.

VENOUS OCCLUSION TEST[5,7]

Principle. Localized venous occlusion of an arm for a standardized period of time is used as a stimulus for release of t-PA from the vessel wall. Pre- and post-occlusion lysis times, using the above-described euglobulin lysis or the fibrin plate lysis tests, are measured. In normal subjects fibrinolysis is greatly enhanced by occlusion.

Method

Withdraw blood from the arm to be tested

without stasis, place it in a citrate-containing tube and keep in an ice-bath. Inflate the sphygmomanometer cuff to a pressure midway between the systolic and diastolic (measured on the other arm). Leave the inflated cuff on for 10 min. Take a sample of venous blood from below the cuff immediately before deflation and place on ice. Measure the lysis in both samples as described previously. This test is uncomfortable and some patients may not be able to tolerate as much as 10 min occlusion.

Results

The post-occlusion lysis times should be shorter than the pre-occlusion times. Shortening by at least 30 min is found in most normal subjects.

Interpretation

Failure to enhance lysis is found in some cases of recurrent venous thrombosis, in obese people and after surgery, trauma or severe illness. It may also be due to a failure to release the activator because insufficient pressure was applied or the occlusion time was too short. Normal people vary in the degree of response: 'good' responders increase the concentration of t-PA by 3–4 fold, whereas 'poor' responders may consistently show only a very slight enhancement of fibrinolysis even with longer occlusion times.

TISSUE PLASMINOGEN ACTIVATOR (t-PA) AMIDOLYTIC ASSAY[10,13]

Principle. Different amidolytic assays for t-PA have been described. One relies on the activation of purified plasminogen to plasmin in the presence of fibrinogen fragments which stimulate the t-PA activity in the test plasma. The plasma is measured using a specific chromogenic substrate. In the second method, t-PA is captured on specific antibodies bound to a solid phase matrix such as a microtitre plate; plasminogen is added together with a stimulator of t-PA activity, and the plasmin produced measured with chromogenic substrates. Alternatively, chromogenic substrates specific for t-PA may be used, but there are specificity problems especially in the plasma assays.

Tissue plasminogen activator can also be measured by ELISA using monoclonal antibodies on microtitre plates.

PLASMINOGEN ACTIVATOR INHIBITOR (PAI-1) ASSAY

Principle. A fixed amount of t-PA is added in excess to undiluted plasma. Part of it rapidly complexes with the t-PA inhibitor (PAI). Plasminogen in plasma is then activated into plasmin by the residual, uncomplexed t-PA. The amount of plasmin formed is directly proportional to the residual t-PA activity and inversely proportional to the PAI activity of the sample. The amount of plasmin generated is measured using a plasmin-specific substrate.

Reagents are available in a kit form and the manufacturer's instructions must be closely followed. The normal range is as yet poorly defined, and each laboratory should establish its own range until reliable normal values become available.

The time of sampling must be standardized. Early morning (7 a.m.) samples have much greater levels of activity then those later in the day. The increase in PAI-1 following venous occlusion may be more informative than basal levels. An ELISA assay is also available to measure the total PAI-1 which is present.

α_2-ANTIPLASMIN AMIDOLYTIC ASSAY

Principle. Plasma dilutions are incubated with excess plasmin, a proportion of which will be inhibited by antiplasmins. The residual, uninhibited plasmin is measured using a specific chromogenic substrate. α_2-Antiplasmin is the major circulating inhibitor of plasmin and forms complexes much faster than other inhibitors: if the reaction times are short, the assay effectively measures α_2-antiplasmin only.

Different commercial kits are available containing all the necessary reagents. The manufacturer's instructions should be carefully followed.

The usual normal range is between 80 and

120%. Congenital α_2-antiplasmin deficiency is associated with a severe bleeding tendency. A reduced concentration is also found in liver disease, DIC and during thrombolytic therapy.

α_2-antiplasmin increases with age and is higher in Caucasians than in Africans.

Tests for fibrin and fibrinogen degradation products are described in Chapter 17.

INVESTIGATION OF PLATELET 'HYPERREACTIVITY'

Platelets may be more reactive than normally as a consequence of in-vivo activation by thrombin or non-endothelial surfaces, such as prosthetic valves or Dacron grafts. This can sometimes be detected by a lowered threshold (increased sensitivity) for aggregating agents. Because there is considerable variation in response to aggregating agents in normal people, the attempts to show platelet hyperaggregability are rarely successful and the results are frequently inconsistent. Spontaneous aggregation of platelets in the blood can also be demonstrated.[24]

Platelets which have formed a part of a platelet thrombus and have been released into the circulation may show a measurable decrease in aggregability due to a loss of some of the granular content. The released contents can be measured in plasma: the α-granule proteins, β-thromboglobulin and platelet factor 4 are the constituents most commonly measured.[25] Shortened platelet survival using [111]Indium-labelled platelets can also be used as a marker of platelet activation by a thrombotic process (see p. 413).

β-THROMBOGLOBULIN (β-TG) AND PLATELET FACTOR 4 (PF4) ASSAYS

Principle. ELISA and RIA methods are available for the measurement of these proteins using specific antisera. In the former, a double antibody sandwich technique is used, in which the surface of a tube or microplate is coated with antibody against β-TG or PF4, and plasma is added. Protein is then bound to the antibody, and may be detected by the binding of a second antibody carrying an enzyme tag. In the RIA methods, there is competition between β-TG or PF4 from the test sample and radiolabelled (usually ^{125}I) tracer protein for binding to a specific antibody. A high plasma concentration of the protein released from the platelets displaces the tracer from the immune complex.

Sample collection

Blood has to be collected and handled carefully to avoid artefactual release of β-TG and PF4 from the platelets. Samples are collected from free-flowing blood, drawn without venous stasis, and the first 2–3 ml discarded. Blood is immediately added to a tube chilled in a beaker filled with melting ice, which contains a special mixture of inhibitors of platelet activation, as well as calcium chelators. Plasma must be separated strictly at 4°C.

Reagents and method

Sample collection tubes and reagents are provided with the commercial kits used for the two tests. It is important to follow the manufacturer's instructions carefully.

The calculation of results depends on whether an ELISA or a RIA method is used.

Interpretation

The normal concentration of β-TG is less than 50 ng/ml and that of PF4 less than 10 ng/ml. Falsely high results may be encountered in RIA methods if diagnostic isotope techniques (such as leg scanning for thrombosis using ^{125}I fibrinogen) have been used in the patient. The tests cannot be performed for a week or so after the scanning or until ^{125}I is cleared from the patient's plasma.

PF4 is rapidly cleared from plasma by the vascular endothelium; it may be displaced from the endothelial binding by heparin. Thus a high

PF4 concentration may be found in patients receiving heparin. β-TG is cleared from plasma by the kidney, and its concentration is commonly high in renal failure. In patients without these clinical problems, both proteins should be measured in order to distinguish in-vivo release from an in-vitro artefact. With in-vivo activation of platelets, the plasma concentration of both proteins rises, but the concentration of β-TG remains much higher owing to the rapid endothelial clearance of PF4. The ratio of β-TG to PF4 is usually greater than 5:1. If venepuncture has been difficult or sample handling inadequate, in-vitro platelet release occurs and the concentration of both proteins is high (ratio less than 2:1).

PLATELET HYPERREACTIVITY

The problems associated with these tests of platelet activation have been circumvented to some extent by the application of flow cytometric analysis of platelets in whole blood samples. The activation of platelets is associated with the appearance of new antigenic determinants on the platelet surface. These can by detected using fluorescein-conjugated antibodies and the degree of expression quantified by flow cytometry. This then gives a measure of platelet activation with a much greater degree of sensitivity than PF4 or β-TG estimation. These tests have not yet entered routine laboratory practice but are proving increasingly useful in research.[1]

INVESTIGATION OF SUSPECTED INHERITED THROMBOTIC SYNDROMES

The prevalence of inherited thrombotic syndromes in the general population may be as high as 1 in 2500 or 1 in 5000.[15] It is becoming increasingly important to screen for such disorders. Screening must start by excluding the common causes of an acquired thrombotic tendency as described above. A careful family history must be taken next; however, a negative history does not exclude an inherited thrombotic tendency because the defects have a low penetration or a fresh mutation may have been responsible. As with a bleeding tendency, laboratory investigation is a step-wise procedure, starting with the simpler, first-line tests (as shown in Table 18.1) The key tests at each step are described below.

MEASUREMENT OF ANTITHROMBIN III

Antithrombin III is the major physiological inhibitor of thrombin, and factors Xa, IXa and XIa and XIIa.[19] It is also known as heparin cofactor I since its inhibitory action is potentiated and accelerated in the presence of heparin. Antithrombin III deficiency is not uncommon and may be acquired (see Table 18.2) or congenital.

A variety of methods are available for measuring either functional or antigenic activity of anti-

thrombin III. The functional methods are based on the reaction with thrombin or factor Xa; they can be coagulation or chromogenic assays. A chromogenic and a thrombin-based coagulation assay are described below.

ANTITHROMBIN III ASSAY USING THROMBIN

Principle. Antithrombin III is a progressive inhibitor. If serum is incubated with excess thrombin, any residual thrombin remaining at the end of incubation will reflect the concentration of antithrombin III in the serum.

Reagents

Thrombin. c 50 u/ml.

Reptilase-R.

Citrate-glyoxaline buffer. Add 1 volume of tri-sodium citrate to 5 volumes of glyoxaline buffer. The pH should be 7.4.

Bovine fibrinogen solution. Make according to the manufacturer's instructions.

Normal platelet-poor plasma. From the normal pool.

Patient's plasma.

Method

Clot 1 ml of patient's and of the normal plasma at 37°C for 10 min with 0.1 ml of Reptilase to remove fibrinogen. Gently remove the clots by winding onto a wooden applicator stick. Then dilute the serum as shown in Table 18.3.

Incubate 0.8 ml of each dilution for 4 min at 37°C with 0.1 ml of thrombin solution. The thrombin should be adjusted initially to give a clotting time of about 15–17 s with the blank. At 4 min pipette two 0.1 ml sub-samples into pre-warmed volumes of fibrinogen solution and note the clotting time.

Results

Plot the clotting times against the concentration of antithrombin III on semi-log graph paper. Draw best-fit straight lines and calculate the ATIII concentration in the patient's sample by reading off at various points along the line and averaging the results.

Normal range

Between 75 and 125 u/dl.

ANTITHROMBIN III MEASUREMENT USING A CHROMOGENIC ASSAY[5,18]

Principle. In the presence of heparin, antithrombin III reacts rapidly to inactivate thrombin by forming a 1:1 complex. Chromogenic antithrombin III assay is a two-step procedure. In the first step the plasma sample is incubated with a fixed quantity of thrombin and heparin. The amount of thrombin inactivated is then proportional to the ATIII concentration in the plasma. In the second step the residual thrombin is measured spectrophotometrically by its action on a synthetic chromogenic substrate which results in the release of para-nitroaniline dye (PNA).

Method

Carry out the procedure on dilutions of a standard plasma so as to construct a standard graph. Then test dilutions of the test plasma in an identical manner and read the results directly from the standard graph.

The reagents provided and details of the method vary from manufacturer to manufacturer and should be closely followed. There may also be variation between different batches of the same reagent.

Normal range

Generally between 75 and 125 u/dl. Some manufacturers, however, recommend a slightly narrower range, i.e. 80–120 u/dl. Repeated freezing and thawing of samples, as well as a storage at or above −20°C result in a reduction in ATIII concentration. It is also important to remember that oral anticoagulant therapy raises the ATIII concentration by *c* 10 u/dl in cases of congenital deficiency.

Interpretation

In an inherited deficiency, the ATIII concentration is usually <70 u/dl. Similar values are seen in acquired deficiencies; very low values are sometimes encountered in fulminant DIC. Normal newborns have a lower ATIII concentration (60–80 u/dl) than adults. In congenitally deficient neonates, very low values (30 u/dl and lower) may be found. Very high values are encountered after myocardial infarction and in some forms of vascular disease.

Further investigations

If an inherited ATIII deficiency is suspected more than one functional ATIII assay should be performed and the antigenic activity also determined. Family studies should always be performed.

The chromogenic method described above is to be preferred because it also measures the heparin cofactor activity of ATIII. Some mutant forms (Type IIc) are deficient only in this respect.

INVESTIGATION OF PROTEIN C DEFICIENCY

Protein C (PC) is a vitamin-K-dependent protein.

After thrombin activation which is accelerated in the presence of thrombomodulin on the vascular endothelium, PC complexes with phospholipids and protein S (PS) to degrade factors Va and VIII:C. Inherited protein C deficiency accounts for some 5–7% of all recurrent thrombo-embolic episodes in young adults.[2,15]. Most such individuals are heterozygotes. The homozygous state has been occasionally reported in the neonate with massive visceral thrombosis and purpura fulminans.[3] Acquired PC deficiency is found in all conditions associated with vitamin-K deficiency or defect, including oral anticoagulant therapy. A low plasma concentration is also found in DIC, liver disease and in the early post-operative period.

PC can be measured using a chromogenic assay, a coagulation assay or an antigenic method.

MEASUREMENT OF FUNCTIONAL PROTEIN C (PC) BY THE PROTAC METHOD[5]

Principle. In the presence of a specific snake venom activator, PC is converted into its active form. Activated PC is measured by its action on one of the specific synthetic substrates (such as S-2366, CBS 65.25). The reaction is stopped by the addition of 50% acetic acid and the *p*-nitroalanine produced measured at 405 nm in a spectrophotometer.

Reagents

Platelet-poor plasma. Standard and test: samples are centrifuged at 1500–2000g for 15 min. After centrifugation, plasma can be stored indefinitely at –40°C or below.

Protac. This is an activator derived from the venom of *Agkistrodon contortix*. This is obtained commercially; each vial contains lyophilized powder which is reconstituted and stored according to the manufacturer's instructions.

Specific chromogenic substrate. Reconstituted and stored according to the manufacturer's instructions.

Barbitone buffered saline. See p. 306.

Acetic acid. 50%.

Method

Construct the standard curve according to the instructions. Some manufacturers recommend the use of commercial calibrators or control plasma in preference to the normal pool.

The assay is carried out by a two-step method. In the first step plasma and activator are incubated for an exact period of time. In the second step the specific chromogenic substrate is added and the reaction is stopped with acetic acid again at a precise point in time. Read the amount of the dye produced at 405 nm against a blank obtained in the following way. Acetic acid, activator and chromogenic substrate are first mixed; then standard or patient's plasma is added to the mixture and the absorbance measured at 405 nm. The manufacturer's instructions must be closely followed. Plot the protein C % activity against the corresponding absorbance reading on linear graph paper.

Normal range

70–140%. Each laboratory should preferably establish its own normal range.

Further investigation

If inherited PC deficiency is suspected, an immunological assay should also be carried out. It is also important to exclude vitamin-K deficiency by assaying other vitamin-K-dependent factors which should be normal. Family studies should be carried out whenever possible.

INVESTIGATION OF PROTEIN S DEFICIENCY

Protein S is also a vitamin-K-dependent protein which acts as a cofactor of the activated PC. In plasma, 60% of PS is bound to C4b-binding

Table 18.3 Dilutions of serum for the antithrombin III assay

Buffern (ml)	Serum (ml)	ATIII (%)
0.8	0	0
0.75	0.05	25
0.70	0.10	50
0.65	0.15	75
0.60	0.20	100
0.55	0.25	125

protein and does not possess any anticoagulant activity; the remaining 40% is free and available to interact with PC. The functional assays of PS are based on the capacity of PS to prolong the one-stage factor Xa time. Measurement of the total PS antigen by an immunoassay is possible using enzyme-linked immunoassays.

ENZYME-LINKED IMMUNOSORBENT ASSAY OF FREE AND TOTAL PROTEIN S

Reagents

Polyethylene glycol (PEG) precipitation solution. Dissolve 100 g of PEG 8000 in 200 ml of sterile water. Prepare approximately 50 ml of working PEG by diluting the stock solution to 18.75% with sterile water. Store in 2-ml aliquots at $-20°C$.

Coating buffer (phosphate buffered saline, pH 7.2). 0.39 g $NaH_2PO_4.2H_2O$, 2.68 g $Na_2HPO_4.12H_2O$, 8.474 g NaCl. Make up to 1 litre and adjust to pH 7.2, store at $4°C$.

Wash buffer. This is the same as the coating buffer, but contains 0.5 M NaCl and 0.2% v/v Tween 20. Add 10.37 g of NaCl to 1 litre of coating buffer and 0.2% Tween 20 (mix well). Store at $4°C$.

Dilution buffer. This is the washing buffer with 30 g/l PEG 8000. Store at $4°C$.

Substrate buffer (citrate phosphate buffer, pH 5.0). 7.3 g citric acid, 23.87 g. $Na_2PHO_4.12H_2O$. Make up to 1 litre with water. Adjust pH to 5.0.

o-phenylenediamine.

Dako anti-Protein S and anti-Protein S peroxidase conjugated.

Sulphuric acid, 1 M.

Microtitre plates. Dynatech M129B.

Standards and controls.

Hydrogen peroxide. '30 vols'.

Methods

Dilute the anti-human protein S immunoglobulin 1:1000 in coating buffer, i.e. 20 µl in 20 ml of buffer. Add 0.1 ml to each well of a microtitre plate, cover with parafilm and leave overnight in a wet box at $4°C$. On the day the assay is to be performed, warm an aliquot of working PEG solution to $30°C$. Accurately pipette 200 µl of standard, patient's and control plasma samples into conical Eppendorf tubes, warm for 5 min at $37°C$. Add exactly 50 µl of warmed PEG, immediately cap and vortex mix twice for 5 s each. Place in water/crushed ice mixture. In turn treat all the sample identically. Leave for 30 min on the melted ice. Centrifuge for 30 s in the Eppendorf centrifuge. Then return to ice and remove 100 µl in a labelled tube (taking care not to remove any precipitate).

Prepare dilutions of control and patient's samples in PEG dilution buffer as follows. For total protein S, dilute 0.05 ml of reference plasma in 8 ml of diluent. Use the PEG precipitated reference plasma for measuring free protein S; add 0.1 ml to 4 ml of dilution buffer.

Prepare a range of standards from these stock solutions using the same dilution schedule for free and total protein S.

A. Stock solution = 1.25 u/ml.
B. 0.8 ml stock + 0.2 ml buffer = 1.0 u/ml.
C. 0.6 ml stock + 0.4 ml buffer = 0.75 u/ml.
D. 0.4 ml stock + 0.6 ml buffer = 0.5 u/ml.
E. 0.2 ml stock + 0.8 ml buffer = 0.25 u/ml.
F. 0.1 ml stock + 0.9 ml buffer = 0.125 u/ml.
G. 0.05 ml stock + 0.95 ml buffer = 0.0625 u/ml.

Control and patient's samples are tested at two dilutions—Total protein S plasma: 1:200 and 1:400; free protein S PEG supernatants: 1:50 and 1:100. Shake out the contents of the previously prepared plate, blot on tissue. Wash the plate three times in wash buffer by filling all the wells, leaving for 2 min, shaking out the contents, blotting and repeating. Add 100 µl of each dilution of standard, control or patient's plasma in duplicate across the plate. Cover and incubate for 3 h in a wet box at room temperature. Wash the plate as described earlier. Dilute 2 µl of peroxidase-labelled antibody in 24 ml of dilution buffer. Add 100 µl of diluted tag (peroxidase-conjugated) antibody to each well and leave in a wet box for 2–3 hours at room temperature. Wash the plate as described earlier. Make up the substrate solution by adding 8 mg of *o*-phenylene diamine to 12 ml of citrate phosphate buffer. Immediately before use add 10 µl of hydrogen peroxide. Add 100 µl of substrate solution to each well. When the weakest standard has a visible yellow colour add 150 µl of 1M sulphuric acid to each well. Read the optical densities on a plate reader at 492 nm. Plot the optical densities against plasma dilutions on double-log graph paper and read the patient's values from the corresponding calibration curve, i.e. total against total and free against free.

Kits for the functional assay of protein S are now commercially available and the tests should be performed according to the manufacturer's instructions.

ACTIVATED PROTEIN C RESISTANCE

Recently, Dahlback and colleagues[6] described an inherited tendency to thrombosis associated with deficiency of a novel cofactor for protein C. Deficiency of this factor can be detected by a relatively simple test based on the APTT. This test has not yet been standardized and the reader is referred to the original publication.

INVESTIGATION OF HEPARIN COFACTOR II (HCII) DEFICIENCY

A deficiency of heparin cofactor II is found in some individuals with recurrent thromboembolism. However, there is no clear evidence that HCII deficiency is more prevalent in this group than in the normal population. Its concentration is measured in the presence of a strong family history if the assays of other physiological inhibitors give normal results.

HEPARIN COFACTOR II ASSAY

Principle. Heparin cofactor II (HCII) present in test and standard plasma is activated by dermatan sulphate and incubated with human thrombin. The residual, uninhibited thrombin is then measured by cleavage of a chromogenic substrate.

Reagents

Reagents are commercially available in a kit form.

Buffer, pH 8.2. 0.05 mol/l Tris, 0.15 mol/l NaCl, 6.8 mmol/l Na_2EDTA, 2 mg/l Polybrene, 10 g/l bovine serum albumin, pH adjusted with HCl.

Dermatan sulphate (free of heparin).
Human thrombin.
Chromogenic substrate for thrombin.

50% Acetic acid.
Pooled normal plasma as standard.
Test plasma.

Method

It is important to follow the manufacturer's instructions which come with the kit. Prepare a range of dilutions of pooled normal plasma in order to construct a calibration curve. Prepare also a single dilution of each test plasma. Incubate the dilutions with dermatan sulphate at 37°C in a plastic tube or a microtitre plate. Then add thrombin, followed, after a further incubation, by the chromogenic substrate. After a suitable reaction time, in accordance with the manufacturer's instructions, add acetic acid to stop the reaction, and measure the absorbance at 405 nm in a spectrophotometer or a microtitre plate reader, as appropriate.

Calculation

Read the absorbance of the test plasma from the calibration curve and express as percentage normal.

Normal range

Generally 55–145%.

Interpretation

The plasma concentration may be increased in healthy women on oral contraceptive pills. HCII is reduced in congenital deficiency, liver disease and DIC.

MARKERS OF COAGULATION ACTIVATION

A number of commercial kits are now available for measuring molecules produced by coagulation activation. These include activation peptides cleaved from the serine proteases of the coagulation cascade such as prothrombin fragment 1+2 and complexes of thrombin and antithrombin (TAT). Others tests will measure cleavage products of fibrinogen such as fibrinopeptide A. These tests are not used routinely and are not required for normal diagnostic work. They often require exceptional care and the use of special anti-coagulants to prevent in-vitro activation of the sample.

REFERENCES

[1]ABRAMS, C. S., ELLISON, N., BUDZYNSKI, A. Z. and SHATTIL, S. J. (1990). Direct detection of activated platelets and platelet derived microparticles in humans. *Blood*, **75**, 128.

[2]BROEKMANS, A. W., VAN DER LINDEN, I. K., JANSEN-KOETER, Y. and BERTINA, R. M. (1986). Prevalence of protein C (PC) and protein S (PS) deficiency in patients with thromboembolic disease. *Thrombosis Research*, Supp **VI**, 135.

[3]BRANSON, H. E., KATZ, MARBLE, R. and GRIFFIN, J. H. (1983). Inherited protein C deficiency and coumarin responsive chronic relapsing purpura fulminans in a newborn infant. *Lancet*, **ii**, 1165.

[4]BRITISH COMMITTEE FOR STANDARDS IN HAEMATOLOGY (1990). Guidelines on the investigation and management of thrombophilia. *Journal of Clinical Pathology*, **43**, 703.

[5]*Coagulation Manual*. Katherine Dormandy Haemophilia Centre, Royal Free Hospital, London. By permission.

[6]DAHLBACK, B., CARLSSON, M. and SVENSSON, P. J. (1993). Familial thrombophilia due to a previously unrecognized mechanism characterised by poor anticoagulant response to activated protein C: Prediction of a cofactor to activated protein C. *Proceedings of the National Academy of Sciences USA*, **90**, 1004.

[7]DAVIDSON, J. F. and WALKER, I. D. (1987). Assessment of the fibrinolytic system. In *Haemostasis and Thrombosis*. Eds. Bloom, A. L. and Thomas, D. P., 2nd edn., p. 953. Churchill Livingstone, Edinburgh.

[8]EXNER, T., RICKARD, K. A. and KRONENBERG, H. (1978). A sensitive test demonstrating lupus anticoagulant and its behavioural patterns. *British Journal of Haematology*, **40**, 143.

[9]HARRIS, E. N., GHARAVI, A. E., PATEL, S. P. and HUGHES, G. R. V. (1987). Evaluation of the anticardiolipin antibody test: report of an international workshop held 4th April 1986. *Clinical and Experimental Immunology*, **68**, 215.

[10]HOLVOET, P., CLEEMPUT, H. and COLLEN, D. (1985). Assay of human tissue type plasminogen activator (t-PA) with an enzyme-linked immunosorbent assay (ELISA) based on three murine monoclonal antibodies. *Thrombosis and Haemostasis*, **54**, 684.

[11]HOWIE, P. W., PRENTICE, C. R. M. and MCNICOL, G. P. (1973). A method of antithrombin III estimation using plasma defibrinated with ancrod. *British Journal of Haematology*, **25**, 101.

[12]LUPUS ANTICOAGULANT WORKING PARTY ON BEHALF OF THE BCSH HAEMOSTASIS AND THROMBOSIS TASK FORCE (1991). Guidelines on testing for the lupus anticoagulant. *Journal of Clinical Pathology*, **44**, 885.

[13]MAHMOOD, M. and GAFFNEY, P. J. (1985). Bioimmunoassay (BIA) of tissue plasminogen activator (t-PA) and its specific inhibitor (t-PA/INH). *Thrombosis and Haemostasis*, **53**, 356.

[14]MANNUCCI, P. M., KLUFT, C. TRAAS, D. W. SEVESO, P. and D' ANGELO, A. (1986). Congenital plasminogen deficiency associated with venous thromboembolism: therapeutic trial with stanozolol. *British Journal of Haematology*, **63**, 753.

[15]MANNUCCI, P. M., and TRIPODI A. (1987) Laboratory screening of inherited thrombotic syndromes. *Thrombosis and Haemostasis*, **57**, 247.

[16]MARSH, N. A. and AROCHA-PINANGO, C. L. (1972). Evaluation of the fibrin plate method for estimating plasminogen activators. *Thrombosis et Diathesis Haemorrhagica*, **28**, 75.

[17]NILSSON, I. M., LJUNGNER, H. and TENGBORN, L. (1985). Two different mechanisms in patients with venous thrombosis and defective fibrinolysis: low concentration of plasminogen activator or increased concentration of plasminogen activator inhibitor. *British Medical Journal*, **290**, 1453.

[18]ODEGARD, O. R., LIE, M. and ABILDGAARD, U. (1976). Heparin cofactor activity measured with an amidolytic method. *Thrombosis Research*, **6**, 287.

[19]SALEM, H. H. (1986). The natural anticoagulants. *Clinics in Haematology*, **15**, 371.

[20]THIAGARAJAN, P., PENGO, V. and SHAPIRO, S. S. (1986). The use of the dilute Russell Viper Venom time for the diagnosis of lupus anticoagulants. *Blood*, **68**, 869.

[21]THIAGARAJAN P. and SHAPIRO, S. S. (1983). Disorders of thrombin formation: lupus anticoagulants. *Methods in Hematology*, 7, 121.

[22]VON KAULLA, K. N. (1963). *Chemistry of Thrombolysis: Human Fibrinolytic Enzymes*. Thomas, Springfield, IL.

[23]WIMAN, B., LJUNGEBERG, B., CHMIELEWSKA, J., URDEN, J., BLOMBACK, M. and JOHNSSON, H. (1985). The role of fibrinolytic system in deep vein thrombosis. *Journal of Laboratory and Clinical Medicine*, **105**, 265.

[24]WU, K. K. and HOAK, J. C. (1976). Spontaneous platelet aggregation in arterial insufficiency: mechanisms and implications. *Thrombosis and Haemostasis*, **46**, 702.

[25]YARDUMIAN, D. A., MACKIE, I. J. and MACHIN, S. J. (1986). Laboratory investigation of platelet function: a review of methodology. *Journal of Clinical Pathology*, **39**, 701.

19. Laboratory control of anticoagulant, thrombolytic and anti-platelet therapy

Revised by M. A. Laffan and A. E. Bradshaw

Oral anticoagulant treatment   367
One-stage prothrombin time   368
  Standardization of commercial thromboplastins   368
  Calibration of thromboplastins   369
Therapeutic range   370
Capillary reagent   371
Heparin treatment   372
  Laboratory control   372
  APTT   373

Thrombin time   374
Anti-Xa assay   374
Protamine neutralization test   374
Anti-Xa assay, low dose heparin   376
Thrombolytic therapy   377
  Titration of initial streptokinase dose   378
  Laboratory control   378
Anti-platelet therapy   379

Anticoagulant therapy prevents thrombosis or the further propagation of an existing thrombus. Anticoagulant drugs have little if any effect upon an already formed thrombus. There are three main classes of anticoagulant drugs:

1. The oral anticoagulants, coumarins and indanediones, which act by interfering with the γ-carboxylation step in the synthesis of the vitamin-K-dependent factors (see p. 301).

2. Heparin and heparinoids (low molecular weight and synthetic compounds) which have a complex action on haemostasis, the main effect being the potentiation and acceleration of the effect of antithrombin III on thrombin and factor Xa.

3. Defibrinating agents such as ancrod (Arvin) and Reptilase which induce hypocoagulability by the removal of fibrinogen from the blood.

4. Hirudin (natural or recombinant). Hirudin was originally extracted from the medicinal leech. It is a highly specific inhibitor of thrombin and thus a potent anticoagulant. It has not yet entered general clinical practice but when used the most appropriate measure of action appears to be the APTT. The target range is the same as for heparin.[8]

The anticoagulant drugs may be used to treat an acute episode of thrombosis or to prevent its onset in cases where there is a high risk of thrombosis, e.g. post-operatively or in pregnancy. Heparin may also be used to treat some patients with DIC and some types of renal failure, as well as during haemodialysis and cardiopulmonary bypass.

ORAL ANTICOAGULANT TREATMENT

It is not possible to produce a therapeutic derangement of haemostasis without increasing the risk of haemorrhage. The purpose of laboratory control is to maintain a level of hypocoagulability—the therapeutic range—which is effective in preventing thrombosis but does not cause spontaneous bleeding. Oral anticoagulant treatment must be regularly and frequently controlled by laboratory tests to ensure that the results of the test remain within the therapeutic range.

Selection of patients

Haemostasis is not as a rule investigated before

starting oral anticoagulant treatment but it is advisable to perform the first-line coagulation screen (PT, APTT, thrombin time and platelet count) before commencing treatment.

A prolongation of these tests must be investigated as a contra-indication to the use of oral anti-coagulants may be revealed.

Methods used for the laboratory control of oral anticoagulant treatment

The one-stage prothrombin time of Quick is the most commonly used test. However, lack of standardization of the thromboplastin prep-arations used in this simple test has caused great discrepancies in the results. In addition, different methods of expressing the prothrombin time results have led to varying intensities of treatment in different parts of the world. The use of ISI, the International Sensitivity Index, to assess the sensitivity of any given thromboplastin, and the use of INR, the International Normalized Ratio, which is the prothrombin time ratio expressed in terms of a common international reference thromboplastin, should minimize these difficulties and ensure uniformity of anticoagulation and interpretation throughout the world (see later).

The Thrombotest of Owren[10] is a test popular in the Scandinavian countries. The results are expressed as a percentage which can in turn be transformed into INR.

The activated partial thromboplastin time is occasionally used to assess the effects of long-term anticoagulant treatment especially before a surgical procedure. It cannot be used alone for safe anticoagulant control; it remains an additional test to be used in special circumstances only.

Chromogenic substrates have been used for the control of anticoagulant treatment in factor X, VII or II assays. Although it is possible to use such a single factor measurement, it must be remembered that the one-stage prothrombin time and the Thrombotest measure three vitamin-K-dependent factors (factors VII, X and II) and are also affected by the presence of PIVKAs* or the acarboxy forms of vitamin-K-dependent factors. This makes them safer and more sensitive tests in

---

*PIVKAs: Proteins induced by Vitamin K antagonists.

the control of this potentially dangerous treatment. Amidolytic versions of the prothrombin time using thromboplastin, calcium and a chromogenic substrate for thrombin have also been introduced recently and may prove a viable alternative.

The prothrombin and proconvertin (P & P) method or Owren and Aas[11] was introduced in an attempt to make the prothrombin time more sensitive to vitamin-K-dependent factors. It was described in previous editions of this book.

CONTROL OF ORAL ANTICOAGULANT TREATMENT BY THE ONE-STAGE PROTHROMBIN TIME

Principle. The test is carried out as described in Chapter 16, p. 307. It is, however, essential to use a thromboplastin standardized by the com-mercial supplier or according to a local, regional or national procedure. To ensure safety and uni-formity of anticoagulation, the results should be reported in INR either alone or in parallel with the locally accepted method of reporting.

Standardization of thromboplastin

There are a number of commercial thromboplastins of animal origin. Human brain thromboplastin is no longer used for the prothrombin time because of the potential danger of the transmission of retroviruses. Each thromboplastin gives different results with the same test and control plasma; even different batches of the same thromboplastin behave differently. It is not possible to define the therapeutic range unless the thromboplastin used is also specified or calibrated in terms of the International Sensitivity Index (ISI).

The calibration of thromboplastins is achieved by comparing the results from the test thromboplastin with those given by a reference thromboplastin calibrated in accordance with the method recommended by the WHO Expert Committee on Biological Standardization.

Reference thromboplastins may be the WHO Reference Preparations or certified reference materials from the European Union Bureau of Reference (BCR). The first are obtained from the National Institute for Biological Standards and Control, and are usually only issued for the calibration and standardization of national or secondary WHO standards. The European reference materials are available to manufacturers and individual laboratories from the European Union.[4] (see p. 36). All the reference preparations have been calibrated in terms of a primary WHO human brain thromboplastin established in 1967 which is no longer available. Rabbit and bovine reference preparations are also available from both sources.

The following terms are employed in the calibration procedure which is described below:

International Sensitivity Index (ISI).[9] This is the slope of the calibration line obtained when the logarithms of the prothrombin times obtained with the reference preparation are plotted on the vertical axis of log-log paper and the logarithms of the prothrombin times obtained by the test thromboplastin are plotted on the horizontal axis. The same normal and anticoagulated patient's plasma samples are used.

International Normalized Ratio (INR). This is the prothrombin time ratio which, by calculation, would have been obtained had the original primary, human reference thromboplastin been used to perform the prothrombin time.

CALIBRATION OF THROMBOPLASTINS

Principle. The test thromboplastin must be calibrated against a reference thromboplastin of the same species (rabbit v rabbit, bovine v bovine). All reference preparations are calibrated in terms of the primary material of human origin and have an ISI which is assigned after a collaborative trial involving many laboratories from different countries.

Reagents

Normal citrated plasma. From 20 healthy donors.
Anticoagulated plasma. From 60 patients stabilized on oral anticoagulant treatment for at least 6 weeks.

The tests need not all be done at the same time but may be carried out on freshly collected samples on successive days.
Reference and test thromboplastins.
CaCl₂. $CaCl_2$. 0.025 mol/l.

Method

Carry out prothrombin time (PT) tests as described in Chapter 16, p. 307. Allow the plasma and

thromboplastin to warm up to 37°C for at least 2 min before adding $CaCl_2$. Test each plasma in duplicate with each of the two thromboplastins in the following order with minimum delay between tests:

	Reference thromboplastin	Test thromboplastin
Plasma 1	Test 1	Test 2
	Test 4	Test 3
Plasma 2	Test 5	Test 6
	Test 8	Test 7 etc

Record the mean time for each plasma. If there is a discrepancy of more than 10% in the clotting times between duplicates, repeat the test on that plasma.

Calibration

Plot the prothrombin times (PTs) on log-log graph paper, with results using the reference preparation (y) on the vertical axis and results with the test thromboplastin (x) on the horizontal axis (Fig. 19.1). On arithmetic graph paper it is necessary to plot the logarithms of the PTs (Fig. 19.2). The relationship between the two thromboplastins is determined by the slope of the line (b).

A rough estimate of the slope can be obtained as shown in Figs 19.1 and 19.2; this can then be used to obtain an approximation of the ISI of the test thromboplastin.

Whenever possible however, to obtain a reliable measurement, the following more complicated calculation should be used instead.

Calculation of ISI

Calculate the slope of the line (1) as follows:

1. Convert all measurements of PTs into their logarithms; thus, x = log PT with test thromboplastin and y = log PT with reference thromboplastin.
2. $\Sigma x = A$; $\Sigma x^2 = B$; $\Sigma y = C$; $\Sigma y^2 = D$; $\Sigma xy = E$.
3. $F = \dfrac{D - C^2}{n}$, $G = \dfrac{B - A^2}{n}$ and $H = \dfrac{E - AC}{n}$

   where n = No. of PTs with each thromboplastin.
4. $m = \dfrac{F - G}{2H}$

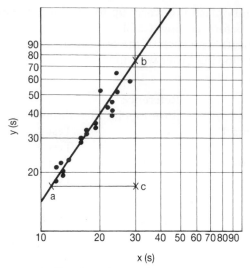

Fig. 19.1 Calibration of thromboplastin. The PTs (in seconds) with the test thromboplastin are plotted on the horizontal axis (x) and with the reference thromboplastin on the vertical axis (y) on double log graph paper. The best-fit line is drawn by eye, and the slope is obtained as follows: Points (a) and (b) are marked on the line just below the lowest recorded PT and just above the longest recorded PT, respectively. (c) is a point where a horizontal line through (a) and a vertical through (b) meet. The distance between (b) and (c) is measured accurately in mm. The slope

$$b = \frac{[(b)-(c)]}{[(a)-(c)]}.$$ In this example (b)–(c) = 55 mm,

(a)–(c) = 35 mm, b = 55/35 = 1.57. The ISI of the reference thromboplastin was 1.11. Therefore, the ISI of the test thromboplastin = 1.11 × 1.57 = 1.74.

5. Slope (b) = $m + \sqrt{m^2 + 1}$
6. ISI of test thromboplastin = ISI of reference thromboplastin × slope.

Calculation of the INR[9, 12, 14]

This is the prothrombin ratio which would have been obtained on the particular plasma had the original primary human reference material been used to perform the prothrombin time. If the ISI of the thromboplastin used is known the INR can be calculated from the following formula:

INR = Prothrombin time ratio obtained using the test thromboplastin to the power of the ISI of the test reagent.

For example a ratio of 2.5 using a thromboplastin with ISI of 1.4 can be calculated from the formula to be:

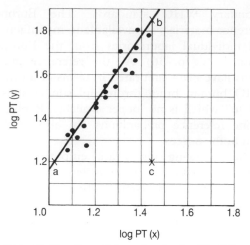

Fig. 19.2 Calibration of thromboplastin. The PTs (in seconds) are converted to their logarithms which are plotted on arithmetic graph paper. The slope is calculated as in Fig. 19.1. In this example, (a)–(c) = 42 mm, (b)–(c) = 65 mm, b = 65/42 = 1.54. Therefore, ISI = 1.11 × 1.54 = 1.71.

$2.5^{1.4} = 3.61$

which is either read from a logarithmic table or calculated on an electronic calculator.

In this way the level of anticoagulation in all plasma samples regardless of the thromboplastin used can be compared and a meaningful therapeutic range established.

THERAPEUTIC RANGE AND CHOICE OF THROMBOPLASTIN

Several different authorities have now published recommended therapeutic ranges denoting the appropriate degree of anticoagulation in different clinical circumstances.[5] These are only to a

Table 19.1 Therapeutic ranges equivalent to an INR of 2.0–4.0 using different commercial thromboplastins. (Modified from Poller.[12])

Thromboplastin	ISI	Ratios equivalent to INR 2.0–4.0
Thrombotest	1.03	2.0–3.8
Thromborel	1.23	1.7–3.1
Dade FS	1.35	1.65–2.8
Simplastin	2.0	1.3–2.0
Boehringer	2.1	1.35–1.9
Ortho	2.3	1.3–1.8

ISI, International Sensitivity Index; INR, International Normalized Ratio.

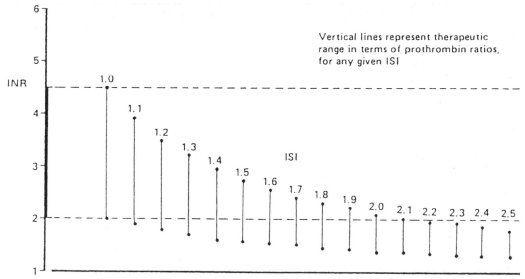

Fig. 19.3   The ratios obtained with thromboplastins with given ISI values equivalent to INR therapeutic range of 2.0–4.5. (Slightly modified, from Poller.[12] With the permission of publisher and editors.)

limited degree based on controlled clinical trials but to a large extent represent a consensus on practice that has emerged over many years.

The choice of thromboplastin greatly determines the accuracy with which anticoagulant control can be maintained. If the ISI of the thromboplastin is high then a small change in PT represents a large change in the degree of anticoagulation. This affects the precision of the analysis and the coefficient of variation for the test increases with the ISI. Moreover, the prothrombin ratio range becomes very small for any given range of INR. This is illustrated in Fig. 19.3 and Table 19.1. For these reasons it is strongly recommended that a thromboplastin with a low ISI is used (i.e. close to 1).

CAPILLARY REAGENT

Principle. Reagents are commercially available for monitoring the INR using samples of capillary blood. These are usually a mixture of thromboplastin, calcium and absorbed plasma so that when whole blood is added the reagent measures the overall clotting activity; it is sensitive to deficiency of factors II, VII, IX and X. The reagents have an ISI assigned to them in the same way as individual thromboplastins and the INR is calculated from

the PT ratio. These reagents are frequently used in anticoagulant clinics when a large number of INRs need to be performed rapidly.

INVESTIGATION OF A PATIENT WHO BLEEDS

The tests commonly used when investigating bleeding by a patient on oral anticoagulants, and their interpretation are shown in Table 19.2.

Table 19.2   Investigation of bleeding in a patient receiving an oral anticoagulant

Test	Result	Comment
PT	INR 2.0–4.5, Fibrinogen and platelets normal	Non-haemostatic cause of bleeding
PT	INR over 4.5, Fibrinogen and platelets normal	Overanticoagulated. Stop or reduce oral anticoagulant
PT	INR over 4.5, Fibrinogen and/ or platelets low	DIC? Liver or renal disease? Stop or reduce oral anticoagulant

PT, prothrombin time; INR, International Normalized Ratio.

HEPARIN TREATMENT

The anticoagulant action of heparin is primarily due to its ability to bind to antithrombin III (ATIII), thereby accelerating and enhancing the latter's rate of inhibition of the major coagulation enzymes, i.e. factors IIa and Xa and to a lesser extent IXa, XIa and XIIa. The two main effects of heparin, the anti-thrombin and the anti-Xa effects, are differentially dependent on the size of the heparin molecule. The basic minimum sequence needed to obtain anticoagulant activity has been identified as a pentasaccharide unit. Of the molecules containing this pentasaccharide, those comprising less than 18 saccharide units and of molecular weight less than 5000 have inhibitory activity against Xa only. In contrast, longer chains have anti-thrombin activity as well. The explanation for this difference appears to be that the inhibition of thrombin requires the formation of a tertiary complex and therefore larger molecules to bridge both ATIII and thrombin.

Attempts have been made to exploit these differences and produce heparin preparations with lower average molecular weight and hence relatively more anti-Xa and less anti-thrombin effect. Evidence indicated that this would result in less haemorrhagic side effects for a given degree of anticoagulation. The preparations remain heterogeneous however, and the two effects have not been entirely separated. Low molecular weight heparins (LMWH) have an average molecular weight of 5000 Da and a ratio of anti-Xa to anti-thrombin effect of 2–5 compared to approximately 1 for unfractionated heparin (UFH). A number of synthetic heparin analogues or heparinoids have been developed with the same intent.

Heparin also has a number of other effects: interaction with histidine-rich glycoprotein in plasma and an effect on the plasma lipases, as well as various interactions with platelets and the products of platelet activation such as PF4.

Because of the variable effects of different preparations, it has been important to measure the in-vivo effect of heparin therapy in terms of its anticoagulant effect. For UFH this has traditionally been performed by the APTT. However, low dose heparin therapy and LMWH produce relatively little effect on the APTT. It then becomes necessary to use a specific heparin assay. The result will then be reported as heparin activity in u/ml. In general, unless stated otherwise, this is in terms of anti-Xa activity. An international standard for LMWH is now available.[1]

Selection of patients

Treatment with heparin carries a high risk of bleeding even in haemostatically normal people and it is advisable to perform the first-line tests of haemostasis as described in Chapter 16 before starting treatment. In the presence of a reduced platelet count or deranged coagulation, heparin may be contra-indicated or if used the dose must be reduced.

LABORATORY CONTROL OF HEPARIN TREATMENT

The laboratory control of heparin treatment will be considered under two headings: therapeutic and prophylactic.

The pharmacokinetics of heparins are extremely complicated; this is partly because of the variation in molecule size. This is one of the reasons why heparin therapy must be so closely monitored. However, the relationship between dose and effect is much more predictable for the LMWHs. For this reason some manufacturers have been able to recommend a simple units per kilogram dosage system for prophylaxis using LMWH that does not require monitoring. This is in some ways similar to low-dose therapy with UFH. The longer half-life of LMWH has also led to suggestions that once daily dosing may be adequate. This has not been fully accepted. When monitoring therapy with LMWH it is most appropriate to use an anti-Xa assay.

THERAPEUTIC HEPARIN TREATMENT

For treating an established thrombotic or embolic event heparin can be administered intravenously (i.v.), preferably as a continuous infusion, or on occasions as intermittent intravenous injections. Patients also may be treated by subcutaneous (s.c.) injection, usually twice daily. The half-life of intravenously administered unfractionated heparin is about 1.5 h; after s.c. injection, heparin is slowly released into the circulation and is present in plasma for on average 12 h. Thus the timing of the blood sample in relation to the heparin injection is important if heparin is not given by continuous infusion. For those receiving intermittent s.c. heparin, standard practice is to collect samples at the mid-point between doses; usually this will be 6 h after twice daily doses. Heparin is a powerful anticoagulant and its use carries a high risk of bleeding. To minimize this risk, its effect on the coagulation should be monitored every 24 h while the patient is on treatment.

The following tests are available for the control of heparinization: whole-blood clotting time, thrombin time, accelerated partial thromboplastin time with kaolin (APTT) on plasma or whole blood, anti-Xa assays using either coagulation or amidolytic methodology, and the protamine neutralization test. The advantages and disadvantages of the various tests are shown in Table 19.3. Measurement of the whole-blood coagulation time, as described in the 5th edition of this book (p. 328), was widely used in the past in the control of heparin therapy. The test is time-consuming, must be performed at the bedside one test at a

Table 19.3   Tests used in the laboratory control of heparin treatment

Test	Advantages	Disadvantages
Whole blood clotting time	Simple, inexpensive, no equipment needed	Time consuming, can only be carried out at the bedside, one at a time, insensitive to <0.4 IU, and to LMW heparins
APTT	Simple, many tests can be carried out in parallel	Not all reagents sensitive to heparin, insensitive to <0.2 IU and to LMW heparins, affected by variables other than heparin
Thrombin time	Simple, many tests can be carried out in parallel	Insensitive to <0.2 IU and to LMW heparins
Protamine neutralization	Sensitive to all concentrations	Time consuming and insensitive to LMW heparins
Anti-Xa assays	Sensitive to all concentrations and to LMWT heparins	Expensive if commercial kits used; time consuming if home-made reagents used

APTT, activated partial thromboplastin time; LMW, low molecular weight.

time, and is also relatively insensitive to the lower concentrations of heparin. The APTT, anti-Xa assay and the protamine neutralization test are described here.

ACTIVATED PARTIAL THROMBOPLASTIN TIME (APTT)*

Principle. This test can be performed on citrated plasma or on whole citrated blood. The test on plasma is currently the most widely used test for monitoring heparin therapy.[6] It is very sensitive to heparin but has a number of shortcomings which must be kept in mind: firstly, different commercial phospholipids (platelet substitutes) have different sensitivities to heparin and with some there is no linear relationship between clotting times and heparin concentration in the therapeutic range (0.2–0.6 IU/ml). Such reagents are not suitable for the control of heparinization.

If a phospholipid reagent carries no manu-

facturer's information on its sensitivity to heparin, or is home-made, it is necessary to establish whether it is a reliable guide to plasma heparin concentration. A crude test for linearity can be made by adding known concentrations of heparin to a normal plasma pool and measuring the APTT immediately after the addition. The APTT is expressed as a ratio of the time obtained with the normal pool containing no heparin. An example of different responses is shown in Fig. 19.4.

---

*Also known as partial thromboplastin time with kaolin (PTTK).

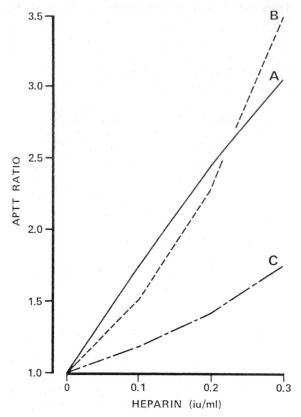

Fig. 19.4   APTT response to heparin added to plasma in vitro. APTT response expressed as ratio (APTT of heparinized plasma/APTT of plasma without heparin). Three different reagents and methods shown. (Slightly modified, from Tomenson and Thomson.[14] With the permission of publisher and editor.)

The second shortcoming of the APTT in the control of heparin treatment is that the APTT is affected by a number of variables not related to heparin (see p. 308). The most important of these are fibrinogen and factor VIII:C concentration and the presence of FDP. In patients with DIC, liver disease or renal disease,[7] heparinization should be controlled using one of the other tests described below.

Reagents and method

The reagents and method are described on p. 308.

Therapeutic range

0.2–0.6 IU/ml.

The prolongation of the APTT achieved with these concentrations varies between reagents according to the sensitivity of the phospholipid used. The results may be expressed as clotting time in seconds or as a ratio. For the majority of sensitive reagents ratios of 1.5–3.0 cover the therapeutic range.

THROMBIN TIME

This test is simple and popular, since it can be performed on batches of plasma in the laboratory. The therapeutic range depends on the strength of the thrombin solution used for the test. When using a concentration of 10 NHS units with a control time of *c* 15 s, the therapeutic range lies between 25 and 100 s. For details of the test see p. 309.

ANTI-Xa ASSAY FOR HEPARIN

Principle. Plasma anti-Xa activity is enhanced by the addition of heparin, and a coagulation or amidolytic (chromogenic) assay of anti-Xa activity can be adapted to measure heparin. The anti-Xa assays are generally used to measure the low concentrations of heparin obtained after the prophylactic administration of low dose or low molecular weight heparins. However, the anti-Xa assay can also be used to measure the higher concentrations of heparin in plasma if a different standard curve is constructed. A number of commercial kits such as Heptest and Hepaclot, as well as various kits based on chromogenic substrates, are in use and give linear and reproducible responses.

A coagulation anti-Xa assay is described under the section on *Prophylactic heparin treatment* (p. 375).

Therapeutic range

0.2–0.6 IU/ml.

The concentration of heparin is read off a standard curve constructed according to the manufacturer's instructions.

PROTAMINE NEUTRALIZATION TEST[2]

Principle. This test is an extension of the thrombin time, various amounts of protamine sulphate being added to the plasma before the addition of thrombin. When all the heparin present in plasma has been neutralized, the clotting time should become normal. From the amount of protamine sulphate required to produce this effect, the concentration of heparin in the plasma can be calculated. The protamine neutralization test is used mainly to calculate the dose of protamine sulphate needed to neutralize circulating heparin after cardiopulmonary surgery and haemodialysis, but it is also used to control treatment or to calculate the dose of protamine to be administered if the patient needs quick reversal of heparinization.

Reagents

Protamine sulphate. Prepare dilutions (0–50 mg/ml) in barbitone buffer, pH 7.4. Dilute 5 ml of protamine sulphate (10 g/l) 1 in 20 with buffer to give 1 dl of a stock solution containing 500 µg/ml. Then make working solutions to cover the range of 0–500 µg/ml in 50 µg steps from the stock solution by dilution with buffer. The solutions keep indefinitely at 4°C.

Thrombin. Dilute thrombin in barbitone buffer to a concentration of about 20 NIH units/ml. Adjust the concentration so that 0.1 ml of thrombin clots 0.2 ml of normal plasma at 37°C in 10 ±1 s. Keep the thrombin in a plastic tube in melting ice during the assay.

Plasma. Citrated platelet-poor plasma from the patient.

Method

Place 0.2 ml of test plasma and 20 µl of barbitone buffer in a glass tube kept in a water bath at 37°C. Allow the mixture to warm and then add 0.1 ml of thrombin. Record the clotting time. If this is *c* 10 s there is no demonstrable heparin in the plasma. If the thrombin time is prolonged, repeat the test using 20 µl of the 500 µg/ml protamine solution instead of buffer. Repeat the test if necessary, until a concentration of protamine is found which gives a clotting time of *c* 10 s.

Calculation

If 20 µl of 150 µg/ml protamine sulphate produce

a normal thrombin time (whereas the clotting time is prolonged with 100 µg/ml protamine), then the concentration of 15 µg of protamine is sufficient to neutralize the heparin in 1 ml of plasma. Assuming weight for weight neutralization, the patient's plasma contains 15 µg of heparin per ml or 1.5 IU, assuming that 1 mg of heparin is equivalent to 100 IU. This figure can be further converted to concentration of heparin per ml of whole blood by multiplying by 1–PCV.

In the above example, for in-vivo neutralization of heparin by protamine sulphate, assuming a total blood volume of 75 ml per kg body weight, the required dose of protamine would be:

$$\frac{15 \times \text{total blood volume}}{1 \div (1 - \text{PCV})} \text{ mg}$$
$$= \frac{15 \times 75 \times \text{body weight} \times (1 - \text{PCV})}{1000} \text{ mg}$$

PROPHYLACTIC HEPARIN TREATMENT

Heparin is administered prophylactically in a much lower dosage than that used therapeutically, usually as a subcutaneous (s.c.) injection. The low concentrations achieved (0.05 to 0.2 IU/ml) are sufficient to increase the anti-Xa activity of the plasma and prevent the onset of thrombosis. The derangement of haemostasis is minimal and in most instances monitoring is not required. However, in patients on long-term s.c. heparin, such as pregnant women, and those about to undergo major surgery, as well as in some special cases (i.e. patients undergoing hip replacement, the elderly, those with splenomegaly and/or a marginally reduced platelet count, etc.) it may be necessary to confirm that the heparin concentration is sufficient to prevent thrombosis yet not so high as to cause haemorrhage. The heparin concentration and its effect must also be monitored if one of the newer low molecular weight heparins with improved bio-availability is used. The peak plasma concentration after a s.c. injection of conventional unfractionated heparin occurs approximately 2 h later and an estimation at this time indicates the probable maximum effectiveness of the treatment. With low molecular weight heparins the plasma concentration reaches a peak within 1–2 h and remains at this level for up to 24 h.

An anti-Xa assay is the method of choice for measuring the effect of low dose or low molecular weight heparin. The APTT test can also be used but only to assess whether the concentration of heparin is unacceptably high. The majority of commercial APTT reagents are not sensitive to heparin concentrations below 0.15 IU/ml and it is generally accepted that the patient's APTT should be within 8 s of the control time. If the clotting time is longer, the plasma heparin concentration is in excess of 0.2 IU/ml and the patient may bleed if haemostatically challenged.

ANTI-Xa ASSAY FOR MONITORING LOW-DOSE SUBCUTANEOUS HEPARIN[3]

Principle. The anti-Xa activity of antithrombin III is enhanced by the addition of heparin. A standard curve is constructed by adding varying amounts of heparin to a normal plasma pool which provides the source of the antithrombin III. The inhibition of factor Xa by heparin is measured in a modified factor-X assay.

Reagents

Pooled normal plasma. From 20 normal donors, see p. 327.

Patient's plasma. Citrated platelet-poor plasma should be collected between 2 and 4 h after the injection of heparin; it should be tested as soon as possible after the collection and kept at +4°C or on crushed ice until tested.

Buffer. Trisodium citrate 30 volumes, glyoxaline buffer (p. 306) 150 volumes, and 20% bovine albumin 1 volume.

Commercially prepared artificial factor-X-deficient plasma.★ Reconstitute according to instructions.

Platelet substitute. Mix equal volumes of factor-X-deficient plasma and platelet substitute.★ This is the working reagent and is kept at 37°C.

Factor Xa. Reconstitute as instructed by the manufacturer. Dilute further in the buffer to give a 1 in 100 dilution. Keep on crushed ice until used.

Heparin. 1000 IU/ml. Dilute in saline to 10 IU/ml. Ideally, the same batch of heparin as the patient is receiving should be used.

$CaCl_2$. 0.025 mol/l.

Method

A standard curve is constructed as shown in Table 19.4. Add 0.05 ml of each dilution to 0.45 ml of the normal plasma pool. This will give final concentrations of heparin from 0.05 to 0.30 IU/ml in 0.05 IU steps.

Pipette 0.3 ml of diluted factor Xa into a large glass tube at 37°C.

Add 0.1 ml of the first standard dilution. Start the stop-watch. At 1 min and 30 s exactly transfer duplicate 0.1 ml volumes of the mixture into two tubes each containing 0.1 ml of pre-warmed $CaCl_2$.

At 2 min after sub-sampling add 0.2 ml of the mixture of factor-X-deficient plasma and platelet substitute, start the stop-watch, mix and record the clotting time.

Repeat for each dilution of standard. The patient's sample is tested undiluted in pooled normal plasma if the clotting time is longer than the times used to construct the standard curve.

Calculation

Plot the clotting times against the heparin concentration on log-linear paper, with the clotting times on the linear axis. The concentration of heparin in the patient's sample can be read directly from the standard curve. It is multiplied by the dilution factor if necessary.

Comment

Anti-Xa assay for measuring low concentrations of heparin can be carried out using commercial

Table 19.4 Preparation of a standard curve for an anti-Xa assay

Reagent	Tube					
	1	2	3	4	5	6
Heparin (10 IU/ml)	0.05	0.10	0.15	0.20	0.25	0.30
Saline (ml)	0.95	0.90	0.85	0.80	0.75	0.70
Concentration of heparin (IU/ml)	0.5	1.0	1.5	2.0	2.5	3.0
Final conc. of heparin after addition to normal plasma pool	0.05	0.10	0.15	0.20	0.25	0.30

★Diagen, Diagnostic Reagents Ltd, Thame, Oxon.

kits based on the coagulation of plasma or on chromogenic substrates. Such assays are technically simple and give reliable results.

INVESTIGATION OF A PATIENT WHO BLEEDS WHILE RECEIVING HEPARIN

Minor bleeding (microscopic haematuria, bruising, bleeding from venepuncture sites, etc.) is common during treatment with heparin and may herald a more serious haemorrhagic episode. A potentially serious side effect to the use of heparin, heparin-associated thrombocytopenia, also presents with bleeding. For this reason every episode of bleeding should be investigated. A suggested plan of investigation is shown in Table 19.5.

Side-effects of heparin therapy

From the laboratory point of view the most difficult complication is that of heparin-induced thrombocytopenia and thrombosis (sometimes

Table 19.5 Investigation of a patient who is bleeding while on heparin treatment

Test	Result	Comment
APTT	2–3 × normal	Excessive heparin dose.
Platelets	Normal	Reduce or stop heparin
Fibrinogen	Normal	
APTT	Within range or long	Heparin-associated
Platelets	Low	thrombocytopenia.
Fibrinogen	Normal	Stop heparin
APTT	Very long	DIC, liver or renal
Platelets	Low	disease. If heparin is to
Fibrinogen	Low	be continued, determine conc. using protamine neutralization or anti-Xa assay. Modify dose

called the HITT syndrome). This complication, which is antibody mediated, can be tested for in the laboratory in a number of ways. Perhaps the simplest is to perform a modified form of the platelet aggregation studies described in Chapter 17 using heparin as the agonist. More involved tests such as the serotonin uptake and release assay have been described.[13]

THROMBOLYTIC THERAPY

The thrombolytic agents currently in use are: urokinase, streptokinase, streptokinase-plasminogen complex and acylated compounds (APSAC), and the tissue type plasminogen activator (t-PA) obtained by recombinant technology or from tissue culture. Single chain urokinase and various activator molecules modified through recombinant techniques are also being developed and studied.

Urokinase. This is a trypsin-like protease found in urine. Urokinase directly converts plasminogen into plasmin by cleaving a single Arg-Val bond. The active enzyme is isolated in either a two-chain or a one-chain form. Both forms have been cloned and can be used therapeutically; they are administered intravenously in doses between 2500 and 4450 units per kg body weight.

Streptokinase. This is a purified fraction of the filtrate from cultures of *Str. haemolyticus.* Streptokinase interacts with plasminogen or plasmin to form a plasminogen activator; the activator complex in turn cleaves a bond in the

plasminogen molecule to give rise to plasmin. Streptokinase is a foreign protein and induces antibody production in man. It also cross-reacts with anti-streptococcal antibodies and this may cause a resistance to therapy. Streptokinase treatment is often started with a loading dose of between 250 000 and 500 000 units and continued at 100 000 units per hour for up to 72 h. A single very high dose (usually over 1 000 000 u) is administered to achieve thrombolysis in myocardial infarction.

Biochemical manipulations have resulted in the preparation of a number of forms of the streptokinase-plasminogen complex, including complexes with the acylated forms of plasmin and plasminogen which have strong fibrin-binding characteristics. These complexes are used for coronary thrombolysis.

The fibrinolytic state induced by urokinase and streptokinase is short-lived once the infusion has been stopped. While the infusion lasts there is fibrinolysis at the site of thrombosis as well as systemic fibrinolysis. The fibrinogen and plasminogen concentrations in plasma fall and the FDP concentration rises.

Tissue-type plasminogen activator (t-PA). This is a single- or double-chain polypeptide obtained by recombinant techniques or from tissue cultures. It is a potent activator of plasminogen and induces a thrombolytic state of a longer duration then either streptokinase or urokinase infusion. t-PA has a strong affinity for fibrin-bound plasminogen and causes less fibrinogenolysis than any of the previously mentioned agents.

Selection of patients

Thrombolytic treatment carries a serious risk of bleeding and thrombolytic agents should not be given to individuals suffering from a variety of illnesses where there is a high risk of bleeding. In addition, each patient should have his haemostatic function and platelet count measured before treatment is started.

TITRATION OF THE INITIAL DOSE OF STREPTOKINASE

Principle. Different amounts of streptokinase are added to patient's plasma in vitro and the samples clotted with thrombin. The smallest amount of streptokinase which causes the clot to lyse within 10 min is multiplied by the presumed plasma volume to give the titrated dose of streptokinase.

Reagents

Patient's plasma. Citrated platelet-poor plasma (see p. 305).

Streptokinase. Vials containing the freeze-dried material to be given to the patient are suitable. Open the vial and add sufficient 9 g/l NaCl to make a solution containing 2000 IU/ml. From this initial solution, make further dilutions containing 1500, 1000 and 500 IU/ml.

Thrombin. A solution containing *c* 50 NIH units per ml of 9 g/l NaCl.

Method

Place four glass tubes in the water-bath at 37°C. Pipette 1 ml of plasma into each tube followed by 0.1 ml of the four streptokinase dilutions and add 0.1 ml of thrombin. Mix the contents of the tubes by inversion and start the stop-watch when clotting has taken place. Lysis will commence first in the tube with 2000 IU/ml of streptokinase. Note the tube containing the smallest amount of streptokinase which will cause clot lysis in 10 min.

Calculation of the dose

Suppose that the clot lysed in the three tubes containing 1000, 1500 and 2000 IU/ml. The least amount of streptokinase able to induce lysis in 1 ml of plasma was 100 IU. If the patient is an adult with a presumed plasma volume of 50 ml per kg body weight and if he weighs 60 kg, the presumed total plasma volume is 3000 ml. The necessary initial dose of streptokinase would be $100 \times 3000 = 300\,000$ IU.

LABORATORY CONTROL OF THROMBOLYTIC THERAPY

Many laboratory tests are abnormal during thrombolytic therapy, but the perfect and specific procedure for monitoring is not available. All screening tests of coagulation are prolonged reflecting the hyperplasminaemic state with the reduction in the fibrinogen concentration and the presence of FDP. The prolongation is most marked with streptokinase and streptokinase-plasminogen complex; it is less marked with urokinase and least with t-PA. The fibrinogen concentration commonly falls to below 0.05 g/l and the FDP concentration may rise to over 1000 ng/l.

Monitoring in venous thrombosis. The thrombin time is commonly used to monitor therapy. A few hours after the start of the infusion, the thrombin time is prolonged to 40 s or more (control 15±1 s); it then settles to approximately 20–30 s. Very long thrombin times carry a high risk of bleeding and are indicative of severe hyperplasminaemia. Many centres use a standard streptokinase and urokinase regime without any laboratory control and carry out laboratory tests only if the patient bleeds.

Monitoring in coronary thrombolysis. This is carried out to ensure that the patient is not at risk of bleeding or to establish that the thrombolysis is proceeding satisfactorily. In the first case, the APTT or thrombin time are sometimes carried out; in the second, one of the tests for the lysis of fibrin (as distinct from fibrinogen) is performed. The two commonest tests are the measurement of cross-linked D-dimer using a monoclonal antibody and the measurement of a fibrin-specific early FDP called Bβ 15–42. Both tests are available as commercial kits and are usually performed as a part of pharmacological studies or therapeutic trials.

Timing the start of anticoagulant therapy. Heparin and oral anticoagulants are started within hours of stopping the infusion of the thrombolytic agent. The timing of anticoagulation is crucial; if it is given too soon, while the fibrinogen concentration is very low, the risk of bleeding is substantial. It is usually considered safe to start anticoagulants when the fibrinogen concentration exceeds 0.05 g/l of plasma. If the fibrinogen concentration is 0.05 g/l and the prolongation of APTT does not exceed twice the base line clotting time, heparin treatment can be safely given and monitored. This usually occurs 4–6 h after streptokinase and urokinase infusion and sooner after t-PA. However,

Table 19.6 Investigation of a patient who is bleeding while on thrombolytic treatment

Timing	Test	Result	Comment
During infusion	TT or APTT Fibrinogen	Very long Low	Hyperplasminaemia. Stop infusion, transfuse (FFP)
Before heparin	TT or APTT Fibrinogen	Very long Very low	Hypofibrinogenaemia. DO NOT give heparin, transfuse if necessary
While on heparin	APTT	Very long	
	a. Fibrinogen Platelets	Normal Normal	Excess heparin, reduce dose
	b. Fibrinogen Platelets	Low Normal	Heparin given too soon*
	c. Fibrinogen Platelets	Low Low	DIC, liver or renal disease*. Investigate

APTT, activated partial thromboplastin time; TT, thrombin time.
*Use anti-Xa assay to measure heparin concentration.

after streptokinase infusion occasional patients may show persistent hypofibrinogenaemia for up to 24 h. Such individuals must be monitored at 4 h intervals and not given heparin and warfarin until their APTT is at least twice the baseline clotting time.

INVESTIGATION OF A PATIENT WHO BLEEDS WHILE ON THROMBOLYTIC AGENTS OR IMMEDIATELY AFTERWARDS

The tests, the timing and the likely mechanism of bleeding are shown in Table 19.6.

ANTI-PLATELET THERAPY

Many drugs inhibit platelet function in vitro but only a few have anti-platelet activity in acceptable doses. Each category of drugs has a different pharmacological action and requires different methods to demonstrate its effect on platelets. Anti-platelet agents are used in primary and secondary prevention of coronary heart disease, in unstable angina, in certain forms of cerebrovascular disease, to prevent thrombo-embolism associated with valvular disease and prosthetic

heart valves, and to prevent thrombosis in arteriovenous shunts. Haematologists are only exceptionally asked to monitor these aspects of anti-platelet therapy. Indeed, it is said that the advantage of these agents is the lack of any need to monitor therapy.

A proportion of patients with thrombocytosis or thrombocythaemia experience episodes of arterial thrombosis. Such patients are often given anti-platelet drugs and the effect of these drugs is sometimes monitored. Three techniques are available for monitoring: prolongation of the bleeding time (see p. 318), inhibition of platelet aggregation response to standard agonists (see p. 320) and normalization of platelet survival using [111]Indium-labelled platelets (p. 413). Such monitoring is usually tailored to the individual patient and the choice of test depends on the drug used, on the abnormalities detectable in the patient, and on the laboratory facilities available. Thus aspirin affects both bleeding time and platelet aggregation, whereas the effect of dipyridamole on platelet aggregation is unpredictable, and can only be reliably shown by measuring platelet survival.

REFERENCES

[1]BARROWCLIFFE, T. W., CURTIS, A. D. and JOHNSON, E. A. (1988). An international standard for low molecular weight heparin. *Thrombosis and Haemostasis*, **60**, 1.

[2]DACIE, J. V. and LEWIS, S. M. (1975). *Practical Haematology*, 5th edn, p. 413. Churchill Livingstone, Edinburgh.

[3]DENSON, K. W. E. and BONNAR, J. (1973). The measurement of heparin. A method based on the potentiation of antifactor Xa. *Thrombosis et Diathesis Haemorrhagica*, **30**, 471.

[4]COMMISSION OF EUROPEAN COMMUNITIES (1982). *BCR Information: Certification of Three Reference Materials for Thromboplastins*. EEC, Brussels

[5]DAVIDSON, J. F., COLVIN, B. T., BARROWCLIFFE, T. W, KERNOFF, P. B. A., MACHIN, S. T., POLLER, L., PRESTON, F. E. and WALKER, I. D. on behalf of the British Society for Haematology (1990). Guidelines on oral anticoagulation: second edition. *Journal of Clinical Pathology*, **43**, 177.

[6]FENNERTY, A. G, RENOWDEN, S., SCOLDING, N., BENTLEY, D. P., CAMPBELL, I. A. and ROUTLEDGE, P. A. (1986). Guidelines to control heparin treatment. *British Medical Journal*, **292**, 579.

[7]FEY, M. F., LANG, M., FURLAN, M. and BECK, E. A. (1987). Monitoring heparin therapy with the activated partial thromboplastin time and chromogenic substrate assays. *Thrombosis and Haemostasis*, **58**, 853.

[8]HOET, B., CLOSE, P., VERMYLEN, J. and VERSTRAETE, M. (1991). In *Recent Advances in Coagulation*, Ed. L Poller, Vol 6. Churchill Livingstone, Edinburgh.

[9]KIRKWOOD, T. B. L. (1983). Calibration of reference thromboplastins and standardization of the prothrombin ratio. *Thrombosis and Haemostasis*, **49**, 238.

[10]OWREN, P. A. (1959). Thrombotest: a new method of controlling anticoagulant therapy. *Lancet*, **ii**, 754.

[11]OWREN, P. A. and AAS, K. (1951). The control of dicoumarol therapy and the quantitative determination of prothrombin and proconvertin. *Scandinavian Journal of Clinical and Laboratory Investigation*, **3**, 201.

[12]POLLER, L. (1987). Oral anticoagulant therapy. In *Haemostasis and Thrombosis*. Eds. Bloom, A. L. and Thomas, D. P., 2nd edn, p. 870. Churchill Livingstone, Edinburgh.

[13]SHERIDAN, D., CARTER, C. and KELTON, J. G. (1986). A diagnostic test for heparin induced thrombocytopenia. *Blood*, **67**, 27.

[14]TOMENSON, J. A. and THOMSON, J. M. (1985). Standardization of the prothrombin time. In *Blood Coagulation and Haemostasis. A Practical Guide*. Ed. Thomson, J. M., p. 370. Churchill Livingstone, Edinburgh.

20. Use of radionuclides in haematology

Revised by M. J. Myers

Forms of radiation   381
Radiation dosage   381
Radiation protection   383
Sources of radionuclides   383

Apparatus used for measuring radioactivity   384
In-vivo measurement of radioactivity   386
Measurement of radioactivity by means of a scintillation
    counter   387

In this chapter a brief general account will be given of the methods of using radionuclides* in haematological diagnosis. For a more complete account of the theory and practice of nuclear medicine techniques the reader is referred to reviews by Sorenson and Phelps,[9] Bowring,[1] Lewis and Bayly,[6] and Maisey. The main properties of the radionuclides useful in diagnostic haematology are summarized in Tables 20.1 and 20.2. Specific instructions for their use are given in Chapter 21.

FORMS OF RADIATION

Radioactivity results from the spontaneous decay of unstable atomic nuclei; this may be accompanied by the emission of charged particles (electrons, α, β^+ or β^- rays) or electromagnetic radiation (γ or X-rays).

Radionuclides which emit γ rays are particularly useful as they have the advantage that their emissions penetrate tissues well so that they can be detected at the surface of the body when they have originated within organs. The radiation from α- and β-ray emitters has little tissue penetration; these are less useful for certain clinical purposes and are potentially more harmful than γ-ray emitters. The different types of radiation can be detected and distinguished by their ionization effect, by chemical and photochemical effects and by the production of scintillations in certain materials. The systems used for measuring radioactivity are described on p. 384.

RADIATION DOSES

When using radionuclides, account must be taken of their potential risk for the recipient and the laboratory worker. The extent of radiation hazard in relation to the small amount of radionuclide employed in diagnostic work depends on a number of factors: e.g. the energy and range of the radiations; whether the radionuclide is widely distributed in the body or becomes localized in specific organs; the physical half-life of the radionuclide and its biological half-time in the body. The radionuclide should, as a rule, have as short a half-life as is compatible with the duration of the test. A radionuclide with a very short half-life can be administered in much higher amounts than those which are likely to remain active in the body for a considerably longer time.

Formerly, radioactivity was expressed in curies (Ci); 10^{-3} Ci = 1mCi and 10^{-6} Ci = 1 μCi. The preferred SI unit of radioactivity is the bequerel (Bq). 1 Bq corresponds to one disintegration per second, so that 1 Ci = 3.7×10^{10}Bq. 1 millicurie (mCi) = 3.7×10^7 Bq or 37 megabequerels (MBq), and 1 microcurie (μCi) = 3.7×10^4 Bq or 0.037 MBq; 10^3 MBq = 1 gigabequerel (GBq).

The effect of radiation on the body depends, essentially, on the amount of energy deposited. This is expressed in grays (Gy). 1 Gy is the dose of

---

*This is the correct usage, but also commonly referred to as 'radioisotopes'.

Table 20.1   Radionuclides used in haematological diagnosis

Element	Physical half-life	Principal radiations	Mean Energies (MeV)	Availability
^{57}Co	270 days	γ	0.122, 0.136	**
^{58}Co	71.3 days	β+ γ	0.20 0.811, 0.511	**
^{51}Cr	27.8 days	γ	0.320	**
^{52}Fe*	8.2 h	β+ γ	0.34 0.511, 0.165	Cyclotron
^{59}Fe	45 days	β− γ	0.15, 0.08 1.09, 1.29	**
^{125}I	60 days	γ X-rays	0.035 0.027	**
^{131}I	8.05 days	β− γ	0.19 0.364, 0.637	**
^{111}In	2.81 days	γ	0.247, 0.173	**
^{113m}In	1.67 h	γ	0.393	**
^{32}P	14.3 days	β−	0.69	**
^{99m}Tc	6 h	γ	0.141	**

*Decays to ^{52}Mn ($T_{1/2}$ = 21 min; 1.4 MeV γ-rays).
**Commercial suppliers, e.g. Amersham International.

Table 20.2   Application of radionuclides in haematological diagnosis

Element	Radiopharmaceutical	Application	Usual dose (MBq)	Effective dose (mSv)
^{57}Co ^{58}Co	Vitamin B12	Investigation of megaloblastic anaemias	0.02–0.04 0.02–0.04	0.2 0.3
^{51}Cr	Sodium chromate Sodium chromate Sodium chromate Sodium chromate Sodium chromate Sodium chromate Sodium chromate	Red cell volume Red cell life-span Sites of red cell destruction Measurement of gastro-intestinal bleeding Platelet life-span Spleen scan Spleen pool	0.4–0.8 1–2 4 4 1–2 3.5–5.5 9	0.2 0.5 1.0 1.0 0.5 1.5 2.5
^{52}Fe	Ferric chloride or citrate	Ferrokinetics	3.5	2.5
^{59}Fe	Ferric chloride or citrate	Absorption of iron (oral) Ferrokinetics and erythropoiesis (intravenous)	0.2–0.8 0.2–0.4	2.0 5.0
^{125}I	Iodinated human serum albumin	Plasma volume	0.08–0.2	2.0
^{111}In	Indium chloride (→ oxine or tropolone)	Platelet life-span Red cell volume Spleen scan, platelets, granulocytes	4 1–2 4	3.0 1.5 3.0
^{99m}Tc	Pertechnetate	Red cell volume Spleen scan Spleen pool	2 100 100	0.02 4.0 1.0

radiation which deposits 1 joule of energy per kg of tissue. In the past this has been expressed in rads (1 Gy = 100 rads). The reaction of the body to the radiation is also affected by the type of the particular ionizing ray, and the biological effect of the radiation is calculated from the amount in Gy (or rad) multiplied by an ionization quality factor; this factor varies with the type of ray and is 20 times more for α-rays than for β- and γ-rays. The unit for describing the biological effect of radiation, i.e. the unit of 'effective dose', is the Sievert (Sv). The annual dose limit for the whole body for somebody working with radionuclides is 50 mSv, with a larger amount for individual organs. Lower dose limits, of 5 mSv, apply to members of the public. Radionuclides should not be given to pregnant women unless the investigation is considered imperative.

RADIATION PROTECTION

The quantity of radioactivity used in diagnostic work is usually small and good laboratory practice is all that is necessary for safe working. However, before using radionuclides, workers should familiarize themselves with the problem of radiation protection for themselves, their fellow workers and patients. In Britain there is an approved Code of Practice and also Guidance Notes which describe the procedures which must be followed in medical and dental practice.[3,7] An important recommendation is that radionuclides should be handled only in approved laboratories. They must be used only under the direction of an authorized person and the amount administered to patients must not exceed the limits laid down by the Administration of Radioactive Substances Advisory Committee.[2]

The greatest danger to individuals in handling diagnostic radionuclides is from ingestion, inhalation or by skin contact, while contamination of apparatus and working area will affect the validity of tests. Working with radionuclides requires the same order of technical competence, experience, discipline and precautions as are needed in handling infective materials.

To monitor the radiation dose received, each designated radiation worker must wear a personal dosemeter. This is usually in the form of a photographic film badge or a thermo-luminescent dose-meter (TLD) badge*. The laboratory should be equipped with at least one suitable portable radiation monitor to detect contamination in the working area, including sinks and drains. In general, the radioactive waste from radionuclides used in haematological diagnostic procedures

may be poured down a single designated laboratory sink. It should be washed down with a large quantity of running water. If the waste material exceeds the amount allowed for disposal in this way, it should be stored in a suitable place until its radioactivity has decayed sufficiently for it to be disposed of via the refuse system. All working and storage areas and disposal sinks should be clearly labelled with the internationally recognized trefoil symbol.

Decontamination of working surfaces, walls and floors can usually be achieved by washing with a detergent such as Decon 90 (Decon Laboratories Ltd). Glassware can be decontaminated by soaking in Decon 90 and plastic laboratory ware by washing in dilute (e.g. 1%) nitric acid.

Protective gloves must always be worn when handling radionuclides; any activity which does get on to the hands can usually be removed by washing with soap and water, or if that fails, with a detergent solution. For each laboratory in which isotopes are used, a radiological safety officer should be nominated to supervise protection procedures.

A good account of the general procedures to be followed in handling radioactive materials is given in a monograph published by the International Atomic Energy Agency.[4]

SOURCES OF RADIONUCLIDES

The longer-lived radionuclides, which are used for haematological investigations are generally available from commercial suppliers. The usual way of obtaining certain short-lived radionuclides is by means of a radionuclide generator, in which a moderately long-lived parent radionuclide decays to produce the required short-lived isotope. The parent radionuclide is adsorbed onto a support material such as an ion exchange resin, surrounded by an aqueous buffer. The daughter nuclide appears in the buffer as it forms, and may be obtained by elution of the generator column. In this way ^{99m}Tc ($T_{1/2}$ = 6 h) can be derived from ^{99}Mo ($T_{1/2}$ = 66 h).

Radioactive elements are often produced as a mixture with a proportion of a non-radioactive but chemically identical element which is known

---

*The National Radiological Protection Board, Harwell, Didcot, provides a film or TLD badge service.

as 'carrier'. The specific activity is a measure of the radioactivity per unit mass of total material. A compound which is carrier-free offers the highest attainable specific activity. As a radionuclide decays, the specific activity decreases. The activity of the radionuclide which is administered is chosen in order to have sufficient radioactivity for the subsequent sample measurements; it is important to ensure that the concentration of the chemical element is not so great as to be non-physiological or even toxic.

APPARATUS FOR MEASURING RADIOACTIVITY

Scintillation detectors

These are by far the most widely used detectors for measuring radiation. Detection is based on the fact that certain crystals (phosphors) have the property of emitting a flash of light (a scintillation) when radiation energy (photons) enters them. Sodium iodide activated with thallium is used in nearly all detectors. The scintillations produced are too weak to be seen directly. Instead, the light is detected by the photocathode of a photomultiplier tube which produces a response to this light by emitting electrons. The electrons are accelerated towards a series of metal grids ('dynodes'), each held at a higher positive voltage than the previous dynode. For each electron striking a dynode several electrons are emitted. The number of electrons is thus progressively increased at each dynode; they accumulate at the anode where they constitute a small electrical pulse, the size of which is proportional to the total energy absorbed by the crystal. The pulses are amplified and are counted in a scaler or ratemeter (see below).

The magnitude of the pulses from the scintillation detector is proportional to the energy of the rays which give rise to the scintillations. In a spectrometer the pulses are sorted by an analyser with respect to their height (Fig. 20.1). The number of pulses within a selected window are counted. By selecting a part of the spectrum in which energies produced by other radionuclides are either not counted or are minimized, a selected radionuclide can be counted when present in a mixture. Pulse selection also enables background

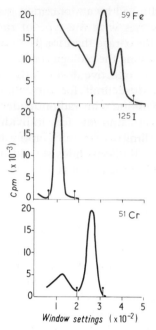

Fig. 20.1   Spectra of ^{59}Fe, ^{125}I and ^{51}Cr obtained on a scintillation spectrometer. The radionuclides should be counted with the window set within the limits indicated by the vertical lines.

noise to be minimized. Care must be taken in in-vivo counting to exclude components of a spectrum which result from scattered radiation arising from activity not within the required field of view.

Thallium-activated sodium iodide crystals are available in various shapes and sizes. A 'well-type' crystal contains a cavity into which is inserted a small container or test-tube holding up to 5 ml of fluid. Since the sample is almost surrounded by the crystal, counting is achieved with high efficiency. As the geometric efficiency of a well-type counter depends on the position of the sample in relation to the crystal, it is important to use the same volume for each sample in a series. Another form of crystal detector is a solid circular cylinder, 2.5–10 cm in diameter. In this form it is used for in-vivo measurements and occasionally for the measurement of bulky samples, e.g. 24 h urine specimens.

Ionization chambers

A known volume of air or other gas is subjected to

irradiation by a radioactive material. Ions produced in the gas are collected on a pair of electrodes and this collection of ions results in the flow of a very small current in an external circuit. This current, which is proportional to the intensity of radiation passing through the chamber, is measured by an electrometer. This type of apparatus is used for the measurement of comparatively large quantities of radioactivity (>37 MBq or 1 mCi); its main use is for the measurement of the activity of a stock radionuclide.

Geiger-Müller counters (GM tubes)

GM tubes are used in survey meters for radiation protection and to detect contamination. An end-window type of tube is usually used to detect contamination with instruments which are calibrated in counts/s. The window is a thin layer of mica which is sufficiently thin to permit the passage of α and β particles into the counter. Special tubes are used in instruments designed to assess radiation dose levels and are calibrated in dose rate units of microsieverts per hour (μSv/h).

Liquid scintillation counters

Low-energy β-emitters can be counted with high efficiency in a liquid scintillator in which the radioactive material is mixed with an organic scintillator in a solvent. The scintillations produced are then measured between a pair of photo-multiplier tubes. The apparatus is usually operated in a refrigerated unit at 4°C to reduce spurious electrical signals. Liquid scintillation solutions have three components:

1. A solvent (e. g. xylene or toluene).
2. A primary solute such as p-terphenyl-1-phenyl-4-phenyloxazole (PPO), and various conjugated phenyls.
3. A secondary solute such as 1,4-di (2,5-phenyloxazole)benzene (POPOP), which traps the excitation energy from the primary solute, emitting photons of a longer wavelength which are measured more efficiently.

A problem of liquid scintillation which is particularly pertinent to haematological work is that a quenching effect with a decrease in counting efficiency is caused by material which is coloured or contains proteins or insoluble substances which are likely to absorb light. To count such material accurately requires careful preparation and the adoption of special procedures to correct for the quenching effect.

Measurement of radioactivity in bulky material

By using two opposed detectors in a single counting system, it is possible to measure, with relative precision, the radioactivity in an organ or in a sample of faeces without the necessity for homogenization. Similarly, the radioactivity in a large volume of urine or other fluid can be measured without the necessity of concentrating to a smaller volume. The sample is placed in a 450 ml waxed cardboard carton with a screw-top lid, and positioned between two counters, placed above and below it, respectively. It is supported over the lower counter by a plastic ring to ensure that the specimen in the carton is approximately equidistant from both crystals. The counting system is surrounded by lead and the responses of both crystals are counted together. If a single detector system is used it is essential to homogenize the samples.

Scalers, timers and ratemeters

These instruments record the output signals from radiation detection after the pulse-height analysis of the signals. A device that only counts pulses is called a scaler and an auxiliary device that controls the scaler counting time is called a timer. Rate-meters record the mean rate of arrival of pulses from the analyser from which extraneous pulses are excluded.

Associated with the scaler or ratemeter is a high voltage unit. Its function is to supply the high voltage necessary to operate the radiation detector. In addition, each counter has a pulse amplifier, the function of which is to increase the voltage of the pulse produced to a size suitable for operating the scaler or ratemeter.

As a rule all the devices are incorporated in one unit to which the detector is connected. Recording of data is increasingly being carried out by means of a computer.

Dead-time

After each pulse there is a short period during which the apparatus cannot respond to a further stimulus. This is the 'dead-time', during which any signal entering the counter will not be registered.

Dead-time losses also occur in pulse-height analysers and scalers. In modern instruments the dead-time is short and correction is unnecessary in clinical investigations unless the count is more than about 3×10^5 counts/min.

IN-VIVO MEASUREMENT OF RADIOACTIVITY

Surface counting

This depends on shielding the crystals by means of a lead collimator to exclude as far as possible the radiation from outside a well defined area of the body.[5] It is thus possible to measure the radioactivity in individual organs. Positioning of the counter in relation to the patient is critical, and if the collimation is sufficiently narrow it is possible by counting over individual organs to detect sites of concentration of radioactivity. For most purposes a crystal with a diameter of 5–7 cm is suitable, but increased sensitivity, as well as more reliable positioning, can be achieved by using a dual counting system, with two opposed counters positioned above and below the patient, who is lying down.

Imaging

Radionuclide imaging has become the most important application of radioactivity in clinical medicine. Its purpose is to obtain a picture of the distribution of a labelled substance within the body after it has been administered. This requires a radionuclide which emits γ-rays, the energies of which are sufficient for the rays to penetrate body tissues and allow deep-lying organs to be imaged. The most widely used method for imaging is by the γ camera. This consists of a large diameter (usually about 40 cm), 10–12 mm thick, thallium-activated sodium iodide detector crystal, an array of photomultiplier tubes, electronics for positioning the scintillations and for pulse-height analysis, a collimator with multiple parallel holes, a video-display unit for image display and a computer system to analyse, store and display the data.

Scanning camera

The gamma camera will normally visualize a circumscribed area of the body. To obtain a whole-body image on a single sheet of film a modification of the gamma camera, called the scanning camera, is used. The detector passes linearly head to foot over the patient's body, recording and displaying the image on a computer screen. The image moves on the display in synchrony with the movement of the detector head, so that the whole-body image is built up and recorded.

The gamma camera can be used not only to obtain the image but also to measure the quantity of the isotope in various parts of the body. This requires determining a calibration factor which relates the number of counts recorded in the scan area to the activity obtained from a physical model ('phantom') containing a known amount of the radionuclide.[8]

Whole-body counting

It is possible by means of a whole-body counter consisting of a number of thallium-activated sodium iodide scintillators to measure the fraction of an administered radionuclide still present in the body with the passing for time. The technique is particularly useful in studying retention and turnover, as it overcomes the problems of collecting and measuring excreta. As the distribution of a radionuclide in the patient's body may vary during the course of an investigation, it is necessary to use several large crystals capable of receiving radiation pulses from the entire body area and to apply careful calibration procedures. Extensive shielding around the detector ('shadow shield') is required to reduce background counts, or if very long-term studies are envisaged, a shielded low background room must be used.

MEASUREMENT OF RADIOACTIVITY BY MEANS OF A SCINTILLATION COUNTER

Standardization of working conditions

Four controls require adjustment:

1. High voltage applied to the photomultiplier.
2. Amplifier gain applied to the incoming pulses before they reach the pulse-height analyser.
3. Analyser threshold.
4. Analyser window.

The pulse-height analyser threshold and window are arbitrary settings and for simplification it is convenient to make the analyser setting correspond to the energy of the γ-rays. Thus, a threshold scale of 0–100 can be made to correspond to a range of 0–1000 keV* by simply varying the amplifier gain.

The procedure is as follows: a radionuclide of known γ-emission, preferably one with a single energy such as ^{99m}Tc (0.140 MeV) or ^{51}Cr (0.320 MeV) is placed in front of the detector. The high voltage is fixed at a convenient level (e.g. 1000 V). The threshold scale is then set to correspond to the photo-peak of the radionuclide (i.e. the energy at which the maximum number of pulses in the pulse-height spectrum are emitted) and the window is set at about 10% of the threshold reading. The amplifier gain is varied until the spectrometer's ratemeter shows a definite peak. It should be established that the peak corresponds to the photopeak of the radionuclide and is not a scattered peak by starting with a high analyser setting and then gradually reducing it. The settings may be checked by means of another radionuclide of different energy when the analyser threshold should yield a maximum ratemeter deflection at a scale reading corresponding to the new energy. Examples of spectra and selected settings are illustrated in Fig. 20.1.

The setting of the apparatus, once determined, should remain constant for many months. The threshold and sensitivity of the equipment should be checked from time to time using a known standard. Ideally, this should be a sample of the radionuclide that is being measured. With a short-lived radionuclide this is not practical, and, instead, an isotope with a long half-life and comparable emission, e.g. ^{57}Co (120 keV, 270 day half-life), can be used.

Counting technique

Measurement of radioactivity

Measurements are usually carried out for a fixed period of time, the results being recorded as counts per s (cps) or counts per min (cpm). Radioactivity is subject to random but statistically predictable variation. The accuracy of the count depends upon the total number of the counts recorded as the variance (σ) of a radioactive count = $\sqrt{}$total count and the coefficient of variation (CV) is given by:

$$\frac{SD}{Count} \times 100\%.$$

Thus, on a count of 100 the inherent error is 10%; it is 1% on a count of 10 000. Any measured activity represents the difference between the sample count and the background count, in which the errors of both counts are cumulative. Other errors include those related to the calibration of the apparatus and those related to techniques, so that in-vivo radioactive measurements rarely have a CV<5% unless the count-rate is very high or the counting time unusually prolonged. In practice, a net count of 2500 over background is adequate for the accuracy required in in-vivo clinical studies.

---

*eV = electron volt, 10^3 eV = 1 keV, 10^3 keV = 1 MeV.

Background counts should be measured alongside that of the radioactive material. If the count rate of the sample is not much above background, then the background should be counted for as long a time as the sample. If the sample-count rate is less than the background, accurate measurement requires extremely long counting times.

Correction for physical decay

As physical decay is a continuous process which proceeds at an exponential rate and is specific for each particular radionuclide it is possible to correct mathematically for the loss of radioactivity with time and so convert any measurement back to that on day 0. This is necessary when successive observations made at different times after the administration of a radionuclide to a patient are compared. An alternative method is to prepare a standard from an accurately measured sample of the originally administered material and to compare the sample measurements with the measurements of the standard at the same time. The loss of radioactivity due to physical decay can then be ignored as both are decaying at identical rates.

Correction for dead-time

If the count rate is so high that the interval between counts is shorter than the dead-time, some counts will not be recorded. The extent of dead-time error can be estimated and a calibrated chart prepared from the expected and corresponding measured counts on samples in various known dilutions or by counting a high activity short-lived radionuclide at various times as it decays. When the solution being measured has a count-rate near to the instrument limit it should be diluted to a known amount or allowed to decay for a known period until the count-rate decreases to a level where loss due to dead-time becomes negligible.

DOUBLE RADIONUCLIDE MEASUREMENTS

If more than one radionuclide is present in a sample, it is possible to measure the radioactivity of each radionuclide separately by one of several techniques:

Mechanical separation

When plasma is labelled with ^{131}I and red cells with ^{51}Cr, the separation of the two components is simple. For example:

(a) Counts per ml whole blood
     = Activity of ^{131}I + ^{51}Cr per ml of blood;

(b) Counts per ml plasma × (1 − PCV)
     = Activity of ^{131}I per ml of blood;

(a) − (b) = Activity of ^{51}Cr per ml of blood

Differential decay

This is of value especially when one of the radionuclides has a very short half-life (e.g. ^{99m}Tc, half-life 6 h). The method is to count the activity in the mixture twice, with the time interval between the counts chosen to allow for the decay of five or more half-lives of the short-lived radionuclide.

Physical separation

When the two radionuclides produce γ-rays of widely different energies they can be counted separately at different settings in a γ-ray spectrometer, as determined by pulse-height analysis. If there is interference of one radionuclide by the other because of overlap of the spectra a correction can be applied by establishing a ratio of counts from a standard of the particular radionuclide measured at the setting for the other one. For example, to separate ^{99m}Tc and ^{51}Cr in a mixture, a ^{51}Cr source is counted in window 1 (optimal for Tc) and window 2 (optimal for Cr). The ^{51}Cr ratio (R) is calculated as counts of ^{51}Cr source in window 1 divided by counts of ^{51}Cr source in window 2. Then, when the mixture is measured, the counts due to ^{51}Cr interference in window 1 (N_1) = R × ^{51}Cr counts in window 2, and the true ^{99m}Tc count in window 1 = total count in window 1 − N_1.

REFERENCES

1. BOWRING, C. S. (1981). *Radionuclide Tracer Techniques in Haematology.* Butterworth, London.

2. DEPARTMENT OF HEALTH AND SOCIAL SECURITY (1979). *Health Service Management: Administration of Radioactive Substances to Persons.* HC (79)17. DHSS, London.

3. HEALTH AND SAFETY COMMISSION (1985). *Approved Code of Practice: The Protection of Persons Against Ionising Radiation Arising from any Work Activity. The Ionising Radiations Regulations 1985.* HMSO, London.

4. INTERNATIONAL ATOMIC ENERGY AGENCY (1973). *Safe Handling of Radionuclides.* IAEA Safety Series No. 1. IAEA. Vienna.

5. INTERNATIONAL COMMITTEE FOR STANDARDIZATION IN HAEMATOLOGY (1975). Recommended methods for surface counting to determine sites of red-cell destruction. *British Journal of Haematology,* **30,** 249.

6. LEWIS, S. M. and BAYLY, R. J. (Ed) (1986). *Radionuclides in Haematology.* Churchill Livingstone, Edinburgh.

7. NATIONAL RADIOLOGICAL PROTECTION BOARD (1988). *Guidance Notes for the Protection of Persons Against Ionising Radiations Arising from Medical and Dental Use.* HMSO, London.

8. SHORT, M. D., RICHARDS, A. R. and GLASS, H. I. (1972). The use of a gamma camera as a whole-body counter. *British Journal of Radiology,* **45,** 289.

9. SORENSON, J. A. and PHELPS, M. E. (1986). *Physics in Nuclear Medicine,* 2nd edn. Grune & Stratton, New York.

10. MAISEY, M. N., BRITTON, K. E. and GILDAY, D. L. (Eds.) (1991). *Clinical Nuclear Medicine,* 2nd edn. Chapman and Hall, London.

21. Blood volume, erythrokinetics and platelet kinetics

Methods of measurement of blood volume   392
Determination of red cell volume   392
   Radioactive chromium method   392
   Technetium method   393
   Indium method   393
Repeated measurements   394
Plasma volume, ^{125}I or ^{131}I-HSA method   394
Total blood volume   395
Splenic red cell volume   397
Radioactive iron   398
Iron absorption   398
Iron distribution   399
   Plasma iron clearance   399

Plasma iron turnover   400
   Iron utilization   400
Surface counting of ^{59}Fe   402
Gastro-intestinal blood loss   403
Red cell life-span in vivo   404
Radioactive chromium(^{51}Cr) method   404
   Compatibility test   409
Sites of red cell destruction   410
Visualization of spleen by scanning   412
Damaged red-cell clearance   413
Platelet life-span   413
   ^{111}In method   414

BLOOD VOLUME

The haemoglobin content, total red cell count and PCV do not invariably reflect the total red cell volume. Whilst in most cases for practical purposes there is adequate correlation between peripheral blood values and (total) red cell volume,[4] there will be a discrepancy if the plasma volume is reduced or increased disproportionately. Fluctuation in plasma volume may result in haemodilution or conversely in haemoconcentration, giving rise to pseudoanaemia or pseudopolycythaemia, respectively.

An increase in plasma volume occurs in pregnancy, returning to normal soon after delivery. Increased plasma volume may also be found in patients with cirrhosis, nephritis, congestive cardiac failure and when there is marked splenomegaly. Reduced plasma volume occurs in stress, oedema, dehydration and following the administration of diuretic drugs. It also occurs during prolonged bed rest.

In contrast to the fluctuations in plasma volume, red cell volume does not fluctuate to any extent if erythropoiesis is in a steady state.

Blood volume should thus be measured whenever the PCV is persistently higher than normal; demonstration of an absolute increase in red cell volume is necessary to diagnose polycythaemia and to assess its severity. The component parts of the blood volume (i.e. red cell and plasma volume) should also be measured, separately, in the elucidation of obscure anaemias when the possibility of an increase in plasma volume cannot be excluded.

MEASUREMENT OF BLOOD VOLUME

Principle. The principle is that of dilution analysis. A small volume of a readily identifiable radionuclide is injected intravenously either bound to the red cells or to a plasma component and its dilution is measured after time has been allowed for the injected material to become thoroughly mixed in the circulation, but before significant quantities have left the circulation or become unbound. The most practical method now available is to use a small volume of the patient's red cells labelled with radioactive chromium (^{51}Cr), technetium (pertechnetate) (^{99m}Tc) or indium (^{113m}In or ^{111}In). The relative advantages and disadvantages of each radionuclide are discussed later.

The labelled red cells are diluted in the whole blood of the patient and from their dilution the total blood volume can be calculated; the red cell volume, too, can be deduced from knowledge of the PCV. The plasma volume can be measured directly by injecting human albumin labelled with radioactive iodine (^{125}I or ^{131}I): the albumin is diluted in the plasma compartment only and thus gives a value for plasma volume only.

In contrast to measurement of red cell volume, plasma-volume measurements are only approximations as the labelled albumin undergoes continuous slow interchange between the plasma and extravascular fluids, even during the mixing period. For this reason it is undesirable to attempt to calculate red cell volume from plasma volume, on the basis of the observed PCV. On the other hand, as the red cell volume is generally more stable, calculation of total blood volume from red cell volume is usually more reliable, provided that the difference between whole body and venous PCV is appreciated and allowed for (see p. 395). Measurement of red cell and plasma volumes separately by direct methods is to be preferred.

DETERMINATION OF RED CELL VOLUME[24]

Radioactive chromium method

Add approximately 10 ml of blood to 1.5 ml of sterile NIH-A acid-citrate dextrose (ACD) solution (see p. 575), in a sterile bottle with a screw cap. Centrifuge at 1200–1500g for 5 min. Discard the supernatant plasma and buffy coat and slowly add to the cells, with continuous mixing, 4–8 × 10^{3}Bq (0.1–0.2 μCi) of Na$_2$^{51}CrO$_4$ per kg of body weight. The sodium chromate should be in a volume of at least 0.2 ml, being diluted in 9 g/l NaCl (saline). Allow the blood to stand for 15 min at 37°C for labelling to take place. Wash the red cells twice in 4–5 volumes of sterile saline*. Finally, resuspend the cells in a volume of sterile saline sufficient for an injection of about 5 ml and the preparation of a standard. Take up the appropriate volume into a syringe which is weighed before and after the injection. The volume injected is calculated from the following formula:

Volume injected (ml)
$$= \frac{\text{Weight of suspension injected (g)}}{\text{Density of suspension (g/ml)}}$$

where

Density of suspension =
$$1.0 + \frac{\text{Hb conc. of suspension (g/l)} \times 0.097}{340}$$

(This assumes that packed red cells have a MCHC of 340 g/l and a density of 1.097.)

Inject the suspension intravenously without delay and note the time; at 10, 20 and 30 min later, collect 5–10 ml of the patient's blood and add it to the appropriate amount of a solid anticoagulant (e.g. K$_2$EDTA). This blood should preferably be withdrawn from a vein other than that used for the injection. However, it is often convenient to insert a self-retaining (e.g. butterfly) needle; in this case care must be taken to ensure that the isotope is well dispersed into the blood stream when injected by flushing through with 10 ml of sterile saline. When the

---

*12 g/l NaCl should be used when red cell osmotic fragility is greatly increased, e.g. in cases of hereditary spherocytosis.

mixing time is likely to be prolonged as in splenomegaly, cardiac failure or shock, another sample should be taken 60 min after the injection.

Measure the PCV of each sample. Deliver 1 ml volumes into counting tubes and lyse with saponin; a convenient method is to add 2 drops of 2% saponin. Measure their radioactivity in a scintillation counter. Then dilute an aliquot of the original suspension which was not injected 1 in 500 in water (for use as a standard) and determine the radioactivity of a 1 ml volume. Then:

Red cell volume (RCV) (ml) =

$$\frac{\text{Radioactivity of standard (cpm/ml)} \times \text{Diln. of standard} \times \text{Volume injected (ml)}}{\text{Radioactivity of post-injection sample (cpm/ml)}} \times \text{PCV}^\star$$

The total blood volume (BV) can be calculated by multiplying the value for RCV by 1/(whole-body PCV) (see p. 395). Plasma volume can be calculated by subtracting RCV from BV.

If a sample has been taken at 60 min in cases where delayed mixing is suspected and there is a significant difference between the measurements at 10–30 min and 60 min, the 60 min measurement should be used for calculating the red cell volume.

TECHNETIUM METHOD[38]

^{99m}Tc is available as sodium pertechnetate. This passes freely through the red cell membrane and will become attached to the cells only if it is present in a reduced form as it enters the cells when it binds firmly to β-chains of haemoglobin. For this to occur, the red cells require to be treated with a stannous (tin) compound by the following in-vivo procedure. Dissolve a vial of Stannous Reagent** (Amerscan, Amersham International) in 6 ml of sterile saline and inject

intravenously 0.03 ml/kg body weight. After 15 min, collect 5 ml of blood into a sterile container to which has been added 200 IU of liquid heparin. Add 2–3.5 MBq (c 50–100 μCi) of freshly generated ^{99m}Tc in approximately 0.2 ml of saline or 75 MBq (c 2 mCi) if measurement of splenic red cell pool and scanning are also required. Allow to stand at room temperature for 20 min (or at 37°C for 10 min). Centrifuge; wash twice in cold sterile saline and resuspend in a sufficient volume of cold sterile saline for an injection of 5–10 ml. Take up c 5 ml in a syringe which is weighed before and after injection and carry out subsequent procedures as for the chromium method. Because of the short half-life of ^{99m}Tc, radioactivity must be measured on the day of the test. Because 5–10% of the radio-activity is eluted from the red cells within 1 h,[15] the method is less suitable than are the chromium and indium methods when there is splenomegaly or another cause of delayed mixing is suspected.

Indium is available as ^{111}In chloride or it can be produced as ^{113}In in a generator by elution from ^{113}Sn. The labelling procedure is simpler than with ^{99m}Tc and there is less elution during the first hour. It is thus particularly suitable for delayed sampling. For labelling blood cells, the indium is complexed with oxine[18], acetylacetone[52] or tropolone.[12,37] The latter two are easier to prepare, and their use is described below.

INDIUM METHOD

1. Preparation of acetylacetone complex

Take approximately 5 ml of blood into a sterile bottle or tube containing 100 IU of liquid heparin. Wash once in sterile saline. To the packed cells, add 10 ml of 1.9 g/l acetylacetone (2,4-pentanedione) in HEPES or Tris buffer, pH 7.6 (p. 578). The acetylacetone should be stored at 4°C but brought to room temperature before use. Mix gently for 1 min, then add 2–3.5 MBq (c 50–100 μCi) of freshly generated ^{113}In or ^{111}In. Mix on a roller mixer for 5 min, then wash twice in saline. Resuspend in a sufficient volume of saline for an injection of 10 ml and preparation of a standard.

---

*As measured on the blood sample by an electronic counting system or by microhaematocrit (see Chapter 5).
**Stannous fluoride and sodium medronate.

2. *Preparation of tropolone complex*

Prepare a solution of 2.5 mg/ml of tropolone (2-hydroxy-2,4,6-cycloheptatrien-1-one) in HEPES saline buffer pH 7.6 (p. 578). Filter through a 0.22 μm Millipore filter. This solution can be used for up to 3 months if kept at 4°C. Take approximately 5 ml of blood into a sterile container containing 100 IU of liquid heparin, or 10 ml into 1.5 ml of ACD (see p. 575). With heparin as anticoagulant, add *c* 50 μg (20 μl) of the tropolone solution per ml of blood; with ACD add *c* 10 μg (4 μl) per ml of blood.[37] Mix gently for 1 min, then add 2–3.5 MBq (*c* 50–100 μCi) of freshly generated ^{113m}In or ^{111}In chloride. Mix on a roller mixer for 5 min, then wash twice in saline. Resuspend in a sufficient volume of saline for an injection of 10 ml and preparation of a standard.

Repeated blood-volume measurements

When repeated blood-volume measurements are required within a few days, the ^{51}Cr method can be used if the residual radioactivity is measured in the blood immediately before each test. However, the residual radioactivity increases the counting error and it may be necessary to increase the amount of tracer injected. The short-lived radionuclides (^{99m}Tc, ^{113m}In) have the advantage that they can be used for repeated tests without this problem and also that the patient will be subjected to lower doses of radioactivity. The radionuclides are slowly eluted in vivo and in vitro. With ^{99m}Tc, elution is slight within the first 10–20 min; it gives results which compare closely with those of ^{51}Cr but because of progressively increasing elution the method is less satisfactory when delayed mixing necessitates sampling at 60 min post-injection.

The labelling procedure using indium is much simpler than with technetium and, as elution is less than with ^{99m}Tc during the first hour, it is particularly suitable for delayed sampling.[49]

DETERMINATION OF PLASMA VOLUME

^{125}I- or ^{131}I-human serum albumin (HSA) method[24]

Human serum albumin (HSA) labelled with ^{125}I or ^{131}I is available commercially. The albumin concentration should not be less than 20 g/l. The user must be reassured that only HIV antibody negative and hepatitis antigen-negative donors have been used as the source of albumin. ^{125}I has the advantage over ^{131}I in that it is readily distinguishable from ^{51}Cr, ^{99m}Tc and ^{113m}In, and this makes possible the simultaneous direct determination of red cell volume and plasma volume (see p. 395).

Withdraw *c* 20 ml of blood into a syringe containing a few drops of sterile heparin solution and transfer to a 30 ml sterile bottle with a screw cap. After centrifuging at 1200–1500***g*** for 5–10 min, transfer *c* 7 ml of plasma to a second sterile bottle and add 2×10^3 Bq (*c* 0.05 μCi) of the radionuclide-labelled HSA per kg body weight. Inject a measured amount (e.g. 5 ml) and retain the residue for preparation of a standard.

After 10, 20 and 30 min, withdraw blood samples from a vein other than that used for the original injection (or after flushing through with 10 ml of sterile 9 g/l NaCl (saline) if a butterfly needle has been used) and deliver into bottles containing EDTA or heparin.

Measure the PCV, centrifuge the sample and separate the plasma. Prepare a standard by diluting part of the residue of the uninjected HSA 1 in 100 in saline.

Measure the radioactivity of the plasma samples in a scintillation counter, and by extrapolation on semilogarithmic graph paper calculate the radioactivity of the plasma at zero time. If only a single sample is collected 10 min after the injection, the radioactivity at zero time may be obtained approximately by multiplying by 1.015 to allow for early loss of the radionuclide from the circulation. Reliance on a single 10 min sample will lead to error if the mixing of the albumin in the plasma is delayed.[31] After measuring the radioactivity of the standard, the plasma volume (ml) is calculated as follows:

$$\frac{\text{Radioactivity of standard (cpm/ml)} \times \text{Diln. of standard} \times \text{Vol. injected (ml)}}{\text{Radioactivity of post-injection sample (cpm/ml, adjusted to zero time)}}$$

DETERMINATION OF TOTAL BLOOD VOLUME

As has already been indicated, the total blood volume is frequently calculated from the red cell volume and PCV. But before this can be done the observed PCV has to be corrected for the difference between the whole-body and venous PCV. The reason for this difference is described below.

Whole-body and venous PCV ratio

It is well known that the PCV measured on venous blood is not identical with the average PCV of all the blood in the body. This is mainly because the red cell : plasma ratio is less in small blood vessels (capillaries, arterioles and venules) than in large vessels. The ratio between the whole-body PCV and venous-blood PCV is normally about 0.9[24] and it is thus necessary in the calculation of total blood volume from measurements of red cell volume to multiply the observed PCV by 0.9. Thus total blood volume is given by:

$$\text{Red-cell volume} \times \frac{1}{\text{PCV} \times 0.9}.$$

However, the ratio varies in individuals, especially in splenomegaly, and it is better to estimate red cell volume and plasma volume by separate measurements rather than to attempt to calculate one of these from an estimate of the other.

Simultaneous measurement of red cell volume and plasma volume

Collect blood and label the red cells by one of the methods described above. If ^{99m}Tc is used it is necessary first to inject stannous reagent (p. 393). Then add ^{125}I HSA (see p. 394) and mix it with the labelled red cell suspension. Inject an accurately measured amount and dilute the remainder 1 in 500 in water for use as a standard. Collect three blood samples at 10, 20 and 30 min, respectively, after the administration of the labelled blood and estimate the radioactivity of a measured volume of each sample and a similar volume of the standard.

When ^{99m}Tc or ^{113m}In has been used in combination with ^{125}I, count on the same day; then leave for 2 days to allow the ^{99m}Tc or ^{113m}In to decay and count again for ^{125}I activity.

As the radioactivity in the preparation due to ^{125}I is much smaller than that from ^{99m}Tc or ^{113m}In, the count from the cells is not likely to be significantly affected by interference from ^{125}I in the initial count. However, if necessary, a correction can be made by subtracting the ^{125}I counts on day 2 (corrected for decay) from the original counts to obtain a measurement of the counts due only to the ^{99m}Tc or ^{113m}In.

When ^{51}Cr has been used in combination with ^{125}I, and a multi-channel counter is available, measure the radioactivity due to the ^{51}Cr and ^{125}I at the appropriate settings for ^{51}Cr and ^{125}I.

Calculate the radioactivity due to ^{51}Cr, ^{99m}Tc or ^{113}In in the blood from the mean of the 10, 20 and 30 min samples, and obtain that due to ^{125}I from the value extrapolated to zero time. Calculate red cell volume as described on p. 393.

Plasma volume is calculated from the formula:

$$\frac{\begin{array}{c}\text{Radioactivity of standard (cpm/ml)}\\ \times \text{Dil. of standard} \times \text{Vol. injected (ml)}\end{array}}{\begin{array}{c}\text{Radioactivity of post-injection sample}\\ \text{(cpm/ml, corrected to zero time).}\end{array}} \times (1 - \text{PCV})$$

Total blood volume = red cell volume
                    + plasma volume.

Expression of results of blood-volume estimations

Red cell volume, plasma volume and total blood volume are usually expressed in ml/kg of body weight. Because fat is relatively avascular, low values are obtained in obese subjects and the relation between blood volume and body weight varies according to body composition. Blood volume is more closely correlated with lean body mass.[21,35] Earlier methods for determination of lean body mass were not practical as a routine procedure, but there are now available instruments that are simple to use for estimating body composition by the different response of fat and other tissues to electrical impedance**.[32]

Discounting excess fat by using an estimate of so-called 'ideal weight' by reference to standard tables which are based on height, age, build and sex is somewhat arbitrary and tends to over-correct for the avascularity of fat. More complicated formulae have been proposed for predicting normal blood volume. Nadler's method[36] was based on measurements of plasma volume in normal men and women, from which

were derived the following formulae for predicting normal blood volume (in ml):

Men $\quad$ 366.9 H^3 + 32.19 W + 604
Women $\quad$ 356.1 H^3 + 33.08 W + 183

where H = height (m), and W = weight (kg).

Hurley's method[20] which relates both red cell and plasma volume to surface area is derived from a relatively large series of measurements (Table 21.1). In practice the diagnosis of absolute polycythaemia can be made with confidence

Table 21.1 Mean values for red cell mass (RCM) and plasma volume (PV) (in ml) related to body surface area (SA in m^2) for men and women

SA	Men RCM	Men PV	Women RCM	Women PV	SA	Men RCM	Men PV	Women RCM	Women PV
1.39	–	–	1136	1964	1.77	1907	2922	1588	2666
1.40	–	–	1148	1982	1.78	1917	2940	1599	2682
1.41	–	–	1162	2000	1.79	1927	2958	1610	2702
1.42	–	–	1172	2018	1.80	1938	2976	1622	2720
1.43	–	–	1184	2039	1.81	1951	2994	1634	2740
1.44	–	–	1196	2058	1.82	1964	3013	1645	2760
1.45	–	–	1208	2076	1.83	1977	3031	1657	2778
1.46	–	–	1220	2094	1.84	1990	3050	1670	2796
1.47	–	–	1232	2112	1.85	2003	3069	1681	2815
1.48	–	–	1242	2132	1.86	2016	3087	1692	2838
1.49	–	–	1254	2148	1.87	2029	3106	1704	2854
1.50	1684	2498	1268	2168	1.88	2042	3125	–	–
1.51	1692	2513	1280	2184	1.89	2055	3144	–	–
1.52	1699	2529	1291	2204	1.90	2070	3164	–	–
1.53	1707	2544	1302	2222	1.91	2087	3183	–	–
1.54	1715	2560	1315	2252	1.92	2104	3202	–	–
1.55	1722	2575	1326	2258	1.93	2112	3222	–	–
1.56	1730	2591	1338	2278	1.94	2138	3242	–	–
1.57	1737	2606	1349	2296	1.95	2156	3261	–	–
1.58	1745	2621	1362	2314	1.96	2173	3280	–	–
1.59	1752	2637	1376	2336	1.97	2191	3299	–	–
1.60	1760	2652	1386	2354	1.98	2208	3318	–	–
1.61	1768	2667	1398	2374	1.99	2226	3337	–	–
1.62	1776	2682	1408	2392	2.00	2244	3358	–	–
1.63	1784	2697	1421	2410	2.01	2266	3390	–	–
1.64	1792	2712	1434	2428	2.02	2288	3402	–	–
1.65	1800	2727	1445	2444	2.03	2310	3424	–	–
1.66	1809	2742	1458	2462	2.04	2332	3446	–	–
1.67	1817	2757	1468	2480	2.05	2354	3468	–	–
1.68	1826	2772	1480	2500	2.06	2375	3490	–	–
1.69	1834	2787	1492	2520	2.07	2397	3513	–	–
1.70	1842	2802	1504	2538	2.08	2419	3536	–	–
1.71	1851	2819	1516	2558	2.09	2441	3558	–	–
1.72	1861	2837	1527	2576	2.10	2463	3580	–	–
1.73	1870	2854	1540	2592	2.11	2486	3604	–	–
1.74	1880	2871	1552	2612	2.12	2510	3628	–	–
1.75	1889	2888	1563	2630	2.13	2535	3653	–	–
1.76	1898	2905	1576	2648	2.14	2560	3679	–	–
					2.15	2586	3704	–	–

Reproduced with permission from Hurley.[20]

***

**Holt body composition analyser, Holtain Ltd, Crosswell, Dyfed, Wales.

by either method if the red cell volume is >125% of the predicted normal value; the plasma volume is accepted as reduced if it is <80% of the predicted normal value.[31,40]

Range in health

Red cell volume: men, 30 ± 5 ml (2 SD)/kg; women, 25 ± 5 ml (2 SD)/kg.

> Plasma volume: 40–50 ml/kg.
> Total blood volume: 60–80 ml/kg.

The total blood volume is 250–350 ml at birth. After infancy the volume increases gradually until adult life. As a rule, the blood volume remains remarkably constant in an individual and rapid adjustments take place within a few hours after blood transfusion or intravenous infusion.

In pregnancy both the plasma volume and total blood volume increase. The plasma volume increases especially in the first trimester, the total volume later,[15] and by full term the plasma volume will have increased by c 40% and total blood volume by c 32% or even more. The blood volume returns to normal within a week post partum.

Bed rest causes a reduction in plasma volume[53] and muscular exercise and changes in posture cause transient fluctuations. In practice, the patient should always be allowed to rest in a recumbent position for 15 min prior to measuring the blood volume.

SPLENIC RED CELL VOLUME

The red cell content of the normal spleen (the red cell 'pool') is less than 5% of the total red cell volume (i.e. <100–120 ml in an adult). In spleno-megaly the pool is increased, e.g. by perhaps as much as 5–10 times in myelofibrosis, poly-cythaemia, hairy cell leukaemia and lympho-proliferative disorders.[47] Increase in the volume of the splenic red cell pool may by itself be a cause of anaemia; measurement of the pool is thus useful in the investigation of anaemia in these conditions. It is also useful in determining the cause of erythrocytosis as the expanded pool in polycythaemia vera contrasts with that in secondary polycythaemia in which it is normal.[2]

An approximate estimate of the splenic red cell volume can be obtained from the difference between the apparent red cell volume, as measured 2–3 min after the injection of radio-nuclide-labelled cells, and that measured after mixing has been completed, i.e. after a delay of c 20 min,[48] or from the difference in surface counts over the spleen before and after mixing has been completed.[54] The splenic red cell volume can be estimated more accurately by quantitative scanning, after injecting viable red cells labelled with ^{99m}Tc or ^{113m}In (p. 393).[19] The blood volume is measured in the usual way using c 2 mCi (74 MBq) of ^{99m}Tc or 1 mCi (37 MBq) of ^{113m}I. The splenic area is scanned 20 min after the injection or after 60 min when there is splenomegaly. To delineate the spleen more precisely, it may be necessary to carry out a second scan after an injection of heat-damaged labelled red cells (see p. 412). From the radioactivity in the spleen, relative to that in a standard, and knowledge of the total red cell volume, the proportion of the total red cell volume contained in the spleen can be calculated. This technique has also been used for demonstrating localized accumulation of blood in haemangiomas in the liver,[34] telangiectasia and other vascular abnormalities.[17]

ERYTHROKINETICS

Whilst much can be learnt about the rate and efficiency of erythropoiesis from the red cell count, reticulocyte count, blood film and bone marrow, studies of iron metabolism and measure-ment of red cell life-span with radioactive isotopes may provide useful additional information. Radioactive iron (^{59}Fe) has been used in clinical investigations to measure:

1. The absorption of iron following an oral dose;
2. The distribution of radioactivity after an intravenous injection;
3. Imaging of radioactive iron uptake.

This isotope has a moderately short half-life, 45 days, and labels haemoglobin after ingestion or injection. If injected intravenously, it labels, too, the plasma iron pool and this allows the measurement of iron clearance and calculation of plasma-iron turnover. Its subsequent appearance in haemoglobin permits the assessment of the rate of haemoglobin synthesis and the completeness of the utilization of iron. Since it is a γ-ray emitter, radioactivity can be measured in vivo by surface counting, and the sites of distribution of the administered iron and the probable sites of erythropoiesis can thus be determined.

IRON ABSORPTION

Principle. A small amount of isotope-labelled inorganic iron is administered by mouth and the amount of radioactivity subsequently eliminated in the faeces is measured. The difference between the radioactivity administered and that excreted is taken as the amount absorbed.

Method

Prepare the test dose within 30 min of its administration. Add 18 mg of ascorbic acid to 15 mg of iron sulphate (FeSO$_4$.7H$_2$O) in a beaker containing 10 ml of 1 mmol/l HCl. Add 0.1–0.2 MBq (*c* 3–5 µCi) of ^{59}Fe in the form of ferric chloride in 10 mmol/l HCl. Make up the solution to *c* 25 ml with water. Keep 1 ml as a standard. Measure an exact volume of the remainder. The patient takes this by mouth in the early morning after an overnight fast, and is not allowed to eat for a further 3 h. The faeces passed during the following 5–7 days (see below) are collected in plastic or cardboard cartons.

Count each sample in a large-volume scintillation counter against 1 ml of the standard diluted in *c* 100 ml of water in a similar carton.

Calculation

% excreted

$$= \frac{\text{cpm/ml of sample}}{\text{cpm/ml of standard} \times \text{Volume administered (ml)}} \times 100.$$

Stool collections are continued until <1% of the administered dose is excreted in a 24 h collection.

Interpretation of results

Iron absorption is a complex process (for reviews, see Bothwell et al[7]), and a test based on the absorption of a small dose of a soluble iron salt is not a reliable indicator of the ability of the gastrointestinal tract to absorb less available forms of iron from different foods. The situation is further complicated by the role of ascorbic acid and chelators in the diet, the presence or absence of achlorhydria, dietary food interactions and the fact that iron may be absorbed but retained in the epithelial cells of the intestine and lost subsequently by the normal process of desquamation. An iron absorption test is thus of very limited value.

In normal subjects the absorption averages about 15–30% of a test dose of a soluble iron salt, but it varies enormously: in iron-deficiency anaemia, absorption depends on the degree of iron deficiency and transferrin saturation, but it is usually in the range 50–80%. Absorption is decreased in the malabsorption syndromes (e.g. in sprue and 'idiopathic' steatorrhoea).

Because of the variation in normal subjects it is difficult to conclude from a single test dose that absorption is impaired. The test is of more use in demonstrating normal absorption (i.e. >10% of the test dose absorbed) in a patient suspected of having an absorption defect. However, the validity of the result depends on the completeness of the faecal collection.

In iron deficiency, in which absorption of iron from a test dose is generally greater than normal, almost all of the administered radioactivity may be expected to appear in the peripheral blood if the patient is absorbing iron normally. Blood radioactivity figures can thus be used in such cases as a simple test of iron absorption obviating the necessity of stool collection. In other cases, an oral dose of $^{131}BaSO_4$ given with the ^{59}Fe will serve as a marker of the passage of the iron through the intestinal tract and thus distinguish between absorbed iron and iron which is retained but not absorbed. This has some value in distinguishing between primary and secondary iron overload.[6]

IRON DISTRIBUTION

Principle. Iron for incorporation into erythroblasts is transported to the bone marrow bound to transferrin. At the surface of the erythroblasts the complex releases its iron which enters the cell to be incorporated into haem, leaving the transferrin free for recycling. Iron not bound to transferrin finds its way to the liver and to other organs rather than to the bone marrow, whilst colloidal particles of iron are rapidly removed by phagocytic cells.

The ferrokinetic studies with ^{59}Fe which provide information on erythropoiesis include the rate of clearance of the radioiron from the plasma, plasma iron turnover, iron incorporation into circulating red cells (iron utilization) and surface counting to measure the uptake and turnover of iron by organs. These are relatively simple procedures which provide clinically useful information. They do not, however, take account of the recirculation of iron which returns to the plasma from tissues, nor of iron turnover resulting from dyserythropoiesis or haemolysis. To take account of these factors requires much more detailed analysis of the iron kinetics with multiple sampling over an extended period.[9,10] These more complex and time-consuming procedures are essential for the quantitative measurement of effective and ineffective erythropoiesis and to provide data on non-erythroid iron turnover. Even so, their interpretation depends on a model which does not necessarily correspond to reality.

In ferrokinetic studies it is important to ensure that any iron administered is bound to transferrin. As a rule, normal (or patient's) plasma has an adequate amount of transferrin. The unsaturated iron-binding capacity (UIBC) or transferrin concentration of the patient's plasma should be measured before the test is carried out and, if the UIBC is <1 mg/l (20 µmol/l) or the transferrin concentration is <0.6 g/l, normal donor plasma (HIV antibody and hepatitis antigen (HBs)-negative) should be used instead of that of the patient for the subsequent labelling procedure. Some workers recommend passing the labelled plasma through an exchange resin to ensure removal of non-transferrin-bound iron prior to injection.[8]

Method

Under sterile conditions, obtain 5–10 ml of plasma from freshly collected heparinized blood. Add 0.3–0.4 MBq (c 7–10 µCi) of ^{59}Fe ferric citrate (specific activity >0.2 MBq/µg). Incubate at room temperature for 15 min. Fill a syringe with all but 1 ml of the mixture. Weigh the syringe to the nearest 10 mg. Inject its content intravenously into the patient, starting a stopwatch at the mid-point of the injection. Reweigh the empty syringe and calculate the volume injected:

$$\text{Volume of plasma (ml)} = \frac{\text{Wt of plasma (g)}}{1.015}.$$

Dilute the residual portion of the dose (1 ml) 1 in 100 in water and use as a measure of the total amount of radioactivity and as a standard in subsequent measurements.

PLASMA-IRON CLEARANCE

Take a sample at 3 min and four or five further samples over a period of 1–2 h, collecting them into heparin or EDTA. Retain a portion of one sample for measurement of plasma iron. Measure the radioactivity in unit volumes of plasma from the samples and plot the values obtained on log-linear graph paper. A straight line will usually be obtained for the initial slope. The radioactivity at the moment of injection is inferred by extrapolation back to zero time and the time taken for the plasma radioactivity to decrease to half its initial value ($T_{1/2}$-plasma clearance) is read off the graph (Fig. 21.1).

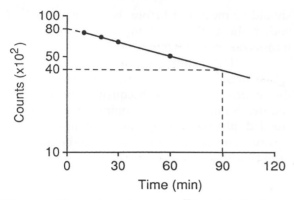

Fig. 21.1   Plasma iron clearance. ^{59}Fe activity in plasma at 10, 20, 30 and 60 min extrapolated to the vertical axis to obtain activity at zero time. The $T_{1/2}$ was 90 min.

Range of $T_{1/2}$-plasma clearance in health.

60–140 min.

The clearance rate is influenced by the intensity of erythropoiesis and also by the activity of the macrophages of the reticulo-endothelial system, especially in the liver, spleen and bone marrow, where the iron is retained as storage iron. Also, to a lesser extent, circulating reticulocytes may take up some of the iron. A rapid clearance indicates hyperactivity of one or more of these mechanisms, as for instance in iron-deficiency anaemias, haemorrhagic anaemias, haemolytic anaemias and polycythaemia vera. The clearance rate is decreased in aplastic anaemia. In leukaemia and in myelosclerosis the results are variable, depending upon the amount of erythropoietic marrow and the extent of extramedullary erythropoiesis; in myelosclerosis, however, rapid clearance is by far the more common finding. In dyserythropoiesis the clearance may be normal or accelerated.

PLASMA-IRON TURNOVER (PIT)

When the plasma-iron clearance is related to the iron content of the plasma, a value can be obtained for plasma-iron turnover in mg/l or μmol/l of blood per day.

PIT (mg/l/day) is calculated from the formula:

$$\text{Plasma iron (mg/l)}^{\star} \times 0.693^{\star\star}$$

$$\times \frac{(60 \times 24)}{T_{1/2}\text{ (min)}} \times (1 - \text{PCV}),$$

which may be simplified to:

$$\frac{\text{Plasma iron (mg/l)} \times 10^3}{T_{1/2}\text{ (min)}} \times (1 - \text{PCV}).$$

PIT (μmol/l/day) is calculated from the formula:

$$\frac{\text{Plasma iron (μmol/l)} \times 10^3}{T_{1/2}\text{ (min)}} \times (1 - \text{PCV}).$$

The range in normal subjects is 4–8 mg/l/day or 70–140 μmol/l/day.

The PIT is increased in iron-deficiency anaemia, haemolytic anaemias and myelosclerosis. It is increased also in ineffective erythropoiesis, particularly so in thalassaemia. In aplastic anaemia the PIT is normal or decreased, but when the plasma iron is raised, the PIT may be above normal. The calculation of PIT assumes a constant rate of iron transport and, while it is an indicator of total erythropoiesis, it does not distinguish between effective and ineffective erythropoiesis. For the reasons discussed earlier and because the findings in health and disease overlap, measurement of the PIT has only limited clinical usefulness.

IRON UTILIZATION

Collect blood samples daily or at least on alternate days for a period of about 2 weeks after the administration of the ^{59}Fe. Measure the radioactivity per ml of whole blood and calculate the percentage utilization on each day from the formula:

$$\frac{\text{cpm/ml daily whole blood sample} \times 100 \times f}{\text{cpm/ml whole blood sample at zero time}}$$

where f is a PCV correction factor, i.e.

$$f = \frac{0.9\text{ PCV}}{1 - 0.9\text{ PCV}}.$$

When there is reason to suspect that the body:venous PCV ratio is not 0.9 (see p. 395), measure the red cell volume by a direct method

---

*Because of marked diurnal variation, the plasma iron should be measured on a sample of blood collected during the plasma clearance study.
**Natural log of 2.

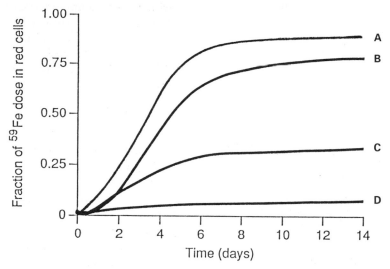

Fig. 21.2   Iron utilization. Red-cell uptake of ^{59}Fe in (A) iron deficiency and polycythaemia, (B) a normal subject, (C) dyserythropoiesis, and (D) severe aplastic anaemia.

(p. 392)* and calculate the percentage utilization on each day from the formula:

Percentage utilization =

$$\frac{\text{Red cell volume (ml)} \times \text{cpm/ml red cells} \times 100}{\text{Total radioactivity injected (cpm)}^{**}}$$

Plot the daily measured percentages against time on arithmetic graph paper. Record the maximum utilization (Fig. 21.2).

The calculation gives a measure of effective erythropoiesis. In normal subjects red cell radioactivity rises steadily from 24 h, and reaches a maximum of 70–80% utilization on the 10th–14th day.

A rapid plasma clearance is usually associated with early and relatively complete utilization and the converse also applies. The results are inconsistent in megaloblastic anaemias and in haemoglobinopathies in which there is ineffective erythropoiesis; and also in myelofibrosis, depending on the extent of extramedullary erythropoiesis

and whether the red cell life-span is reduced. If there is rapid haemolysis, the utilization curve will be distorted by destruction of some of the labelled red cells; this may be recognized if frequent (daily) samples are measured. In aplastic anaemia the utilization is usually 10–15%; in ineffective erythropoiesis it is as a rule 30–50%.

If the iron utilization is known, it is possible to determine the red cell iron turnover expressed as mg/l blood per day (PIT × % maximum utilization). This provides a measure of effective erythropoiesis. In normal subjects it is about 5 mg/l, but it gives an underestimate if there is increased haemolysis. In normal subjects the ratio of plasma iron turnover to red cell iron turnover is 1.2–1.3:1.0.[16]

The ferrokinetic patterns in various diseases are shown in Table 21.2.

Marrow transit time

This can be determined from the red cell utilization data and is the time taken to reach one-half the maximum red cell uptake of the radioiron. It is normally about 80 h. It is thought, to some extent, to reflect the effectiveness of erythropoiesis.[29]

---

*Calculation of plasma volume from extrapolation of the ^{59}Fe disappearance curve is often unreliable and the figure for plasma volume should not be used as the basis for the calculation of red cell volume.
**The radioactivity is adjusted for physical decay up to the day of measurement.

Table 21.2 Ferrokinetic patterns in various diseases

	Plasma clearance T$_{1/2}$	Plasma iron turnover	Red cell utilization
Normal	60–140 min	70–140 µmol/l/d	70–80%
Iron deficiency	↓	N	↑
Aplastic anaemia	↑	N	↓
Chronic infection	Slightly ↓	N	N
Dyserythropoiesis	Slightly ↓	↑	↓
Myelofibrosis	↓	↑	↓
Haemolytic anaemia	↓	↑	↑

↓, Shortened/decreased. ↑, Prolonged/increased.

SURFACE COUNTING OF ^{59}FE

The technique of surface counting is similar to that with ^{51}Cr, as described on p. 410. In addition to measurements over the heart, liver and spleen, the ^{59}Fe activity in the marrow can be measured by placing a collimated counter over the upper portion of the sacrum with the patient lying prone. In order to obtain a pattern of the distribution of the radioactive iron, count the sites mentioned as soon as possible after the intravenous administration of the isotope, as described on p. 399. Count again after 5, 20, 40 and 60 min, and hourly for 6–10 h. Then make measurements daily or on alternate days for the next 10 days or so. In order to compare the pattern in different patients express the initial counts at each site as 100% and convert subsequent counts proportionately after correction for the physical decay of the isotope. The results obtained in a normal subject and in various diseases are illustrated in Fig. 21.3.

Surface counting after the administration of ^{59}Fe is laborious, but the technique has a place in the investigation of patients thought to be suffering from aplastic anaemia, myelofibrosis or 'refractory' anaemia.

(a)

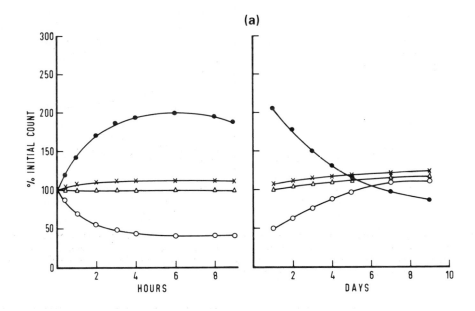

(b)

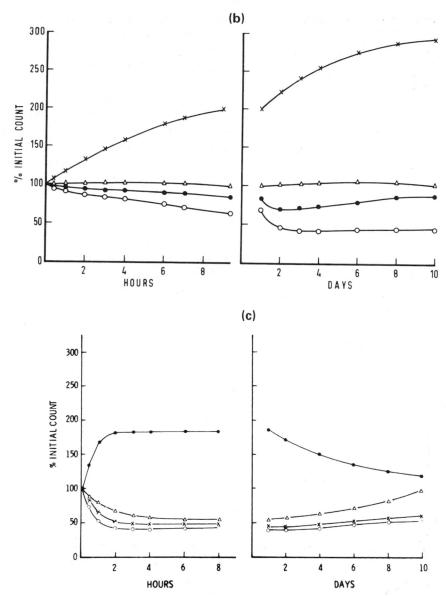

(c)

Fig. 21.3 Surface-counting patterns following an intravenous injection of ^{59}Fe. (a) Normal subject, (b) aplastic anaemia, and (c) dyserythropoiesis. Radioactivity was measured over the heart (O), sacrum (●), spleen (△) and liver (×). In aplastic anaemia the bulk of ^{59}Fe is taken up by the liver where it is stored; in dyserythropoiesis there is active uptake by the bone marrow where much of it is retained, indicating ineffective erythropoiesis.

MEASUREMENT OF BLOOD LOSS FROM THE GASTRO-INTESTINAL TRACT USING ^{51}Cr

The ^{51}Cr method of red cell labelling can be used to measure quantitatively blood lost into the gastro-intestinal tract, as ^{51}Cr is neither excreted nor more than minimally reabsorbed[51].

Accordingly, when the blood contains ^{51}Cr-labelled red cells faecal radioactivity is at a very low level unless bleeding has taken place somewhere within the gastro-intestinal tract. Measurement of the faecal radioactivity then gives a reliable indication of the extent of the blood loss.

Method

Label the patient's own blood with approximately 3.5 MBq (*c* 100 μCi) of ^{51}Cr, as described on p. 392. On each day of the test collect the faeces in plastic or waxed cardboard cartons. Prepare a standard by adding a measured volume (3–5 ml) of the patient's blood, collected on each day, to approximately 100 ml of water in a similar carton. Compare the radioactivity of the faecal samples

and the corresponding daily standard in a large-volume counting system (see p. 385). Then:

$$\text{Volume of blood in faeces (in ml)} = \frac{\text{cpm/24 h faeces collection}}{\text{cpm/ml standard}}.$$

Blood loss from any other source, e.g. surgical operation or menstruation, can be measured in a similar way by counting swabs, dressings, etc., placed in a carton. It is not, however, possible to measure blood or haemoglobin loss in the urine (haematuria or haemoglobinuria) by this method as free ^{51}Cr is normally excreted in the urine.

ESTIMATION OF THE LIFE-SPAN OF RED CELLS IN VIVO

The first practical method of estimating red cell life-span was the differential agglutination method of Ashby. This has been replaced by the use of radionuclide labelling of red cells, and there have been extensive studies of, and a vast literature on, the survival of red cells in haemolytic anaemias by this method (see review by Bentley and Miller[5]). Although now undertaken less frequently than in the past, measurement of red cell survival can still provide important data in cases of anaemia in which increased haemolysis is suspected but not clearly demonstrated by other tests. The majority of studies are carried out using the patient's own red cells which are labelled in vitro before reinjection. Donor red cells are, however, sometimes used to distinguish between an intrinsic and an extrinsic red cell defect.

In this procedure a population of circulating red cells of all ages is labelled ('random labelling'). In 'cohort labelling' an isotope is incorporated into haemoglobin during its synthesis by erythroblasts and radioactivity is measured in red cells which appear in the circulation as a cohort of closely similar age. Red cell life-span can be calculated from measurements of red cell iron turnover obtained with ^{59}Fe,[50] but the results have to be interpreted with caution because of the reutilization for haem synthesis of iron derived from red cells at the end

of their life-span. Random labelling is a much more practical method than cohort labelling.

RADIOACTIVE CHROMIUM (^{51}Cr) METHOD

^{51}Cr is a γ-ray emitter with a half-life of 27.8 days. As a red cell label it is used in the form of hexavalent sodium chromate. After passing through the surface membrane of the red cells, it is reduced to the trivalent form which binds to protein, preferentially to the β-polypeptide chains of haemoglobin.[39] In this form it is not reutilized nor transferred to other cells in circulation.

The main disadvantage of ^{51}Cr is that it gradually elutes from red cells as they circulate; there may be, too, an increased loss over the first 1–3 days, and uncertainty as to how much has been lost makes it impossible to measure red cell life-span accurately. Chromium, whether radioactive or non-radioactive, is toxic to red cells probably by its oxidizing actions; it inhibits glycolysis in red cells when present at a concentration of 10 μg/ml or more[26] and blocks glutathione reductase activity at a concentration exceeding 5 μg/ml.[27,28] Blood should thus not be exposed to more than 2 μg of chromium per ml of packed red cells.

$Na_2{}^{51}CrO_4$ is available commercially at a specific activity of 13–22 GBq/mg Cr (350–

600 mCi/mg); it is usually dissolved in 9 g/l NaCl (saline). It is convenient to dilute the stock in saline and to dispense 2–5.5 MBq (50–150 µCi) amounts in ampoules which can then be sterilized by autoclaving. ACD must not be used as a diluent as this reduces the chromate to the cationic chromic form.

Care must be taken to avoid lysis when the red cells are washed; and it may be necessary, especially if the blood contains spherocytes, to use a slightly hypertonic solution, e.g. 12 g/l NaCl. This should certainly be used if an osmotic-fragility test has demonstrated lysis in 9 g/l NaCl. In patients whose plasma contains high-titre, high-thermal-amplitude cold agglutinins the blood must be collected in a warmed syringe, delivered into ACD solution previously warmed to 37°C and the labelling and washing in saline carried out in a 'warm room' at 37°C.

Method

The technique of labelling red cells is the same as for blood-volume measurement (see p. 392). To ensure as little damage to red cells as possible, with subsequent minimal early loss and later elution, it is important to maintain the blood at an optimal pH. This can be achieved by adding 10 volumes of blood to 1.5 volumes of the recommended (NIH–A) ACD solution[23] (see p. 575).

For a red cell survival study 0.02 MBq (c 0.5 µCi) of $Na_2{}^{51}CrO_4$ per kg body weight is recommended. But if surface counting is to be carried out also, a higher dose (e.g. 0.04 MBq or 1 µCi/kg) should be used, bearing in mind that <2 µg of chromium should be added per ml of packed red cells.

After injection, allow the labelled cells to circulate in the recipient for 10 min (or for 60 min in patients with cardiac failure or splenomegaly in whom mixing may be delayed). Then collect a sample of blood from a vein other than that used for the injection (or after washing the needle through with saline if a butterfly needle is used) and mix with EDTA anticoagulant. The radioactivity in this sample provides a base line for subsequent observations. Retain part of the labelled cell suspension which was not injected into the patient to serve as a standard. This enables the blood volume to be calculated if required.

Take further 4–5 ml blood samples from the patient 24 h later (day 1) and subsequently at intervals, the frequency of the samples depending on the rate of red cell destruction. The recommended procedure is to take three specimens between day 2 and day 7, and then two specimens per week for the duration of the study.[23] Measurements should be continued until at least half the radioactivity has disappeared from the circulation.

Measure the haemoglobin or PCV in a part of each sample; then lyse the samples with saponin, mix well and deliver 1 ml into counting tubes, if possible in duplicate.

Measurement of radioactivity

Estimate the percentage survival (of ^{51}Cr) on any day (t) by comparing the radioactivity of the sample taken on that day with that of the day 0 sample, i.e. the sample withdrawn 10 (or 60) min after the injection of the labelled cells. Thus ^{51}Cr survival on day t (%) is given by:

$$\frac{\text{cpm/ml of blood on Day t}}{\text{cpm/ml of blood on Day 0}} \times 100.$$

No adjustment is necessary for the physical decay of the isotope, provided that the standard is counted within a few minutes of the day t sample.

Carry out the measurements in any high quality scintillation counter, at least 2500 counts being recorded in order to achieve an accuracy of ±2%.

Processing of radioactivity measurements

Before the data can be analysed and interpreted, factors, other than physical decay, which are involved in the disappearance of radioactivity from the circulation have to be considered. There are two processes: ^{51}Cr-labelled cells are lost from the circulation by lysis, phagocytosis or haemorrhage and, in addition, ^{51}Cr is eluted from intact red cells which still circulate.

Elution

The rate of elution differs to a small extent from one individual to another. It is thought to vary to a greater extent between different diseases,[11] especially when the red cell life-span is considerably reduced. However, in such cases elution and variation in the rate of elution become unimportant. The rate of elution is also influenced by technique, especially by the anticoagulant solution into which the blood is collected prior to labelling. With the NIH-A ACD solution the rate of elution is c 1% per day.[23]

Early loss

Sometimes, in addition to the elution that occurs continuously and at a relatively low and constant rate, up to 10% of the ^{51}Cr may be lost within the first 24 h. The cause of this major early loss is obscure and several components may be involved. If this major loss does not continue beyond the first 2 days, it is often looked upon as an artefact, in the sense that it does not denote an increased rate of lysis in vivo, and it can be and usually is ignored by replotting the figures as described on p. 409. This procedure is acceptable, at least for clinical studies, but it does not take into account the possibility that a small proportion of red cells are present that are unusually prone to lysis and the rate of elimination of the rest of the labelled

Table 21.3 Normal range for ^{51}Cr survival curves with correction for elution[23]

Day	% ^{51}Cr (corrected for decay; *not* corrected for elution)	Elution correction* factors
1	93–98	1.03
2	89–97	1.05
3	86–95	1.06
4	83–93	1.07
5	80–92	1.08
6	78–90	1.10
7	77–88	1.11
8	76–86	1.12
9	74–84	1.13
10	72–83	1.14
11	70–81	1.16
12	68–79	1.17
13	67–78	1.18
14	65–77	1.19
15	64–75	1.20
16	62–74	1.22
17	59–73	1.23
18	58–71	1.25
19	57–69	1.26
20	56–67	1.27
21	55–66	1.29
22	53–65	1.31
23	52–63	1.32
24	51–60	1.34
25	50–59	1.36
30	44–52	1.47
35	39–47	1.53
40	34–42	1.60

*To correct for elution, multiply the % ^{51}Cr by the elution factor for the particular day.

cells is not representative of the entire cell population. Even when the ^{51}Cr data are cor-

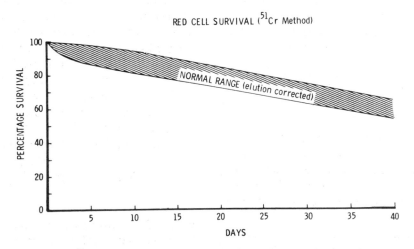

RED CELL SURVIVAL (^{51}Cr Method)

Fig. 21.4 ^{51}Cr red cell survival. The hatched area shows the normal range.

rected for elution the survival curve may not be strictly comparable with an Ashby survival curve. This is, however, not of great importance provided the findings are compared with ^{51}Cr survival curves obtained in strictly normal subjects by an identical technique (see Table 21.3 and Fig. 21.4). It is common practice to calculate the $T_{50}Cr^{\star}$, i.e. the time taken for the concentration of ^{51}Cr in the blood to fall to 50% of its initial value, after correcting the data for physical decay but not for elution. The chief objection to the use of $T_{50}Cr$ is that it may be misleading without additional information on the pattern of the survival curve. Moreover, the mean red cell life-span cannot be directly derived from it. With the technique described above, the mean value of T_{50} in normal subjects is c 30 days, range 25–33 days.

Correction for elution

When haemolysis is marked, elution is of minor importance and can be ignored. When haemolysis is not greatly increased, it is essential to correct for elution. This can be done by multiplying the measured survival by the factors given in Table 21.3.

Drawing survival curves and deriving the mean red cell life-span

Plot the % radioactivity figures or count-rates per ml of whole blood (corrected for physical decay and for elution) on arithmetic and semi-logarithmic graph paper and attempt to fit straight lines passing through the data points.

1. If a straight line *can* be fitted to the arithmetic plot, the mean red cell life-span is given by the point in time at which the line or its extension cuts the abscissa (Fig. 21.5).
2. As a rule, however, a straight line is better fitted to the semi-logarithmic plot; the mean red cell life-span can be read as the exponential e^{-1}; i.e. the time when 37% of the cells are still surviving (Fig 21.6) or calculated by multiplying

the half-time of the fitted line by the reciprocal of the natural log of 2 (0.693), i.e. multiplying by 1.44.

With a computer the mathematical analysis can be readily automated and a program can be prepared for a more precise curve-fitting procedure. However, the more complex procedure is not likely to improve overall accuracy of the results for clinical purposes.[3,23]

Interpretation of survival curves

In the auto-immune haemolytic anaemias, the slope of elimination is usually markedly curvilinear when the data are plotted on arithmetic graph paper. Red cell destruction is typically random and the curve of elimination is thus exponential, and the data give a straight line when plotted on semi-logarithmic graph paper.

In some cases of haemolytic anaemia (? only when there are intracorpuscular defects) the survival curve appears to consist of two components, an initial steep slope being followed by a much less steeply falling slope. This suggests the presence of cells of widely varying life-span. This type of 'double population' curve is seen in paroxysmal nocturnal haemoglobinuria and in sickle-cell anaemia, and in some cases of hereditary enzyme-deficiency haemolytic anaemia, and when the labelled cells consist of a mixture of transfused normal cells and short-lived patient's cells. The mean cell life-span of the entire cell population can be deduced by plotting the points on semilogarithmic graph paper, as described above. The proportion of cells belonging to the longer-lived population can be estimated by plotting the data on arithmetic graph paper and extrapolating the less steep slope back to the ordinate; the life-span of this population can be estimated by extending the same slope to the abscissa (Fig. 21.7). The life-span of the short-lived cells can be deduced from the formula:

$$MCL_s = \frac{\%S}{\dfrac{100}{MCL_T} - \dfrac{\%L}{MCL_L}}$$

where S = short-lived population, L = longer-lived population, T = entire cell population, and MCL = mean cell life-span.

$^{\star}T_{50}$ is used rather than $T_{1/2}$ when the fractional rate of elimination is not constant.

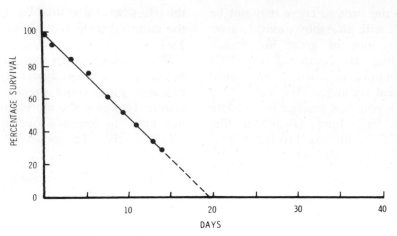

Fig. 21.5 **^{51}Cr red cell survival curve.** Patient with hereditary spherocytosis. The results give a straight line when plotted on arithmetic graph paper. The mean cell life-span is indicated by the point at which its extension cuts the abscissa (20 days).

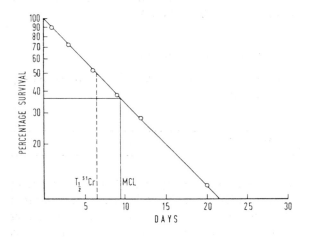

Fig. 21.6 **^{51}Cr red cell survival curve.** Patient with auto-immune haemolytic anaemia. The results have been plotted on semi-logarithmic graph paper and the mean cell life-span was read as the time when 37% of the cells were still surviving (9–10 days). The T_{50}Cr was 6–7 days. MCL, mean cell life-span.

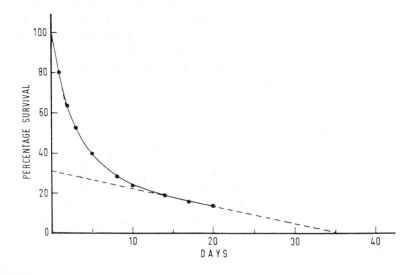

Fig. 21.7 **^{51}Cr red cell survival curve showing a 'double population'.** By plotting the data on semilogarithmic graph paper as described in Fig. 21.6 and on p. 407, the mean cell life-span (MCL) of the entire cell population was deduced as 5 days. When plotted on arithmetic graph paper, by extrapolation of the less steep slope to the ordinate it was deduced that approximately 30% of the red cells belonged to one population, and by extrapolation of the same slope to the abscissa the MCL of this population was deduced as 35 days. The life-span of the remaining 70% of cells was calculated to be 3.6 days (see formula on p. 407). The T_{50}Cr was 3–4 days.

Correction for early loss

The simplest method is to ignore the early loss by taking as 100% the radioactivity still present at the end of 24–48 h. Alternatively, the following method can be employed; it has the advantage that the slope of the survival curve is not altered. The data are plotted on arithmetical graph paper, the line of the slope beyond the initial steep part is extrapolated back to the ordinate and the point of intersection is taken as 100% and the ordinate scale recalibrated accordingly.

Blood-volume changes

There is no need to correct the measurements of radioactivity per ml of whole blood for alterations in PCV provided that the total blood volume remains constant throughout the study. However, if it is suspected that the blood volume may be changing, e.g. in patients suffering from haemorrhage or being transfused, serial determinations of blood volume should be carried out and the observed radioactivity should be multiplied by the observed blood volume and divided by the initial blood volume. In practice, if a patient receives a blood transfusion during a survival study, it can, as a general rule, be assumed that the blood volume will have returned to its pre-transfusion level within 24–48 h.

Correction of survival data for blood loss

When there is a relatively constant loss of blood during a red cell survival study, the true mean red cell life-span can be obtained by the following equation:

$$\text{True MCL} = \text{Ta} \times \frac{\text{RCV}}{\text{RCV} - (\text{Ta} \times \text{L})}$$

where Ta = apparent time of MCL (days), RCV = red cell volume (ml), and L = mean rate of loss of red cells (ml/day).

Normal red cell life-span

The mean red cell life-span in health is usually taken as 120 days.

COMPATIBILITY TEST

The behaviour of ^{51}Cr- (or ^{113m}In-) labelled donor cells in a recipient will provide important information on the compatibility or otherwise of the donor blood:

1. When serological tests suggest that all normal donors are incompatible.
2. When in the presence of an allo-antibody no non-reacting donor can be found.
3. When the recipient has had an unexplained haemolytic transfusion reaction.
4. When the viability of the donor cells may possibly have been affected by suboptimal storage conditions.

Method[23]

Remove 1–2 ml of blood from the donor bag using a sterile technique. Label 0.5 ml of the red cells with 0.8 MBq (c 2 μCi) of ^{51}Cr, ^{111}In, ^{113m}In or ^{99m}Tc in the standard way (p. 392) and administer to the recipient. Collect 5–10 ml of blood into EDTA or heparin at 3, 10 and 60 min after the injection from a vein other than that used for the injection. Prepare 1 ml samples in counting vials. Centrifuge the remainder of the specimens and pipette 1 ml of the plasma into counting vials. Measure the radioactivity in the usual way. Calculate the activity in the blood and plasma samples as a percentage of the 3 min blood sample.

Interpretation

With compatible blood the radioactivity in the 60 min sample is, on average, 99% of that of the 3 min sample, but it may vary between 94% and 104%. If the blood radioactivity at 60 min is not less than 70% and the plasma activity is not more than 3%, the donor cells may be transfused with minimal hazard.[23]

DETERMINATION OF SITES OF RED CELL DESTRUCTION USING ^{51}Cr

As ^{51}Cr is a γ-ray emitter, the sites of destruction of red cells, with special reference to the spleen and liver, can be determined by in-vivo surface counting using a shielded scintillation counter placed, respectively, over the heart, spleen and liver.

A collimated scintillation detector with a crystal of not less than 7.5 cm diameter and not less than 3.75 cm thickness is required.[22] The collimator should exclude radiation from extraneous sources and should be capable of surveying a representative area of the organ being studied. A cylindrical-hole collimator about 7 cm deep, 5 cm internal hole diameter and 10 cm external diameter is suitable. However, more reliable results are probably obtained by using two counters, 25–30 cm apart, positioned above and below the counting couch. It is essential when counting on successive days to make the measurements over the chosen points under standardized conditions. Thus, the patient should always be supine in the same position.

Mark the following selected points with marking ink and cover by a layer of transparent dressing:

Heart: third interspace at left sternal border.
Liver: halfway between mid-clavicular and anterior axillary lines on the right side of the body, 3–4 cm above the costal margin.
Spleen: select the site of maximum activity on the first occasion by means of a preliminary count for a few seconds over each of several adjacent sites; then mark this position as the point for subsequent counting.

To ensure that the scanned area consists of the spleen some workers recommend that the spleen should first be visualized by injecting ^{99m}Tc-labelled heat-damaged red cells (see p. 412); this will not interfere with subsequent surface counting if 24 h are allowed to elapse.

If a single detector is used, this should be placed directly over the liver, heart and splenic counting points, just touching the skin. Dual counters, if used, should be placed above and below the selected point in the same vertical axis, and at a fixed distance from each other.

In haemolytic anaemias the first measurements are normally made 30–60 min after injection of the ^{51}Cr-labelled red cells and they are usually made thereafter daily or on alternate days depending on the rate of haemolysis. At least 2500 counts should be recorded at each site, and it is convenient to count at each site for two periods of 1 min and to average the counts. The measurements should be repeated if there is a difference of more than 2% between the counts. After Day 0, the counts have to be corrected for physical decay of the isotope by reference to a standard counted on each occasion under conditions of constant geometry.

In order to compare the results in different patients irrespective of the amount of isotope administered, the initial count over the heart is taken as the base-line. This is recorded as '1000 counts', irrespective of the actual number of counts recorded, and all the other counts at every site are adjusted ('normalized') proportionately. The fall in heart counts parallels the loss of the labelled red cells from the circulation, although the actual counts usually fall off more slowly than the radioactivity of the blood measured in vitro, probably because ^{51}Cr is deposited in all tissues before it is excreted. Alternatively, the changes in blood radioactivity (measured in vitro) can be used to 'normalize' the observed count-rate over liver and spleen. This may at times give more consistent results. Theoretically, the counts over the spleen and the liver should fall at the same rate as the heart and blood counts unless lysis or sequestration of red cells is taking place within the organ(s) or unless ^{51}Cr eluted from red cells in the blood stream accumulates in the organ(s). When the counts over the liver or spleen exceed the calculated amount (based on the fall in heart or blood count), the excess radioactivity is recorded by subtracting the expected counts from the counts actually obtained. The counts recorded in a patient suffering from haemolytic anaemia are illustrated in Table 21.4.

Table 21.4   Example of method for calculation of surface counting data

Day	0	1	2	5	8	10	12	14
Heart	1000	850	780	720	670	600	500	370
Liver								
Actual counts	670	670	660	560	640	630	550	530
Expected counts		570	522	482	449	402	335	248
Excess		100	138	78	191	228	215	282
Spleen								
Actual counts	970	1265	1490	1800	2130	2370	2210	2020
Expected counts		825	756	698	650	582	485	359
Excess		440	734	1102	1480	1788	1725	1661
Spleen:liver ratio								
Actual*	1.45	1.89	2.26	3.21	3.33	3.76	4.02	3.81
Adjusted	1.00	1.30	1.56	2.21	2.30	2.59	2.77	2.62

The actual count rate over the heart on day 0 was 7500 counts per min. This was recorded as 1000 and all other counts were adjusted proportionately.
*Obtained from the actual counts of the organs. The ratio on day 0 was recorded as 1.00 and the results on subsequent days were adjusted proportionately.

It is useful to calculate an index, the Spleen:Liver Ratio, which reflects the relative accumulation of ^{51}Cr in the spleen and liver. The ratio between the counts on Day 0 is recorded as 1.00 and all subsequent ratios are related to this.

Normal surface-counting patterns are illus-trated in Fig. 21.8. The interrupted lines indicate the limits of accumulation observed in normal subjects. In haemolytic anaemias the results differ from case to case. Four patterns can be distinguished:[30]

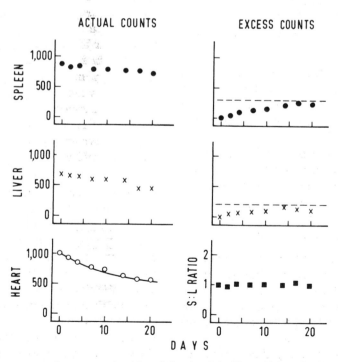

Fig. 21.8   Surface-counting pattern in a normal subject following labelling of his red cells with ^{51}Cr. The interrupted lines indicate the limits of accummulation in normal subjets.

1. Excess accumulation in the spleen, as in hereditary spherocytosis (HS) and hereditary elliptocytosis and some cases of auto-immune haemolytic anaemia (AIHA).

2. Excess accumulation chiefly in the liver; seen only in sickle-cell anaemia, especially in older patients.

3. Little or no excess accumulation in either spleen or liver, as in some hereditary enzyme-deficiency haemolytic anaemias and in paroxysmal nocturnal haemoglobinuria.

4. Excess accumulation in both liver and spleen, as in some cases of AIHA.

Clinical experience has shown that splenectomy usually benefits patients giving pattern (1) and to a more limited degree, in parallel with the Spleen:Liver Ratio, patients giving the pattern (4). The degree of improvement is not, however, closely correlated with the magnitude of the ^{51}Cr accumulation in the spleen.[1]

Surface-counting studies have their limitations. Even minor alterations in the conditions of counting and positioning of the patient may produce significant changes. Isolated readings may, therefore, be misleading. Amongst the variables which affect the count-rate are the volume of the organ counted in relation to its total volume, the distance of the organ from the surface of the body, the absorption of radiation by the overlying tissues and the rate of loss of deposited ^{51}Cr from the organ. Nevertheless, despite these difficulties, surface counting has proved to be of value in the management of patients with some types of haemolytic anaemia when used in conjunction with other clinical and laboratory investigations.[1,14,26]

VISUALIZATION OF THE SPLEEN BY SCINTILLATION SCANNING

This procedure is a development and extension of the techniques of surface counting described above. It has been used:

1. To demonstrate enlargement or abnormal position of the spleen or accessory splenic tissue.

2. To identify the nature of a mass in the left hypochondrium.

3. To demonstrate the presence of space-occuping lesions within the spleen.

4. To assess splenic function and to demonstrate splenic atrophy.

Red blood cells labelled with ^{51}Cr, ^{199m}Tc or ^{111}In are heat-damaged to ensure that after re-injection they are selectively removed by the spleen. The accumulation of radioactivity within the spleen provides a means of demonstrating its size and position. The rate and extent of uptake of the isotope by the spleen is a measure of its function.

Scintillation scanning is usually started about 1 h after the injection of the damaged cells, but it can be performed up to 3–4 h later; satisfactory scans can also be obtained with ^{51}Cr and ^{111}In up to 24 h after the injection.

Methods

With ^{51}Cr as the label[33]

Deliver approximately 10 ml of the patient's blood into 1.5 ml of sterile ACD solution. Centrifuge the sample at 1200–1500g for 5–10 min. Keep the plasma in a sterile container. Label the red cells with $Na_2^{51}CrO_4$, using 0.06–0.08 MBq (c 1.5–2.0 µCi) per kg body weight. Wash the labelled cells three times in sterile 9 g/l NaCl (saline). Place the packed cells in a sterile 30 ml glass bottle with a screw cap. Heat the bottle in a water-bath at a constant temperature of 49.5–50°C for exactly 20 min with occasional gentle mixing. Resuspend the cells in their own plasma and inject intravenously as soon as possible. Follow a standardized technique meticulously. It is important to use a glass bottle as some plastic containers take considerably longer than glass to reach the required temperature.

With ^{99m}Tc as the label

Carry out pretinning in vivo by an injection of a

stannous compound as described on p. 393. Then collect 5–10 ml of blood into a sterile bottle containing 100 IU of heparin. Wash twice in sterile 9 g/l NaCl (saline), centrifuging at 1200–1500g for 5–10 min. Transfer 2 ml of the packed red cells to a 30 ml glass bottle with a screw cap; heat the bottle in a water-bath at a constant temperature of 49.5–50°C for exactly 20 min with occasional gentle mixing. Wash the cells in saline until the supernatant is free from haemoglobin and discard the final supernatant. Label with 35 MBq (c 1 mCi) of ^{99m}Tc by the method as described on p. 393. After standing for 5 min, wash twice in saline. Resuspend in about 10 ml of saline and inject as soon as possible.

With ^{111}In or ^{113m}In as the label

Prepare 2 ml of heat-damaged red cells as for the ^{99m}Tc method. Wash twice in sterile 9 g/l NaCl (saline). Add 9 MBq (c 250 µCi) of ^{111}In or ^{113}In, as described on p. 393–394. Then wash twice in saline. Resuspend in about 10 ml of saline and inject as soon as possible.

RATE OF CLEARANCE OF DAMAGED RED CELLS

Information on splenic activity may be obtained by measuring the rate of clearance of heat-damaged labelled red cells from the circulation. A blood sample is taken exactly 3 min after the mid-point of the injection and further samples are collected at 5 min intervals for 30 min at 45 min and a final sample at 60 min. The radioactivity in each sample is measured and expressed as a percentage of the radioactivity in the 3 min sample. The results are plotted on semilogarithmic graph paper, the 3 min sample being taken as 100% radioactivity.

For constant results a carefully standardized technique is necessary to ensure that the red cells are damaged to the same extent.

The disappearance curve is, as a rule, exponential. The initial slope reflects the splenic blood flow; the rate of blood flow is calculated as the reciprocal of the time taken for the radioactivity to fall to half the 3 min value, i.e. $0.693/T_{1/2}$, where 0.693 is the natural log of 2.

When the spleen is functioning normally the $T_{1/2}$ is 5–15 min and fractional splenic blood flow is 0.05–0.14 ml/min, i.e. 5–14% of the circulating blood per min. The clearance rate is considerably prolonged in thrombocythaemia and in conditions associated with splenic atrophy such as sickle-cell anaemia, coeliac disease and dermatitis herpetiformis.[47] It thus provides some indication of spleen function. However, the disappearance curve is a complex of at least two components. The first (mentioned above) reflects the splenic blood flow, and the second component mainly measures cell trapping, the consequence of both transient sequestration and phagocytosis with irreversible extraction of the cells from circulation.[42,43] Measurement of phagocytosis is obtained more reliably with IgG (anti-D) coated red cells.[41,46]

MEASUREMENT OF PLATELET LIFE-SPAN

Principle. The procedure for measuring platelet life-span is broadly similar to that for red cell survival (see p. 404). A method using ^{51}Cr-labelled platelets, recommended by the International Committee for Standardization in Haematology, was described in the 5th edition of this book. More recently ^{111}In has been recommended as an alternative label.[25] It has several advantages over ^{51}Cr: a shorter half-life, higher photon emissions and a greater affinity for platelets. It is thus possible to carry out a survival study on patients with low platelet counts and to combine this with measurement of platelet pooling and identification of sites of platelet destruction. A modification of this method is described below.

Method[13]

Collect 51 ml of blood into 9 ml of NIH-A ACD (p. 575). Distribute equally into three 30 ml polystyrene tubes containing 2 ml of 60 g/l hydroxyethyl starch (Hespan, Dupont). Mix and immediately centrifuge at 150*g* for 10 min. Transfer the supernatant platelet-rich plasma (PRP) into clean centrifuge tubes and add ACD, 1 volume to 10 volumes of the PRP, to prevent platelet aggregation. If necessary centrifuge again at 150*g* for 5 min to remove residual red cells.

Centrifuge the PRP at 640*g* for 10 min to obtain a platelet pellet. Carefully remove the supernatant platelet-poor plasma (PPP) but do not discard. Add 1 ml of the PPP to the platelet pellet, and gently tap the tube to resuspend.

Prepare a solution of tropolone, 4.4 mmol/l (0.54 mg/ml), in HEPES-saline buffer, pH 7.6 (p. 578). Mix 0.1 ml with *c* 8 MBq (250 µCi) of ^{111}InCl, in < 50 µl of 40 mmol/l HCl. Add the platelet suspension with gentle mixing and leave at room temperature for 5 min. Add 5 ml of PPP. Centrifuge at 640*g* for 10 min. Remove the supernatant and resuspend the platelet pellets in 5 ml of PPP. Take up the platelet suspension into a 10 ml plastic syringe.

Add 0.5 ml of the platelet suspension to 100 ml of water in a volumetric flask as a standard. Weigh the syringe, inject the platelets into the patient through a butterfly needle and reweigh.

$$\text{Volume injected} = \text{wt (g)} \times \frac{1}{1.015}$$

where 1.015 = sp gr of plasma.

Collect blood samples in EDTA at 20 min, 2 h, 3 h and 4 h after injection and thereafter daily for up to 10 days.

Lyse the samples with 2 drops of 2% saponin and measure the radioactivity of 1–2 ml volumes of each and a similar volume of the diluted standard.

Calculation

% Platelets surviving at each sampling time =

$$\frac{\text{cpm/ml blood sample}}{\text{Total radioactivity *injected}} \times \text{Blood volume (ml)}.$$

Analysis of data

Plot the % survival against time on arithmetic graph paper and estimate the survival time as for red cell survival (see p. 407).

Normal mean platelet life-span: 8–10 days.

The validity of the analysis is based on the assumption that the blood volume is constant and the pattern of disappearance of platelets from the circulation remains constant during the course of the study.

This analysis is adequate when the platelet life-span is markedly shortened, as in most of the clinical situations in which the survival study is likely to be undertaken. When more precise assessment and analysis of the shape of the survival curve is required, more complex procedures have to be carried out. The International Committee for Standardization in Haematology has published computer programs for obtaining estimates of mean platelet survival based on a 'multiple hit'.[25]

Platelet survival in disease

In idiopathic thrombocytopenia purpura (ITP) platelet life-span is considerably reduced, and the measurement may have diagnostic and prognostic importance. The platelet life-span is shortened, too, in consumption coagulopathies, and in thrombotic thrombocytopenic purpura. In thrombocytopenia due to defective production of platelets the life-span should be normal provided that platelets are not being lost by bleeding during the course of the study. In thrombocytopenia associated with splenomegaly the recovery of injected labelled platelets is low, but their survival is usually almost normal. Surface counting of radioactivity over the spleen and liver in ^{51}Cr studies has given inconsistent results and has not proved helpful in ITP in determining which patients will benefit from splenectomy. By quantitative scanning with ^{111}In, it is possible to measure the splenic platelet pool and to distinguish the relative importance of pooling and destruction of platelets in the spleen.[44,45] It must be recognized, however, that platelet kinetic

---

*cpm/ml std × diln. of std × vol injected.

studies are often difficult to interpret, and are only occasionally helpful in the management of patients with thrombocytopenia.

The splenic platelet pool is normally about 30% of the total platelet population, and it is thought that each platelet spends a third of its life-span in the spleen.[45] The size of the pool is increased in splenomegaly, resulting in thrombocytopenia but not necessarily in a reduced mean platelet life-span. In immune thrombocytopenias antibody-coated platelets may be destroyed in the liver (whilst only the normal pool is present in the spleen) or they may be destroyed in the liver and in the spleen.

REFERENCES

[1] AHUJA, S., LEWIS, S. M. and SZUR, L. (1972). Value of surface counting in predicting response to splenectomy in haemolytic anaemia. *Journal of Clinical Pathology*, **25**, 467.

[2] BATEMAN, S., LEWIS, S. M., NICHOLAS, A. and ZAAFRAN, A. (1978). Splenic red cell pooling: a diagnostic feature in polycythaemia. *British Journal of Haematology*, **40**, 389.

[3] BENTLEY, S. A. (1977). Red cell survival studies reinterpreted. *Clinics in Haematology*, **6**, 601.

[4] BENTLEY, S. A. and LEWIS, S. M. (1976). The relationship between total red cell volume, plasma volume and venous haematocrit. *British Journal of Haematology*, **33**, 301.

[5] BENTLEY, S. A. and MILLER, D. T. (1986). Radionuclide blood cell survival studies. *Methods in Hematology*, **14**, 245.

[6] BOENDER, C. A. and VERLOOP, M. C. (1969). Iron absorption, iron loss and iron retention in man: studies after oral administration of a tracer dose of $^{59}FeSO_4$ and $^{131}BaSO_4$. *British Journal of Haematology*, **17**, 45.

[7] BOTHWELL, T. H., CHARLTON, R. W., COOK, J. D. and FINCH, C. A. (1979). *Iron Metabolism in Man*. Blackwell Scientific Publications, Oxford.

[8] CAVILL, I. (1971). The preparation of ^{59}Fe-labelled transferrin for ferrokinetic studies. *Journal of Clinical Pathology*, **24**, 472.

[9] CAVILL, I. (1986). Plasma clearance studies. *Methods in Hematology*, **14**, 214.

[10] CAZZOLA, M., BAROSI, G., ORLANDI, E. and STEFANELLI, M. (1980). The plasma ^{59}Fe clearance curve in man; an evaluation of methods of measurement and analysis. *Blut*, **40**, 325.

[11] CLINE, M. J. and BERLIN, N. I. (1963). The red cell chromium elution rate in patients with some hematologic diseases. *Blood*, **21**, 63.

[12] DANPURE, H. J., OSMAN, S. and BRADY, F. (1982). The labelling of blood cells in plasma with ^{111}In-tropolonate. *British Journal of Radiology*, **55**, 247.

[13] DANPURE, H. J., OSMAN, S. and PETERS, A. M. (1990). Labelling autologous platelets with ^{111}In tropolonate for platelet kinetic studies: limitations imposed by thrombocytopenia. *European Journal of Haematology*, **45**, 223.

[14] FERRANT, A., CAUWE, J. L., MICHAUX, C., BECKERS, C., VERWILGHEN, R. and SOKAL, G. (1982). Assessment of the sites of red-cell destruction using quantitative measurement of splenic and hepatic red-cell destruction. *British Journal of Haematology*, **50**, 591.

[15] FERRANT, A., LEWIS, S. M. and SZUR, L. (1974). The elution of ^{99m}Tc from red cells and its effect on red cell volume measurement. *Journal of Clinical Pathology*, **27**, 983.

[16] FINCH, C. A., DEUBELBEISS, K., COOK, J. D., ESCHBACH, J. W., HARKER, L. A., FUNK, D. D., MARSAGLIA, G., HILLMAN, R. S., SLICHTER, S., ADAMSON, J. W., GANZONI, A. and GILBERT, E. R. (1970). Ferrokinetics in man. *Medicine*, **49**, 17.

[17] FRONT, D. and ISRAEL, O. (1981). Tc-99m-labelled red blood cells in the evaluation of vascular abnormalities. *Journal of Nuclear Medicine*, **22**, 149.

[18] GOODWIN, D. A. (1978). Cell labelling with oxine chelates of radioactive metal ions: techniques and clinical implications. *Journal of Nuclear Medicine*, **19**, 557.

[19] HEGDE, U. M., WILLIAMS, E. D., LEWIS, S. M., SZUR, L., GLASS, H. I. and PETTIT, J. E. (1973). Measurement of splenic red cell volume and visualization of the spleen with ^{99m}Tc. *Journal of Nuclear Medicine*, **14**, 769.

[20] HURLEY, P. J. (1975). Red cell and plasma volumes in normal adults. *Journal of Nuclear Medicine*, **16**, 46.

[21] HUFF. R. L. and FELLER, D. D. (1956). Relation of circulating red cell volume to body density and obesity. *Journal of Clinical Investigation*, **35**, 1.

[22] INTERNATIONAL COMMITTEE FOR STANDARDIZATION IN HAEMATOLOGY (1975). Recommended methods for surface counting to determine sites of red-cell destruction. *British Journal of Haematology*, **30**, 249.

[23] INTERNATIONAL COMMITTEE FOR STANDARDIZATION IN HAEMATOLOGY (1980). Recommended methods for radioisotope red-cell survival studies. *British Journal of Haematology*, **45**, 659.

[24] INTERNATIONAL COMMITTEE FOR STANDARDIZATION IN HAEMATOLOGY (1980). Recommended methods for measurements of red-cell and plasma volume. *Journal of Nuclear Medicine*, **21**, 793.

[25] INTERNATIONAL COMMITTEE FOR STANDARDIZATION IN HAEMATOLOGY (1988). Recommended method for ^{111}In platelet survival studies. *Journal of Nuclear Medicine*, **29**, 564.

[26] JANDI, J. H., GREENBERG, M. S., YONEMOTO, R. H. and CASTLE, W. B. (1956). Clinical determination of the sites of red cell sequestration in hemolytic anemias. *Journal of Clinical Investigation*, **35**, 842.

[27] KOUTRAS, G. A., HATTORI, M., SCHNEIDER, A. S., EBAUGH, F. G. and VALENTINE, W. N. (1964). Studies of chromated erythrocytes. Effect of sodium chromate on erythrocyte glutathione reductase. *Journal of Clinical Investigation*, **43**, 323.

[28] KOUTRAS, G. A., SCHNEIDER, A. S., HATTORI, M. and VALENTINE, W. N. (1965). Studies of chromated erythrocytes. Mechanisms of chromate inhibition of glutathione reductase. *British Journal of Haematology*, **11**, 360.

[29] LABARDINI, J., PAPAYANNOPOULOU, T., COOK, J. D., ADAMSON, J. W., WOODSON, R. D., ESCHBACH, J. W., HILLMAN, R. S. and FINCH, C. A. (1973). Marrow radioiron kinetics. *Haematologia*, **7**, 301.

[30] LEWIS, S. M., SZUR, L. and DACIE, J. V. (1960). The pattern of erythrocyte destruction in haemolytic anaemia, as studied with radioactive chromium. *British Journal of Haematology*, **6**, 122.

[31] LEWIS, S. M. and LIU YIN, J. A. (1986). Blood volume studies. *Methods in Hematology*, **14**, 198.

[32] LUKASKI, H. C. (1987). Methods for the assessment of human body composition: traditional and new. *American Journal of Clinical Nutrition*, **46**, 537.

[33] MARSH, G. W., LEWIS, S. M. and SZUR, L. (1966). The use of ^{51}Cr-labelled heat-damaged red cells to study splenic function. I. Evaluation of method. *British Journal of Haematology*, **12**, 161.

[34] MILLER, J. H. (1987). Technetium-99m-labelled red blood cells in the evaluation of the liver in infants and children. *Journal of Nuclear Medicine*, **28**, 1412.

[35] MULDOWNEY, F. P. (1957). The relationship of total red cell mass to lean body mass in man. *Clinical Science*, **16**, 163.

[36] NADLER, S. B., HIDALGO, J. U. and BLOCH, T. (1962). Prediction of blood volume in normal human adults. *Surgery*, **51**, 224.

[37] OSMAN, S. and DANPURE, H. J. (1987). A simple in vitro method of radiolabelling human erythrocytes in whole blood with ^{113m}In-tropolonate. *European Journal of Haematology*, **39**, 125.

[38] PAVEL, D. G., ZIMMER, A. M. and PATTERSON, V. N. (1977)). In vivo labelling of red blood with ^{99m}Tc: a new approach to blood pool visualization. *Journal of Nuclear Medicine*, **18**, 305.

[39] PEARSON, H. A. (1963). The binding of ^{51}Cr to hemoglobin. I. In vitro studies. *Blood*, **22**, 218.

[40] PEARSON, T. C. and GUTHRIE, D. L. (1984). The interpretation of measured red cell mass and plasma volume in patients with elevated PCV values. *Clinical and Laboratory Haematology*, **6**, 207.

[41] PETERS, A. M. (1983). Splenic blood flow and blood cell kinetics. *Clinics in Haematology*, **12**, 421.

[42] PETERS, A. M., RYAN, P. F. J., KLONIZAKIS, I., ELKON, K. B., LEWIS, S. M. and HUGHES, G. R. V. (1981). Analysis of heat-damaged erythrocyte clearance curves. *British Journal of Haematology*, **49**, 581.

[43] PETERS, A. M., RYAN, P. F. J., KLONIZAKIS, I., ELKON, K. B., LEWIS, S. M., HUGHES, G. R. V. and LAVENDER, J. P. (1982). Kinetics of heat damaged autologous red blood cells. *Scandinavian Journal of Haematology*, **28**, 5.

[44] PETERS, A. M., SAVERYMUTTU, S. H., BELL, R. N. and LAVENDER, J. P. (1958). The kinetics of short-lived indium-111 radiolabelled platelets. *Scandinavian Journal of Haematology*, **34**, 137.

[45] PETERS A. M., SAVERYMUTTU, S. H., WONKE, B., LEWIS, S. M. and LAVENDER, J. P. (1984). The interpretation of platelet kinetic studies for the identification of site of abnormal platelet destruction. *British Journal of Haematology*, **57**, 637.

[46] PETERS, A. M., WALPORT, M. J., ELKON, K. B., REAVY, H. J., FERJENCIK, P. P., LAVENDER, J. P. and HUGHES, G. R. V. (1984). The comparative blood clearance kinetics of modified radiolabelled erythrocytes. *Clinical Science*, **66**, 55.

[47] PETTIT, J. E. (1977). Spleen function. *Clinics in Haematology*, **6**, 639.

[48] PRYOR D. S. (1967). The mechanism of anaemia in tropical splenomegaly. *Quarterly Journal of Medicine*, **36**, 337.

[49] RADIA, R., PETERS, A. M., DEENMAMODE, M., FITZPATRICK, M. L. and LEWIS, S. M. (1981). Measurement of red cell volume and splenic red cell pool using ^{113m}indium. *British Journal of Haematology*, **49**, 587.

[50] RICKETTS, C., CAVILL, I. and NAPIER, J. A. F. (1977). The measurement of red cell lifespan using ^{59}Fe. *British Journal of Haematology*, **37**, 403.

[51] ROCHE, M. and PÉREZ-GIMÉNEZ, M. E. (1959). Intestinal loss and reabsorption of iron in hookworm infection. *Journal of Laboratory and Clinical Medicine*, **54**, 49.

[52] SINN, H. and SILVESTER, D. J. (1979). Simplified cell labelling with indium-111-acetylacetone. *British Journal of Radiology*, **52**, 758.

[53] TAYLOR, H. L., ERICKSON, L., HENSCHEL, A. and KEYS, A. (1945). The effect of bed rest on the blood volume of normal young men. *American Journal of Physiology*, **144**, 227.

[54] TOGHILL, P. J. (1964). Red-cell pooling in enlarged spleens. *British Journal of Haematology*, **10**, 347.

22. Investigation of megaloblastic anaemia

By B. F. A. Jackson and A. V. Hoffbrand

Principle of microbiological assays   418
Microbiologicol assay of serum and red cell folate   418
Chloramphenicol-resistant *L. casei* method   419
   Normal reference range   420
   Effect of drugs on the serum folate (*L. casei*) assay   420
Measurement of serum B_{12} by radioassay   420
Measurement of serum folate by radioassay   422
Measurement of red cell folate by radioassay   423
Automated non-isotopic methods   423
Quality control of B_{12} and folate assays   425
Deoxyuridine suppression test   426
Investigation of the absorption of B_{12} 427

Urinary excretion (Schilling) test   428
Estimation of intrinsic factor (IF) in gastric juice   429
Intrinsic factor antibodies   430
   Estimation of Type I intrinsic factor antibody   430
   Estimation of Type II (precipitating or
   co-precipitating)   431
Parietal cell antibodies   432
Plasma (or serum) B_{12} binding capacity   432
   Estimation of UBBC   432
   Transcobalamin separation   433
Response to treatment as an aid to diagnosis   434

Megaloblastic anaemia can be suspected from the presence in a blood film of macrocytes, oval red cells, pear-shaped poikilocytes and neutrophils with hypersegmented (>5 lobes) nuclei. The first indication in many cases is the finding of a raised MCV, often without anaemia. The diagnosis may be confirmed by finding megaloblasts and giant metamyelocytes in the marrow. Assay of serum cobalamin (B_{12}) and serum and red cell folate can provide the additional evidence for a firm diagnosis to be made. Serum B_{12} assay is particularly important in the diagnosis of B_{12} neuropathy, as this is often associated with little haematological abnormality.

B_{12} in serum is predominantly methylcobalamin bound to carrier proteins, transcobalamins (TCs). A fall in the serum B_{12} is an early sign of deficiency and may be found before the cellular changes in the marrow and blood. A low serum level is not, however, specific for B_{12} deficiency and may be found in severe folate deficiency, normal pregnancy, myelomatosis, TC I deficiency and sometimes for no apparent reason.

On the other hand, megaloblastic anaemia due to B_{12} deficiency or failure in metabolism can occur in the presence of a normal serum B_{12} level with TC II deficiency, with elevated TC I levels, as in chronic myeloid leukaemia, and with nitrous oxide anaesthesia. Depletion of B_{12} bound to TC II occurs early in B_{12} deficiency[41] and a TC II assay may help to clarify equivocal serum B_{12} levels. Assay of serum methylmalonic acid and homocysteine may reveal early B_{12} deficiency,[51] but their estimation is not suitable for general laboratory use and will not be described here.

Serum folate (5-methyltetrahydrofolate, methyl-THF) falls with a reduction in folate intake or with negative folate balance and may be low without significant body deficiency.[13e] The red cell folate (largely folate polyglutamates) concentration shows better correlation with megaloblastic change,[42] though it is not a specific sign of folate deficiency. It is also low in about half the patients with severe B_{12} deficiency[13f] due to the requirement for B_{12} in the provision of tetrahydrofolate (THF) which is needed rather than methyl-THF as substrate for folate polyglutamate synthesis.[16,43,49] The red cell folate may be normal despite folate deficiency when there is reticulocytosis,[42] following a recent blood transfusion or when anaemia is absent.[42] Vitamin assays should not therefore be interpreted in isolation.

The deoxyuridine suppression test is a sensitive test of both B_{12} and folate deficiency[79] and may be abnormal before obvious morphological changes develop.[12] It may also be used to determine which deficiency is present.

The elucidation of the cause of deficiency of B_{12} and folate depends both on the clinical picture and on laboratory tests. For B_{12} deficiency, tests include measurement of the absorption of B_{12}, other intestinal absorption tests, demonstration of antibodies to intrinsic factor or gastric parietal cells, and measurement of gastric secretion of intrinsic factor. The estimation of serum B_{12} binding capacity and transcobalamins are of occasional help. For folate deficiency, the diet history and if malabsorption

is suspected, jejunal biopsy to exclude gluten-induced enteropathy are important tests. Features of splenic atrophy in the blood film, in the absence of splenectomy suggest gluten-induced enteropathy.

In this chapter we first consider microbiological assays, then the more widely used radioisotope assays for B_{12} and folate and the recently available automated non-radionuclide assays. The deoxy-uridine suppression test is given next and finally some of the tests to determine the cause of either deficiency.

A recent review by the British Committee for Standards in Haematology provides guidelines for the investigation of cobalamin and folate deficiencies.[80]

PRINCIPLE OF MICROBIOLOGICAL ASSAYS

Certain micro-organisms (e.g. *Euglena gracilis* and *Lactobacillus casei*) require specific factors for growth which they cannot synthesize. The assay medium for *Euglena* contains all the essentials with the exception of B_{12} which is provided by standards and sera. The growth is directly proportional to the concentration of B_{12}. Likewise *Lactobacillus casei* requires folate which is provided by standards and test sera.

MICROBIOLOGICAL ASSAY OF B_{12} IN SERUM

Several methods are available, using *Euglena gracilis*, *Lactobacillus leichmannii*, *Escherichia coli* and *Ochromonas malhamensis*. The *E. gracilis* method is sensitive, accurate and especially suitable for the assay of a large number of specimens though it has been largely confined to use in centres with a particular interest in B_{12} metabolism. It was the assay method[2] chosen to assign a potency value to the British Standard for human serum B_{12}[20] and is described in the 6th edition of this book. Microbiological assays are used with decreasing frequency because of the greater convenience of radionuclide, immuno-logical and other non-radioisotopic methods for routine work.[64]

MICROBIOLOGICAL ASSAY OF SERUM AND RED CELL FOLATE

The folate activity of serum is due mainly to the presence of methyl-THF. Because this compound is a growth requirement for *Lactobacillus casei,* this organism is used for the assay of naturally-occurring folates in serum and in red cells.

Methyl-THF is labile, but can be protected during assay with ascorbic acid.[76] Serum to which 5 mg/ml of ascorbic acid have been added can be stored at $-20°C$ for up to 2 months. Haemolysis must be avoided because of the high folate concentration in red blood cells. For assay of red cell folate, whole blood anticoagulated with EDTA can be stored for up to 1 week at $4°C$. A lysate is prepared by adding 0.1 ml of whole blood (of known PCV) to 1.9 ml of 10 g/l freshly prepared aqueous ascorbic acid, with incubation for at least 10 min at room temperature before assay. This allows for polyglutamate forms of folate to be deconjugated by plasma folate polyglutamate hydrolase at the low pH (approximately 4.6) of the ascorbate solution. The lysate may be stored for up to 5 months at $-20°C$.

A protein-free extract was originally used for serum and red cell assays.[42,76] An aseptic technique without protein precipitation[38] simplified the assay and the use of a *L. casei* strain resistant to chloramphenicol permits automated and semi-automated methods.[21,55]

CHLORAMPHENICOL-RESISTANT
L. Casei METHOD

Reagents and materials

Glassware. Carry out the assays in 100 × 16 mm (disposable) glass tubes.

Water. Use glass-distilled water throughout.

Organism. Chloramphenicol-resistant *Lactobacillus casei* NCIB 10463.

Chloramphenicol solutions.

A. 1 g/l. Dissolve 100 mg of chloramphenicol base B.P. in 1 ml of absolute ethanol and make up to 100 ml with water.

B. 3 g/l. Dissolve 300 mg of chloramphenicol base B.P. in 1 ml absolute ethanol and make up to 100 ml with water.

Maintenance medium. Bacto *Lactobacillus* Broth AOAC (Difco 0901-15-3). Suspend 19 g of dehydrated medium in 450 ml of water and dissolve by boiling for 2 min, protected from light. To 180 ml of broth add 20 ml of chloramphenicol solution A. Distribute 10-ml volumes into screw-capped glass bottles and autoclave at 121°C for 15 min. Store in the dark at 4°C. Use the stronger chloramphenicol broth for the stock culture and subculture the organism for assay in the weaker chloramphenicol broth.

Preparation of inoculum. Transfer the freeze-dried culture to 10 ml of maintenance medium containing 300 µg/ml chloramphenicol and incubate at 37°C for 48 h. Transfer 1.0 ml of the 48 h culture into 4 bottles of maintenance medium containing 100 µg/ml chloramphenicol and incubate at 37°C for 24 h. Centrifuge, discard supernatant and wash twice with single strength assay medium. Add 2 ml of single strength assay medium to each bottle and pool contents. Adjust the absorbance of the suspension to read 0.8–0.9 at 530 nm. Distribute 0.2 ml volumes into freezing vials and store in liquid nitrogen. This inoculum remains viable for at least 1 yr.

Washing in bulk and storage of washed organisms saves time and improves precision between assays.

Should there be difficulty in gaining access to liquid nitrogen the stock culture and inoculum may be prepared and stored as follows.

Following the reconstitution of the freeze-dried culture as above, transfer 1.0 ml to one bottle of maintenance medium containing 100 µg/ml chloramphenicol and 1.0 ml into maintenance medium containing 300 µg/ml chloramphenicol (stock culture) and incubate both at 37°C for 24 h. Store the stock culture at 4°C and use the culture in 100 µg/ml chloramphenicol for preparation of the inoculum. Wash twice with single strength medium, resuspend with 2 ml of medium and adjust absorbance as described previously.

Subculture the stock culture every 7–10 days into maintenance medium containing 300 µg/ml chloramphenicol as above. The day before setting up the assay subculture 1.0 ml of the stock culture into maintenance medium containing 100 µg/ml chloramphenicol and incubate at 37°C for 24 h. Wash and prepare inoculum as before.

Assay medium. Prepare Folic Acid Casei Medium Difco 0822 by adding 500 ml of distilled water to 47 g of dry medium, boiling for 2 min, cooling and adding a further 500 ml of distilled water. Protect it from light during heating and use, to avoid destruction of riboflavin.[3] Add 10 ml of chloramphenicol solution A, 250 mg of ascorbic acid and a 0.1 ml inoculum to each litre of single-strength medium.

Preparation of standards

Dry folic (pteroylglutamic) acid powder (SIGMA) at 100°C for 2 h.

Stock solution A. Prepare an aqueous folic acid solution (1 g/l) by bringing the folic acid into solution with a few drops of 0.2 mol/l NaOH. Store at –20°C in 1.5 ml volumes.

Solution B. Dilute the stock solution A 1 in 100 in 20% ethanol to give a solution of 10 mg/l. Store in a dark bottle at 4°C.

Solution C. Dilute solution B 1 in 100 with water to give a solution of 100 µg/l.

Standard curve. Dilute solution C in water according to Table 22.1.

Store in aliquots at –20°C, use a fresh set for each assay.

Table 22.1   Preparation of standard solutions for the *L. casei* method for assay of serum and red cell folate

Folic acid solution C 100 µg/l (ml)	0	0.1	0.2	0.4	0.6	0.8	1.0	1.2	1.4
Water (ml)	5	4.9	4.8	4.6	4.4	4.2	4.0	3.8	3.6
Concentration of standard (µg/l)	0	2.0	4.0	8.0	12.0	16.0	20.0	24.0	28.0

Method

Mix inoculated assay medium continuously on a magnetic stirrer. Set up 0.05 ml volumes of sera and lysates in duplicate and standards in triplicate. Add 4.95 ml of assay medium to each tube. Cover the tubes and incubate at 37°C for 20–24 h.

Reading the assay

Remove the tubes from the water-bath and cool at 4°C for 30 min. Mix on a vortex mixer and read the turbidity at 620 nm in a spectrophotometer, preferably with a flow-through cell and recorder, first setting the instrument to zero with the standard tubes containing no folic acid.

Calculation

Plot the absorbance against the folic acid concentration in µg/l on arithmetic graph paper to prepare a standard curve. Read the serum and haemolysate folates directly from the curve. Correct the lysate for the dilution factor of 20 and divide by the haematocrit to obtain the red cell folate. It is not usually necessary to correct the lysate for the small amount of serum folate present, though the following formula can be used:

Red cell folate µg/l =

$$\frac{(\text{Whole blood folate} \times 20) - (\text{Serum folate} \times (1 - \text{PCV}))}{\text{PCV}}$$

Normal reference range

Serum folate. 3–20 µg/l (7–46 nmol/l); mean 10 µg/l (23 nmol/l)

Red cell folate. 160–640 µg/l (365–1460 nmol/l); mean 316 µg/l (720 nmol/l).

In the series reported by Waters and Mollin,[76] patients with megaloblastic anaemia due to folate deficiency had serum folate levels of <4.0 µg/l and patients with pernicious anaemia had levels of 4.0–27 µg/l (mean 16.6 µg/l). In patients with megaloblastic anaemia due to folate deficiency the red cell folate was 8–143 µg/l, mean 79 µg/l, and in pernicious anaemia 26–395 µg/l, mean 146 µg/l.[42]

Effect of drugs on the serum folate (*L. casei*) assay[13d]

The growth of *L. casei* is inhibited by penicillins, tetracycline, erythromycin, streptomycin, lincomycin, rifampicin, trimethoprim and sulphonamides. Methotrexate and pyrimethamine also inhibit the assay. Alkylating agents do not usually inhibit the assay at conventional dosage whereas some anti-metabolites, e.g. cytosine arabinoside and hydroxyurea do. Drug inhibition will depend on the dosage given as well as on the nature of the drug. Serious inhibition is evident if the growth of the organism is less in the test serum than in the blank (zero folic acid) standard tube and inhibition can also be detected by assay of a mixture of the patient's serum and a normal serum, or of a higher dilution of the patient's serum. Inhibition is rarely observed with haemolysate assays because of their higher dilution.

MEASUREMENT OF SERUM B$_{12}$ BY RADIOASSAY

Assay of serum B$_{12}$ by radionuclide dilution (competitive binding) was first described over 30 years ago.[6] Many variations have since been reported and commercial kits have extended the use of the test. Radioimmunoassay which is sensitive and specific has been developed[68] using antibodies raised in rabbits against the mono-carboxylic acid derivative of cyanocobalamin conjugated to human serum albumin. Donkey anti-rabbit gamma globulin coated magnetic particles used to separate the bound from free B_{12} are an improvement.[61] Radionuclide methods have the advantage over microbiological assays in that they are simpler and more rapid and the results are unaffected by antibiotics and other drugs which may affect a microbiological assay organism. However, the strict regulations involving storage use and disposal of radioactivity are a disadvantage.

Principle of radioisotope dilution assay

A known amount of radioactive 'hot' B_{12} is diluted with the non-radioactive 'cold' B_{12} in the test serum which is released from the serum binders by heat or chemical means. A measured volume of the mixture of hot and cold B_{12} is bound to a binding protein which is added in an amount insufficient to bind all the 'hot' B_{12}. The bound B_{12} is separated from the free and its radioactivity counted. This count will be inversely proportional to the B_{12} concentrations in the test serum, as the higher the serum B_{12} the greater will be the dilution of the radioactive cobalamin and thus less radioactivity will be attached to the binding protein. By comparison with standards of known B_{12} content, the B_{12} content of the serum can be calculated. Variations at each assay step that can affect the results include:

1. Extraction of B_{12} from serum transcobalamins

Boiling or autoclaving at an acid pH with removal of the protein precipitate by filtration or centri-fugation, as for *L. leichmannii*, was first used and is the most satisfactory method of extraction.[17,28] The pH of the extract does not require adjustment for a subsequent binding stage by intrinsic factor (IF). Denaturation of the binders by boiling at a pH of 9.2–11.7 or at room temperature at pH 12.9–13.0, without removal of the protein products, is used in many commercial methods, but with both techniques the residue gives a varying amount of non-specific binding (NSB) which may be excessive with certain sera (e.g.

those with high transcobalamin levels as in chronic myeloid leukaemia). Dithiothreitol (DTT) reduces NSB.[50] The effect of NSB on the apparent serum levels depends on the separation stage (see below). Alkaline extraction will require subsequent adjust-ment of the pH to that optimal for the binding stage. Intrinsic factor antibodies do not appear to affect the assays.[28] In many assays only 200 µl of test material are required and it is possible to use serum or plasma from heparinized or EDTA anticoagulated blood.

2. Binding agent

IF of human or porcine origin is commonly used. The IF may be purified (e.g. by affinity chroma-tography), contaminating R binder may be rendered inactive (blocked) by the addition of excess analogue (e.g. cobinamide)[4] or the IF may be coupled to a solid phase carrier, prior to the assay, at a pH which prevents R binder uptake.[73] Carriers used include polyacrylamide beads, glass particles, microcrystalline cellulose and magnetic particles. The specificity of pure and blocked IF can be demonstrated by the addition of 10 µg/l cobinamide dicyanide (Sigma) to sera; cross-reactivity should be minimal with no significant increase in the assay value.

Other binders used include normal human serum[63] (essentially transcobalamin II), unsaturated TCI,[67] and the R binders of saliva[11] and of chicken serum[36] which give higher results, estimating both B_{12} and the microbiological inert analogues, i.e. total corrinoids. B_{12} (cobalamin) contains a nucleotide, 5,6-dimethylbenzimidazole, which is attached to the corrin ring through a ribose group and directly to the central cobalt atom. Corrinoids are compounds containing the corrin ring with either altered side chains and/or lacking the specific B_{12} nucleotide. They are commonly called B_{12} analogues and are essentially microbiologically inactive. Pure IF binds only cobalamins whereas other binding proteins may bind analogues.[40] The first commercial kits used crude IF preparations and sometimes gave falsely normal results[18,47] attributed to such analogues.

3. B_{12} standards

For non-commercial methods, the pharmaceutical

preparation of cyanocobalamin, Duncan Flockhart), 250 µg/ml, is satisfactory. The cobalamins of the sera are converted to the cyano form during the extraction. The standards usually range from 50 or 100 to 2000 µg/l. With heat extraction, aqueous standards are usually satisfactory, but a protein matrix, to 'balance' that of the test serum, is required for alkaline extracts. The *Biorad* standards containing B_{12} and folic acid in human serum albumin are suitable (see p. 425).

4. Radioisotope tracer

^{57}Co-labelled cyanocobalamin is used in all methods. CN(^{57}Co) cobalamin, 0.05 µg in 1 ml with activity 370–740 kBq, is available from Kodak Clinical Diagnostics Ltd. (product number CT2). Good precision is required to diagnose B_{12} deficiency at the lower end of the normal reference range, and the amount of tracer added should be such that 40–50% is bound at this level.[66]

5. Separation of free from bound B_{12}

Charcoal coated with albumin or haemoglobin is used although it is messy and invariably takes up some bound B_{12}.[1] Alternative agents are Sephadex gel and DEAE-cellulose.[29,75] Following centrifugation, the supernatant containing the bound B_{12} is decanted into counting tubes without disturbing the deposit. Centrifugation in solid phase methods leaves the free B_{12} in the supernatant; the deposit in the assay tube is counted, sometimes after washing.[57] The removal of the supernatant calls for care and a standard technique. Tween 20 may enhance the pelleting of the deposit.[57] Bound ^{57}Co-B_{12} gives the higher counts at the lower B_{12} concentrations. B_{12} bound non-specifically remains in the supernatant in the liquid systems, adds to the counts of that specifically bound and gives apparently lower serum B_{12} levels, whereas in solid phase systems the NSB-B_{12} is discarded, giving apparently higher serum B_{12} levels. The zero standard will allow correction for NSB only when the protein content of the standards is the same as in the test material.

6. Calculation of results

The bound B_{12} in the standards and sera are counted in a γ counter, a curve relating counts to B_{12} concentration in the standards is drawn and the unknowns are read from this. However, with the usual workload this needs to be done automatically or semi-automatically. Computerized programs are available with modern counters. The choice of methods for expressing results has been reviewed by Ekins[26]; the most popular is the percentage binding (B/B_0 × 100, where B is the count of the test and B_0 the count of the zero standard) on the log ordinate axis and the B_{12} concentration on the log abscissa axis.

MEASUREMENT OF SERUM FOLATE BY RADIOASSAY

The development of commercial radioisotope dilution (RID) kits followed upon the discovery of suitable folate binders and the production of γ-emitting iodinated folate compounds. The principle of the assay is the same as for serum B_{12} and the procedures are similar.

1. Extraction of folate from the serum binder

In contrast to microbiological assay the folate has to be released by heat or alkaline denaturation of the endogenous binder. Ascorbic acid must not be added to sera for preservation of folate during extraction (and storage) if the sample is also to be used for B_{12} assay because it destroys B_{12}. Dithiothreitol (DTT) is used in most combined B_{12} and folate assays to keep the folate in the reduced, stable form. Without it, stored sera may give low results.[22]

2. Binding agent

β-Lactoglobulin isolated from cow's milk[31] is

commonly used. At pH 9.3 ± 0.1 the binding affinities of the serum methyl-THF and the folic acid of the standards are similar. It is essential that the pH at this stage is strictly maintained.[34] Porcine serum is a less satisfactory binder. There is cross-reactivity with methotrexate and folinic acid.

3. Folate standards

Methyl-THF is unstable and the majority of assay methods use folic acid standards, which may cause under-estimation of serum folate.[56]

4. Radioactive tracer

[125]I-labelled folic acid is generally used.

5. Separation of free from bound folate

The liquid and solid phase methods used for B_{12} are satisfactory for folate assays. Many of the assay kits measure both B_{12} and folate.

MEASUREMENT OF RED CELL FOLATE BY RADIOASSAY

Whereas *L. casei* responds equally to both tri- and mono-glutamates, the affinity of the binder for folates varies with the number of glutamate residues. Reproducible assays can only be obtained by release and conversion of the protein-bound folate polyglutamates, mainly methyl-THF with four or five additional glutamate moieties, to a monoglutamate. Adequate dilution of the red cells,[5] a pH between 3 and 6,[60] plasma folate polyglutamate hydrolase, and ascorbic acid to preserve the reduced form,[42] are required. Sodium ascorbate does not lyse the red cells completely. Inadequate lysis and deconjugation give falsely low results.[58,72]

To prepare the lysate, dilute $100\,\mu l$ of whole blood (of known PCV) in $1.9\,ml$ of *freshly* prepared 1% aqueous ascorbic acid and leave at room temperature for at least 10 min. Assay immediately or store at $-20°C$. Some kits use different concentrations of ascorbic acid, require the addition of protein diluent before assaying and use a different dilution.

AUTOMATED NON-ISOTOPIC METHODS

BAXTER STRATUS AUTOMATED FLUOROMETRIC ENZYME-LINKED IMMUNOASSAY FOR VITAMIN B_{12} AND FOLATE

The B_{12} assay uses the principle of sequential binding between natural B_{12} in the sample, or an enzyme-linked B_{12} to porcine intrinsic factor (pIF). Cyanocobalamin is used for calibration and enzyme labelling and potassium cyanide to convert sample B_{12} to the more stable cyanocobalamin. Endogeneous B_{12} binders are denatured at alkaline pH and the treated sample is neutralized in the presence of pIF:mouse anti pIF complex, and reacts on glass fibre paper with immobilized goat anti-mouse immunoglobulin. Conjugase consisting of alkaline phosphatase-labelled B_{12} is added and it reacts with unoccupied sites on the immobilized pIF. Enzyme substrate 4 methylumbelliferyl phosphate is added and the reaction rate which is inversely proportional to the concentration of B_{12} in the sample is measured by an optical system that monitors the reaction rate by fluorimetry. The first result is obtained in 6–8 min and thereafter at 1-min intervals. Statistical evaluation and graphics of control values are easily obtained using the software on the microprocessor.

The folate assay employs the principle of sequential binding of natural sample folate and an enzyme-linked folate conjugate to bovine milk-derived folate binding protein (FPB). A stable form of folate, folic acid, is used for calibrators and enzyme labelling. The serum folate is reduced and extracted from endogenous serum binders at alkaline pH eliminating the necessity of boiling. The extracted sample is neutralized and then adjusted to a pH which facilitates equal folate affinity for immobilized mouse monoclonal anti-FBP/FBP complexed with goat anti-mouse IgG, Fc fragment specific, on glass fibre paper. Free folate combines with folate binding proteins. Alkaline phosphatase conjugase covalently linked to folate is added and combines with unoccupied binding sites on the FBP. The substrate 4-methylumbelliferyl phosphate initiates enzyme activity and the reaction rate is measured by fluorimetry. The rate is inversely proportional to the concentration of folate present in the sample; the first result is obtained in 6–8 min and thereafter at 1-min intervals.

CIBA CORNING ACS:180 ASSAY

This is a fully automated random access system allowing the use of primary bar coded collection tubes with a 15-min assay time using the same Ciba Corning Magic Lite chemiluminescent reaction as is used in their manual Magic Lite assays available since 1986. The B_{12} and folate assays are competitive assays in which B_{12} or folate from the sample competes with the Lite reagent, which is B_{12} or folate bound to acridinium ester, for a limited amount of purified intrinsic factor/purified bovine milk binding protein covalently coupled to paramagnetic particles (Solid Phase). Sodium hydroxide and DTT release the B_{12}/folate from endogenous binding proteins in the sample. The chemiluminescent reaction is measured and the photon output (relative light units) quantitated. An indirect relationship exists between the amount of B_{12}/folate and the relative light units detected. Quality control statistics and charts are produced automatically.

ABBOTT FLUORESCENT MICROPARTICLE ENZYME ASSAY USING ABBOTT IMX ANALYSER

B_{12} assay[48]

The sample is treated at pH >12.5 to release bound B_{12} and to convert all forms to cyanocobalamin. The analyte is bound at a lower pH by purified porcine IF immobilized to a solid phase of polymeric microspheres. Alkaline phosphatase conjugate binds to the B_{12}/IF complex. A substrate of 4-methylumbelliferyl phosphate is converted by alkaline phosphatase to form a fluorescent product, methylumbelliferone, which is generated in inverse proportion to the amount of B_{12} in the original sample. The fluorescence is read by the IMX. 24 samples can be assayed in 60 min.

Several other manufacturers intend releasing automated non-isotopic methods on to the market.

Which method?

The choice should be based upon the technical performance, clinical value and compatibility with current laboratory procedures, and with the user. Consideration may need to be given to the turn around time required by the requesting clinicians and the requirement to be efficient in cost, speed and accuracy of service.

A laboratory setting up B_{12} assays would not now normally introduce a microbiological method since radioassays are generally satisfactory and more convenient. The automated non-radioactive methods, although expensive, produce results quickly, some providing random access and requiring less highly trained personnel for routine operation. The accuracy of a B_{12} assay can be judged by assay of reference sera and by its performance in external quality assessment schemes, in which the mean from a large number of participants appears to be the true value.[22] The accuracy of most radioassay kits is acceptable. A satisfactory assay gives a CV of 5% or less with within-batch duplicates and of 10% or less with between-batch assays. All manufacturers claim that these levels can be reached. A laboratory carrying out other in-house B_{12} investigations may wish to establish its own method. The solid phase boil technique of Muir and Chanarin[57] (though the bead preparation is both time-consuming and not inexpensive) and the boil technique with charcoal separation of Gutcho and Mansbach[37] are recommended.

The present unavailability of a standard reference preparation limits technical assessment of folate assays. Both the serum and red cell folate assays show considerable variation in accuracy, though the correlation between them is reasonable.[33] Some laboratories may wish to measure only serum or red cell folate, but because of the limitations of both (see p. 417) it is advisable to assay both, or to do the red cell assay whenever the serum folate is low.

Table 22.2 lists the kits in use in the United Kingdom. Kits using solid phase binders for B_{12} and folate assays are preferable since they reduce the number of assay steps and are as satisfactory as charcoal separation. A boil technique with a solid phase binder was generally considered the best for detecting B_{12} deficiency.[17] However, good correlation is obtained using both an established radioassay and the new non-isotopic methods, all the latter being no-boil. Table 22.3 lists the automated non-isotopic methods. Whichever method is chosen, each laboratory should establish its own normal reference range. The features mentioned previously which affect radioassays and the references to their performance should help in the choice of an appropriate kit. The protocol should be studied before a trial kit is obtained. A new kit requires full evaluation including the assay of sera of low B_{12} and folate content.

QUALITY CONTROL AND REFERENCE MATERIALS FOR B_{12} AND FOLATE ASSAYS

Sera and haemolysates of known B_{12} and folate content must be included in each assay. For quality control it is usual to collect pools of low, intermediate and normal values, to store these in 1 ml volumes at $-20°C$ and to thaw one for each assay. Their vitamin content is determined by assay alongside samples of known concentration from another laboratory or samples from previous external quality assessment surveys. An international reference reagent for human serum B_{12} has been developed by ICSH[45] and established by WHO; an equivalent British Standard is also available for checking the accuracy of an assay*. Recovery

*From National Institute for Biological Standards and Control, P.O. Box 1193, Potters Bar, EN6 3QH, UK.

Table 22.2 Commercial kits for B_{12} and folate radioassays

Manufacturer	Kit		Extraction pH	Binding pH	Separator	Relative accuracy[22] (microbiological assay = 100%)			Selected references
							Folate		
						B_{12}	Serum	Red cell	
Kodak Clinical Diagnostics Ltd	B_{12}/folate+	A	12.9	9.5	Charcoal	90		155	17,22,32,33
Becton-Dickinson	B_{12}	B	9.3	9.3	Charcoal				4,62,65
	Simultrac B_{12}/folate	B	9.3	9.3	Charcoal	93	80	115	14,17,22,28,32
	Simultrac-S B_{12}/folate	B	9.3	9.3	Solid phase	99	82	85	22
	Simultrac-SNB B_{12}/folate	A	12–13	9.3	Solid phase	94	96	104	22
	Folic acid	B	9.3	9.3					
Biorad	Quantaphase B_{12}/folate+	B	11.7	9.2	Polymer beads	100	98	73	22,32,33,62,65
Diagnostic Products Corp.	Dualcount SP	A	13.0	9.3	Cellulose	92	96	135	22,62,65
	Dualcount SP	B	9.4		Particles				14,62,65
Ciba-Corning	Magic B_{12}/folate	B	9.2		Paramagnetic particles				33
	Magic B_{12}/folate	A	12–13	9.3	Paramagnetic particles				
	**Magic Lite B_{12}	A	12–13	9.3	Paramagnetic particles				
	**Magic Lite folate	A	12–13	9.3	Paramagnetic particles				

A, alkaline denaturation; B, boil. The binder in all kits is IF, purified except in Simultrac kits when R is blocked by analogue in tracer.
+Reagents for a single B_{12} or folate assay are available.
**Non isotopic.

Table 22.3   Automated non-isotopic no-boil B_{12} and folate assays

Manufacturer	Assay system	Principle
Ciba-Corning	ACS: 180	Chemiluminescence using intrinsic factor/milk binder coupled to paramagnetic particles
Baxter	STRATUS	Fluorometric enzyme linked immunoassay
Abbott Laboratories	IMX (B_{12} only at present)	Micro-particle enzyme intrinsic factor assay
Biorad	RADIAS	ELISA based immunoassay

experiments with the addition of B_{12} and folic acid to normal samples are of some value, although they do not assess the extraction stage in B_{12} assays or the haemolysate preparation in folate assays. The repeat assay of three to five sera from the previous batch and plotting the mean or median of each batch (providing the samples come from an unchanging population) help to assure reproducibility of the assay.

Commercial controls are widely available, several companies offering free statistical analysis on an individual basis as well as a comparison with laboratories world-wide.

Participation in an external quality assessment scheme is essential to monitor technical performance.

DEOXYURIDINE SUPPRESSION TEST[79]

Principle. Pre-incubation of normal bone marrow with an appropriate concentration of deoxyuridine (dU) suppresses the subsequent incorporation of tritiated thymidine (^{3}H-TdR) into DNA. This suppression is less in patients with B_{12} or folate deficiency. This is due to failure of the thymidylate synthesis reaction in which deoxyuridine monophosphate (dUMP) is methylated to thymidine monophosphate (dTMP), the methyl donor being the folate co-enzyme 5,10-methylene tetrahydrofolate (in the polyglutamate form). dU suppression is normal when the cause of the megaloblastic anaemia is neither B_{12} nor folate deficiency, nor any other defect in thymidylate synthesis.[30,54]

Materials

Bone marrow. $10–50 \times 10^6$ nucleated cells or 0.5–2.0 ml of aspirated marrow, in EDTA. It is preferable to test the marrow freshly but it can be left overnight at 18–25°C without affecting the results significantly.

Blood. 10 ml of heparinized blood.

Reagents

Hanks balanced salt solution (GIBCO Cat. No. 041-4020) ready for use.

KCl 0.6 mol/l. 4.473 g in 100 ml of water.

Phosphate buffered saline, pH 7.4. Add 90 ml of 0.15 mol/l, $NaH_2PO_4.H_2O$ (23.4 g/l) and 410 ml of 0.15 mol/l Na_2HPO_4 (21.3 g/l) to 500 ml of 9.0 g/l NaCl (saline).

Perchloric acid, 0.5 mol/l. Make up 20.8 ml of concentrated perchloric acid to 500 ml with water.

Hydroxocobalamin, 1000 µg/ml.

Folinic acid (calcium leucovorin) (Lederle), 3 mg/ml.

5-Methyltetrahydrofolic acid (Sigma), 1 mg. Reconstitute with 33 µl of saline immediately before use.

Tritiated thymidine TRA 120 (Amersham), 185 GBq/mmol. Dilute 100 µl to 10 ml with saline (1 µCi/0.2 µmol/100 µl).

Deoxyuridine (Sigma), 100 mmol/l. Prepare a working solution of 11.4 mg in 0.5 ml of saline. This is stable at 4°C.

Scintillation fluid, e.g. Packard emulsifier scintillator 299™ Cat. No. 6013079.

Method

Whenever possible, except when stated, carry out all procedures at 4°C.

Table 22.4 Preparation of assay tubes for the deoxyuridine suppression test

Tubes	Saline (μl)	Vitamin B_{12} (μl)	Folinic acid (μl)	5-Methyl-THF (μl)	Cells* (ml)	dU* (μl)	^{3}H-TdR** (μl)
1 & 2	20	–	–	–	1	–	100
3 & 4	10	–	–	–	1	10	100
5 & 6	–	10	–	–	1	10	100
7 & 8	–	–	10	–	1	10	100
9 & 10	–	–	–	10	1	10	100

*Mix and incubate all tubes at 37°C for 15 min with shaking.
**Mix and incubate all tubes at 37°C for 1 h with shaking.

Wash marrow once in buffered Hanks solution, centrifuging at 4°C at 1000**g** for 5 min.

Lyse the red cells by adding 3 ml of cold water; mix for 30 s; add 1.0 ml of 0.6 mol/l KCl; add 1–2 ml of buffered Hanks solution to maintain the pH, and then centrifuge at 1000**g** for 5 min.

Wash the deposit with buffered Hanks solution, centrifuging at 1000**g** for 5 min. Discard the supernatant. Repeat the lysing process if a visible button of red cells remains.

Suspend the pellets in 1 ml of Hanks solution, checking that there are no clumps in the final suspension. If necessary, pass the suspension through a 19-gauge needle attached to a 1 ml syringe.

Count the number of cells present and express the number as ×10^6/ml.

Add 1 volume of autologous plasma to 4 volumes of Hanks solution and dilute the cells with this solution to obtain 1–3 ×10^6 cells/ml.

Set up the plastic centrifuge tubes as shown in Table 22.4.

Transfer the tubes into an ice-bath.

Centrifuge at 1000**g** for 5 min and discard the supernatant.

Vortex-mix and wash the pellets once with 2.0 ml of cold phosphate buffered saline. Discard the supernatant.

Mix and add 2 ml of the perchloric acid to each pellet.

Mix and stand in the ice-bath for 10 min. Centrifuge and discard the supernatant. If necessary, the pellets can be left overnight at this stage.

Mix, add 0.5 ml of the perchloric acid, mix and place the tubes in a water-bath at 80°C for 20 min.

Centrifuge at 18–25°C and 1000**g** for 5 min.

Transfer 100 μl of the supernatant into counting vials. Add 5 ml of scintillation fluid, allow to equilibrate for 30 min and count for 200 s.

Calculate % counts per min using the counts of ^{3}H-TdR alone as 100%.

Interpretation

1. Deoxyuridine suppression in normal marrow <8%.
2. Deoxyuridine suppresion in megaloblastic marrow >8%.
3. Correction, partial or complete, with added B_{12} but not with methyl-THF, in B_{12} deficiency.
4. Correction with added folinic acid (5-formyl THF) to <5% in both B_{12} and folate deficiencies.
5. Correction, partial, with added methyl-THF in folate deficiency.
6. There may be partial correction with both B_{12} and methyl-THF in mixed B_{12} and folate deficiency.
7. A microtitre plate method is reported to be less cumbersome and more economic in sample requirement, thus allowing more replicate tests.[53] The use of peripheral blood lymphocytes has been criticized since normal cultured cells develop folate deficiency.[79]

INVESTIGATION OF THE ABSORPTION OF B_{12}

An important step in the study of a patient suffering from B_{12} deficiency is to establish whether or not he or she has the capacity to absorb the vitamin normally. This is best accomplished with the aid of B_{12} labelled by a radioactive isotope of cobalt. Originally, ^{60}Co was employed, but the shorter-lived isotopes, ^{58}Co (half-life 71 days) and ^{57}Co (half-life 270 days) are more suitable. ^{57}Co emits γ-rays of several energies, the most important being of 122 keV, and no particulate energies are emitted. It can be used in larger tracer doses than ^{58}Co and is the isotope of choice when a well-type scintillation counter is used. ^{58}Co can be used with all counting methods, but its counting efficiency is low and relatively large amounts must be given to obtain adequate count-rates, especially for measuring blood radioactivity. Labelled cyano-cobalamin is used routinely.

Method

Give an oral dose of 1 µg (37 kBq) of ^{57}Co- or ^{58}Co-B_{12}* in about 200 ml of water to a subject who has fasted overnight, no food being taken for a further 2 h. Prepare a standard from a similar dose of radioactive B_{12} suitably diluted in water.

Either the urinary excretion or whole-body counting test is then utilized to assess the absorption of the test dose.[19,57] The hepatic uptake and faecal excretion methods are obsolete and the estimation of plasma radioactivity is unreliable. These previously used methods are not described here. The urinary-excretion test has been recommended by the International Committee for Standardization in Haematology as being the most convenient and reliable in practice.[44]

If absorption is found to be subnormal, the test can be repeated with the simultaneous administration of intrinsic factor mixed with the liquid dose.[52]

Urinary excretion (Schilling) test[69]

Give 1.0 µg of radioactive B_{12} (^{57}Co or ^{58}Co) by mouth to the fasting patient and at the same time give 1 mg of non-radioactive hydroxocobalamin intramuscularly (a flushing dose). Collect the urine for 24 h. Measure the radioactivity of this urine and of a standard. Calculate the percentage dose excreted in the urine as follows:

$$\frac{\text{Total cpm in 24 h urine}}{\text{cpm in standard (= test dose)}} \times 100.$$

---

*E.g., Amersham International:
    Co^{57}-B_{12}, Code CR51P; Co^{58}-B_{12} Code CR3P.

It is, however, both more convenient and cheaper to prepare 10 test doses at one time. Vial CT3P* contains c 10 µg of B_{12} with activity c 0.37 MBq (10 µCi). Using sterile containers, dilute the contents to 100 ml in water. Take 100 µl for the standard. Dispense the remainder in 10 ml volumes. Dilute the 100 µl standard to 100 ml in water. Store doses and standard at 4°C. This standard is a 1 in 10 000 dilution of the test dose.

Mix the 24 h urine collection well and estimate the radioactivity in equal volumes of urine and standard. Calculate the percentage of the test dose excreted as follows:

$$\frac{\text{Urine cpm} \times \text{Urine volume (ml)}}{\text{Standard cpm} \times \text{Dilution of standard}} \times 100.$$

A dual isotope (Dicopac) kit of free ^{58}Co-B_{12} and ^{57}Co-B_{12} bound to intrinsic factor is available (Amersham International). The dual test can be used with whole-body counting.

Interpretation of results

The normal urinary excretion is >10% of the test dose in the first 24 h; in patients with pernicious anaemia or with B_{12} deficiency associated with intestinal malabsorption, the excretion is usually <5%. This can be increased in pernicious anaemia by the simultaneous administration of intrinsic factor, whereas absorption remains sub-normal if the malabsorption is due to an intestinal defect. The second test dose, with intrinsic factor, can be given 48 h after the first, provided that an additional flushing injection is given 24 h after the first oral dose. Low results may be found in patients with renal disease, when excretion may be delayed. In such cases urine should be collected for 48 h.

The method is generally reliable (except in renal disease); the results are clear-cut and the technique is simple. The need for large flushing doses of B_{12} is a disadvantage in that they may interfere with other studies, and the tests depend on a complete collecton of urine.

Deficiency of B_{12} and of folate may cause temporary malabsorption of B_{12}[39]. It is advisable to repeat the tests which have given discrepant results after replacement therapy for 2 months.

With the Dicopac test the results differ from those of separately performed tests,[27] partly because of the difference in the size of oral doses and partly because some exchange of radionuclides occurs in the combined test. In normal subjects the quoted figures are [58]Co 11–28% and [57]Co 12–30%; and in pernicious anaemia they are [58]Co 0–5.5% and [57]Co 5–14%. A ratio of % [57]Co excreted/[58]Co excreted may be calculated and this may be of value if the urine collection is incomplete.[13c] Normal subjects and patients with intestinal malabsorption give a ratio of 0.7–1.5, whereas patients with pernicious anaemia usually give ratios >1.8.

Achlorhydria due to atrophic gastritis and following partial gastrectomy may be associated with normal absorption of aqueous B_{12} but malabsorption of protein-bound B_{12}.[24] Tests with B_{12} attached to binders in egg yolk[25] and in chicken serum[23] have been described. The 'food Schilling test' may help to diagnose malabsorption of dietary B_{12} when normal Schilling tests results are found in patients with atrophic gastritis or other conditions with otherwise unexplained low serum B_{12} levels.

Whole body counting

The advantage of this method is that a 'flushing' dose of B_{12} is not given so that the patient's B_{12} metabolism is not affected, though the necessity to withhold treatment may sometimes be a disadvantage.[9] It requires specialized equipment and, normally, a low background room. Initial counting (100% value) is performed 1 h after swallowing the dose. Repeat counting is done after 7 days to establish how much has been retained. A system has been described which can be used in the absence of a low-background room and fairly accurate measurements of [58]Co absorption have been reported.[9] [57]Co-B_{12} can also be used[74] and a double isotope test has been described.[8]

Results

Normal subjects absorb >30% and usually >50% of a 1 μg dose. Patients with PA absorb <20%.

ESTIMATION OF INTRINSIC FACTOR (IF) IN GASTRIC JUICE[7]

Direct estimation of the IF content of gastric juice is useful in the diagnosis of PA, particularly when there is associated small intestinal disease which complicates the interpretation of B_{12} absorption studies.

Principle

B_{12} binding by the gastric juice is due to its content of IF and R proteins (salivary and gastric). Normally more than 90% is due to IF. Estimation of this may be done by determining the difference in the binding capacity of the gastric juice with and without neutralization of the IF by serum IF antibody (IFA).[35] An assay in which the non-IF binding is neutralized by the addition of B_{12} analogue (e.g. cobinamide) gives comparable results, does not depend upon the availability of IFA of certain potency and is simpler.

This technique is described here.

Reagents

Buffer. 0.01 mol/l Tris-HCl, pH 8.0 containing 0.15 mol/l NaCl and 50 μg/ml 22% bovine albumin.

Activated albumin-coated charcoal (25 g/l). Heat 2.5 g of activated charcoal (Norit A*) at 110°C overnight. Suspend in 50 ml of water. Add 6.8 ml of 22% bovine albumin in 50 ml of water and mix well for 10 s. The coating is done immediately before use.

Vitamin B_{12}. Dilute [57]Co-B_{12} (Code CT2), 45–85 ng B_{12}, 370–740 kBq (10–20 μCi)**, with water to 1 ng/l. Store in the dark at 4°C. This is stable for 3 months. For the assay add non-radioactive cyanocobalamin to give a solution containing 200 ng/l.

Cobinamide. Make up a stock solution of 10 mg/l. Store at 4°C. For use dilute to give 50 ng in 100 μl.

Collection of gastric juice. Collect into an icecooled container the basal secretion for 1 h followed by a further hour collection after subcutaneous administration of pentagastrin as a

---

*Merck; Sigma.
**Lifescreen, Watford, UK.

Table 22.5 Preparation of control and sample tubes for the estimation of intrinsic factor in gastric juice

Tube	Buffer (ml)	Gastric juice (µl)	Cobinamide (µl)
A Untreated	3.7	0	0
B Charcoal control	2.2	0	0
C Standard	2.0	100	100
D Test	2.0	100	100

stimulus (8 µg/kg body weight). Centrifuge at 1000g for 15 min to separate the mucus. Record the pH. Take clear juice, add sufficient 5 mol/1 NaOH to obtain a pH of 11.0, stand for 20 min at room temperature to inactivate peptidases and then neutralize to pH 7.0 with 1 mol/l HCl. Measure the volume. It may be stored for some months at −20°C without loss of activity.

Method

Set up controls and samples, in duplicate, as shown in Table 22.5. Mix and incubate at c 20°C for 30 min. Add 100 µl of ^{57}Co-B$_{12}$ to each tube. After mixing, again leave at c 20°C for 10 min. Add 1.5 ml of coated charcoal suspension to all tubes except A. Mix and incubate for 10 min. Centrifuge the tubes and deliver 2 ml into counting vials. Measure the radioactivity and average the counts.

Calculation

By definition 1 unit (u) of IF binds 1 ng of B$_{12}$.

$$\text{Units IF/ml gastric juice} = \frac{D - B}{C - A} \times 10 \times 20$$

The total binding capacity of a gastric juice may be determined by omitting the cobinamide in the assay.

Interpretation

The normal range varies widely from 15 to 115 u/ml with a total secretion per hour of 500 to several thousand units.[13b] In females the concentration is the same as in males, but because of a smaller volume of gastric juice, there is only half the total secretion. The concentration in PA is usually zero and never more than 10 u/ml, with a total secretion of less than 250 u in 1 h.

INTRINSIC FACTOR ANTIBODIES[13g]

Two types of antibody to IF have been detected in the sera of patients with PA. Type I (blocking antibody) prevents the attachment of B$_{12}$ to IF, while Type II (precipitating antibody) prevents the attachment of IF or the IF-B$_{12}$ complex to the ileal receptors. Type I antibody is present in over two-thirds of cases of PA; Type II probably occurs with equal frequency[15] and has been reported to be even more frequent.[77] The presence of antibodies in a patient under investigation for PA confirms the diagnosis and renders an absorption test unnecessary. The antibodies occur only rarely in conditions other than PA, e.g. they have been described in a few patients with thyroid disorders, diabetes mellitus and the Eaton-Lambert myasthenic syndrome. The gastric juice in PA usually contains IF antibodies, but tests for these are not carried out routinely and will not be described here.

ESTIMATION OF TYPE 1 INTRINSIC FACTOR ANTIBODY

Reagents

Normal gastric juice. Determine the IF content. Dilute in 0.154 mol/l NaCl to give a solution containing 25 µ/ml. Store at −20°C in volumes suitable for a batch of tests.

Normal serum. Pool the sera from six or more normal subjects.

^{57}Co-B$_{12}$. 50 µg/l. Code CT2*.

Albumin-coated charcoal. 25g/l (p. 429).

Method

Set out a series of tubes, in duplicate, as shown in Table 22.6. Mix and incubate at room temperature

---

*Lifescreen, Watford, UK.

Table 22.6 Estimation of Type I intrinsic factor antibody. Preparation of control and sample tubes

Tube	0.154 mol/l NaCl (ml)	Gastric juice (µl)	Normal serum (µl)	Test serum (µl)
A Radioactive control	3.7	0	0	0
B Charcoal control	2.2	0	0	0
C Normal serum pool	1.85	50	300	0
D Positive serum	1.85	50	0	300
E Test serum	1.85	50	0	300

for 30 min with periodic mixing. Add 5ng of ^{57}Co-B$_{12}$ in 100 µl volumes to all tubes. Incubate at room temperature for 10 min. Add 1.5 ml of charcoal suspension to tube B onwards. Mix and incubate at room temperature for 5 min. Centrifuge at 1500g for 15 min and transfer 2 ml of the supernatant to counting vials. Measure the radioactivity and calculate the ratio of normal to test serum counts.

Interpretation

Negative sera, ratio <1.02; positive sera, ratio >1.10. Ratios between these figures are termed indeterminate and the test should be repeated using 500 µl volumes of the test and normal sera. These ratios are given as guidelines, and each laboratory should determine its own normal range.

In this method the proportion of ng IF to ml serum is 4:1.[71] The sensitivity of the test can be enhanced by reducing this proportion but preliminary treatment of the sera with a microfine silica QUSO is required to neutralize the effect of their transcobalamins.[59]

ESTIMATION OF TYPE II (PRECIPITATING OR CO-PRECIPITATING) INTRINSIC FACTOR ANTIBODY

Reagents

Barbitone buffer, pH 8.3. 0.04 mol/l sodium diethyl barbitone 100 ml; 0.2 mol/l HCl 6.21 ml. Make up the solution freshly every 4 weeks, and keep at 4°C.

Anhydrous sodium sulphate. 300 g/l and 150 g/l.

Albumin-coated charcoal. (See p. 429).

Gastric intrinsic factor/^{57}Co-B$_{12}$ complex. For every 1 ml of normal gastric juice add an excess of ^{57}Co-B$_{12}$, e.g. 200 ng. Leave at c 20°C for 30 min, and then remove excess (free) B$_{12}$ by adding 1 ml of charcoal suspension. After a further 10 min at c 20°C, centrifuge the suspension for 15 min at 1500g; dispense the supernatant in 2 ml volumes and store at −20°C.

Method

Place 0.3 ml of serum, including negative and positive control sera, in 10 ml centrifuge tubes. Add 0.5 ml of barbitone buffer and 1.0 ml of IF/^{57}Co-B$_{12}$ complex, diluted 1 to 5 with saline. Incubate at 37°C for 30 min. Add 2 ml of 300 g/l sodium sulphate, warmed to 37°C. After mixing, incubate for a further 10 min, and then centrifuge the suspensions at 1500g for 15–20 min. Discard the supernatant and add 1 ml of 150 g/l sodium sulphate and centrifuge twice. After discarding the supernatant, add 3.5 ml of saline to each tube to dissolve the precipitate. Place 3 ml volumes from each tube in counting vials and count the radioactivity. A radioactive control containing 1.0 ml of the diluted IF/^{57}Co-B$_{12}$ complex and 2.0 ml of water is also set up and counted.

Interpretation

Precipitating antibodies are indicated by a high count in the precipitate, usually ten times higher than that of the negative controls. A sensitive radioimmune assay using ^{125}I-labelled IF[15] and an ELISA technique[78] for the simultaneous detection of Types I and II antibodies have been reported recently. Using this technique,[77] Type-II antibodies were detected in 39 of the 40 sera containing Type-II antibodies only, suggesting that the occurrence of Type-II antibodies both alone and in combination with Type I is a more common feature than has been previously recognized.

Intrinsic factor antibody kits

A radioisotope competitive binding assay kit which detects binding antibodies only is available from Diagnostic Products Corporation Ltd. An ELISA kit which detects both Type-I and Type-II antibodies is available from Cambridge Life Sciences.

PARIETAL CELL ANTIBODIES

These are present in the sera of about 90% of patients with PA but also occur in other conditions and with increasing frequency with age so that about 15% of elderly individuals may exhibit them. They are usually detected by an immunofluorescence technique, using human or rat stomach.

PLASMA (OR SERUM) B_{12} BINDING CAPACITY[13a,35]

The total binding capacity (TBBC) of plasma comprises the sum total of the serum B_{12} concentration and the plasma unsaturated binding capacity (UBBC). 80% or more of the serum B_{12} is bound to transcobalamin I (TC I). A small fraction is bound to TC II, and TC III is virtually unsaturated. TC I and TC III (R binders) are both glycosolated proteins and differ only in their sugar moiety. Congenital absence of R binders results in a very low serum B_{12}, normal TBBC, no evidence of B_{12} deficiency and no adverse effects. It is suggested that some 'idiopathic' low B_{12} levels may be due to a decrease in R binder concentration.[10]

TC II delivers B_{12} to the tissues. Rare congenital absence or functional abnormality results in a fulminating pancytopenia and megaloblastosis usually within 2 months of birth. The serum B_{12} is normal, the UBBC is reduced, B_{12} absorption is reduced and the deoxyuridine suppression test is abnormal and corrected by B_{12}.

Estimation of the unsaturated binding capacity of the individual TCs requires a separation technique; the adsorption of TC II to silica powder[46] is a suitable procedure. Estimation of the UBBC and of its components needs care in the collection of the sample. To minimize release of TC I and TC III from granulocytes blood should be added to an anticoagulant mixture of 1 mg EDTA and 2 mg sodium fluoride per ml blood.[70] If serum is used, this should be separated within 2 h of collection.

ESTIMATION OF UBBC

Requirements

^{57}Co B_{12} Code CT2 (Lifescreen, Watford, UK). Dilute ^{57}Co B_{12} specific activity c 6.6–8.1 MBq/µg in non-radioactive cyanocobalamin (Duncan Flockhart) to give a concentration of 2 µg/l as follows:

Dilute cyanocobalamin 1000 µg/ml 1 in 100 in water and add 50 µl to 1 ml ^{57}Co B_{12}. Make this up to 5 ml, mix and aliquot into 0.3 ml amounts and store at −20°C. On day of assay thaw, add 14.7 ml of water and mix.

Albumin-coated charcoal

Suspend 1 g of activated charcoal (DARCO G60)* in 20 ml water and dispense 0.67 ml of 30% bovine serum albumin in a further 20 ml of water. Add the albumin to the charcoal suspension with constant mixing for 10 s. Prepare fresh for each assay.

Method

Set up a series of conical centrifuge tubes containing plasma or 9 g/l NaCl as shown in Table 22.7. Add 1 ml of ^{57}Co-B_{12} to each tube. After mixing and incubating at c 20°C for 30 min, add 2 ml of

---

*Merck Ltd.

Table 22.7 Preparation of tubes for the estimation of plasma B_{12} binding capacity

Tube	Saline (ml)	Plasma (ml)
A Standard	2.5	0
B Supernatant control	0.5	0
C Test	0	0.5

charcoal suspension to each tube except A. After standing for 10 min, centrifuge the tubes at 1500g for 10 min. Pipette 3 ml volumes of the supernatant into counting vials. Measure the radioactivity and correct for background counts.

Calculation

$$UBBC \ (ng/l) = \frac{C-B}{A} \times ng/l \ ^{57}Co\text{-}B_{12} \times Plasma \ dilution$$

If the UBBC is equal to or greater than the amount of ^{57}Co-B_{12} added, the test should be repeated after appropriately diluting the plasma with saline.

Normal range

The normal range for serum UBBC is 670–1200 ng/l; that of plasma collected into EDTA-sodium fluoride is 505–1208 ng/l[70].

TRANSCOBALAMIN SEPARATION

A variety of techniques are available for the separation and measurement of transcobalamin I, II and III, each being based on some physico-chemical difference between them. The method described here[46] is simple to perform and reliable. It should be noted, however, that as cobalamin is added to a volume of serum to saturate available binders a functionally ineffective TC II would not be detected.

SEPARATION OF TRANSCOBALAMIN II FROM TRANSCOBALAMINS I AND III

Requirements

Microfine precipitated silica (non crystalline) QUSO (Croxton and Garry, Surrey).

Method

After counting the UBBC add 90 mg of QUSO to each sample and blank, mix, centrifuge at 1500g for 10 min and remove the supernatant into a 10 ml flat bottomed polystyrene tube. Count both sets of tubes on a γ-counter. Calculations for separated TC II and TC I + III are the same as for the UBBC.

TRANSCOBLAMIN I AND III SEPARATION

Requirements

1. Diethylaminoethyl cellulose (DE23) Whatman (Fibrous anion exchanger).
2. 0.06 M Phosphate buffer pH 6.3.
3. Stock solution (A) KH_2PO_4 8.165 g in 1 litre distilled water.
4. Stock solution (B) Na_2HPO_4 8.517 g in 1 litre distilled water.
5. To prepare buffer for assay mix 162 ml (A) with 38 ml (B).
6. 0.02 M Phosphate buffer pH 6.3.
7. Add 10 ml of 0.06 M buffer as prepared above to 20 ml of water mix and discard 2 ml.
8. Add 2.4 g of DE23 to 28 ml of 0.02 M buffer and allow to equilibrate for at least 10 min.

Method

TC I and III are taken up by DE23. TC III is eluted off by the 0.06 M buffer leaving TC I on the DE23.

To each tube containing supernatant after removal from TC II, add 2 ml of pre-wetted DE23 and leave the tubes to mix on a rotary mixer for 10 min. Add 5 ml of 0.06 M buffer and continue mixing for a further 10 min. Centrifuge at 1500g for 10 min; discard supernatant. Add 5 ml of fresh 0.06 M buffer, mix for 10 min, centrifuge, discard supernatant and repeat once more. Count the tubes containing TC I on a γ-counter and calculate as before. The TC III values are obtained by subtracting TC I from the TC I and III result.

Normal range
UBBC 520–1132 ng/l
TC I 49–132 ng/l.
TC II 402–930 ng/l.
TC III 80–280 ng/l.

RESPONSE TO TREATMENT AS AN AID TO DIAGNOSIS

Assessment of response to treatment should be an integral part of the diagnosis of a mega-loblastic anaemia. An optimum response is shown by the red cell count rising, depending upon the severity of the anaemia, to 3.0×10^{12}/l and by at least 1.0×10^{12}/l, or to normal by the 15th day after the start of therapy. A maximum reticulocyte count occurs on the 6th or 7th day of therapy. In patients with little or no anaemia, therapeutic doses of the deficient vitamin should normalize the MCV within 3–4 months. This response confirms former deficiency but is not specific for either vitamin and depends upon other causes for macrocytosis, especially alcohol intake and smoking, and also iron status, remaining unaltered.

A haematological response to pharmacological doses of folic acid (5 mg daily) occurs in B_{12} deficient megaloblastic anaemia. However, B_{12} neuropathy is aggravated or may even be precipitated, so B_{12} deficiency should be excluded before folic acid is given.

REFERENCES

[1] ADAMS, J. F. and McEWAIN, F. C. (1974). The separation of free and bound vitamin B_{12}. *British Journal of Haematology*, **26**, 581.

[2] ANDERSON, B.B. (1964). Investigations into the Euglena method for the assay of vitamin B_{12} in serum. *Journal of Clinical Pathology*, **17**, 14.

[3] ANDERSON, B. and COWAN, J. D. (1968). Effect of light on the *Lactobacillus casei* microbiological assay. *Journal of Clinical Pathology*, **21**, 85.

[4] BAIN, B., BROOM, G. W., WOODSIDE, J., LITWINCZUK, R. A and WICKREMASINGE, S. N. (1982). An assessment of a radioisotope assay for vitamin B_{12}, using an intrinsic factor preparation with R protein blocked by cobinamide. *Journal of Clinical Pathology*, **35**, 1110.

[5] BAIN, B. J., WICKREMASINGHE, S. N., BROOM, G. W., LITWINCZUK, R. A. and SIMS, J. (1984). Assessment of the value of a competitive protein binding radioassay of folic acid in the detection of folic acid deficiency. *Journal of Clinical Pathology*, **37**, 888.

[6] BARAKAT, R. M. and EKINS, R. P. (1961). Assay of vitamin B_{12} in blood. *Lancet*, **ii**, 25.

[7] BEGLEY, J. A. and TRACHTENBERG, A. (1979). An assay for intrinsic factor based on blocking of the R binder of gastric juice by cobinamide. *Blood*, **53**, 788.

[8] BRIEDIS, D., McINTYRE, P. A., JUDISCH, J. and WAGNER, H. N. (1973). An evaluation of a dual isotope method for the measurement of vitamin B_{12} absorption. *Journal of Nuclear Medicine*, **14**, 135.

[9] CALLENDER, S. T., WITTS, L. J., WARNER, G. T. and OLIVER, R. (1966). The use of a simple wholebody counter for haematological investigations. *British Journal of Haematology*, **12**, 276.

[10] CARMEL, R. (1988). R-binder deficiency. A clinically benign cause of cobalamin deficiency. *Journal of the American Medical Association*, **250**, 1886.

[11] CARMEL, R. and COLTMAN, C. A. (1969). Radioassay for serum vitamin B_{12} with the use of saliva as the vitamin B_{12} binder. *Journal of Laboratory and Clinical Medicine*, **74**, 967.

[12] CARMEL, R, and KARNAZE, D. S. (1985). The deoxyuridine suppression test identifies subtle cobalamin deficiency in patients without typical megaloblastic anemia. *Journal of the American Medical Association*, **253**, 1284.

[13] CHANARIN, I. (1979). *The Megaloblastic Anaemias*, 2nd edn, (a) p. 59, (b) p. 87, (c) p. 121, (d) p. 190, (e) p. 193, (f) p. 194, (g) p. 362. Blackwell Scientific Publications, Oxford.

[14] CHEN, I. W., SILBERSTEIN, E. S., MAXON, H. R., SPERLING, M. and BARNES, E. (1981). Clinical significance of serum vitamin B_{12} measured by radioassay using pure intrinsic factor. *Journal of Nuclear Medicine*, **22**, 447.

[15] CONN, D. A. (1986). Detection of Type I and Type II antibodies to intrinsic factor. *Medical Laboratory Sciences*, **43**, 148.

[16] COOK, T. D., CICHOWICZ, D. J., GEORGE, S., LAWLER, A. and SHANE, B. (1987). Mammalian folipolyglutamate synthetase. 4. In vitro and in vivo metabolism of folates and analogues and regulation of folate homeostasis. *Biochemistry*, **26**, 530.

[17] COOPER, B.A., FEHEDY, V. and BLANSHAY, P. (1986). Recognition of deficiency of vitamin B_{12} using measurement of serum concentration. *Journal of Laboratory and Clinical Medicine*, **107**, 447.

[18] COOPER, B. A. and WHITEHEAD, V. M. (1978). Evidence that some patients with pernicious anaemia are not recognised by radiodilution assay for cobalamin in serum. *New England Journal of Medicine*, **299**, 816.

[19] COTTRALL, M. F., WELLS, D. G., TROTT, N. G. and RICHARDSON, N. E. G. (1971). Radioactive vitamin B_{12}

absorption studies: comparison of the whole-body retention, urinary excretion and eight-hour plasma levels of radioactive vitamin B_{12}. *Blood*, **38**, 604.

[20]CURTIS, A. D., MUSSETT, M. V. and KENNEDY, D. A. (1986). British Standard for human serum vitamin B_{12}. *Clinical and Laboratory Haematology*, **8**, 135.

[21]DAVIS, R. E., NICOL, D. J. and KELLY, A. (1970). An automated method for the measurement of folate activity. *Journal of Clinical Pathology*, **23**, 47.

[22]DAWSON, D. W., FISH, D. I., FREW, I. D. O., ROOME, T. and TILSTON, I. (1987). Laboratory diagnosis of megaloblastic anaemia: current methods assessed by external quality assurance trials. *Journal of Clinical Pathology*, **40**, 393.

[23]DAWSON, D. W., SAWERS, A. H. and SHARMA, R. K. (1984). Malabsorption of protein bound vitamin B_{12}. *British Medical Journal*, **288**, 675.

[24]DOSCHERHOLMEN, A., McMAHON, J. and RIPLEY, D. (1978). Inhibitory effect of eggs in vitamin B_{12} absorption: description of a simple ovalbumin ^{57}Co-vitamin B_{12} absorption test. *British Journal of Haematology*, **33**, 261.

[25]DOSCHERHOLMEN, A., SILVIS, S. and McMAHON, J. (1983). Dual Schilling test for measuring absorption of food-bound and free vitamin B_{12} simultaneously. *American Journal of Clinical Pathology*, **80**, 490.

[26]EKINS, R. P. (1974). Radioimmunoassay and saturation analysis. Basic principles. *British Medical Bulletin*, **30**, 3.

[27]ENGLAND, J. M., SNASHALL, E. A. and DE SILVA, P. M. (1981). Comparison of the DICOPAC with the conventional Schilling test. *Journal of Clinical Pathology*, **34**, 1191.

[28]FISH, D. I. and DAWSON, D. W. (1983). Comparison of methods used in commercial kits for the assay of serum vitamin B_{12}. *Clinical and Laboratory Haematology*, **5**, 271.

[29]FRENKEL, E. P., WHITE, J. D., REISCH, J. S. and SHEENAN, R. G. (1973). Comparison of two methods of the radioassay of vitamin B_{12} in serum. *Clinical Chemistry*, **19**, 1327.

[30]GANESHAGURU, K. and HOFFBRAND, A. V. (1978). The effect of deoxyuridine, vitamin B_{12}, folate and alcohol on the uptake of thymidine and on the deoxyuridine triphosphate concentration in normal and megaloblastic cells. *British Journal of Haematology*, **40**, 29.

[31]GHITIS, J. (1966). The labile folate of milk. *American Journal of Clinical Nutrition*, **18**, 452.

[32]GILOIS, C. R., BEATTIE, G. and MILLS, S. P. (1986). Measurement of vitamin B_{12} and serum folic acid; a comparison of methods. *Medical Laboratory Sciences*, **43**, 140.

[33]GILOIS, C. R. and DUNBAR, D. R. (1987). Measurement of low serum and red cell folate levels; a comparison of analytical methods. *Medical Laboratory Sciences*, **44**, 33.

[34]GIVAS, J. and GUTCHO, S. (1975). pH dependence of the binding of folate to milk binder in radioassay of folates. *Clinical Chemistry*, **21**, 427.

[35]GOTTLIEB, C., LAU, K. S., WASSERMAN, L. R. and HERBERT, V. (1965). Rapid charcoal assays for intrinsic factor (IF), gastric juice unsaturated B_{12} binding capacity, antibody to IF and serum unsaturated B_{12} binding capacity. *Blood*, **25**, 6.

[36]GREEN, R., NEWARK, P. A., MUSSO, A. M. and MOLLIN, D. L. (1974). The use of chicken serum for the measurement of serum vitamin B_{12} by radioisotope dilution. Description of method and comparison with microbiological assay results. *British Journal of*

Haematology, **27**, 507.

[37]GUTCHO, S. and MANSBACH, L. (1977). Simultaneous radioassay of serum vitamin B_{12} and folic acid. *Clinical Chemistry*, **23**, 1609.

[38]HERBERT, V. (1966). Aseptic addition method for *Lactobacillus casei* assay of folate activity in human serum. *Journal of Clinical Pathology*, **19**, 12.

[39]HERBERT, V. (1969). Transient (reversible) malabsorption of vitamin B_{12}. *British Journal of Haematology*, **17**, 213.

[40]HERBERT, V., COLMAN, N., PALAT, D. et al (1984). Is there is a 'gold standard' for human serum, vitamin B_{12} assay? *Journal of Laboratory and Clinical Medicine*, **104**, 829.

[41]HERZLICH, B. and HERBERT, V. (1988). Depletion of serum holotranscobalamin II. An early sign of negative vitamin B_{12} balance. *Laboratory Investigations*, **58**, 332.

[42]HOFFBRAND, A. V., NEWCOMBE, B. F. A. and MOLLIN, D.L. (1966). Method of assay of red cell folate activity and the value of the assay as a test for folate deficiency. *Journal of Clinical Pathology*, **19**, 17.

[43]HOFFBRAND, A. V. and JACKSON, B. F. A. (1993). Correction of the DNA synthesis depletion in vitamin B_{12} deficiency by tetrahydrofolate: evidence in favour of the methyl-folate trap hypothesis as the cause of megaloblastic anaemia in vitamin B_{12} deficiency. *British Journal of Haematology*, **83**, 643.

[44]INTERNATIONAL COMMITTEE FOR STANDARDIZATION IN HAEMATOLOGY (1981). Recommended method for the measurement of vitamin B_{12} absorption. *Journal of Nuclear Medicine*, **22**, 1091.

[45]INTERNATIONAL COMMITTEE FOR STANDARDIZATION IN HAEMATOLOGY (1981). Proposed serum standard for human serum vitamin B_{12} assay. *British Journal of Haematology*, **64**, 809.

[46]JACOB, E. and HERBERT, V. (1975). Measurement of unsaturated 'granulocyte-related' (TCI and TCIII) and 'liver-related' (TCII) B_{12} binders by instant batch separation using a microfine precipitate of silica (QUSO G32). *Journal of Laboratory and Clinical Medicine*, **88**, 505.

[47]KOLHOUSE, J. F., KONDO, H., ALLEN, N. C., PODELL, E. and ALLEN, R. H. (1978). Cobalamin analogues are present in human plasma and can mask cobalamin deficiency because current radioisotope dilution assays are not specific for true cobalamin. *New England Journal of Medicine*, **299**, 785.

[48]KUEMMERIE, G. L., BOLTINGHOUSE, G. L., DELBY, S. M., LANE, T. L. and SIMONDSEN, R. P. (1992). Automated assay of vitamin B_{12} by the Abbott IMX analyser. *Clinical Chemistry*, **38**, 2073.

[49]LAVOIE, A., TRIPP, E. and HOFFBRAND, A. V. (1974). The effect of vitamin B_{12} deficiency on methylfolate metabolism and pteryolpolyglutamate synthesis in human cells. *Clinical Science and Molecular Medicine*, **47**, 617.

[50]LEE-OWEN, V., BOLTON, A. E. and CARR, P. J. (1979). Formation of a vitamin B_{12}-serum complex on heating at alkaline pH. *Clinica Chimica Acta*, **93**, 239.

[51]LINDENBAUM, J., HEALTON, E. B., SAVAGE, D. G. et al (1988). Neuropsychiatric disorders caused by cobalamin deficiency in the absence of anaemia or macrocytosis. *New England Journal of Medicine*, **318**, 1720.

[52]McDONALD, J. W. D. and BARTON, W. B. (1975). Spurious Schilling test results obtained with intrinsic factor enclosed in capsules. *Annals of Internal Medicine*, **83**, 827.

[53]MATTHEWS, J. and WICKREMASINGHE, S. N. (1986). A method for performing deoxyuridine suppression on microtitre plates. *Clinical and Laboratory Haematology*, **8**, 61.

[54]METZ, J., KELLY, A., SWETT, V. C., WAXMAN, S. and HERBERT, V. (1968). Deranged DNA synthesis by bone marrow from vitamin B_{12}-deficient humans. *British Journal of Haematology*, **14**, 575.

[55]MILLBANK, L., DAVIS, R. E., RAWLINS, N. and WATERS, A. H. (1970). Automation of the assay of folate in serum and whole blood. *Journal of Clinical Pathology*, **23**, 54.

[56]MITCHELL, G. A., POCHRON, S. P., SMUTNY, P. V. and GUTTY, R. (1976). Decreased radioassay values for folate after serum extraction when pteroylglutamic acid standards are used. *Clinical Chemistry*, **22**, 647.

[57]MUIR, M. and CHANARIN, I. (1983). The assay of serum cobalamin by solid phase saturation analysis. In *Methods in Hematology, Vol. 10: The Cobalamins*. Ed. C.A. Hall, p. 85. Churchill Livingstone, Edinburgh.

[58]NETTELAND, B. and BAKKE, O. M. (1977). Inadequate sample-preparation technique as a source of error in determination of erythrocyte folate by competitive binding of radioassay. *Clinical Chemistry*, **23**, 1505.

[59]NIMO, R. E. and CARMEL, R. (1987). Increased sensitivity of detection of the blocking (type I) anti-intrinsic factor antibody. *American Journal of Clinical Pathology*, **88**, 729.

[60]OMER, A. (1969). Factors influencing the release of assayable folate from erythrocytes. *Journal of Clinical Pathology*, **22**, 217.

[61]O'SULLIVAN, J. J., LEEMING, R. J., LYNCH, S. S. and POLLOCK, A. (1992). Radioimmunoassay that measures serum vitamin B_{12}. *Journal of Clinical Pathology*, **45**, 328.

[62]OXLEY, D. K. (1984). Serum vitamin B_{12} assays. *Archives of Pathology Laboratory Medicine*, **108**, 277.

[63]PALTRIDGE, G., RUDZKI, Z. and RYALL, R. G. (1980). Validity of transcobalamin II-based radioassay for the determination of serum vitamin B_{12} concentrations. *Annals of Clinical Biochemistry*, **17**, 287.

[64]RAVEN, J. L., ROBSON, M. B., MORGAN, J. O. and HOFFBRAND, A. V. (1972). Comparison of three methods for measuring vitamin B_{12} in serum: radioisotopic, *Euglena gracilis* and *leichamannii*. *British Journal of Haematology*, **22**, 21.

[65]REYNOSO, G. and MACKENZIE, J. R. (1982). Are ligand assay methods specific for cobalamin? *American Journal of Clinical Pathology*, **78**, 621.

[66]ROBARD, D. (1978). Data processing for radioimmunoassays; an overview. In *Clinical Immunochemistry*. Eds. Natelson, S., Pesce, A. and Dietz, A., p. 477. American Association for Clinical Chemistry, Washington.

[67]ROTHENBERG, S. P. (1968). A radioassay for serum B_{12} using unsaturated transcobalamin I as the binding protein. *Blood*, **31**, 44.

[68]ROTHENBERG, S. P., MARCOULIS, G. P., SCHWARZ, S. and LADER, E. (1984). Measurement of cyanocobalamin in serum by a specific radioimmunoassay. *Journal of Laboratory and Clinical Medicine*, **103**, 959.

[69]SCHILLING, R. F. (1953). Intrinsic factor studies. II. The effect of gastric juice on the urinary excretion of radioactivity after the oral administration of radioactive vitamin B_{12}. *Journal of Laboratory and Clinical Medicine*, **42**, 860.

[70]SCOTT, J. M., BLOOMFIELD, F. J., STEBBINS, R. and HERBERT, V. (1974). Studies on derivation of transcobalamin III from granulocytes. Enhancement by lithium and elimination by fluoride of *in vitro* increments in vitamin B_{12}-binding capacity. *Journal of Clinical Investigation*, **53**, 228.

[71]SHACKLETON, P. J., FISH, D. I. and DAWSON, D. W. (1989). Intrinsic factor antibody tests. *Journal of Clinical Pathology*, **42**, 210.

[72]SHANE, B., TAMURA, T. and STOKSTAD, E. L. R. (1980). Folate assay: a comparison of radioassay and microbiological methods. *Clinica Chimica Acta*, **100**, 13.

[73]SHUM, R. Y., O'NEILL, B. J. and STREETER, A. M. (1971). Effect of pH changes on the binding of vitamin B_{12} by intrinsic factor. *Journal of Clinical Pathology*, **24**, 239.

[74]TAIT, C. E. and HESP, R. (1976). Measurement of [57]Co-vitamin B_{12} uptake using a static whole-body counter. *British Journal of Radiology*, **49**, 948.

[75]TIBBLING, G. (1969). A method for determination of vitamin B_{12} in serum by radioassay. *Clinica Chimia Acta*, **23**, 209.

[76]WATERS, A. H. and MOLLIN, D. L. (1961). Studies on the folic acid activity of human serum. *Journal of Clinical Pathology*, **14**, 335.

[77]WATERS, H. M., DAWSON, D. W., HOWARTH, J. E. and GEARY, C. G. (1993). High incidence of Type II auto-antibodies in pernicious anaemia. *Journal of Clinical Pathology*, **46**, 45.

[78]WATERS, H. M., SMITH, C., HOWARTH, J. E., DAWSON, D. W. and DELAMORE, I. W. (1989). A new enzyme immunoassay for the detection of total Type I and Type II intrinsic factor antibody. *Journal of Clinical Pathology*, **42**, 307.

[79]WICKRAMASINGHE, S. N. and MATTHEWS, J. H. (1988). Deoxyuridine suppression: biochemical basis and diagnostic applications. *Blood Reviews*, **2**, 168.

[80]AMOS, R. J., DAWSON, D. W., FISH, D. I., LEEMING, R. J. and LINNELL, J. C. (1994) Guidelines on the investigation and diagnosis of cobalamin and folate deficiencies. *Clinical and Laboratory Haematology*, **16**, 101.

23. Iron deficiency anaemia

By M. Worwood

Serum iron   437
Iron-binding capacity   438
Serum transferrin   439

Serum ferritin   439
Enzyme immunoassay   440

ESTIMATION OF SERUM IRON

The method below is a modification[15] of that recommended by the International Committee for Standardization in Haematology (ICSH) and is based on the development of a coloured complex when ferrous iron is treated with a chromagen solution.[12]

Reagents and materials

All reagents must be of analytical grade with the lowest obtainable iron content.

Protein precipitant. 100 g/l trichloracetic acid and 30 ml/l thioglycollic acid in 1 mol/l HCl. This solution may be stored in a dark brown bottle for 2 months.

Chromogen solution. 1.5 mol/l sodium acetate containing 0.025% ferrozine (monosodium 3-(2-pyridil)-5,6-bis(4-phenylsulphonic acid)-1, 2, 4-triazine). Store in a dark brown bottle wrapped in aluminium foil for up to 2 weeks.

Iron standard; stock. Dissolve 100 mg of freshly cleaned pure iron wire in 4 ml of 7 mol/l HCl (overnight) and make up the volume to 1 litre with water.

Iron standard; working. Dilute 2 ml of the stock iron standard in 100 ml water with 5 mmol/l of HCl (= 2 mg/l; 35.8 μmol/l).

Preparation of glassware. It is essential to avoid contamination by iron. Wash all glassware, including reagent bottles, in a detergent solution; soak in 2 mol/l HCl for 24 h and finally rinse in iron-free water. If possible use plastic tubes and bottles.

Iron-free water. Use de-ionized, double-distilled water for the preparation of all solutions and for rinsing glassware.

Method

Place 0.5 ml of serum (free of haemolysis), 0.5 ml of working iron standard and 0.5 ml of iron-free water (as a blank), respectively, in three separate iron-free test-tubes. Add 0.5 ml of protein precipitant to each. Mix the contents vigorously, e.g. with a vortex mixer, and allow to stand for 5 min. Centrifuge the tube containing the serum at 1500g for 15 min to obtain an optically clear supernatant. To 0.5 ml of this supernatant, and to 0.5 ml of each of the other mixtures, add 0.5 ml of the chromogen solution with thorough mixing. After standing for 10 min, measure the absorbance in a spectrophotometer against water at 562 nm.

If EDTA-plasma is used, the colour develops more slowly and the preparation should be allowed to stand for at least 15 min before measuring the absorbance. Iron chelators such as desferrioxamine also delay colour development.[6]

Calculation

Serum iron (µmol/l) =

$$\frac{A^{562} \text{ test} - A^{562} \text{ blank}}{A^{562} \text{ standard} - A^{562} \text{ blank}} \times 35.8$$

AUTOMATED METHODS

A similar procedure may be used, with absorbance measured in a microtitre plate, in which 0.2 ml of serum is required.[30] Methods that do not require centrifugation have obvious advantages in terms of automation, and techniques in which iron is released from transferrin without precipitating serum proteins are widely applied[21] despite considerable problems caused by the high absorbance contributed by the serum.[6] Procedures for measuring serum iron are available for most clinical chemistry analyzers. Serum iron concentrations may also be measured by atomic absorption spectroscopy but this has the disadvantage of measuring any form of iron present.

Serum iron concentrations in health and disease[6]

The mean serum iron concentration of 20 µmol/l is similar in adult males and females. Serum iron concentrations approximate to a normal distribution and the standard deviation is approx 7 µmol/l. This figure does not refer to 'iron replete' subjects, as the groups studied often included subjects with absent iron stores or with frank anaemia (see for example Jacobs et al[16]). However, an upper limit of normal is approximately 32 µmol/l. Mean concentrations of serum iron are higher (22 µmol/l) than the adult mean during the first month of life and fall to the lower mean value of about 12 µmol/l found throughout childhood by the age of 1 year.[18,24]

Measurement of the serum iron concentration alone provides little useful clinical information because of the considerable variation from hour to hour and day to day in normal individuals. Low concentrations (below 13 µmol/l) are found in patients with iron-deficiency anaemia and as responses to inflammation, infection, surgery or chronic disease. Low serum iron concentrations do not, however, necessarily indicate an absence of storage iron. High concentrations are found in liver disease, hypoplastic anaemias, ineffective erythropoiesis and iron overload.

IRON-BINDING CAPACITY

In the plasma, iron is bound to transferrin and the total iron-binding capacity is a measure of this protein. The additional iron-binding capacity of transferrin is known as the 'unsaturated iron-binding capacity'. The serum-iron concentration plus the unsaturated iron-binding capacity together give total iron-binding capacity.

Iron-binding capacity is usually measured by adding an excess of iron and measuring the iron retained after the action of a suitable reagent such as light magnesium carbonate, an ion-exchange resin, haemoglobin-coated charcoal or Sephadex G-25. All methods are empirical, and none is completely satisfactory. That described below is reliable.[13]

ESTIMATION OF TOTAL IRON-BINDING CAPACITY (TIBC)

Principle. Excess iron as ferric chloride is added to serum. Any iron which does not bind to transferrin is removed with excess magnesium carbonate. The iron concentration of the iron-saturated serum is then measured.

Reagents

Basic magnesium carbonate, $MgCO_3$, 'light grade'.
Ferric chloride, $FeCl_3.6H_2O$. A stock iron solution is made by placing 300 mg of ferric chloride and 4 ml of concentrated HCl in a

volumetric flask and making up to 1 litre with water. Make a 1 in 10 dilution with iron-free water on the day of each assay. The 'saturating iron solution' contains 6.2 µg Fe/ml.

Method

Place 1 ml of plasma or serum in an iron-free tube and add 1 ml of saturating iron solution. Mix carefully by hand and leave at room temperature for 15 min. Use a plastic scoop or tube to add 200 mg ($\pm$ 25 mg) of light magnesium carbonate and cap the tube with a rubber stopper covered with Parafilm. Shake vigorously and allow to stand for 30 min with occasional mixing. Centrifuge at 1500g for 30 min. If the supernatant contains traces of magnesium carbonate, remove the supernatant and recentrifuge. Carefully remove 1 ml of the supernatant and treat as serum for the iron estimation described above. Multiply the final result by $\times$ 2.

DETERMINATION OF UNSATURATED IRON-BINDING CAPACITY (UIBC) AND TRANSFERRIN CONCENTRATION

The unsaturated iron-binding capacity may be determined by methods which detect iron remaining, and able to bind to chromogen, after adding a standard and excess amount of iron to the serum.[21] The problems inherent in these direct assays have been summarized.[6] An alternative technique involves the addition of radioactive iron in order to saturate the binding sites followed by measurement of the radioactivity present in the supernatant after treatment with $MgCO_3$ and centrifugation.[6] As for the serum-iron determination, protocols for clinical chemistry analysers often include a method for UIBC. An alternative approach is to measure transferrin directly by an immunological assay. This avoids some of the spuriously high values of TIBC found when the transferrin is saturated and non-transferrin iron is measured.[15] Rate immuno-nephelometric methods are rapid and precise[4] and there is generally a good correlation between the chemical and immunological TIBC.[11] However, Bandi et al[3] reported great variability among a number of immunochemical assays for transferrin.

Normal range of transferrin and total iron-binding capacity

In health the serum transferrin is c 2.0–3.0 g/l, and 1 mg of transferrin binds 1.4 µg of iron. The normal serum total iron-binding capacity is 45–70 µmol/l (250–390 µg/dl), with about 33% saturation.

The iron-binding capacity is raised in iron-deficiency anaemia, and in pregnancy; it is lower then normal in infections, malignant disease and renal disease. In pathological iron overload the iron-binding capacity of the serum is reduced and the serum is completely saturated with iron.

Transferrin saturation

The transferrin saturation is the ratio of the serum iron concentration and the total iron-binding capacity expressed as a percentage. A transferrin saturation of <16% is usually considered to indicate an inadequate iron supply for erythropoiesis.[2] The most valuable use of calculating transferrin saturation is for the detection of genetic haemochromatosis. Even in the early stages of the development of iron overload an elevated transferrin saturation (>60% for men and > 50% for women) is indicative of the disorder.[8]

ASSAY OF SERUM FERRITIN

With the recognition that the small quantity of ferritin in human serum (normal 15–300 µg/l in men) reflects body iron stores, measurement of serum ferritin has been widely adopted as a test for iron deficiency and iron overload.

The first reliable method to be introduced was an immunoradiometric assay[1] in which excess radiolabelled antibody is reacted with ferritin and the excess antibody removed with an immuno-adsorbent. This assay was supplanted by the two-site immunoradiometric assay[19] which is sensitive and convenient but suffers from the 'high-dose hook' effect (see later). This means that at high concentrations of ferritin the amount of labelled antibody bound to the tube or bead begins to decrease instead of continuing to increase. Since then the principle of the two-site immunoradiometric assay has been extended to non-isotopic labelling, including enzymes. ELISA methods and the method described below are of this type.

ENZYME IMMUNOASSAY FOR FERRITIN

The technique is based on well-known principles and is one developed by the International Council for Standardization in Haematology (Expert Panel on Iron).[31]

Reagents and materials

Ferritin. This may be prepared from human liver or spleen, either normal or iron-loaded and obtained at operation (spleen) or post mortem. The permission of the patient or the patient's relatives should be obtained before the tissue is removed. Tissue should be obtained as soon as possible after death and may be stored at −20°C for 1 yr. Remember the risk of infection when handling tissues and extracts. Ferritin is purified by methods which exploit its stability at 75°C. Further purification is obtained by chromatography and either by ultracentrifugation[27] or by precipitation from cadmium sulphate solution.[14] Purity should be assessed by polyacrylamide gel electrophoresis[27] and the protein content determined by the method of Lowry et al as described in ref.[27] Human ferritin may be stored in solution at 4°C, at 1–4 mg protein/ml, in the presence of sodium azide as a preservative, for up to 3 years.

Antibodies to human ferritin. High affinity antibodies to human liver or spleen ferritin are suitable. Polyclonal antibodies may be raised in rabbits or sheep by conventional methods[10] and the titre checked by precipitation with human ferritin.[27] An IgG enriched fraction of antiserum is required for labelling with enzyme in the assay. The simplest method is to precipitate IgG with sodium sulphate.[9] Monoclonal antibodies which

are specific for 'L' subunit rich ferritin (liver or spleen ferritin) are also suitable. Ascitic fluid preparations should be purified by sodium sulphate precipitation to obtain an IgG fraction for labelling with enzyme and for coating plates. Store in water at 10 mg protein/ml at −20°C*.

Conjugation of antiferritin IgG preparation to horseradish peroxidase[25]

1. Dissolve 4 mg of horseradish peroxidase (Sigma Type VI P-8375) in 1 ml of water and add 200 µl of freshly prepared 0.1 mol/l sodium periodate solution. The solution should turn greenish-brown. Mix gently by inverting and leave for 20 min at room temperature, mixing gently every 5 min. Dialyse overnight against 1 mmol/l sodium acetate buffer, pH 4.4.

2. Add 20 µl of 0.2 mol/l sodium carbonate buffer, pH 9.5 to a solution of antiferritin IgG fraction (8 mg in 1 ml). Add 20 µl of 0.2 mol/l sodium carbonate buffer, pH9.5 to the horseradish peroxidase solution to raise the pH to 9.0–9.5 and immediately mix the two solutions. Leave at room temperature for 2 h and mix by inversion every 30 min.

3. Add 100 µl of freshly prepared sodium borohydride solution (4 mg/ml in water) and stand at 4°C for 2 h. Dialyse overnight against 0.1 mol/l borate buffer pH 7.4.

4. Add an equal volume of 60% glycerol in borate buffer to the conjugate solution and store at 4°C.

Assay reagents

Buffer A. Phosphate buffered saline, pH 7.2, containing 0.05% Tween 20. Prepare a 10 times concentrated (1.5 mol/l) stock solution by dissolving sodium chloride, 80 g; potassium chloride, 2 g; anhydrous disodium phosphate, 11.5 g and anhydrous potassium phosphate (KH_2PO_4), 2 g in 1 litre of water. Store at room temperature. Prepare Buffer A by diluting 100 ml of stock solution to 1 litre with water and adding

---

*Suitable antibodies (including a preparation labelled with horseradish peroxidase) may also be obtained from Dako Ltd, High Wycombe, Bucks, UK.

0.5 ml of Tween 20. Store at 4°C for up to 2 weeks.

Buffer B. Prepare by dissolving 5 g of bovine serum albumin (BSA) in 1 litre of buffer A. Store at 4°C for up to 2 weeks.

Buffer C. Carbonate buffer, 0.05 mol/l, pH 9.6. Dissolve sodium carbonate, 1.59 g and sodium bicarbonate, 2.93 g in 1 litre of water and store at room temperature.

Buffer D. Citrate phosphate buffer, 0.15 mol/l, pH 5.0. Dissolve 21 g of citric acid monohydrate in 1 litre of water and store at 4°C. Dissolve 28.4 g of anhydrous disodium phosphate in 1 litre of water and store at room temperature. Prepare fresh buffer on the day of assay by mixing 49 ml of citric acid solution with 51 ml of phosphate solution.

Substrate solution. Prepare immediately before use by adding 33 µl of hydrogen peroxide, 30%, to 100 ml of buffer and mixing well. Add 1 tablet containing 30 mg of *o*-phenylenediamine dihydrochloride (Sigma) and mix.

Preparation and storage of a standard ferritin solution. Dilute a solution of human ferritin to approximately 200 µg/ml in water. Measure the protein concentration by the method of Lowry after diluting further to 20–50 µg/ml.[27] Then dilute the ferritin solution (approx. 200 µg/ml) to a concentration of 10 µg/ml in 0.05 mol/l sodium barbitone solution containing 0.1 mol/l NaCl, 0.02% NaN_3, bovine serum albumin (5 g/l) and adjusted to pH 8.0 with 5 mol/l HCl. Deliver 200 µl into small plastic tubes, cap tightly and store at 4°C for up to 1 yr. For use, dilute in Buffer B to 1000 µg/l, then prepare a range of standard solutions between 0.2 and 25 µg/l. Calibrate this working standard against the 2nd WHO standard for the assay of serum ferritin (reagent 80/578, human spleen ferritin)★.

Coating of plates. 96-well microtitre plates for immunoassay are required. Do not use the outer wells until you have established the assay procedure and can check that all wells give consistent results. Coat the plates by adding to each well 200 µl of antiferritin IgG preparation diluted to 2 µg/ml in Buffer C. Seal the plate or cover with 'parafilm' or 'cling-film' and leave overnight at 4°C. On the day of the assay empty the wells by sharply inverting the plate and dry by tapping briefly on paper towels. Block unreacted sites by adding 200 µl of 0.5% (w/v) bovine serum albumin (Sigma, A-7030) in Buffer C. After 30 min at room temperature wash each plate three times by filling each well with Buffer A (using a syringe and needle) and emptying and draining as described above.

Preparation of test sera. Collect venous blood and separate the serum. Samples may be stored at 4°C for 1 week or for 2 yr at –20°C. Plasma obtained from heparinized blood is also suitable. For assay, dilute 50 µl of serum to 1 ml with Buffer B. Further dilutions may be made in the same buffer if required.

Assay procedure

The use of a multi-channel pipette for rapid addition of solutions is recommended. Standards and sera, in duplicate, should be added to each plate within 20 min.

Add 200 µl of standard solution or diluted serum to each well. Cover the plate and leave at room temperature on a draught-free bench away from direct sunlight for 2 h. Empty the wells by sharply inverting the plate and dry by draining on paper towels. Wash three times by filling each well with Buffer A, leaving for 2 min at room temperature and draining as described above. Dilute the conjugate in 1% bovine serum albumin in Buffer A. The optimal dilution (of the order of 10^3–10^4 times) must be ascertained by experiment.

Add 200 µl of diluted horseradish peroxidase conjugate to each well and leave the covered plate for a further 2 h at room temperature. Wash three times with Buffer A. Add 200 µl of substrate solution to each well. Incubate the plate for 30 min in the dark. Stop the reaction by adding 50 µl of 25% (v/v) sulphuric acid to each well. Read the absorbance at 492 nm within 30 min using an automatic plate reader. Alternatively, transfer 200 µl from each well to a tube containing 800 µl of water and read the absorbance in a spectrophotometer.

★Available from National Institute for Biological Standards and Control (NIBSC), South Mimms, Herts EN6 3QG, UK.

Calculation of results

Calculate the mean absorbance for each point on the standard curve and plot against ferritin concentration using semilogarithmic paper. Read concentrations for the serum from this curve. If results are calculated with a computer program the log-logit plot provides a linear dose response. For serum ferritin concentrations >200 μg/l, reassay at a dilution of 100 times or greater. Control sera should be included in each assay.

Selecting an assay method

The following notes may be of use for those considering introducing the ferritin assay into a clinical laboratory by purchasing a commercially available kit.

1. Limit of detection. Two-site immunoradiometric assays are intrinsically more sensitive than radioimmunoassays. For example, concentrations of ferritin in buffer solution as low as 0.01 μg/l may be detected. Avoidance of serum effects (see below) requires dilution of samples, however, and, for practical purposes, the lower limit of detection is of the order of 1 μg/l. For some radioimmunoassays the limits of detection may approach 10 μg/l and this may cause difficulties in using the assay for detection of iron deficiency. This point should be considered carefully. The detection limits for enzyme-linked assays are gradually improving.

2. The 'high-dose hook'. This is a problem peculiar to labelled antibody assays, particularly two-site immunoradiometric assays.[20,22] Two causes have been suggested: (a) heterogeneity of the solid phase antiserum, and (b) incomplete washing after the first reaction (binding) of ferritin to the solid phase. Exhaustive washing may move the 'hook' to higher ferritin concentrations but does not usually eliminate it. The only safe method is to assay all serum samples at two dilutions to ensure that both dilutions are on the 'ascending' part of the dose response curve. In view of the wide range of serum ferritin concentrations which may be encountered in hospital patients (0–40 000 μg/l) this is, in any case, a good practice.

3. Interference by non-ferritin proteins in serum. This may occur with any method but particularly with labelled antibody assays. Serum proteins may inhibit the binding of ferritin to the solid when compared with the binding in buffer solution alone. Such an effect may be avoided by diluting the standards in a buffer containing a suitable serum or by diluting serum samples as much as possible. For example, for two-site immunoradiometric assays, the sample may be diluted 20 times with buffer while the standards are prepared in 5% normal rabbit serum in buffer (if antibodies have been raised in rabbits). Further dilutions of the sera are carried out with this solution. A much more serious cause of error, and difficult to detect, is interference by anti-immunoglobulin antibodies.[5] This possibility has received little attention in the literature on ferritin assays. These antibodies bind to the animal immunoglobulins used to detect the antigen and form artefactual "sandwiches". Such antibodies are found in about 10% of patients and normal subjects. Interference may be reduced by adding the appropriate species of animal immunoglobulins to block the cross-reaction but this is not always successful.[32] One solution is to use antibodies from different species as solid-phase and labelled antibodies. Thus one may use a polyclonal, rabbit antiferritin to coat plates in the ELISA with a polyclonal sheep antiferritin labelled with horse-radish peroxidase as the second antibody. Rabbit serum (0.5%) replaces bovine serum albumin in buffer B.

4. Reproducibility. Most assays are satisfactory, but this must always be established for any method introduced into the laboratory. Particular problems (different readings in the outer wells for example) may be encountered with enzyme-linked assays which have microtitre plates as the solid phase.

5. Dilution of serum samples. It should be established that both standard and serum samples dilute in parallel over at least a 10-fold range.

6. Accuracy. The use of reference ferritin preparation is recommended (see above).

Interpretation of results

The use of serum ferritin for the assessment of iron stores has become well-established.[28] In most normal adults serum ferritin concentrations lie within the range 15–300 µg/l. During the first months of life mean serum ferritin concentrations change considerably, reflecting changes in storage iron concentration. Concentrations are lower in children than in adults and from puberty to middle life are higher in men than in women. In adults concentrations of <15 µg/l indicate an absence of storage iron but in children the lower limit of normal is lower and the assay is less valuable for detecting iron deficiency. The interpretation of serum concentration in many pathological conditions is less straightforward, but concentrations of less than 15 µg/l indicate depletion of storage iron.

Iron overload causes high concentrations of serum ferritin but these may also be found in patients with liver disease, infection, inflammation or malignant disease. Careful consideration of the clinical evidence is required before it is concluded that a high serum ferritin concentration is primarily the result of iron overload and not due to tissue damage or enhanced synthesis of ferritin. However, a normal ferritin concentration provides good evidence against iron overload.

Serum ferritin concentrations are high in patients with advanced haemochromatosis but the serum ferritin estimation should not be used alone to screen the relatives of patients or to assess re-accumulation of storage iron after phlebotomy. This is because in many patients the early stages of iron accumulation (when total iron stores are not much elevated) are detected by an increased serum-iron concentration and transferrin saturation even when the serum ferritin concentration is within the normal range. This is one of the few instances where the measurement of serum iron and total iron-binding capacity provides useful information not given by the ferritin assay.

In patients with acute or chronic disease, interpretation of serum ferritin concentrations is less straightforward[26] and patients may have serum ferritin concentrations of up to 100 µg/l despite an absence of stainable iron in the bone marrow. There is evidence that ferritin synthesis[23] is enhanced by interleukin-1 — the primary mediator of the acute phase response. In patients with chronic disease the following approach should be adopted: low serum ferritin concentrations indicate absent iron stores, values within the normal range either low or normal levels, and high values indicate either normal or high levels. In terms of adequacy of iron stores for replenishing haemoglobin in anaemic patients the degree of anaemia must also be considered. Thus a patient with a haemoglobin concentration of 100 g/l may benefit from iron therapy if the serum ferritin concentration is <100 µg/l, as below this level there is unlikely to be sufficient iron available for full regeneration.

Immunologically, plasma ferritin resembles the 'L-rich' ferritins of liver and spleen and only low concentrations are detected with antibodies to heart or HeLa cell ferritin, ferritins rich in 'H' subunits. The heterogeneity of serum ferritin on isoelectric focusing is largely due to glycosylation and the presence of variable numbers of sialic acid residues and not variation in the ratio of H to L subunits.[29] Attempts to assay for 'acidic' (or 'H'-rich) isoferritins in serum as tumour markers have not been successful.[7,17]

REFERENCES

[1] ADDISON, G. M., BEAMISH, M. R., HALES, C. N., HODGKINS, M., JACOBS, A. and LLEWLLIN, P. (1972). An immunoradiometric assay for ferritin in the serum of normal subjects and patients with iron deficiency and iron overload. *Journal of Clinical Pathology*, **25**, 326.

[2] BAINTON, D. F. and FINCH, C. A. (1964). The diagnosis of iron deficiency anemia. *American Journal of Medicine*, **37**, 62.

[3] BANDI, Z. L., SCHOEN, I. and BEE, D. E. (1985). Immunochemical methods for measurement of transferrin in serum: effects of analytical errors and inappropriate reference intervals on diagnostic utility. *Clinical Chemistry*, **31**, 1601.

[4] BEILBY, J., OLYNYK, J., CHING, S., PRINS, A., SWANSON, N., REED, W., HARLEY, H. and CARCIA-WEBB, P. (1992). Transferrin index: an alternative method for calculating the iron saturation of transferrin. *Clinical Chemistry*, **38**, 2078.

[5] BOSCATO, L. M. and STUART, M. C. (1988). Heterophillic antibodies: a problem for all immunoassays. *Clinical Chemistry*, **34**, 27.

[6] BOTHWELL, T. H., CHARLTON, R. W., COOK, J. D. and FINCH, C. A. (1979). *Iron Metabolism in Man*. Blackwell Scientific Publications, Oxford.

[7] CAVANNA, F. RUGGERi, G., IACOBELLO, C., CHIEREGATTI, G., MURADOR, E., ALBERTINI, A. and AROSIO, P. (1983). Development of a monoclonal antibody against human

heart ferritin and its application in an immunoradiometric assay. *Clinica Chimica Acta*, **134**, 347.

[8] EDWARDS, C. Q. and KUSHNER, J. P. (1993). Current concepts — screening for hemochromatosis. *New England Journal of Medicine*, **328**, 1616.

[9] HEIDE, K. and SCHWICK, J. G. (1978). Salt fractionation of immunoglobulins. In *Handbook of Experimental Immunology*. Ed. D. M. Weir, Vol. 1, p. 7.1. Blackwell Scientific Publications, Oxford.

[10] HERBERT, W. J. (1978). Laboratory animal techniques for immunology. In *Handbook of Experimental Immunology* Ed. Weir, D. M. Vol. 3, p. 4.1. Blackwell Scientific Publications, Oxford.

[11] HUEBERS, H. A., ENG, M. J. JOSEPHSON, B. M. et al (1987). Plasma iron and transferrin iron-binding capacity evaluated by colorimetric and immunoprecipitation methods. *Clinical Chemistry*, **33**, 273.

[12] INTERNATIONAL COMMITTEE FOR STANDARDIZATION IN HAEMATOLOGY (1978). Recommendations for measurement of serum iron in human blood. *British Journal of Haematology*, **38**, 291.

[13] INTERNATIONAL COMMITTEE FOR STANDARDIZATION IN HAEMATOLOGY (1978). The measurement of total and unsaturated iron-binding capacity in serum. *British Journal of Haematology*, **38**, 281.

[14] INTERNATIONAL COMMITTEE FOR STANDARDIZATION IN HAEMATOLOGY (Expert Panel on Iron) (1985). Proposed international standard human ferritin for the serum ferritin assay. *British Journal of Haematology*, **61**, 61.

[15] INTERNATIONAL COMMITTEE FOR STANDARDIZATION IN HAEMATOLOGY (EXPERT PANEL ON IRON) (1990). Revised recommendations for the measurement of serum iron in human blood. *British Journal of Haematology*, **75**, 615.

[16] JACOBS, A., WATERS, W. E., CAMPBELL, H. and BARROW, A. (1969) A random sample from Wales. III. Serum iron, iron binding capacity and transferrin saturation. *British Journal of Haematology*, **17**, 581.

[17] JONES, B. M., WORWOOD, M. and JACOBS, A. (1980). Serum ferritin in patients with cancer: determination with antibodies to HeLa cell and spleen ferritin. *Clinica Chimica Acta*, **106**, 2003.

[18] KOERPER, M. A. and DALLMAN, P. R. (1977) Serum iron concentration and transferrin saturation in the diagnosis of iron deficiency in children: normal developmental changes. *Journal of Pediatrics*, **91**, 870.

[19] MILES, L. E. M., LIPSCHITZ, D. A., BIEBER, C. P. and COOK, J. D. (1974). Measurement of serum ferritin by a 2-side immunoradiometric assay. *Analytical Biochemistry*, **61**, 209.

[20] PERERA, P. and WORWOOD, M. (1984). Antigen binding in the two-site immunoradiometric assay for serum ferritin: the nature of the hook effect. *Annals of Clinical Biochemistry*, **21**, 393.

[21] PERSIJN, J.–P., VAN DER SLIK, and W. RIETHORST, A. (1971) Determination of serum iron and latent iron-binding capacity (LIBC). *Clinical Chimica Acta* **35**, 91.

[22] ROBARD, D., FELDMAN, Y., JAFFE, M. L. and MILES, L. E. M. (1978). Kinetics of two-site immunoradiometric ('sandwich') assays — II. Studies on the nature of the 'high-dose hook' effects. *Immunochemistry*, **15**, 77.

[23] ROGERS, J. T., BRIDGES, K. R., DURMOWIEZ, G. P., GLASS, J., AURON, P. E. and MUNRO, H. N. (1990) Translational control during the acute phase response. *Journal of Biological Chemistry*, **265**, 14572.

[24] SAARINEN, U. M. and SIIMES, M. A. (1977). Developmental changes in serum iron, total iron-binding capacity, and transferrin saturation in infancy. *Journal of Pediatrics*, **91**, 875.

[25] WILSON, M. B. and NAKANE, P. K. (1978). Recent developments in the periodate method of conjugating horseradish peroxidase (HRPO) to antibodies. In *Immunofluorescence and Related Staining Technique*s. Eds. W. KNAPP, K. HOLUBAR, G. WICK, p. 215–24. Elsevier/North-Holland, Amsterdam.

[26] WITTE, D. L. (1991). Can serum ferritin be effectively interpreted in the presence of the acute-phase response? *Clinical Chemistry*, **37**, 484.

[27] WORWOOD, M. (1980). Iron: serum ferritin. *Methods in Hematology*, **1**, 59.

[28] WORWOOD, M. (1982). Ferritin in human tissues and serum. *Clinics in Haematology*, **11**, 275.

[29] WORWOOD, M. (1986). Serum ferritin (Editorial review). *Clinical Science*, **70**, 215.

[30] WORWOOD, M. and DARKE, C. (1993). Serum ferritin, blood donation, iron stores and haemochromatosis. *Transfusion Medicine*, **3**, 21.

[31] WORWOOD, M., THORPE, S. J. HEATH, A., FLOWERS, C. H. and COOK, J. D. (1991). Stable lyophilized reagents for the serum ferritin assay. *Clinical and Laboratory Haematology*, **13**, 291.

[32] ZWEIG, M. H., CSAKO, G., BENSON, C. C., WEINTRAUB, B. D. and KAHN, B. B. (1987). Interference by anti-immunoglobulin G antibodies in immunoradiometric assays of thyrotropin involving mouse monoclonal antibodies. *Clinical Chemistry*, **33**, 840.

24. Red cell blood-group antigens and antibodies

Revised by A. H. Waters

Red cell blood groups   445
ABO system   446
Rh system   448
Other blood-group systems   449
Mechanisms of immune destruction of blood cells   450
Antigen-antibody reactions   451
Serological technique and quality control   452
Enzyme-treated red cells   453

Agglutination of red cells by antibody   455
  Reading results   455
Demonstration of lysis   456
Antiglobulin test   457
  Antiglobulin reagents   458
  Recommended test procedure   459
Assessment of worker performance   461
Titration of antibodies   461
Test for secretion of A and B substances   463

In one short chapter it is impossible to give a detailed survey of the human blood groups. Facts basic to an understanding of clinical blood-group serology are given together with a description of important serological techniques.

In recent years platelet and leucocyte antigens and antibodies have been extensively studied. These are discussed in Chapter 25. The present chapter deals exclusively with red cell antigens and antibodies.

RED CELL BLOOD GROUPS

Since Landsteiner's discovery in 1901 that human blood groups existed, a vast body of serological, genetic and more recently biochemical data on red cell blood-group antigens have been accumulated.

About 200 red cell antigens have been described, most of which have been antigens to well defined blood-group systems (Table 24.1). A numerical catalogue of red cell blood-group antigens is being maintained by an ISBT Working Party.[7,22] Apart from the ABO system, most of these antigens were detected by antibodies stimulated by transfusion or pregnancy.

Almost all blood-group genes are expressed as co-dominant antigens, i.e. both genes are expressed in the heterozygote. Some blood-group genes have been assigned to specific chromosomes, e.g.

ABO system on chromosome 9, Rh system on chromosome 1 (Table 24.1). For a review of the molecular biology of red cell blood-group genes, see ref 24.

The clinical importance of a blood-group antigen depends on the frequency of occurrence of the corresponding antibody and its ability to haemolyse red cells in vivo. On these criteria, the ABO and Rh systems are of major clinical importance. Anti-A and anti-B occur regularly, and are capable of causing severe intravascular haemolysis after an incompatible transfusion. The Rh D antigen is the most immunogenic red cell antigen after A and B, being capable of stimulating anti-D production after transfusion or pregnancy in the majority of Rh D-negative individuals.

Table 24.1   Major blood-group systems in historical order of discovery

Year	System	Main antigens	Chromosome location
1901	ABO	A, B	9
1927	MNSs	M, N, S, s	4
1927	P	P_1, P, P^k, p	22(?)
1939	Rh	C, c, D, (d), E, e	1
1945	Lutheran	Lu^a, Lu^b	19
1946	Kell	K, k, Kp^a, Kp^b, Js^a, Js^b	7
1946	Lewis	Le^a, Le^b	19
1950	Duffy	Fy^a, Fy^b	1
1951	Kidd	Jk^a, Jk^b	2
1952	Vel	Vel^1, Vel^2	–
1953	Wright	Wr^a, Wr^b	–
1955	Diego	Di^a, Di^b	–
1956	Cartwright	Yt^a, Yt^b	–
1956	I	Ii	–
1962	Xg	Xg^a	X
1962	Scianna	Sc^1, Sc^2	1
1965	Dombrock	Do^a, Do^b	–
1965	Colton	Co^a, Co^b	–

Table 24.2   ABO blood-group system

Blood group	Sub-group	Antigens on red cells	Antibodies in plasma
A	A_1 A_2	$A + A_1$ A	Anti-B (Anti-A_1)*
B	–	B	Anti-A, Anti-A_1
AB	A_1B A_2B	$A + A_1 + B$ A + B	None (Anti-A_1)*
O	–	(H)***	Anti-A, Anti-A_1 Anti-B Anti-A, B**

   * Anti-A_1 found in 1–2% of A_2 subjects and 25–30% of A_2B subjects.

 ** Cross-reacting with both A and B cells.

*** The amount of H antigen is influenced by the ABO group; O cells contain most H and A_1B cells least. Anti-H may be found in occasional A_1 and A_1B subjects (see text).

ABO SYSTEM

Discovery of the ABO system by Landsteiner in 1901 marked the beginning of safe blood transfusion. The ABO antigens, although most important in relation to transfusion, also have variable expression on most tissues and are important histocompatibility antigens.

Antigens (Table 24.2)

There are four main blood groups: A, B, AB and O. There is racial variation in the frequency of these groups; in the British Caucasian population the frequency of group O is 46%, A 42%, B 9% and AB 3%.[27,30]

The presence of A, B or O antigens on red cells is determined by the inheritance of the allelic genes *A*, *B*, and *O* on chromosome 9, which are inherited in pairs as Mendelian dominants. It is likely that the *O* and *B* genes are mutations of the *A* gene. *O* is identical to *A* except for the deletion of a single DNA base pair which causes a frame-shift during transcription and translation resulting in an inactive enzyme, and *B* differs from *A* by four consistent nucleotide substitutions. The cellular expression of A and B antigens is determined by a further gene, the *H* gene, which is inherited independently: this gene codes for an enzyme that converts a carbohydrate precursor

into H substance. The *A* and *B* genes code for specific enzymes (glycosytransferases) which convert H substance into A and B antigens by the terminal addition of *N*-acetyl-D-galactosamine and D-galactose, respectively (Fig. 24.1). The *O* gene produces an inactive transferase, so that H substance persists unchanged in group O. In the extremely rare Oh Bombay phenotype, the *H* genotype is 'silent' (*hh*) and no H-transferase is produced; consequently no H substance is made and therefore *A* and *B* genes, if present, cannot be expressed. These individuals have anti-A, anti-B and anti-H in their blood, all active at

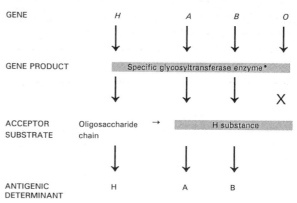

Fig. 24.1   Pathways from HAB blood-group genes to antigens. *Glycosyltransferase H transfers L-fucose; A transfers *N*-acetyl-D-galactosamine; B transfers D-galactose; O is inactive.

37°C, and can only be safely transfused with other Oh blood.

Serologists have defined two common subgroups of the A antigen: about 20% of group 'A' and group 'AB' subjects belong to group A_2 and group A_2B respectively, and the remainder belong to group A_1 and group A_1B. The distinction is most conveniently made using the lectin from *Dolichos biflorus* which only reacts with A_1 cells. The H antigen content of red cells depends on the ABO group and when assessed by agglutination reactions with anti-H, the strength of reaction tends to be graded $O > A_2 > A_2B > B > A_1 > A_1B$. Antigens weaker than A are occasionally found (called A_3, A_x, etc.). These serological variations in the A antigen are due to mutant forms of the glycosyl transferases produced by the *A* gene, which are less efficient at transferring *N*-acetyl-D-galactosamine to C2 in the hexose ring of H substance.

The A, B and H antigens are detectable early in fetal life, but are not fully developed on the red cells at birth. The number of antigen sites reaches 'adult' levels at about 1 year of age and remains the same throughout life until old age when a slight reduction may occur.

Secretors and non-secretors (Table 24.3)

The ability to secrete A, B and H substances in water-soluble form is controlled by a dominant secretor gene *Se* (allele *se*). In a Caucasian population, about 80% are secretors (genotype *SeSe* or *Sese*) and 20% non-secretors (genotype *sese*). Secretors have H substance in the saliva and other body fluids together with A and/or B substances depending on their blood group. Only traces of these substances are present in the secretions of non-secretors, although the antigens are normally expressed on their red cells and other tissues, and the corresponding blood-group substance is present in the plasma.

An individuals's secretor status can be determined by testing for ABH substance in saliva (p. 463).

Antibodies

Anti-A and anti-B. A feature of the ABO system is the regular occurrence of anti-A and anti-B in the absence of the corresponding red cell antigens (Table 24.2). This allows for reverse (serum) grouping as a means of confirming the red cell phenotype.

The antibodies are a potential cause of dangerous haemolytic reactions if transfusions are given without regard to ABO compatibility. Anti-A and anti-B are always, to some extent, naturally occurring and of IgM class. Although they react best at low temperatures, they are nevertheless potentially haemolytic at 37°C. Hyperimmune anti-A and anti-B occur less frequently, usually in response to transfusion or pregnancy, but may also be formed following the injection of some toxoids and vaccines. They are predominantly of IgG class and are usually produced by group-O and sometimes by group-A_2 individuals. Hyperimmune IgG anti-A and/or anti-B from group-O or group-A_2 mothers may cross the placenta and cause haemolytic disease of the newborn (HDN). These antibodies react over a wide thermal range and are more effective haemolysins than the naturally occurring antibodies. Group-O donors should always be screened for hyperimmune anti-A and anti-B antibodies which may cause haemolysis when group-O whole blood is transfused to recipients with A and B phenotypes. These dangerous 'universal' donors should be reserved

Table 24.3 Secretor status

	Genes	Blood group of red cells	ABH substance present in saliva	Incidence (%)
Secretors	*SeSe* or *Sese*	A B AB O	A + H B + H A + B + H H	80
Non-secretors	*sese*	A, B, AB or O	None	20

for group-O recipients only, or the blood should be used as packed red cells.

Anti-A₁ and anti-H. An antibody reacting only with A_1 and A_1B cells, called anti-A_1, is occasionally found in the serum of group-A_2 subjects (1–2%) and not uncommonly in the serum of group-A_2B subjects (25–30%). An antibody reacting most strongly with O and A_2 cells, probably best referred to as anti-H, is sometimes found in the serum of group-A_1, -A_1B or -B subjects (Table 24.2).

These two antibodies normally act as cold agglutinins and rarely react with the appropriate red cell antigens at temperatures over 30°C. They seldom cause haemolytic reactions in vivo, but may be a source of confusion in room temperature compatibility tests. A notable, but rare, exception is the anti-H that occurs in the Bombay phenotype Oh, which is an IgM antibody and causes lysis at 37°C.

Rh SYSTEM

The Rh system was so named because the original antibody that was raised by injecting red cells of rhesus monkeys into rabbits and guinea-pigs reacted with most human red cells. Although the original antibody (now called anti-LW) was subsequently shown to be different from human anti-D, the Rh terminology has been retained for the human blood group system. The clinical importance of this system is due to the fact that Rh-negative individuals are easily stimulated to make Rh antibodies if transfused with Rh-positive blood or, in the case of pregnant women, if exposed to Rh-positive fetal red cells which have crossed the placenta.

Antigens

This is a very complex system. At its simplest, it is convenient to classify individuals as Rh positive or Rh negative depending on the presence of the D antigen. This is largely a preventive measure to avoid transfusing an Rh-negative recipient with the D antigen, which is the most immunogenic red cell antigen after A and B.

At a more comprehensive level, it is convenient to consider the Rh system as a gene complex

Table 24.4 The Rh haplotypes in order of frequency (Fisher nomenclature) and the corresponding short notations

Fisher	Short notations	Approximate frequency (%)
CDe	R^1	41
cde	r	39
cDE	R^2	14
cDe	R^0	3
C^wDe	R^{1w}	1
cdE	r"	1
Cde	r'	1
CDE	R^z	rare
CdE	r^y	rare

which gives rise to various combinations of three alternative antigens C or c, D or d and E or e, as originally suggested by Fisher; the *d* gene was thought to be amorphic without any corresponding antigen on the red cell. Recent observations[3] suggest that the Rh locus on chromosome 1 consists of two closely linked genes, one encoding the D protein, which is absent in Rh-negative individuals, and the other encoding the Cc and Ee proteins. This concept of D and CcEe genes linked closely and transmitted together is consistent with the Fisher nomenclature.

The Rh haplotypes are named either by the component antigens (e.g. CDe; cde) or by a single shorthand symbol (e.g. R^1 = CDe; r = cde). Thus a person may inherit *CDe* (R^1) from one parent and *cde* (*r*) from the other, and have the genotype *CDe/cde* (R^1r). The haplotypes in order of frequency and the corresponding shorthand notation are given in Table 24.4. Although two other nomenclatures are also used to describe the Rh system, namely, Wiener's Rh-Hr terminology and Rosenfield's numerical notation, the CDE nomenclature, derived from Fisher's original theory, is recommended by a WHO Expert Committee[41] in the interest of simplicity and uniformity.

The Rh antigens are defined by corresponding anti-sera, with the exception of 'anti-d' which does not exist. Consequently, the distinction between homozygous DD and heterozygous Dd cannot be made by direct serological testing; this may be resolved by informative family studies, otherwise the genotype can only be predicted from the phenotype on the basis of probability tables for the various Rh genotypes in the population (Table 26.2).

There are racial differences in the distribution of Rh antigens, e.g. Rh D negativity is a Caucasian trait (c 15%), while lower levels of negativity in other ethnic groups are thought to be due to intermingling of Caucasian genes.[27]

The Rh antigens are present only on red cells and are a structural part of the cell membrane.[3] Complete absence of Rh antigens (Rh null phenotype) may be associated with a congenital haemolytic anaemia with spherocytes and stomatocytes in the blood film[1]

Rh antigens are well developed before birth and can be demonstrated on the red cells of very early fetuses.

Antibodies

Fisher's nomenclature is convenient when applied to Rh antibodies, and antibodies acting against all the Rh antigens, except d, have been described, namely anti-D, anti-C, anti-c, anti-E, anti-e.

Rh antigens are restricted to red cells and Rh antibodies are due to allo-immunization by previous transfusion or pregnancy, except for some naturally-occurring forms of anti-E. They are usually IgG (sometimes with an IgM component), react best at 37°C, and do not fix complement. Haemolysis, when it occurs, is therefore extra-vascular and predominantly in the spleen. Anti-D is the most important clinically; it may cause haemolytic transfusion reactions and was a common cause of fetal death resulting from haemolytic disease of the newborn (HDN) before the introduction of anti-D prophylaxis in 1970. The other Rh antibodies, although much less common, may nevertheless cause haemolytic transfusion reactions and HDN.

OTHER BLOOD-GROUP SYSTEM...

Routine Rh D grouping before blood ... and the success of anti-D prophylaxis ... ... D negative mothers bearing Rh D positive infants have greatly reduced the incidence of allo-immunization to the D antigen. At the same time, the increasing use of blood transfusion has meant that more patients are being immunized by other antigens, especially Rh (c, E) and those of the Kell (K), Duffy (Fy[a]) and Kidd (Jk[a]) systems.[14] These antibodies have all been associated with haemolytic transfusion reactions and HDN.

Mollison et al[25a] analysed the prevalence of transfusion-induced red cell allo-antibodies (Table 24.5). Rh antibodies other than anti-D (or -CD or -DE) — mainly anti-c or anti-E — accounted for 53% of the total and anti-K and anti-Fy[a] for a further 38%, leaving only about 9% for all other specificities. A similar distribution of the different red cell antibodies was found in a smaller group of patients who experienced immediate haemolytic transfusion reactions (HTR). On the other hand, the figures for delayed HTR showed a striking increase in the relative frequency of Jk antibodies. This probably reflects two characteristics of Jk antibodies. They are difficult to detect in pretransfusion compatibility tests (p. 457), especially at low concentration, due to the tendency for the antibody to disappear after previous stimulation. However, once boosted by a further transfusion, the antibody may cause severe haemolysis due to the combined effects of both IgG and C3 (p. 450), so that delayed HTR is more readily diagnosed than when caused by some other antibodies.

Table 24.5 Relative frequency of immune red-cell allo-antibodies*

| Patient group | No. studied | Blood group allo-antibodies (% of total) | | | | |
		Rh**	K	Fy	Jk	Other
Transfused (some pregnant)	5228	53.1	28.1	10.2	4.0	4.7
Immediate HTR[†]	142	42.2	30.3	18.3	8.5	0.7
Delayed HTR[†]	82	34.2	14.6	15.9	32.9	2.4

*Excluding antibodies of ABO, Lewis, P systems and anti-M and anti-N.
**Excluding anti-D (or -CD or -DE); almost all were anti-c or anti-E.
[†]Haemolytic transfusion reaction.
Adapted from Mollison et al[25a] based on published data from several sources.

For a more detailed exposition of the blood-group systems the reader is referred to Race and Sanger[30] and Mollison et al.[25]

MECHANISMS OF IMMUNE DESTRUCTION OF BLOOD CELLS[8]

Immune haemolysis may be used as a model to illustrate the mechanisms of immune blood-cell destruction. Immune haemolysis depends on:

1. The *Ig class* of the antibody — for all practical purposes antibodies against red cell antigens are of IgM or IgG class.
2. The ability of the antibody to activate and fix *complement*.
3. Interaction with the *mononuclear phagoyte (MP) system*. The most important phagocyte participating in immune haemolysis is the macrophage, predominantly in the spleen.

The mechanism of immune haemolysis determines the site of haemolysis:

(a) *Intravascular haemolysis* due to complement lysis is characteristic of IgM antibodies; some IgG antibodies also act as haemolysins. Red cells are typically destroyed by intravascular complement lysis in ABO incompatible transfusion reactions (p. 491). Most other allo-immune red cell destruction is extravascular and mediated by the MP system.

Red cell auto-antibodies may also cause intravascular haemolysis, especially the IgG auto-antibody of paroxysmal cold haemoglobinuria (PCH) (p. 522) and some IgM auto-antibodies of the cold-haemagglutinin syndrome (p. 501). Complement-mediated intravascular haemolysis may also occur in drug-induced immune haemolysis (p. 524).

(b) *Extravascular haemolysis* by the MP system is, characteristic of IgG antibodies and occurs predominantly in the spleen. Macrophages have Fcγ receptors for cell-bound IgG, and sensitized red cells may be wholly phagocytosed or lose part of the membrane and return to the circulation as a microspherocyte. Spherocytes are less deformable and more readily trapped in the spleen than normal cells, which shortens their life-span.

In addition to Fc receptor mediated phago-cytosis, *antibody-dependent cell-mediated cytoxicity (ADCC)* may also contribute to cell damage during the phase of close contact with splenic macrophages.[8]

Complement components may enhance red cell destruction. Complement activation by some IgM and most IgG red cell antibodies is not always complete, the red cell thus escaping intravascular haemolysis. The activation sequence stops at the C3 stage, and in these circumstances complement components can be detected on the red cell by the antiglobulin test using appropriate anti-complement reagents (p. 458).

The first activation product of C3 is membrane-bound C3b, which is constantly being broken down to C3bi (see Table 24.7). Red cells with these components on their surface adhere to phagocytes (monocytes, macrophages, granulo-cytes) which have corresponding membrane receptors (CR1 and CR3). These sensitized cells are rapidly sequestered in the liver because of its bulk of phagocytic (Kupffer) cells and large blood flow, but no engulfment occurs. When C3bi is cleaved, leaving only C3dg on the cell surface, the cells tagged with 'inactive' C3dg return to the circulation, as in CHAD (p. 501). However, when IgG is also present on the cell surface, C3b enhances phagocytosis, and under these circumstances both liver and spleen are important sites of extravascular haemolysis.

Macrophage activity is an important component of cell destruction and further study of cellular interactions at this stage of immune haemolysis may provide an explanation for the differing severity of haemolysis in patients with apparently similar antibodies. In-vitro macrophage (mono-cyte) assays are being introduced to supplement conventional serological techniques in order to assess this aspect of immune haemolysis.[9]

Factors that may affect the interaction between sensitized cells and macrophages include:

1. *IgG subclass.* IgG1 and IgG3 antibodies have a higher binding affinity to mononuclear Fcγ receptors than IgG2 and IgG4 antibodies.

2. *Antigen density.* Affects the number of antibody molecules bound to the cell surface.

3. *Fluid-phase IgG.* Serum IgG concentration is a determinant of Fc-dependent MP function.[18] Normal levels of IgG block the adherence of sensitized red cells to monocyte Fc receptors in vitro. Haemoconcentration in the splenic sinusoids is probably a major factor in minimizing this effect in vivo, which may explain why the spleen is about 100 times more efficient at removing IgG-sensitized red cells than the liver, in spite of its greater macrophage mass and higher blood flow.[9]

The initial effect of high-dose intravenous IgG is to cause blockade of macrophage Fcγ receptors.[5,12] This reduces the immune clearance of antibody-coated cells, and has particular application in the management of auto-immune thrombocytopenia and post-transfusion purpura.

4. *Regulation of macrophage activity.* This may depend on specific cytokines which regulate expression of receptors for IgG and complement (phagocytosis) and secretion of cytotoxins (ADCC). Steroids may diminish, and infection may enhance, this phase of immune cell destruction.

The rate of immune cell destruction is therefore determined by antigen and antibody characteristics and MP function. The severity of the resultant cytopenia is a balance between cell destruction and the compensatory capacity of the bone marrow to increase cell production.

ANTIGEN-ANTIBODY REACTIONS

The red cell is a convenient marker for serological reactions and agglutination or lysis (due to complement action) is a visible indication (end-point) of an antigen-antibody reaction. The reaction occurs in two stages: in the first stage, the antibody binds to the red cell antigen (sensitization); the second stage involves agglutination (or lysis) of the sensitized cells.

The *first stage*, i.e. association of antibody with antigen (sensitized), is reversible and the strength of binding (equilibrium constant) depends on the 'exactness of fit' between antigen and antibody. This is influenced by:

1. *Temperature* — cold antibodies (usually IgM) generally bind best to the red cell at a low temperature, e.g. 4°C, whereas warm antibodies (usually IgG) bind most efficiently at body temperature, i.e. 37°C.

2. *pH* — there is relatively little change in antibody binding over the pH range 5.5–8.5, but to ensure comparable results it is preferable to buffer the saline in which serum or cells are diluted to a fixed pH, usually 7.0. Some antibody elution techniques depend on altering the pH to below 4 or above 10.

3. *Ionic strength* of the suspension medium — low ionic strength increases the rate of antibody binding. This is the basis of antibody detection tests using low ionic strength saline (LISS).

The *second stage* depends on various laboratory manipulations to promote agglutination or lysis of sensitized cells. The red cell surface is negatively charged (mainly due to sialic acid residues), which keeps individual cells apart; the minimum distance between red cells suspended in saline is about 18 nm. Agglutination is brought about by antibody cross-linking between cells. The span between antigen binding sites on IgM molecules (30 nm) is sufficient to allow IgM antibodies to bridge between saline suspended red cells (after settling) and so cause agglutination. IgG molecules have a shorter span (15 nm) and are usually unable to agglutinate sensitized red cells suspended in saline; notwithstanding, heavy IgG sensitization due to high antigen density lowers intercellular repulsive forces and is able to promote agglutination in saline (e.g. IgG anti-A, anti-B). However, it is standard procedure to promote agglutination of IgG sensitized red cells by:

1. Reducing intercellular distance by the addition of albumin or pretreatment of red cells with protease enzymes, e.g. papain or bromelin (p. 454).

2. Bridging between sensitized cells with an antiglobulin reagent in the antiglobulin test (p. 457).

Some complement-binding antibodies (especially IgM) may cause lysis in vitro (without noticeable agglutination), which can be enhanced by the addition of fresh serum as a source of complement. On the other hand, complement activation may only proceed to the C3 stage; in these circumstances cell-bound C3 can be detected by the antiglobulin test using an appropriate anti-complement reagent (p. 458).

GENERAL POINTS OF SEROLOGICAL TECHNIQUE AND QUALITY CONTROL

A high standard of proficiency in blood-group serology requires a series of quality control steps each designed to identify any deficiency in reagents, techniques and equipment. This should be combined with the quality control of performance by external quality assessment schemes and 'in-house' exercises. This and the following chapter emphasize the importance of quality control for careful serological work in a hospital blood transfusion laboratory. For a more detailed exposition the reader is referred to the review by Voak and Napier.[40]

Health and safety

Whenever possible use reagents that have been screened for HIV, HBV and HCV. All high-risk samples must be handled according to the laboratory safety code.

Standard operating procedures

All procedures must be detailed in a laboratory manual as standard operating procedures (SOP) which must be readily accessible and regularly reviewed.[2c]

Serum vs plasma

Serum is preferred to plasma for the detection of red cell allo-antibodies. Nevertheless, plasma is being used increasingly for convenience in microplate technology, especially when associated with automation.

When plasma is used, complement is inactivated by the EDTA anticoagulant. This is relevant for the detection of some complement-binding IgG antibodies, e.g. of Kidd specificity, that may be missed or give only one weak reactions with anti-IgG in the routine antiglobulin test, but can be readily detected by anti-complement (p. 458). It is therefore essential, when using plasma, to optimize the sensitivity of techniques for detecting weak IgG antibodies and to validate the procedure (p. 460). For example, in antibody screening, increased sensitivity can be achieved by using panel red cells with homozygous expression of selected antigens (p. 487).

Collection and storage of blood samples

Positive identification of the patient and careful labelling of blood samples are essential to avoid misidentification errors.[2a] Venous blood is desirable for blood-grouping purposes and 5–10 ml of blood should be taken and either allowed to clot at room temperature or anticoagulated with EDTA in a sterile glass tube. This will provide serum or plasma and cells. If serum is required urgently, the specimen may be placed in a 37°C water-bath and centrifuged as soon as the clot can be seen to have started to retract.

STORAGE OF SERA OR PLASMA

Great care must be taken to identify and label correctly any serum or plasma separated from the patient's original blood sample.

Patient's serum or plasma is best stored frozen at −20°C (or better still at −40°C) in 1–2 ml volumes in glass or plastic vials. Repeated thawing of a sample is harmful. If the sera are stored at −20°C or below, no precautions as to sterility are necessary. At 4°C sterility is essential; if this can be maintained, it will be found that the sera will retain their potency for months.

Complement deteriorates quickly on storage, but sera separated from blood as quickly as possible and stored at −20°C retain most of their complement activity for 1–2 weeks. For compatibility tests, samples of serum should be separated from the red cells as soon as possible and stored at −20°C until used, as the content of complement may be important for the detection of some antibodies. In plasma samples EDTA inactivates complement by chelating calcium.

RED CELL SUSPENSIONS

(a) Normal ionic strength saline (NISS)

A 2% suspension of washed red cells in phosphate buffered saline (PBS), pH 7.0, is generally suitable for agglutination tests in tubes. Unless otherwise specified, throughout this text 'saline' or 'buffered saline' refers to 9g/1 NaC1 buffered to pH 7.0 (see p. 579).

(b) Low ionic strength saline (LISS)

It is known that the rate of association of antibodies with red cell antigens is enhanced by lowering the ionic strength of the medium in which the reactions take place. Nevertheless, there has been some reluctance to use low ionic strength media in routine laboratory work for two reasons: first, non-specific agglutination may occur when NaCl concentrations <2 g/1 (0.03 mol/l) are used, and secondly, complement components are bound to the red cells at low ionic strengths.

A number of studies have, however, demonstrated that, provided certain precautions are observed, low ionic strength solutions (LISS) may be safely used in routine laboratory work.[26,37] The LISS solution can be made up in the laboratory (see p. 576) or purchased commercially.

The major advantage of LISS is that the incubation period in the IAT (p. 459) can be shortened whilst maintaining or increasing the sensitivity of detection of the majority of red cell antibodies. LISS is widely used in grouping, antibody screening and identification, and in cross-matching.

To avoid false positives, the following rules should be followed:

1. Red cells resuspended in LISS and serum or plasma should be incubated together in equal volumes: 2 volumes of cells to 2 volumes of serum are recommended to ensure the optimal molarity in the test of the order of 0.09 mol. Doubling the serum to cell ratio (by halving the cell concentration, e.g. from 3% to 1.5%) will enhance the detection of some antibodies, e.g. anti-Kell, that might otherwise be missed.[38]

2. The red cells should be washed in saline (× 2) and then LISS (× 1) before suspending in LISS at 1.5–2.0% cell concentration.

3. The working solution of LISS should be kept at room temperature.

4. Centrifugation force and time should be optimal to give maximum sensitivity with freedom from false positive or negative reactions (p. 460).

Reagent red cells

Red cells of selected phenotypes are needed for ABO and Rh D grouping, Rh phenotyping, and antibody screening and identification (see Chapter 26). Such cells are available commercially or from Blood Transfusion Centres.

USE OF ENZYME-TREATED RED CELLS

Enzyme-treated red cells have proved to be valuable reagents in the detection and investigation of auto- and allo-antibodies. Papain and bromelin are currently used for this purpose. Enzyme treatment is known to increase the avidity of both IgM and IgG antibodies. The receptors of some blood-group antigens, however, may be inactivated by enzyme-treatment, e.g. M, N, S, Fy[b] and Pr.

The most sensitive techniques are those using washed enzyme-pretreated red cells (two-stage techniques) which should match the performance of the spin tube LISS antiglobulin test (p. 459).

One-stage mixture techniques are relatively insensitive and have caused many missed incompatibilities in external proficiency trials.[15,16] A recent one-stage inhibitor papain technique[32] has been shown to be slightly less sensitive than the two-stage technique, but far superior to the traditional Löw's one-stage mixture technique.[33] As such, the papain inhibitor technique is suitable as a supportive test for antibody detection and cross-matching of small batches (e.g. 12–24 tests) in routine hospital transfusion laboratories.

A joint Working Party of the ISBT/ICSH* has addressed the problem of standardization of enzyme techniques, in particular the selection of enzyme reference preparations, assay methods and optimum techniques.[34] The reader should also consult the review of papain techniques in blood-group serology by Scott et al.[33]

Löw's method for the preparation of papain solution[23]

A 1% solution of activated papain is made as follows.

Grind 2 g of papain (Merck) in a mortar in 100 ml of Sörensen's phosphate buffer, pH 5.4 (p. 579). Centrifuge for 10 min and add 10 ml of 0.5 mol/l cysteine hydrochloride to the supernatant to activate the enzyme. Dilute the solution to 200 ml with the phosphate buffer and incubate for 1 h at 37°C. Dispense the enzyme in small volumes (e.g. 0.1–0.2 ml); it will keep satisfactorily for many months at −20°C, but once a tube is unfrozen any of the solution not immediately used should be discarded.

The enzyme activity should be standardized using an azoalbumin assay,[33] as this will determine the incubation time for enzyme treatment of the cells. The enzyme preparation should also be compared with the ISBT/ICSH papain standard using the same batch of azoalbumin, and so serve as an 'in house' standard.[34]

Two-stage papain method[33]

Add 1 volume of 1% papain (activated as described above) to 9 volumes of Sörenson's phosphate buffer, pH 7.0 (p. 579) in a 10 × 75 mm glass tube. Incubate at 37°C equal volumes of the freshly diluted papain and packed washed red cells for a time which must be determined for each batch of papain depending on the azoalbumin activity;[33] this is normally 15–30 min. After incubation, wash the cells in two changes of saline, pH 7.0, then dilute as required — to 3% in NISS or 1.5% in LISS. For NISS tests, add 1 drop of NISS-suspended cells to 1 drop of serum. For LISS tests add 2 drops of LISS-suspended cells to 2 drops of serum. Incubate for 15 min in a 37°C water-bath.

One-stage papain inhibitor method[32,33]

Add 1 drop of papain solution (azoalbumin activity 0.6) to 1 drop of 3% NISS-suspended red cells, or two drops of 1.5% LISS-suspended red cells, in a 10 × 75 mm glass tube. Mix by shaking and incubate for 15 min in a 37°C water-bath. Add 1 drop of a 1 in 10 dilution in PBS of 1 mmol/lE-64, a synthetic peptide papain inhibitor, shake and allow to incubate for a further 2 min for inhibition to occur. Then add 2 drops of serum, shake and incubate for 15 min, also in the 37°C water-bath.

For both methods, after incubation, centrifuge the tubes for 15 s at 500*g*. Read by an appropriate method (p. 455).

Preparation of bromelin solution[29]

Prepare a 0.5% solution by dissolving the bromelin powder in a mixture of 9 volumes of saline and 1 volume of Sörensen's phosphate buffer, pH 5.4 (p. 579). Store the solution in 0.5–1.0 ml volumes at −20°C, at which temperature it will keep for months. As preservatives, add 0.1% sodium azide and 0.5% Actidione (a fungicide). Add the bromelin, as papain is added in Löw's technique, to the serum just before the addition of the red cells. There is no need to pre-treat the red cells with the enzyme. Bromelin activity can be standardized by an azoalbumin assay as for papain.

Controls are particularly important when enzyme-treated cells are being used, and it must be established without question that the altered cells are reacting appropriately with sera of known antibody content. Only in this way can

---

*See p. 463 for an explanation of abbreviations of names which are referred to in this and subsequent Chapters.

the potency of the enzyme and the method of enzyme treatment be checked. Enzyme-treated cells are compared with untreated cells in reactions with a positive control (0.25 IU/ml anti-D) and a negative (inert) control (AB serum or fresh compatible serum).

AGGLUTINATION OF RED CELLS BY ANTIBODY: A BASIC METHOD

Agglutination tests are usually carried out in tubes — either sedimentation tube tests or spin tube tests. Slide tests are sometimes used for emergency ABO and Rh D grouping (p. 482 and 485). For microplate tests, see p. 482.

Tube tests

Add 1 volume of a 2% red cell suspension to 1 volume of serum or serum dilution in a disposable plastic or glass tube. Mix well and leave undisturbed for the appropriate time (see below)

Tubes. For agglutination tests use medium-sized (75 × 10 or 12 mm) disposable plastic or glass tubes. Similar tubes should be used for lysis tests when it is essential to have a relatively deep layer of serum to look through, if small amounts of lysis are to be detected. The level of the fluid must rise well above the concave bottom of the tubes.

Glass tubes should always be used if the contents are to be heated to 50°C or higher, or if organic solvents are being used. Glass tubes, however, are difficult to clean satisfactorily, particularly small bore tubes, and methods such as those given in the Appendix (p. 580) should be followed in detail.

Temperature and time of exposure of red cells to antibody

In blood-group serology tube tests are generally done at 37°C and/or room temperature. There is some advantage in using a 20°C water-bath rather than relying on 'room temperature' which in different countries and seasons may vary from 15°C (or less) to 30°C (or more).

Sedimentation tube tests are usually read after 1–2 h have elapsed. Strong agglutination will, however, be obvious much sooner than this. In spin tube tests agglutination can be read after only 5–10 min incubation if the cell-serum mixture is centrifuged.

Slide tests

Because of evaporation, slide tests must be read within about 5 min. Reagents which produce strong agglutination within 1–2 min are normally used for rapid ABO and Rh D grouping. Since the results are read macroscopically, strong cell suspensions should be used (35–45% cells in their own serum or plasma) (See Fig. 24.2.)

READING RESULTS OF TUBE TESTS

Only the strongest complete (C) grade of agglutination seems to be able to withstand a shake procedure without some degree of disruption which may downgrade the strength of reaction. The BCSH Blood Transfusion Task Force has therefore recommended the following reading procedure.[2b]

(a) Microscopic reading

It is essential that a careful and standardized technique be followed. Lift the tube carefully from its rack without disturbing the button of sedimented cells. Holding the tube vertically, introduce a Pasteur pipette, with its tip cut at 90°. Carefully draw up a column of supernatant about 1 cm in length and then, without introducing an air bubble, draw up a 1–2 mm column of red cells by placing the tip of the pipette in the button of red cells. Gently expel the supernatant and cells on to a slide over an area of about 2 × 1 cm. It is important not to overload the suspension with cells, and the method described above achieves this.

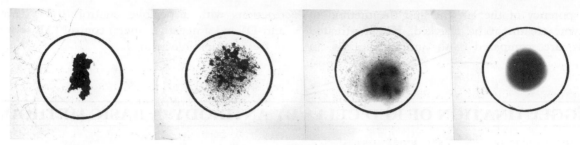

Fig. 24.2   Macroscopic appearances of agglutination in round-bottom tubes or hollow tiles. Agglutination is shown by various degrees of 'graininess'; in the absence of agglutination the sedimented cells appear as a smooth round button, as on the extreme right.

A scheme of scoring the results is given in Table 24.6.

(b) Macroscopic reading

A gentle agitation tip-and-roll 'macroscopic' method is recommended. It is possible to read agglutination tests macroscopically with the aid of a hand reading-glass or concave mirror, but it is then difficult to distinguish reactions weaker than + (microscopic reading) from the normal slight granular appearance of unagglutinated red cells in suspension. Macroscopic reading thus gives lower titration values than does microscopic reading. Follow the system of scoring in Table 24.6.

A good idea of the presence or absence of agglutination can often be obtained by inspection of the deposit of sedimented cells: a perfectly smooth round button suggests no agglutination whilst agglutination is shown by varying degrees of irregularity, 'graininess' or dispersion of the deposit (Fig. 24.2).

DEMONSTRATION OF LYSIS

Many blood-group antibodies lyse red cells under suitable conditions in the presence of complement. This is particularly true of anti-A and anti-B, anti-P, anti-Lewis, anti-P + P_1 + P^k(anti-Tj^a) and certain auto-antibodies (p. 518). If it is necessary to add fresh complement, this should be mixed with the serum being tested before the addition of red cells. Otherwise, agglutination occurs and could block complement access. Lysis should be looked for at the end of the incubation period before the tubes are centrifuged, if the cells have sedimented sufficiently; it may be scored roughly quantitatively after centrifuging the suspensions and comparing the colour of the supernatant with that of the control.

If the occurrence of lysis is of interest, then the final volume of the cell-serum suspension has to be greater than is required for the reading of agglutination. 75 × 10 or 12 mm tubes should be used and the level of the cell-serum suspension must rise well above the concave bottom of the tubes.

Table 24.6   Scoring of results in red cell agglutination tests

Symbol	Agglutination score*	Description
4+ or C (complete)	12	Cell button remains in one clump, macroscopically visible
3+	10	Cell button dislodges into several large clumps, macroscopically visible
2+	8	Cell button dislodges into many small clumps, macroscopically visible
1+	5	Cell button dislodges into finely granular clumps, macroscopically just visible
(+) or w (weak)	3	Cell button dislodges into fine granules, only visible microscopically**
–	0	Negative result — all cells free and evenly distributed

*Titration scores are the summation of the agglutination scores at each dilution.
**May be further classified depending on the number of cells in the clumps, e.g. clumps of 12–20 cells (score 3); 8–10 cells (score 2); 4–6 cells (score 1) — this is the minimum agglutination that should be considered positive.

In testing for lytic activity a high concentration of complement may be required. Therefore, in contrast to tests for agglutination, it is advantageous to use a stronger red cell suspension (c 5%).

Lysis tests are usually carried out at 37°C, but with cold antibodies a lower temperature, e.g. 20°C or 30°C, would be appropriate, depending on the upper thermal range of activity of the antibody, or, in the case of the Donath-Landsteiner antibody, 0°C followed by 37°C (p. 522).

Methods for titrating an antibody to demonstrate its lysis titre are described on p. 520. With certain antibodies, too, the pH of the cell-serum suspension affects the occurrence of lysis (p. 512).

Controls

It is necessary to be sure that any lysis observed is not artefactual, i.e. that lysis is brought about by the serum under test and not by the serum added as complement, and that the added complement is potent. A complement control (no test serum) is thus necessary and also a control using a serum known to contain a lytic antibody.

In lysis tests, great care should be taken to deliver the cell suspension directly into the serum. If the cell suspension comes into contact with the side of the tube and starts to dry, this in itself will lead to lysis.

ANTIGLOBULIN TEST

The antiglobulin test (Coombs test) was introduced by Coombs, Mourant and Race in 1945[6] as a method for detecting 'incomplete' Rh antibodies, i.e. IgG antibodies capable of sensitizing red cells, but incapable of causing agglutination of the same cells suspended in saline, as opposed to 'complete' IgM antibodies which do agglutinate saline-suspended red cells.

Direct and indirect antiglobulin tests can be carried out. In the *direct* test (DAT) the patient's cells, after careful washing, are tested for in-vivo sensitization; in the *indirect* test (IAT) normal red cells are incubated with a serum suspected of containing an antibody and subsequently tested, after washing, for in-vitro bound antibody.

The antiglobulin test is probably the most important test in the serologist's repertoire. The DAT is used to demonstrate in-vivo attachment of antibodies to red cells, as in auto-immune haemolytic anaemia (p. 505), allo-immune haemolytic disease of the newborn (p. 493); and allo-immune haemolysis following an incompatible transfusion (p. 491). The IAT has wide application in blood transfusion serology, including antibody screening and identification and cross-matching.

ANTIGLOBULIN REAGENTS

(a) Polyspecific (broad-spectrum) reagents

These should contain both anti-IgG and anti-complement. If plasma is used, only anti-IgG is necessary as EDTA prevents complement activation (p. 452).

The majority of red cell antibodies are non-complement-binding IgG; anti-IgG is therefore an essential component of any polyspecific reagent. Anti-IgA is not required as IgG antibodies of the same specificity always occur in the presence of IgA antibodies. Anti-IgM is also not required because clinically significant IgM allo-antibodies that do not cause agglutination in saline are much more easily detected by the complement they bind.

Anti-complement is necessary to detect clinically significant antibodies that bind complement, but which may react only weakly in anti-IgG tests.[11] Such antibodies, e.g. anti-Jk[a] which may be barely detectable by anti-IgG with heterozygous Jk(a + b +) red cells, may be readily detected by a polyspecific reagent containing anti-complement.[39]

The question arises as to which anti-complement antibodies are best for the detection

Table 24.7   C3 determinants in various C3 states on red cells[20]

C3 state	C3b complete	→	C3bi	→	C3dg(α_2D)	→	C3d**
Components	c + (g –)*d +		c + g + d +		g + d +		d +
Monoclonal	Anti-C3c		Anti-C3c		Anti-C3g		Anti-C3d
antibody	Anti-C3d		Anti-C3g		Anti-C3d		
reactions			Anti-C3d				

*g is concealed in C3b.
**Red cells treated with trypsin; the final C3 fragment found on red cells in vivo is C3dg.

of complement binding allo-antibodies. If red cells are not lysed immediately, complement activation usually stops at the C3 stage. The first activation product of C3 is C3b which reacts with antibodies against the C3c and C3d parts of the molecule (Table 24.7). Conversion of C3b to C3bi takes place rapidly and exposes another antigenic determinant, C3g[19,20], and red cells at this stage (coinciding with incubation times of 15–45 min) are agglutinated by anti-C3c, anti-C3g and anti-C3d. After further inactivation C3c is split off and reactions with anti-C3g and anti-C3d remain. Conversion of C3bi to C3dg, as determined by loss of reactivity with anti-C3c, may be complete within 2 h in the presence of excess serum at 37°C.[4,35] However, with the amount of serum routinely used in the indirect antiglobulin test and the shorter incubation times which are now used, little C3c is lost.[13] Nevertheless, to cover the wide range of incubation times still being used in antiglobulin tests it would be safer to target C3c and/or C3d with appropriate monoclonal reagents. Such reagents are now available either singly, e.g. BRIC-8 anti-C3d,[17] or as a blend of anti-C3c and anti-C3d. These newer reagents cause fewer false-positive reactions at higher titres and are suitable for mixing with anti-IgG in a polyspecific reagent.

The complement component C4 also accumulates on red cells stored in plasma or serum at 4°C; for this reason the antiglobulin reagent should contain little or no anti-C4 which is a nuisance antibody causing false-positive reactions.

(b) Monospecific reagents

These can be prepared against the heavy chains of IgG, IgM and IgA and are referred to as anti-γ, anti-μ and anti-α; antibodies against IgG subclasses are also available. Specific antibodies against the complement components C4 and C3 and C3 breakdown products can be prepared as mentioned above.

The main clinical application of these mono-specific reagents is to define the immunochemical characteristics of antibodies. This is relevant to the mechanisms of in-vivo cell destruction and, in the case of IgG, the subclasses have different biological properties (p. 451).

QUALITY CONTROL OF ANTIGLOBULIN REAGENTS

The quality control of antiglobulin reagents must always be carried out by the exact technique by which they are to be used. All reagents should be used according to the manufacturer's instructions, unless appropriately standardized for other methods.

The ISBT/ICSH Working Party on the Standardization of Antiglobulin Reagents has recommended the use of polyspecific antiglobulin reagents for compatibility testing by spin-tube techniques.[12]

A conventional polyclonal reference reagent (designated R3P) is available from Dr. M. Overbeeke, CLB, Amsterdam (see p. 590).

The quality control procedure of a new antiglobulin reagent should assess the following qualities of the reagent:

1. *Specificity.* The reagent should only agglutinate red cells sensitized with antibodies and/or coated with significant levels of complement components.

2. *Potency of anti-IgG* by serological titration.

3. *Specificity and potency of anti-complement antibodies.* A polyspecific reagent should contain anti-C3c and anti-C3d at controlled levels to avoid false-positive reactions or a suitable potent monoclonal anti-C3d (e.g. BRIC-8). It should

contain little or no anti-C4. The assessment of these qualities requires red cells specifically coated with C3b, Cb3i, C3d and C4. Details of the procedures recommended for the preparation of such cells have been published by the above Working Party.[39]

It is appreciated that some hospital blood banks will be unable to evaluate an antiglobulin reagent as comprehensively as outlined above. They should, however, carry out the following minimal assessment of all new antiglobulin reagents:

1. Test the antiglobulin reagent for freedom from false positives by simulated cross-match tests.

(a) Test for excess anti-C3d by incubating fresh serum at 37°C by NISS and LISS tests with six ABO compatible cells from CPD-A1 donor unit segments (10–30 days old). This is a critical test for false positives due to C3d uptake by stored blood which is further augmented by incubation with fresh serum.

(b) Tests for contaminating red cell antibodies (against washed A_1, B and O cells) must be negative.

Only proceed further if the antiglobulin reagent passes the above tests.

2. Compare the antiglobulin reagent with the current reagent using a selection of weak antibodies. These antibodies may be selected from those encountered in routine work or can be obtained from a Regional Transfusion Centre or Reference Laboratory. Store such antibodies in small volumes at −4°C for repeated tests.

3. Dilute a weak IgG anti-D (0.8 IU/ml), as used for routine antiglobulin test controls, from undiluted (neat) to 1 in 16 and sensitize R_1r red cells with each dilution of anti-D. These sensitized cells (washed × 4) should then be tested with neat to 1 in 8 dilutions of the antiglobulin reagents. The antiglobulin reagent should not show prozones by immediate spin tests using 2 volumes of antiglobulin per test. The potency of the test antiglobulin should at least match the current antiglobulin reagent.

The ISBT/ICSH antiglobulin reference reagent can be used to calibrate an 'in-house' antiglobulin reagent for use as a routine standard.

The quality control of Ig class and sub-class specific antiglobulin reagents, while following the above general principles, is more complex. Details of the appropriate techniques are beyond the scope of this chapter and the reader should consult the review by Englefriet et al.[10]

RECOMMENDED ANTIGLOBULIN TEST PROCEDURE

A spin tube technique is recommended for the routine antiglobulin test and the procedure described here is based on BCSH *Guidelines for Compatibility Testing in Hospital Blood Banks.*[2b] Reliable performance depends on the correct procedure at each stage of the test and appropriate quality control measures.

The test should be carried out in glass tubes (75 × 10 or 12 mm). Plastic tubes are not recommended as they may adsorb IgG which could neutralize anti-IgG of the antiglobulin reagent.

1. *Sensitize red cells* (not relevant to the direct test) by using the following serum:cell ratios:

(a) For normal ionic strength saline (NISS), use 2 volumes of serum and 1 volume of a 3% suspension of red cells washed (× 3) and suspended in phosphate buffered saline (PBS) or 0.15 mol/l NaCl (p. 579).

(b) For low ionic strength saline (LISS), use 2 volumes of serum and 2 volumes of a 1.5% suspension of red cells washed (× 2) in PBS or 0.15 mol/l NaCl and once in LISS and then suspended in LISS (p. 576).

(c) For commercial low ionic strength additive solutions, the manufacturer's instructions must be followed.

As the volume of 'a drop' varies according to the type of pipette or dropper bottle, a measured or known drop volume should be used to ensure that appropriate serum:cell ratios are maintained.

Mix the reactants by shaking, then incubate at 37°C, preferably in a water-bath, for a minimum period of 15 min for LISS tests and 45 min for NISS tests.

2. *Wash the test cells* 4 times with a minimum of 3 ml of saline per wash. Vigorous injection of saline is necessary to resuspend the cells and

achieve adequate mixing. As much of the supernatant as possible should be removed after each wash to achieve maximum dilution of residual serum.

3. *Add 2 volumes of a suitable antiglobulin reagent* to each test tube and centrifuge without delay after thorough mixing. The combinations of centrifugal force (RCF) and time for spin-tube tests are as follows:

RCF (g)	100	200–220	500	1000
Time (s)	60	25–30	15	8–10

4. *Read agglutination* as previously described (p. 455).

5. *Quality control of the test* should be monitored by:

(a) An IgG anti-D diluted to give 1 + or 2 + reactions with Rh D positive (R_1r) cells as a *positive control*.

(b) An inert group AB serum with the same Rh D positive cells as a *negative control*; this is not essential as most tests are negative.

(c) *The addition of sensitized cells to all negative tests.* This is widely used to detect neutralization of the antiglobulin reagent due to incomplete removal of serum by the wash step. The value of this test as a control depends on the strength of reaction of the sensitized cells. Appropriate control cells sensitized with IgG anti-D should give a 3 + reaction when tested directly with the antiglobulin reagent and should still be positive (if the reagent is potent) when added to negative tests, but downgraded (1+ or 2+) due to the 'pooled-cell' effect of the non-sensitized cells. The reaction will of course be negative if the antiglobulin has been neutralized by residual serum.

The production of satisfactory antiglobulin control cells can be achieved by limiting the level of anti-D sensitization to that which gives a negative test in the presence of 1 in 1000 parts serum in saline.[2b]

The suitability of the antiglobulin control cells can be checked as follows:

i.   Prepare two tubes (10 × 75 mm) with one volume of 3% unsensitized cells; wash four times.

ii. Add two volumes of antiglobulin to each of the tubes, mix well, spin and read the tubes to confirm the tests are negative.

iii. Add one volume of 1 in 1000 serum in saline to one tube and one volume of saline as a control to the other tube. Mix and incubate for 1 min at RT.

iv. Add one volume of control cells to each tube, mix, spin and read the tests.

The test containing 1 in 1000 serum in saline should be negative and the control tube should give at least 2+ reaction. A negative reaction with the control tube suggests a washing deficiency and demands corrective action. If an automated cell washing centrifuge is used, the washing efficiency should be checked: see *Quality Control of Cell Washing Centrifuges.*[2b,28]

TWO-STAGE EDTA-COMPLEMENT INDIRECT ANTIGLOBULIN TEST (IAT)

Stored serum may become anticomplementary. To overcome this, a two-stage method is recommended. Antibody is taken up in the first stage and complement in the second stage.

Add 1 drop of a 3% suspension of red cells to 4 drops of EDTA-treated serum, prepared by adding 0.1 ml of neutral EDTA (i.e. 11 µmol; *c* 4 mg) (p. 576) per ml of serum, and incubate at 37°C for 1 h. Wash the cells 3 times in saline and then reincubate with 2 drops of compatible fresh normal serum for 15 min at 37°C. Finally wash the cells and treat them in the usual manner for the IAT.

NEW TECHNOLOGY FOR ANTIBODY DETECTION BY THE ANTIGLOBULIN TEST

New techniques have emerged that have a simpler reading phase than the manually read spin-tube IAT. These are of two main types: solid phase[31] and gel techniques.[21] Before the introduction of a new technique, it is essential to remember that validation and routine test trials must be performed by competent workers who are fully familiar with the new system, and that it should be carried out strictly according to the manufacturer's instructions.[36] A well-performed spin-tube IAT, as described above, is the standard against which any new system should be compared.

ASSESSMENT OF INDIVIDUAL WORKER PERFORMANCE

It is recommended that all staff (including 'on-call' staff who do not routinely work in the blood bank) should be assessed at regular intervals. A procedure based on 'blind' replicate antiglobulin tests may be used for this purpose.[2b,28]

The procedure is as follows:

1. A low titre (8–16) IgG anti-D, as used for the control of the antiglobulin test, should be titrated against OR_1r or pooled O Rh D-positive cells to find the dilution of anti-D that gives 1+ or 2+ sensitized cells (most workers use around 0.3 IU/ml). A standard BCSH-NIBSC anti-D reference reagent (91/608) is available for this purpose (available from NIBSC, P.O. Box 1193, Potters Bar, Herts EN6 3QG, UK)[28].

2. A batch of sensitized cells is prepared, e.g. by incubating 16 ml of the selected anti-D dilution with 8 ml of of 3% washed OR_1r red cells at 37°C for 45 min.

3. Twelve tubes are labelled for blind tests by another person. One volume of 3% 1+ or 2+ sensitized cells and 2 volumes of group AB inert serum (to simulate the volumes of serum used in routine tests) are placed in nine random tubes, and then 1 volume of unsensitized cells + 2 volumes of group-AB inert serum are placed in the remaining tubes. The position of the various tests is recorded.

4. The cells are washed thoroughly 4 times, antiglobulin is added and the tubes are spun and read.

5. The number of false negative (and false positive) results are recorded for each worker and analysed in relation to reading and/or washing technique. It is advisable to give immediate tuition to any workers with washing or reading test faults, followed by further blind replicate trials to demonstrate improvement in procedure and to restore confidence.

TITRATION OF ANTIBODIES

Preparation of serial dilutions of patient's or other sera

When comparing the effect of different temperatures on agglutination or the different sensitivities of several types of red cells, it is important to make a set of master serial dilutions of the serum being tested and to subsample an appropriate number of small volumes from each dilution as it is made.

Doubling dilutions are usually made and can be prepared by adding an equal volume of serum to the diluent and transferring the same volume of the mixture to the next volume of diluent and so on. The dilutions may be made with a marked glass Pasteur pipette. Commercially available Pasteur pipettes are satisfactory, and provided the ends are not chipped, the pipettes, if held vertically, will deliver 30 ± 1 drops to the ml. Sometimes when the serum is in short supply it is convenient to use fine-bore '50-dropper' pipettes.

The methods of making dilutions, referred to above, suffer from 'carry over' of serum — that is to say, traces of concentrated serum remain in the pipette and tend to increase the concentration of serum in the tubes which should contain only highly-diluted serum. This results in erroneously high titration figures and long drawn-out end-points. However, the titrations are easy to carry out and the results obtained have a relative value and are satisfactory for most clinical purposes. To obtain more accuracy it is necessary to use a separate accurately calibrated pipette for each dilution (Table 24.8).

Four-fold dilutions using a drop method

A method employing fourfold dilutions is economical of time and materials, and Fig. 24.3

Table 24.8   Comparison of titration end-points of a high-titre cold agglutinin using conventional doubling dilution techniques with those obtained by making dilutions with separate pipettes.

Final serum dilution		1 in 1024	1 in 4096	1 in 16 000	1 in 64 000	1 in 256 000	1 in 1 000 000	Control (saline)
1. In doubling dilutions using Pasteur pipette								
(a) no mixing in stem	macro	+	+	+	+⃞	–	–	–
	micro	+	+	+	+	+	+⃞	–
(b) with mixing in stem	macro	+	+	+	weak	–	–	–
	micro	+	+	+	+	+	+⃞	–
2. Doubling dilutions using glass automatic pipette	macro	+	+	+	+⃞	(?)	–	–
	micro	+	+	+	+	+	+⃞	–
3. Dilutions prepared using a separate pipette for each dilution	macro	+	+	+⃞	(?)	–	–	–
	micro	+	+	+	+⃞	–	–	–

The titre read macroscopically was recorded as 32 000.

Only the results of readings made on the last seven alternate tubes of the titrations are recorded. The doubling dilutions were prepared commencing with undiluted serum, and the separate dilutions (3 above) were prepared from an initial serum dilution of 1 in 256.

The titrations were carried out at room temperature (18°C) and the end-points of the titration were determined macroscopically (macro) using a concave mirror, and also microscopically (micro). The end-points are indicated +⃞.

The end-points determined macroscopically using the conventional doubling-dilution techniques give results which closely approximate to those obtained when dilutions of serum are prepared using a separate pipette for each dilution and the result is read microscopically.

illustrates how such a titration can be carried out using a drop technique. The master dilutions can be made by the drop method or if greater accuracy is desired by using separate pipettes for each dilution.

The diluent should be buffered saline, pH 7.0, for agglutination tests; or for lysis tests undiluted ABO-compatible fresh normal human serum acidified so that the pH of the cell-serum mixture is c 6.8. The normal serum serves as a source of complement.

Titrations which involve reading the result by

the antiglobulin method should be carried out in relatively large (e.g. 75 × 10 mm) tubes so that the red cells can be washed thoroughly in the same tubes in relatively large volumes of saline.

Addition of red-cell suspensions to dilutions of serum

It is conventional to add 1 volume of red-cell suspension to 1 volume of serum or serum dilution. This means that each antibody dilution, and hence the 'final' titre, will be twice that of the original serum dilution.

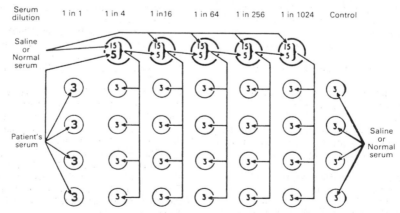

Fig. 24.3   Diagram illustrating method of preparing four sets of four-fold dilutions of a serum. The large circles at the top represent the large tubes in which the primary dilutions are made; the smaller circles represent the tubes in which the titrations are carried out. The figures represent drops or volumes. The patient's serum is indicated by the bold type.

TEST FOR SECRETION OF A AND B SUBSTANCES

Principle. Saliva is serially diluted, then added to anti-A or anti-B serum. The sera are tested with A_2 or B cells to see whether the antibodies have been neutralized. About 20% of persons are non-secretors.

Method

Dilute an anti-A or anti-B serum so that it gives good visible agglutination with A_2 or B cells at the end of 1 h at room temperature, e.g. if the titre of the serum is 128, use it at a dilution of 1 in 16.

Collect several ml of saliva in a centrifuge tube. Place the tube in boiling water for 10 min and then centrifuge. Serially dilute the clear supernatant in saline so as to give dilutions ranging from 1 in 2 to 1 in 32. Use a tube containing saline alone as a control. Add an equal volume of the diluted anti-A (or anti-B) serum to each tube and, after shaking the rack of tubes, allow it to stand for 10–15 min at room temperature. Then add an equal volume of a 2% suspension in saline of A_2 (or B) red cells to each tube. Mix the contents, and allow to stand at room temperature for 1–2 h; then inspect for agglutination. If the saliva contains A or B substances, agglutination is usually inhibited in all the tubes except the saline-control tube. It is desirable to use saliva from a known secretor and non-secretor, respectively, as additional controls.

H substance can be demonstrated in a similar way using an extract of Ulex, eel serum or the naturally occurring 'incomplete' cold antibody as a source of anti-H.

ACKNOWLEDGEMENTS

The author wishes to thank Dr. D. Voak and Mrs. Judith Chapman, FIMLS for advice in the preparation of this chapter and, with respect, to pay tribute to the late Eleanor Lloyd, FIMLS, who was his co-author for the previous edition.

Abbreviations used in this chapter

ICSH	International Council for Standardization in Haematology
ISBT	International Society of Blood Transfusion
BCSH	British Committee for Standards in Haematology
AABB	American Association of Blood Banks
CLB	Central Laboratory of the Netherlands Red Cross Blood Transfusion Service

REFERENCES

[1] ANSTEE, D. J. and TANNER, M. J. A. (1988). Blood group antigen deficiencies associated with abnormal red cell shape. *Blood Reviews*, **2**, 115

[2] BRITISH COMMITTEE FOR STANDARDS IN HAEMATOLOGY (1991). *Standard Haematology Practice*. Ed. Roberts, B., (a) p. 128; (b) p. 150; (c) p. 217. Blackwell Scientific Publications, Oxford.

[3] CARTRON, J. P. and AGRE, P. (1993). Rh blood group antigens: protein and gene structure. *Seminars in Haematology*, **30**, 193.

[4] CHAPLIN, H., MONROE, M. C. and LACHMANN, P. J. (1982). Further studies of the C3g component of the $\alpha_2 D$ fragments of human C3. *Clinical and Experimental Immunology*, **51**, 639.

[5] CLARKSON, S. B., BUSSEL, J. B. and KIMBERLEY, R. P. (1986). Treatment of refractory immune thrombocytopenic purpura with an anti-Fc receptor antibody. *New England Journal of Medicine*, **314**, 1236.

[6] COOMBS, R. R. A., MOURANT, A. E. and RACE, R. R. (1945). A new test of the detection of weak and 'incomplete' Rh agglutinins. *British Journal of Experimental Pathology*, **26**, 255.

[7] DANIELS, G. L. and 25 others (1993). ISBT Working Party on terminology for red cell surface antigens: Sao Paulo Report. *Vox Sanguinis*, **65**, 77.

[8] ENGELFRIET, C. P. (1992). The immune destruction of red cells. *Transfusion Medicine*, **2**, 1.

[9] ENGELFRIET, C. P., OVERBEEKE, M. A. M. and OUWEHAND, W. H. (1988), Detection and characterisation of alloantibodies and autoantibodies. In: Blood Transfusion. Ed. Greenwalt, T. J. *Methods in Haematology*, **17**, 106.

[10] ENGELFRIET, C. P., OVERBEEKE, M. A. M. and VOAK, D. (1987). The antiglobulin test (Coombs test) and the red cell. In *Progress in Transfusion Medicine*. Ed. Cash, J. D., Vol. 2, p. 74–98. Churchill Livingstone, Edinburgh.

[11] ENGELFRIET, C. P. and VOAK, D. (1987). International reference polyspecific anti-human globulin reagents. *Vox Sanguinis*, **53**, 241.

[12] FEHR, J., HOFMANN, V. and KAPPELER, U. (1982). Transient reversal of thrombocytopenia in idiopathic

thrombocytopenia by high dose intravenous gamma globulin. *New England Journal of Medicine*, **306**, 1254.

[13] GARRATTY, G. and PETZ, L. (1976). The significance of red cell bound complement components in development of standards and quality assurance for the anti-complement components in antiglobulin sera. *Transfusion*, **16**, 297.

[14] GIBLETT, E. R. (1977). Blood group alloantibodies: an assessment of some laboratory practices. *Transfusion*, **17**, 299.

[15] HOLBURN, A. M. and PRIOR, D. M. (1986). The UK National External Quality Assessment Scheme in Blood Group Serology. ABO and D grouping and antibody screening 1982–1983. *Clinical and Laboratory Haematology*, **8**, 243.

[16] HOLBURN, A. M. and PRIOR, D. M. (1987). The U.K. National External Quality Assessment Scheme in Blood Group Serology. Compatibility testing 1983–1984: the influence of variables in test procedures on detection of incomplete antibodies. *Clinical and Laboratory Haematology*, **9**, 33.

[17] HOLT, P. D. J., DONALDSON, C., JUDSON, P. A., JOHNSON, P., PARSONS, S. F., ANSTEE, D. J. (1985). NBTS/BRIC 8. A monoclonal anti-C3d antibody. *Transfusion*, **25**, 267.

[18] KELTON, J. G. (1985). The interaction of IgG with reticulo-endothelial cells: biological and therapeutic implications. In *Current Concepts in Transfusion Therapy*. Ed. Garratty, G. p. 51–107. American Association of Blood Banks, Arlington, VA.

[19] LACHMANN, P. J., PANGBURN, H. K. and OLDROYD, R. G. (1982). Breakdown of C3bi to C3c, C3d and a new fragment C3g. *Journal of Experimental Medicine*, **156**, 205.

[20] LACHMANN, P. J., VOAK, D., OLDROYD, R. G., DOWNIE, D. M. and BEVAN, D. C. (1983). The use of monoclonal anti-C3 antibodies to characterise the fragments of C3 that are found on erythrocytes. *Vox Sanguinis*, **45**, 367.

[21] LAPIERRE, Y., RIGEL, D., ADAMS, J., JOSEF, D., MEYER, F., GERBER, S. and DROT, C. (1990). The gel test: a new way to detect red cell antigen-antibody reactions. *Transfusion*, **30**, 109.

[22] LEWIS, M. and 29 others (1990). Blood group terminology. *Vox Sanguinis*, **58**, 152.

[23] LÖW, B. (1955). A practical method using papain and incomplete Rh-antibodies in routine Rh blood-grouping. *Vox Sanguinis*, **5(OS)**, 94.

[24] LUTZ, P. and DZIK, W. H. (1992). Molecular biology of red cell blood group genes. *Transfusion*, **32**, 467.

[25] MOLLISON, P. L., ENGELFRIET, C. P. and CONTRERAS, M. (1993). *Blood Transfusion in Clinical Medicine*, 9th edn., (a) p. 112. Blackwell Scientific Publications, Oxford.

[26] MOORE, H. C. and MOLLISON, P. L. (1976). Use of low ionic-strength medium in manual tests for antibody detection. *Transfusion*, **16**, 291.

[27] MOURANT, A. E., KOPEC, A. C. and DOMANIEWSKA-SOBCZAK, K. (1976). *The Distribution of the Human Blood Groups and Other Biochemical Polymorphisms*, 2nd edn.

Oxford University Press, Oxford.

[28] PHILLIPS, P. K., VOAK, D., WHITTON, C. M., DOWNIE, D. M., BEBBINGTON, C. and CAMPBELL, J.(1993). BCSH-NIBSC anti-D reference reagent for antiglobulin tests: the in-house assessment of red cell washing centrifuges and of operator variability in the detection of weak macroscopic agglutination. *Transfusion Medicine*, **3**, 143.

[29] PIROFSKY, B. (1959). The use of bromelin in establishing a standard cross-match. *American Journal of Clinical Pathology*, **32**, 350.

[30] RACE, R. R. and SANGER, R. (1975). Blood Groups in Man, 6th edn. Blackwell Scientific Publications, Oxford.

[31] SCOTT, M. L. (1991). The principles and applications of solid phase blood group serology. *Transfusion Medicine Reviews*, **1**, 60.

[32] SCOTT, M. L. and PHILLIPS, P. K. (1987). A sensitive two-stage papain technique without cell washing. *Vox Sanguinis*, **52**, 67.

[33] SCOTT, M. L., VOAK, D. and DOWNIE, D. M. (1988). Optimum enzyme activity in blood grouping and a new technique for antibody detection: an explanation for the poor performance of the one-stage mix technique. *Medical Laboratory Sciences*, **45**, 7.

[34] SCOTT, M. L., VOAK, D., PHILLIPS, P. K., HOPPE, P. A. and KOCHMAN SHERYL, A. (1994). Review of the problems involved in using enzymes in blood group serology: provision of 4 freeze-dried ICSH/ISBT protease enzyme and anti-D reference standards. *Vox Sanguinis*, **67**, 89.

[35] STRATTON, F. and RAWLINSON, V. I. (1974). Preparation of test cells for the antiglobulin test. *Journal of Clinical Pathology*, **27**, 359.

[36] VOAK, D. (1992). Validation of new technology for antibody detection by antiglobulin tests. *Transfusion Medicine*, **2**, 177.

[37] VOAK, D., DOWNIE, D. M., DARNBOROUGH, L., HAIGH, T. and FAIRHAM, S. M. (1980). Low-ionic strength media for rapid antibody detection: optimum conditions and quality control. *Medical Laboratory Sciences*, **37**, 107.

[38] VOAK, D., DOWNIE, D. M., HAIGH, T. and COOK, N. (1982). Improved antiglobulin tests to detect difficult antibodies: detection of anti-Kell by LISS. *Medical Laboratory Sciences*, **39**, 363.

[39] VOAK, D., DOWNIE, D. M., MOORE, P. B. L. and ENGELFRIET, C. P. (1986). Anti-human globulin reagent specification: the European and ISBT/ICSH view. *Biotest Bulletin*, **1**, 7.

[40] VOAK, D. and NAPIER, J. A. F. (1990). Quality assurance in the hospital transfusion laboratory: quality control in blood group serology. In *Quality Control in Haematology*. Ed. Cavill, I. *Methods in Haematology*, **22**, 129.

[41] WORLD HEALTH ORGANIZATION (1977). *Twenty-eighth Report of WHO Expert Committee on Biological Standardization*. Technical Report Series, 610. WHO, Geneva.

25. Platelet and neutrophil antigens and antibodies

By A. H. Waters

Allo-antigen systems   465
  Clinical significance   465
Allo-antibodies   465
Iso-antibodies   466
Auto-antibodies   466
Demonstration of platelet and neutrophil antibodies   468
  Allo-antibodies   468
  Auto-antibodies   468
  Drug-induced antibodies   469

Methods of demonstrating antibodies   470
  Fluorescent-labelled antiglobulin methods   470
Platelet and granulocyte immunofluorescence tests (PIFT, GIFT)   471
Chloroquine-treated platelets and granulocytes   473
Monoclonal antibody immobilization of platelet antigens (MAIPA)   474
Other methods   475
Molecular genotyping of platelet allo-antigens   475

ALLO-ANTIGEN SYSTEMS

Platelet and neutrophil allo-antigens may be exclusive to each cell type (cell-specific) or shared with other cells. The currently recognized cell-specific antigen systems are shown in Tables 25.1 and 25.2. Of the shared antigens, the HLA system is the most important clinically; only class 1 antigens (HLA-A, -B, and to a lesser extent -C) are expressed on platelets and neutrophils. ABH antigens (Chapter 24) are also expressed on platelets (in part absorbed from the plasma), but cannot be demonstrated on neutrophils.

CLINICAL SIGNIFICANCE OF PLATELET AND NEUTROPHIL ANTIBODIES

Platelet and neutrophil antibodies may be classified on the basis of the antigenic stimulus, e.g. allo-, iso-, auto- and drug-induced antibodies.

(a) Allo-antibodies

Allo-immunization to platelet and neutrophil

Table 25.1 Platelet allo-antigen systems

System	Antigens		Antigen frequency*(%)	Gene frequency*	GP	Amino acid polymorphism
HPA-1	HPA-1a	Zw^a, P1^{A1}	97.46	0.8340	IIIa	Leucine 33
	HPA-1b	Zw^b, P1^{A2}	30.80	0.1660		Proline
HPA-2	HPA-2a	Ko^b	99.79	0.9399	Ib (α)	Threonine 145
	HPA-2b	Ko^a, Sib^a	11.81	0.0601		Methionine
HPA-3	HPA-3a	Bak^a, Lek^a	86.14	0.6162	IIb (β)	Isoleucine 843
	HPA-3b	Bak^b	62.92	0.3838		Serine
HPA-4	HPA-4a	Yuk^b, Pen^a	>99.9	0.9917	IIIa	Arginine 143
	HPA-4b	Yuk^a	<0.1			Glutamine
HPA-5	HPA-5a	Br^b, Zav^b	98.79	0.8890	Ia (α)	Glutamic acid 505
	HPA-5b	Br^a, Zav^a, Hc^a	20.65	0.1110		Lysine

HPA, human platelet antigen; nomenclature proposed by ICSH Platelet Serology Working Party. Platelet antigen systems numbered in chronological order of discovery; allelic antigens designated alphabetically: a, high frequency; b, low frequency; see also ref. 40.
GP, Glycoprotein location of epitopes
* Frequency in a Caucasian population;[22] see also ref. 50.

Table 25.2   Neutrophil-specific allo-antigen systems[6,9,14]

System	Antigens	Phenotype frequency (%)	Genotype frequency
NA	NA1	61.2	0.32
	NA2	89.6	0.68
NB	NB1	90.8	0.72
	NB2	31.0	0.17
NC	NC1	94.5	0.80
ND	ND1	98.5	0.88
NE	NE1	22.9	0.12

antigens is most commonly due to transfusion or pregnancy. The associated clinical problems depend on the specificity of the antibody, which determines the target cell involved. Cell-specific allo-antibodies are associated with well defined clinical conditions which are summarized in Tables 25.3 and 25.4. HLA allo-immunization is an important cause of refractoriness to platelet transfusion. Primary HLA immunization depends on the presence of contaminating lymphocytes in the transfused blood component; leucocyte-poor transfusions can therefore delay the onset of refractoriness due to HLA antibodies.[13,39] ABO incompatibility has little effect on the survival of transfused platelets, except in patients who have high-titre anti-A or anti-B lytic antibodies.[3]

Table 25.3   Clinical significance of platelet-specific allo-antibodies[57]

1. Neonatal allo-immune thrombocytopenia
   All IgG platelet-specific antibodies

2. Post-transfusion purpura
   ? restricted to antibodies reacting with epitopes on GP IIb/IIIa

3. Refractoriness to platelet transfusion
   Usually due to HLA antibodies.

GP, glycoprotein.

Table 25.4   Clinical significance of neutrophil-specific allo-antibodies[14,28,35]

1. Neonatal allo-immune neutropenia

2. Febrile reactions following transfusion
   (HLA antibodies also involved)

3. Transfusion-related acute lung injury (TRALI)
   (transfusion of high-titre antibody)

4. Poor survival and function of transfused granulocytes
   (HLA antibodies also involved)

5. Auto-immune neutropenia—some auto-antibodies have allospecificity for N system antigens.

(b) Iso-antibodies

Occasionally, after blood transfusion or pregnancy, patients with type I Glanzmann's disease make antibodies which react with platelet glycoprotein (GP) IIb/IIIa not present on their own platelets but present on normal platelets, i.e. isotypic determinants.[2,4,44,53] Similarly, patients with Bernard-Soulier syndrome may make antibodies against isotypic determinants on GP Ib/V/IX not present on their own platelets.[12] This may present a serious clinical problem because no compatible donor platelets can be found to treat severe bleeding episodes. Fortunately the occurrence of such antibodies is rare in these patients.

(c) Auto-antibodies

Auto-immune thrombocytopenia may be primary (idiopathic) or secondary (preceded by or associated with other conditions) (Table 25.5). Diagnosis depends on the exclusion of other causes of thrombocytopenia associated with adequate numbers of megakaryocytes in the bone marrow. Demonstration of a platelet auto-antibody is not mandatory; even with the most suitable techniques now available, platelet auto-antibodies remain elusive in a variable proportion (10–20%) of patients.[60]

In the diagnosis of auto-immune thrombocytopenia it is important to consider and exclude three other immunological conditions:

Table 25.5   Conditions associated with auto-immune thrombocytopenia (AIT)[56,64]

Post-viral infection
   Acute AIT of childhood
   Specific viral infections

Other auto-immune diseases
   Blood (e.g. Evans syndrome)
   Generalized (e.g. SLE, rheumatoid arthritis)
   Organ-specific (e.g. thyroid)

Lymphoproliferative disorders
   Chronic lymphocytic leukaemia
   Lymphoma

Cancer (solid tumours)

Immune system imbalance
   HIV infection
   Chemotherapy or radiotherapy
   Post bone-marrow graft

1. *Post-transfusion purpura (PTP)*—a blood transfusion within 2 weeks will suggest this possibility.[63]

2. *Drug-induced immune thrombocytopenia*—a drug history is essential.[37]

3. *Pseudo-thrombocytopenia*—the patient has an EDTA-dependent platelet antibody which is active only in vitro. The antibody (IgG and/or IgM) reacts with hidden (cryptic) antigens on platelet GP IIb/IIIa, which are exposed due to conformational changes in the complex caused by the removal of Ca^{2+} by EDTA.[42] The antibody causes platelet agglutination in the EDTA blood sample associated with large platelet clumps on the blood film or platelet satellitism around neutrophils, both of which lead to a falsely low platelet count. These effects are not seen when a citrate anticoagulant is used. Similar effects, which are independent of the anticoagulant used, may be produced by a cold platelet auto-antibody.[43,54]

Failure to recognize these conditions may lead to a false diagnosis of auto-immune thrombocytopenia by the unwary, but platelet serology will help to differentiate a platelet auto-antibody from the various antibodies responsible for the above conditions.

Auto-immune neutropenia may be primary (idiopathic) or secondary (Table 25.6). Idiopathic auto-immune neutropenia is more common in infants than in adults, in whom auto-immune neutropenia is usually associated with other disorders which have in common a postulated imbalance of the immune system.[6,26,29,35,48]

Table 25.6 Auto-immune neutropenia[29,35]

1. Primary (idiopathic)

2. Secondary (a) Auto-immune conditions
                    SLE
                    Felty's syndrome
                    AIHA ± thrombocytopenia
                    (Evans syndrome)

            (b) Lymphoproliferative conditions
                    ± chemotherapy and/or radiotherapy

            (c) Immune system imbalance
                    Hypogammaglobulinaemia
                    HIV infection
                    Post bone-marrow graft

Auto-immune neutropenia is the least well studied of the auto-immune cytopenias. This is partly because of the limitations of neutrophil serology, especially in the differentiation of auto-antibodies and circulating immune complexes (see below), and partly because the peripheral neutrophil count is an inadequate reflection of total granulocyte kinetics.

Neutrophil auto-antibodies (which are usually IgG) are unusual in that they often have well defined specificity for neutrophil-specific allo-antigens, especially NA1 or NA2.[6,26,29] However, it is not always possible to demonstrate allo-specificity; such auto-antibodies may have a wider target than mature neutrophils, and are better described as granulocyte auto-antibodies. These auto-antibodies may suppress granulocyte precursors in the bone marrow and cause more severe neutropenia. The investigation of suspected auto-immune neutropenia should, when possible, include serological tests and clonal assays (e.g. CFU-GM) on bone marrow precursors as target cells, especially when antibodies to mature neutrophils are not found.

The relative importance of auto-antibodies, immune complexes and cellular mechanisms in the pathogenesis of auto-immune neutropenia has yet to be resolved and the diagnosis is therefore based on the interpretation of a combination of tests.[29,48,52]

(d) Drug-induced antibodies

Drug-induced antibodies may cause selective haemolytic anaemia (p. 524), thrombocytopenia or neutropenia, or various combinations of these in the same patient.[7,16,37]

A drug may cause an immune cytopenia by stimulating production of either an *auto-antibody* (which reacts directly with the target cell independently of the drug itself) or a *drug-dependent antibody* which destroys the target cell by reacting with a drug-membrane complex on the target cell.[38] Laboratory tests may demonstrate both types of antibody in some patients.[15,45,47]

DEMONSTRATION OF PLATELET AND NEUTROPHIL ANTIBODIES

No single method will detect all types of platelet and neutrophil antibodies equally well. In practice it is useful to have a basic screening method that will detect most commonly occurring antibodies, both cell-bound (direct test) and in serum (indirect test), and to supplement this with other selected methods for demonstrating particular properties of an antibody and for measuring the amount of cell-bound antibody.

Labelled antiglobulin methods are widely used for routine platelet and neutrophil serology; fluorescent, enzyme and neutrophil labelled antiglobulin reagents are available. There is a general trend to introduce microtechnology in order to cope with increasing work loads and to reduce the consumption of reagents. Flow cytometry is also being introduced for reading results in the fluorescence test. For a critical analysis of these and other methods, see refs. 9, 14, 31 and 57.

(a) Allo-antibodies

Reports of recent national and international workshops[10,62] make it possible to formulate guidelines for *platelet serology*. The basic procedure for demonstrating platelet allo-antibodies should include:

(i) A platelet test for platelet-reactive antibodies

The ISBT/ICSH Working Party on Platelet Serology[62] recommended the platelet suspension immunofluorescence test[59] as the standard for assessment of other platelet antibody techniques.

It is important to combine a sensitive binding assay, such as the platelet immunofluorescence test (PIFT), with an antigen capture method, such as the monoclonal antibody immobilization of platelet antigens (MAIPA),[25] to increase the chance of detecting weak antibodies or those that react with relatively few antigen sites.

(ii) A lymphocyte test for detecting HLA antibodies

As HLA antibodies also react with platelets, a lymphocyte cytotoxicity and/or immuno-fluorescence test should be included in the basic antibody screening procedure.

(iii) Tests to differentiate platelet-specific from HLA antibodies

The MAIPA technique using appropriate mono-clonal antibodies is particularly useful for resolving mixtures of platelet-reactive antibodies (p. 474). The chloroquine-'stripping' technique to inactivate HLA Class 1 molecules on platelets[41] is also helpful in this respect (p. 473). Conventional serological techniques (e.g. differential reactions with a panel of normal lymphocytes and platelets; differential absorption of HLA antibodies) can also be used to differentiate cell-specific and HLA antibodies, but these are less suitable for rapid screening than the choroquine-'stripping' technique.

Further characterization of platelet-specific antibodies may require referral to a reference laboratory. Identification of allospecificity is carried out as for red cell antibodies by reaction with a selected panel of group O platelets.

An important consideration in platelet serology is the occasional occurrence of antibodies against hidden (cryptic) antigens of the GP IIb/IIIa complex which are exposed by EDTA and paraformaldehyde (PFA) fixation.[58] These antibodies, which are only active in vitro, are unpredictable, but when suspected can be avoided by using unfixed test platelets from citrated blood.

Neutrophil serology is not so advanced, but the above plan for platelet serology can be used as a provisional guide.

(b) Auto-antibodies

The detection of auto-antibodies and drug-induced antibodies requires special consideration.

It can be misleading, when looking for platelet (or neutrophil) auto-antibodies, only to test the patient's serum against normal platelets (neutrophils), as positive reactions may be due to the presence of allo-antibodies (e.g. HLA or cell-specific) induced by previous transfusion or pregnancy. It is important to show that an auto-antibody in the patient's serum reacts with the patient's own cells. Ideally a direct antiglobulin test (e.g. platelet immunofluorescence test) should be performed before treatment is given to detect antibody bound in vivo. Where a severe cytopenia exists, it may not be possible to harvest enough cells for the test; nevertheless, serum samples should be stored at $-20°C$ and tested retrospectively against the patient's cells when the peripheral platelet (or neutrophil) count has increased in response to treatment.

A major interest in platelet auto-immunity is the quantitative measurement of platelet-associated immunoglobulins as an indication of in-vivo sensitization. A criticism of these quantitative methods is that they detect not only platelet auto-antibody, but also Ig non-specifically trapped or bound to platelets and platelet fragments,[49] and are therefore generally non-specific in the diagnosis of auto-immune thrombocytopenia.[56] On the other hand, the platelet immunofluorescence test (PIFT)[59] avoids the problem of non-specific binding by using PFA fixation to block the platelet Fcγ receptor so that immune complexes and IgG aggregates do not interfere with the test.[17] Moreover, PFA fixation induces platelet swelling with the expulsion of non-specific platelet-associated immunoglobulins.[61] Furthermore, as the test is read by examination of a platelet suspension using fluorescent microscopy, background fluorescence and platelet fragments can be seen and excluded. In a study of 75 patients with ITP, von dem Borne et al[60] found a weak positive (± to +) direct PIFT in 60% of patients and strong reactions (+ + to + + + +) in only 26% of patients. In the same study, the indirect PIFT was positive with the patient's serum in 66% of cases who had a positive direct PIFT, and positive with an ether eluate of the patient's platelets in 94% of the same cases. While these results may be a reflection of the relative insensitivity of the method, they may also be due to a low affinity antibody that is easily eluted during the assay procedure,[49] or indicate an alternative immune mechanism for thrombocytopenia in some cases.

The immunoglobulin (Ig) class of platelet auto-antibodies is similar in idiopathic and secondary auto-immune thrombocytopenia; mostly it is IgG (92%), but often (also) IgM (42%), and sometimes (also) IgA (9%).[60] All IgG subclasses occur, but IgG1 and/or IgG3 are the most frequent.

The main target antigens for platelet auto-antibodies from patients with ITP are the platelet glycoproteins (GP) IIb/IIIa and/or Ib/IX.[24]

A major unresolved problem in *neutrophil serology* is the distinction between positive reactions due to auto-antibodies and circulating immune complexes.[14] This is particularly relevant to laboratory confirmation of the diagnosis of auto-immune neutropenia which may have to rely on other supporting evidence.[29,48,52]

(c) Drug-induced antibodies

The serological investigation of drug-induced immune thrombocytopenia (neutropenia) follows the same pattern as for haemolytic anaemia (p. 503), with the exception that it is not always possible to collect enough cells to test at the nadir of thrombocytopenia or neutropenia. The following blood samples are therefore necessary:

1. *Acute phase blood sample* when the cell count is at the nadir. If there are too few cells to test for cell-bound antibody and complement at this time, it is necessary to test the acute phase serum against the patient's cells during remission. These tests will demonstrate the immune basis of the cytopenia.

If the patient's acute phase serum is tested against *normal* donor cells, it is essential to take account of positive reactions due to HLA or cell-specific allo-antibody in the patient's serum. Furthermore, negative results with normal donor cells may be due to absence of the antigen for the particular drug-dependent antibody, e.g. due to genetic restriction of the antigen concerned.[8]

2. *Subsequent samples after stopping the drug.* Ideally, sampling should be done when the drug has been eliminated and the antibody is still detectable. Tests using this sample with and without the drug in the assay system are necessary to demonstrate the part played by the drug in causing the immune cytopenia. The drug may be added directly to the assay system (and included in the wash solution) or the cells may be pre-

treated with the drug. For some drugs a metabolite and not the native drug is the appropriate antigen for testing; in these cases an 'ex vivo' drug antigen may be used, from urine or plasma.[46]

METHODS OF DEMONSTRATING ANTIBODIES

The basic fluorescent-labelled antiglobulin method and the MAIPA assay will be described in detail. Only brief mention will be made of other methods.

FLUORESCENT-LABELLED ANTIGLOBULIN METHODS

The fluorescent-labelled antiglobulin methods are based on the conventional antiglobulin technique (p. 457) and are suitable for platelet,[59] granulocyte[55] and lymphocyte[11] serology. The platelet immunofluorescence test (PIFT) and granulocyte immunofluorescence test (GIFT)* are described in detail in this chapter.

These tests are read by direct examination of a cell suspension using fluorescence microscopy; this enables false positive fluorescence due to debris or damaged cells to be seen and excluded.

These tests can detect allo-, auto- and drug-induced antibodies and by using appropriate monospecific antiglobulin reagents can determine the Ig class and sub-class of the antibody and cell-bound complement components.

Both tests can be used with chloroquine-treated cells to differentiate cell-specific from HLA antibodies.[32]

Patient's and screening panel cells

Platelets and granulocytes are prepared from venous blood taken into 5% (w/v) Na_2 EDTA in water (9 volumes blood : 1 volume anticoagulant).

Screening panel cells should be obtained from group O donors for platelet serology to avoid positive reactions due to anti-A and anti-B, but this is not necessary for granulocyte serology as A and B antigens cannot be demonstrated on granulocytes. If a patient's serum must be tested with ABO-incompatible platelets, anti-A and/or anti-B can be absorbed with corresponding red cells or A or B substance.

The best results are obtained with the freshest cell preparations, but some delay is tolerable (see below). Neutrophils are more susceptible to storage damage than platelets; cells should be fixed (see below) on the day of collection, but serology may be delayed to the following day. *Platelets* are more resilient and an anticoagulated blood sample may be satisfactory for testing for up to 2 days at ambient temperature (c 20°C). Once fixed, platelets may be kept for up to 3–4 days at 4°C before serological testing. For longer storage, platelet-rich plasma may be kept at –40°C for at least 2 months; however, there is some membrane damage after recovery of frozen platelets, which causes increased background fluorescence that may limit the sensitivity of the test.[1,10,18] For longer-term storage a cryoprotectant, e.g. DMSO, may be used.[18]

Patient's serum

Serum from clotted venous blood should be heated at 56°C for 30 min to inactivate complement, and stored in 1–2 ml volumes (to avoid repeated thawing) at –40°C.

Control sera

Negative control serum is prepared from a pool of 10 sera from normal group AB male donors who have never been transfused. *Positive control* sera containing platelet-specific antibodies (e.g. anti-P1[A1]), neutrophil-specific antibodies, or multi-specific HLA antibodies should be obtained from reference centres.

Eluate from patient's sensitized cells

Elution is important to confirm the antibody nature of cell-bound immunoglobulin and to determine

---

*The general term granulocyte is used throughout this section, although over 90% of the cells separated from blood samples are neutrophils.

the specificity of antibodies. This applies especially when no antibody is demonstrable in the patient's serum, which often occurs in patients with auto-immune thrombocytopenia and neutropenia.

Elution by lowering the pH of the medium, by ether (or DMSO) and by heating to 56°C, has been used.[19] For routine platelet serology, ether elution for platelet auto-antibodies or heating to 56°C for platelet-specific allo-antibodies is most convenient.

Heat eluate. Incubate platelets or granulocytes suspended in 0.5 ml of 0.2% bovine serum albumin (BSA) in phosphate buffered saline (PBS) for 60 min at 56°C. Centrifuge and remove the supernatant which contains the eluted antibody.

Ether eluate. Mix washed packed platelets from 50 ml of EDTA blood with one part of PBS-BSA (0.2%) and two parts of ether, by vigorous shaking for 2 min. Incubate the mixture for 30 min at 37°C in a water-bath with repeated shaking. After centrifugation (2800g, 10 min) three layers are present, consisting of ether, stroma and the eluate. Pipette off the eluate with a Pasteur pipette and test in the indirect PIFT with normal donor platelets as described for serum.

Platelet preparation

1. Prepare platelet-rich plasma (PRP) by centrifugation of anticoagulated blood (200g, 10 min).

2. Wash the platelets × 3 (2500g, 5 min) in PBS/EDTA buffer (8.37 g of Na$_2$EDTA dissolved in 2.5 litres of phosphate buffered saline, pH 7.2); resuspend the platelets thoroughly each time.

3. Fix the platelets in 3 ml of 1% paraformaldehyde (PFA) solution for 5 min at room temperature. (A stock solution of PFA is prepared by dissolving 4 g of PFA (BDH) in 100 ml of PBS by heating to 70°C with occasional mixing. Add 1 mol/l NaOH dropwise with continuous mixing until the solution clears. This 4% stock solution may be stored at 4°C protected from light for several months. Prepare a 1% PFA working solution by adding one volume of the 4% PFA stock solution to three volumes of PBS and by correcting the pH if necessary to 7.2–7.4 with 1 mol/l HCl.)

Wash the platelets twice as before and resuspend in PBS/EDTA buffer at a concentration of 250–500 × 10^9/l for use in the PIFT.

Granulocyte preparation

1. Mix anticoagulated blood or blood retained from platelet preparation after removal of PRP (and made up to its original volume with PBS) with 2 ml of Dextran solution per 10 ml of blood (Dextran 150 injection BP in 5% dextrose)*. Incubate this mixture at 37°C for 30 min at an angle of about 45° to accelerate red cell sedimentation, and then remove the leucocyte-rich supernatant (LRS).

2. Granulocytes can be separated by double density sedimentation (Fig. 25.1). The LRS is underlayered with 2 ml of LSM (Lymphocyte Separating Medium = Ficoll-hypaque sp gr 1.077) which is then underlayered with 2 ml of MPRM (Mono-poly Resolving Medium = Ficoll-hypaque sp gr 1.114)**. The density gradient tube is then centrifuged at 2500g for 5 min. Granulocytes form an opaque layer at the LSM/MPRM interface from which they are harvested by careful pipetting (microscopic examination shows that the cells from this layer are predominantly neutrophil polymorphs). Lymphocytes can similarly be harvested from the plasma/LSM interface, e.g. for use in the lymphocyte immunofluorescence test (LIFT)[11].

3. Wash the granulocytes three times (400g, 5 min) in PBS/BSA buffer (PBS pH 7.2 with 0.2% BSA).

4. Fix the granulocytes in 3 ml of 1% PFA for 5 min at room temperature.

5. Wash the granulocytes twice as before, and resuspend in PBS/BSA buffer at a concentration of about 10 × 10^9/l for use in the GIFT.

PLATELET AND GRANULOCYTE IMMUNOFLUORESCENCE TESTS (PIFT AND GIFT)

The serological methods for testing platelets and granulocytes in the suspension immunofluorescence test are similar, except that platelets are washed throughout in PBS/EDTA buffer, and granulocytes in PBS/BSA buffer. A flow diagram of the PIFT is shown in Fig. 25.2.

---

*Fisons Ltd, Loughborough, UK.
**Both LSM and MPRM supplied by Flow Laboratories Ltd.

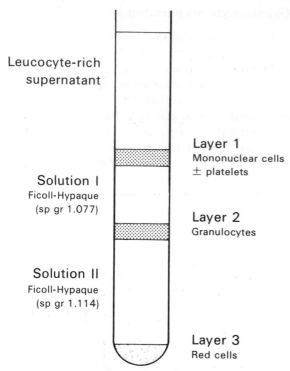

Fig. 25.1 Double density separation of lymphocytes and granulocytes. A leucocyte-rich supernatant is underlayered with Ficoll-Hypaque with a specific gravity of 1.077 (Solution 1) and 1.114 (Solution 2) and then centrifuged at 2500**g** for 5 min. Lymphocytes concentrate in layer 1, granulocytes in layer 2.

Fluorescein-isothiocyanate (FITC) labelled antiglobulin reagents are used as follows: anti-Ig (polyspecific), anti-IgG, anti-IgM and anti-C3. F(ab)$_2$ fragments of these reagents should be used to minimize non-specific membrane fluorescence due to Fc receptor binding, which is a particular problem with granulocytes. The optimal dilution for each reagent should be determined by chequer-board titration. Centrifuge the FITC conjugates at 2500**g** for 10 min before use to remove fluorescent debris and reduce background fluorescence.

Positive and negative controls (as described above) should be included with each batch of tests.

Indirect test

1. In plastic precipitin tubes (7 × 50 mm) mix 0.1 ml of serum and 0.1 ml of the appropriate cell suspension, as prepared above. (The method can also be adapted for use with microtitre plates which has the advantage of using smaller volumes).

2. Incubate for 30 min at 37°C (IgG and C3 tests) and at room temperature (IgM tests). For C3 tests *only*, sediment cells (1000**g**, 5 min), remove the supernatant and resuspend the cell button in 0.1 ml of freshly thawed human serum as a source of complement. Incubate for 30 min at 37°C.

3. Wash the cells three times (1000**g**, 5 min) with appropriate buffer—PBS/EDTA for platelets, PBS/BSA for granulocytes; decant the final supernatant. This and subsequent steps are common for both the *indirect* test (i.e. patient's serum with donor cells) and the *direct* test (i.e. patient's own cells to detect in-vivo sensitization).

4. Add the fluorescent antiglobulin reagent (0.1 ml of the appropriate dilution determined by chequer-board titration), mix with the cell button and leave at room temperature for 30 min in the dark.

5. Wash twice as before, and remove the supernatant.

6. Mix 0.5 ml of glycerol-PBS (3 volumes glycerol:1 volume PBS) with the cell button and mount on a glass slide under a cover-slip.

7. Examine microscopically using × 40 objective and epifluorescent UV illumination.

Scoring results

Reactions in the PIFT and GIFT may be scored on a scale from negative (−) through graded positives + to + + + +. Although subjective, this method of scoring in experienced hands can produce semi-quantitative results in the PIFT[61].

In general, normal platelets and granulocytes incubated with AB serum do not fluoresce after incubation with an appropriately diluted FITC antiglobulin reagent. Sometimes the negative control may show weak fluorescence (up to two fluorescing points on some cells): in these cases the test result is classified as positive only if it is clearly stronger than the negative control (AB serum). Stronger fluorescence in the negative control should raise doubts about the performance of the test.

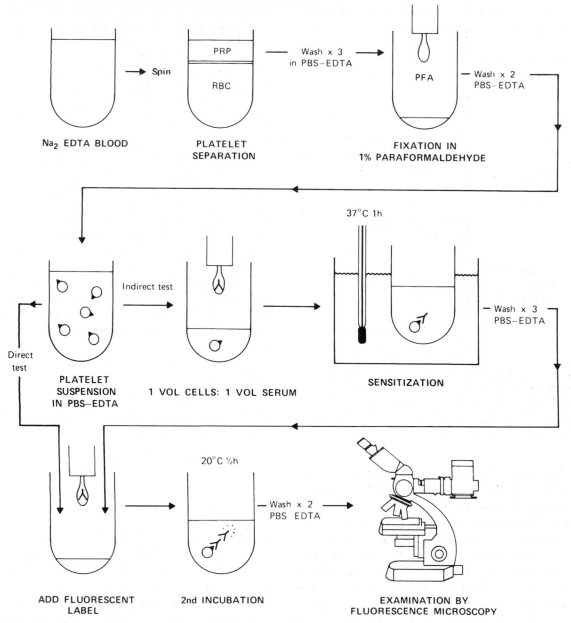

Fig. 25.2 Platelet immunofluorescence test. PRP, platelet-rich plasma; PBS, phosphate buffered saline; PFA, paraformaldehyde.

CHLOROQUINE TREATMENT OF PLATELETS AND GRANULOCYTES[36,41]

Platelets for chloroquine (Cq) treatment should be prepared from fresh blood or blood stored overnight at 4°C; granulocytes are suitable only if freshly prepared. An important consideration is the extent of chloroquine-induced cell membrane damage, which is minimal with fresh cells.

1. Cells are prepared as already described. Two-thirds of the cells are treated with chloroquine; the remaining one-third is not treated. After washing, and before PFA fixation, the cell button

is incubated with 4–5 ml of chloroquine diphosphate in PBS (200 mg/ml, pH adjusted to 5.0 with 1 mol/l NaOH) for 2 h at room temperature with occasional mixing, or overnight at 4°C without mixing, if this is more convenient for the laboratory routine.

2. Wash three times in the appropriate buffer and fix in 1% PFA as previously described. Cell clumping during washing may be a problem after chloroquine treatment, especially with granulocytes; cell clumps should be dispersed by repeated gentle aspiration with a Pasteur pipette. The final cell suspension for serological testing should be prepared as previously described.

When reading the test under fluorescence microscopy, it is important to recognize and allow for any fluorescence due to chloroquine-induced cell damage, which is more likely to occur with granulocytes than platelets. Damaged cells are easily recognized by bright homogeneous fluorescence. Such cells should be excluded from assessment; only cells showing obvious punctate fluorescence should be considered positive.

Chloroquine-treated cells were tested initially in the fluorescent antiglobulin method, but they may also be used in enzyme and radionuclide-labelled antigen methods.

Interpretation of results with chloroquine-treated cells

Typical results with HLA and cell-specific antibodies are shown in Table 25.7. If a serum, which has been shown to contain HLA antibodies by LCT and/or LIFT, gives equal or stronger reactions with chloroquine-treated cells than with untreated cells, then a cell-specific antibody is also present. The Second Canadian Workshop on Platelet Serology[10] concluded that a weaker reaction with chloroquine-treated platelets should be interpreted with caution; this could indicate residual HLA reactivity, especially in the presence of high-titre multispecific HLA antibodies. If a platelet-specific antibody is nevertheless still suspected, other methods should be used to confirm this, e.g. MAIPA using appropriate monoclonal antibodies for capture (see below).

Similar caution should be observed in interpreting the GIFT results with chloroquine-treated cells.

MAIPA ASSAY

The principle of the MAIPA assay is shown in Fig. 25.3. The test is based on the use of monoclonal antibodies, such as anti-IIb/IIIa, anti-Ib/IX, anti-Ia/IIa, anti-HLA class I, to 'capture' specific platelet membrane glycoproteins. The availability of appropriate monoclonal antibodies has led to the wider clinical application of this method.[20] The same principle can be used with granulocytes, depending on the availability of appropriate monoclonal antibodies.[5,20,33]

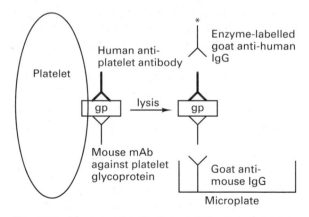

Fig. 25.3   Monoclonal antibody immobilization of platelet antigens (MAIPA): principle of the method. gp, platelet membrane glycoprotein; mAb, monoclonal antibody.

Table 25.7   Platelet and granulocyte antibody reactions using cells prepared with and without treatment with chloroquine

Sera	Untreated cells		Chloroquine-treated cells	
	Platelets	Granulocytes	Platelets	Granulocytes
Negative	−	−	−	−
Multispecific HLA antibodies	+++	++	−	−
Granulocyte-specific antibody	−	++	−	+++
Platelet-specific antibody	+++	−	+++	−

The following assay protocol was developed from the original method described by Kiefel.[20,25]

1. Prepare platelets as for the PIFT (p. 471) except that PFA fixation is omitted.

2. Resuspend a pellet of $50-100 \times 10^6$ platelets in 30 µl of human serum or plasma to be tested and incubate at 37°C for 30 min in a U-well microplate.

3. Wash platelets ×2 in PBS/EDTA buffer (p. 471); resuspend the platelets in 30 µl of mouse monoclonal antibody (anti-Gp IIb/IIIa, Ia/IIa, Ib/IX or HLA at 20 µg/ml), and incubate at 37°C for 30 min.

4. Wash platelets ×2 in PBS/EDTA buffer, lyse by the addition of 100 µl of Tris buffered saline (TBS) containing 0.5% Nonidet P–40 and leave at 4°C for 30 min.

5. Transfer the platelet lysate to a 2 ml conical tube and centrifuge at 11 600g for 30 min at 4°C to remove particulate matter.

6. Dilute 60 µl of the resulting supernatant with 180 µl of TBS wash buffer (0.5% Nonidet P-40, 0.05% Tween 20 and 0.5 mmol $CaCl_2$).

Transfer 100 µl of diluted platelet lysate, in duplicate, to a flat-well microplate previously coated with goat anti-mouse IgG*. Leave at 4°C for 90 min.

7. Wash the microplate wells ×4 with 200 µl of TBS wash buffer and then add 100 µl of alkaline phosphatase labelled anti-human IgG (Jackson, code 109–055–008) diluted 1:4000 in TBS wash buffer.

Leave at 4°C for a further 90 min, then wash the wells ×4 with TBS wash buffer and add 100 µl of substrate solution (1 mg/ml p-nitrophenyl phosphate in diethanolamine buffer, pH 9.8) to each well.

8. Measure the resulting colour change at 30 min using a dual wavelength photometer (e.g. Bio-Rad model 450).

Express results as the mean absorbance at 405 nm of duplicate tests minus the mean of eight blanks containing TBS wash buffer instead of platelet lysate.

Use pooled AB serum as a negative control (p. 470).

OTHER METHODS

A number of other methods for detecting platelet[23,31,57] and granulocyte[9,14,27] antibodies have been described and successfully applied, but they are not in general use mainly because of insufficient standardization.

Several ELISA methods using intact platelets and microtitre plates have been described. These are reviewed by Sintnicolaas et al[51] who describe a method which they have shown to be comparable to the standard PIFT in reproducibility and sensitivity for the detection of platelet allo-antibodies. A more complex two-stage ELISA is suitable for the quantitative measurement of platelet-associated immuno-proteins.[21]

There is little experience of the use of ELISA for the detection of granulocyte antibodies. A two-stage ELISA[21] can be applied for this purpose, and appears to have advantages over the GIFT in the investigation of drug-induced immune neutropenia.[47]

MOLECULAR GENOTYPING OF PLATELET ALLO-ANTIGENS

The application of DNA technology for platelet genotyping is based on recent observations that the platelet antigen systems are due to single DNA base changes which lead to single amino acid polymorphisms in the platelet membrane glycoproteins (Table 25.1).

Molecular genotyping involves amplification of the relevant segments of genomic DNA from any nucleated cell by the polymerase chain reaction (PCR) in combination with sequence-specific primers[34] or by allele-specific restriction enzyme analysis[50] or allele-specific oligonucleotide dot-blot hybridization.[30]

This approach allows the investigation of patients with severe thrombocytopenia and makes it possible

---

*The microplate is prepared by adding to each well 100 µl of goat anti-mouse IgG (Sera-Lab, code SBA 1030-01) at 3 µg/ml in carbonate coating buffer, pH 9.6. Leave the plate to stand overnight at 4°C. Next morning wash the plate ×4 with TBS wash buffer. Leave the last wash supernatant for 30 min to 'block' non-specific protein adsorption to the plastic and then decant.

to determine the fetal platelet genotype in early pregnancy to assess the risk of allo-immune thrombocytopenia.

ACKNOWLEDGEMENT

The author wishes to thank Dr. Paul Metcalfe for assistance in the preparation of this chapter.

REFERENCES

[1] ANDERSEN, E., BASHIR, H. and ARCHER, G. T. (1981). Modification of the platelet suspension immunofluorescence test. *Vox Sanguinis*, **40**, 44.

[2] BIERLING, P., FROMONT, P., ELBEZ, A., DUEDARI, N. and KIEFFER, N. (1988). Early immunization against platelet glycoprotein IIIa in a new born Glanzmann type I patient. *Vox Sanguinis*, **55**, 109.

[3] BRAND, A, SINTNICOLAAS, K., CLASS, F. H. J. and EERNISSE, J. G. (1986). ABH antibodies causing platelet transfusion refractoriness. *Transfusion*, **26**, 463.

[4] BROWN, C. H., WEISBERG, R. J., NATELSON, E. A. and ALFREY, C. P. Jr (1975). Glanzmann's thrombasthenia: assessment of the response to platelet transfusions. *Transfusion*, **15**, 124.

[5] BUX, J., KOBER, B., KIEFEL, V. and MUELLER-ECKHARDT, C. (1993). Analysis of granulocyte-reactive antibodies using an immunoassay based upon monoclonal-antibody-specific immobilization of granulocyte antigens. *Transfusion Medicine*, **3**, 157.

[6] BUX, J. and MUELLER-ECKHARDT, C. (1992). Autoimmune neutropenia. *Seminars in Hematology*, **29**, 45.

[7] CLAAS, F. H. J. (1987). Drug-induced immune granulocytopenia. *Bailliere's Clinical Immunology and Allergy*, **1**, 357.

[8] CLAAS, F. H. J., LANGERAK, J., DE BEER, L. L. and VAN ROOD, J. J. (1981). Drug-induced antibodies: interaction of the drug with a polymorphic platelet antigen. *Tissue Antigens*, **17**, 64.

[9] CLAY, M. E. and KLINE, W. E. (1985). Detection of granulocyte antigens and antibodies: current perspectives and approaches. In *Current Concepts in Transfusion Therapy*. Ed. Garratty, G, p. 183. American Association of Blood Banks, Arlington, VA.

[10] DECARY, F. (1988). Report on the second Canadian workshop on platelet serology. *Current Studies in Hematology and Blood Transfusion*, **54**, p.1. Karger, Basel.

[11] DECARY, F., VERMEULEN, A. and ENGELFRIET, C. P. (1975). A look at HLA antisera in the indirect immunofluorescence technique (IIFT). In *Histocompatibility Testing*, p. 380. Munksgaard, Copenhagen.

[12] DEGOS, L., TOBELEM, G., LETHIELLIUX, P., LEVY-TOLEDANO, S., CEAN, J. and COLOMBANI, J. (1977). A molecular defect in platelets of patients with Bernard-Soulier syndrome. *Blood*, **50**, 899.

[13] EERNESSE, J. G. and BRAND, A. (1981). Prevention of platelet refractoriness due to HLA antibodies by administration of leucocyte-poor blood components. *Experimental Haematology*, **9**, 77.

[14] ENGELFRIET, C. P., TETTEROO, P. A. T., VAN DER VEEN, J. P. W., WERNER, W. F., VAN DER PLAS-VAN DALAN, C. and VON DEM BORNE, A. E. C. Kr. (1984). Granulocyte-specific antigens and methods for their detection. In *Advances in Immunobiology: Blood Cell Antigens and Bone Marrow Transplantation*, p. 121. Liss, New York.

[15] HABIBI, B. (1985). Drug induced red blood cell autoantibodies co-developed with drug specific antibodies causing haemolytic anaemias. *British Journal of Haematology*, **61**, 139.

[16] HABIBI, B. (1987). Drug-induced immune haemolytic anaemias. *Bailliere's Clinical Immunology and Allergy*, **1**, 343.

[17] HELMERHORST, F. M., SMEENK, R. J. T., HACK, C. E., ENGELFREIT, C. P. and VON DEM BORNE, A. E. G. Kr. (1983). Interference of IgG aggregates and immune complexes in tests for platelet autoantibodies. *British Journal of Haematology*, **55**, 533.

[18] HELMERHORST, F. M., TEN BOERGE, M. L., VAN DER PLAS-VAN DALEN, C. M., ENGELFRIET, C. P. and VON DEM BORNE, A. E. G. Kr (1984). Platelet freezing for serological purposes with and without a cryopreservative. *Vox Sanguinis*, **46**, 318.

[19] HELMERHORST, F. M., VAN OSS, C. J., BRUYNES, E. C. E., ENGELFRIET, C. P. and VON DEM BORNE, A. E. G. Kr. (1982). Elution of granulocyte and platelet antibodies. *Vox Sanguinis*, **43**, 196.

[20] KIEFEL, V. (1992). The MAIPA assay and its applications in immunohaematology. *Transfusion Medicine*, **2**, 181.

[21] KIEFEL, V., JAGER, S. and MUELLER-ECKHARDT, C. (1987a). Competitive enzyme-linked immunoassay for the quantitation of platelet-associated immunoglobulins (IgG, IgM, IgA) and complement (C3c, C3d) with polyclonal and monoclonal reagents. *Vox Sanguinis*, **53**, 151.

[22] KIEFEL, V., KROLL, H., BONNERT, J., UNKELBACH, K., KATZMANN, B., NEBENFÜHRER, Z., SANTOSO, S. and MUELLER-ECKHARDT, C. (1993). Platelet alloantigen frequencies in Caucasians: a serological study. *Transfusion Medicine*, **3**, 237.

[23] KIEFEL, V. and MUELLER-ECKHARDT, C. (1993). Report on the Fifth International Society of Blood Transfusion Platelet Serology Workshop. *Transfusion*, **33**, 65.

[24] KIEFEL, V., SANTOSO, S. and MUELLER-ECKHARDT, C. (1992). Serological, biochemical and molecular aspects of platelet autoantigens. *Seminars in Hematology*, **29**, 26.

[25] KIEFEL, V., SANTOSO, S., WEISHEIT, M. and MUELLER-ECKHARDT, C. (1987b). Monoclonal antibody specific immobilization of platelet antigens (MAIPA): a new tool for the identification of platelet-reactive antibodies. *Blood*, **70**, 1722.

[26] LALEZARI, P., KHORSHIDI, M. and PETROSOVA, M. (1986). Autoimmune neutropenia of infancy. *Journal of Pediatrics*, **109**, 764.

[27] LUCAS, G. F. and CARRINGTON, P. A. (1990). Results of the First International Granulocyte Serology Workshop. *Vox Sanguinis*, **59**, 251.

[28] McCULLOUGH, J. (1985). The clinical significance of granulocyte antibodies and in vivo studies of the fate of granulocytes. In *Current Concepts in Transfusion Therapy*. Ed. Garratty, G., p. 125. American Association of Blood Banks, Arlington, VA.

[29] McCULLOUGH, J., CLAY, M. E. and THOMPSON, H. W. (1987). Autoimmune granulocytopenia. *Bailliere's Clinical*

Immunology and Allergy, **1**, 303.

[30] McFarland, J. G., Aster, R. H., Bussel, J. B., Gianopoulos, J. G., Derbes, R. S. and Newman, P. J. (1991). Prenatal diagnosis of neonatal alloimmune thrombocytopenia using allele-specific oligonucleotide probes. *Blood*, **78**, 2276.

[31] McMillan, R. (1983). Immune cytopenias. *Methods in Hematology*, **9**, 1.

[32] Metcalfe, P., Minchinton, R. M., Murphy, M. F. and Waters, A. H. (1985). Use of chloroquine-treated granulocytes and platelets in the diagnosis of immune cytopenias. *Vox Sanguinis*, **49**, 340.

[33] Metcalfe, P. and Waters, A. H. (1992). Location of the granulocyte-specific antigen LAN on the Fc-receptor III. *Transfusion Medicine*, **2**, 283.

[34] Metcalfe, P. and Waters, A. H. (1993). HPA-1 typing by PCR amplification with sequence-specific primers (PCR-SSP): a rapid and simple technique. *British Journal of Haematology*, **85**, 227.

[35] Minchinton, R. M. and Waters, A. H. (1984a). The occurrence and significance of neutrophil antibodies. *British Journal of Haematology*, **56**, 521.

[36] Minchinton, R. M. and Waters, A. H. (1984b). Chloroquine stripping of HLA antigens from neutrophils without removal of neutrophil specific antigens. *British Journal of Haematology*, **57**, 703.

[37] Mueller-Eckhardt, C. (1987). Drug-induced immune thrombocytopenia. *Bailliere's Clinical Immunology and Allergy*, **1**, 369.

[38] Mueller-Eckhardt, C. and Salama, A. (1990). Drug-induced immune cytopenias: a unifying pathogenetic concept with special emphasis on the role of drug metabolites. *Transfusion Medicine Reviews*, **4**, 69.

[39] Murphy, M. F., Metcalfe, P., Thomas, H., Eve, J., Ord, J., Lister, T. A. L. and Waters, A. H. (1986). Use of leucocyte-poor blood components and HLA-matched platelet donors to prevent HLA alloimmunisation. *British Journal of Haematology*, **62**, 529.

[40] Newman, P. J. (1994). Nomenclature of human platelet allo-antigens: a problem with the HPA system? *Blood*, **83**, 1447.

[41] Nordhagen, R. and Flaathen, S. T. (1985). Chloroquine removal of HLA antigens from platelets for the platelet immunofluorescence test. *Vox Sanguinis*, **48**, 156.

[42] Pegels, J. G., Bruynes, E. C. E., Engelfriet, C. P. and von dem Borne, A. E. G. Kr. (1982). Pseudothrombocytopenia: an immunologic study on platelet antibodies dependent on ethylene diamine tetra-acetate. *Blood*, **59**, 157.

[43] Ribera, A., Hernandez, M., Lopez, R., Milla, F., Flores, A., Martinez-Brotons, F. and Roncales, J. (1988a). Pseudothrombocytopenia and platelet cold agglutinin. Abstracts *XX Congress International Society of Blood Transfusion in Association with British Blood Transfusion Society*, BBTS, Manchester, p. 240.

[44] Ribera, A., Martin-Vega, C., Pico M. and Gonzalez, J. (1988b). Sensitization against platelet antigens in Glanzmann disease. Abstracts *XX Congress International Society of Blood Transfusion in Association with British Blood Transfusion Society*, BBTS, Manchester p. 240.

[45] Salama, A. and Mueller-Eckhardt, C. (1986). Two types of nomifensine-induced immune haemolytic anaemias: drug-dependent sensitization and/or autoimmunization. *British Journal of Haematology*, **64**, 613.

[46] Salama, A., Mueller-Eckhardt, C., Kissel, K., Pralle, H. and Seeger, W. (1984). Ex vivo antigen preparation for the serological detection of drug-dependent antibodies in immune haemolytic anaemias. *British Journal of Haematology*, **58**, 525.

[47] Salama, A., Schutz, B., Kiefel, V., Breithaupt, H. and Mueller-Eckhardt, C. (1989). Immune-mediated agranulocytosis related to drugs and their metabolites: mode of sensitization and heterogeneity of antibodies. *British Journal of Haematology*, **72**, 127.

[48] Shastri, K. A. and Logue, G. L. (1993). Autoimmune neutropenia. *Blood*, **81**, 1984.

[49] Shulman, N. R., Leissinger, C. A., Hotchkiss, A. J. and Kautz, C. A. (1982). The non-specific nature of platelet associated IgG. *Transactions of Association of American Physicians*, **95**, 213.

[50] Simsek, S., Faber, N. M., Bleeker, P. M., Vlekke, A. B. J., Huiskes, R., Goldschmeding, R. and von dem Borne, A. E. G. Kr. (1993). Determination of human platelet antigen frequencies in the Dutch population by immunophenotyping and DNA (allele-specific restriction enzyme) analysis. *Blood*, **81**, 835.

[51] Sintnicolaas, K., van der Steuijt, K. J. B., van Putten, W. L. J. and Bolhuis, R. L. H. (1987). A microplate ELISA for the detection of platelet alloantibodies: comparison with the platelet immunofluorescence test. *British Journal of Haematology*, **66**, 363.

[52] van der Veen, J. P. W., Hack, C. E., Engelfriet, C. P., Pegels, J. G. and von dem Borne, A. E. G. Kr. (1986). Chronic idiopathic and secondary neutropenia: clinical and serological investigations. *British Journal of Haematology*, **63**, 161.

[53] van Leeuwen, E. F., von dem Borne, A. E. G. Kr., von Riesz, L. E., Nijenhuis, L. E. and Engelfriet, C. P. (1981). Absence of platelet specific alloantigens in Glanzmann's thrombasthenia. *Blood*, **57**, 49.

[54] van Vliet, H. H. D., Kappers-Klunne, M. C. and Abels, J. (1986). Pseudothrombocytopenia: a cold autoantibody against platelet glycoprotein gpIIb. *British Journal of Haematology*, **62**, 501.

[55] Verheught, F. W. A., von dem Borne, A. E. G. Kr., Decary, F. and Engelfriet, C. P. (1977). The detection of granulocyte alloantibodies with an indirect immunofluorescence test. *British Journal of Haematology*, **36**, 533.

[56] von dem Borne, A. E. G. Kr. (1987). Autoimmune thrombocytopenia. *Bailliere's Clinical Immunology and Allergy*, **1**, 269.

[57] von dem Borne, A. E. G. Kr. and Ouwehand, W. H. (1989). Immunology of platelet disorders. *Bailliére's Clinical Haematology*, **2**, 749.

[58] von dem Borne, A. E. G. Kr., van der Lelie, J., Vos, J. J. E., van der Plas-van Dalen, C. M., Risseeuw-Bogaert, N. J., Ticheler, M. D. A. and Pegels, H. G. (1986). Antibodies against crypt antigens of platelets. Characterisation and significance for the serologist. *Current Studies in Hematology and Blood Transfusion*, **52**, p. 33. Karger, Basel.

[59] von dem Borne, A. E. G. Kr, Verheught, F. W. A., Oosterhof, F., von Reisz, E., Brutel de la Riviere, A. and Engelfriet, C. P. (1978). A simple immunofluorescence test for the detection of platelet antibodies. *British Journal of Haematology*, **39**, 195.

[60] von dem Borne, A. E. G. Kr, Vos J. J. E., van der

LELIE, J., BOSSERS, B. and VAN DALEN, C. M. (1986b). Clinical significance of positive platelet immunofluorescence test in thrombocytopenia. *British Journal of Haematology*, **64**, 767.

[61] VOS, J. J. E., HUISMAN, J. G., WINKEL, I. N., RISSEEUW-BOGAERT, N. J., ENGLEFRIET, C. P. and VON DEM BORNE, A. E. G. Kr. (1987) Quantification of platelet-bound alloantibodies by radioimmunoassay: a study on some variables. *Vox Sanguinis*, **53**, 108.

[62] WATERS, A. H. (1988). Role of platelet serology workshops. Abstracts *XX Congress International Society of Blood Transfusion in Association with British Blood Transfusion Society*, BBTS, Manchester, p. 108.

[63] WATERS, A. H. (1989). Post-transfusion purpura. *Blood Reviews*, Vol. 3, p. 83. Churchill Livingstone, Edinburgh.

[64] WATERS, A. H. (1992). Autoimmune thrombocytopenia: clinical aspects. *Seminars in Hematology*, **29**, 18.

26. Laboratory aspects of blood transfusion

Revised by A. H. Waters

Pre-transfusion compatibility testing   479
ABO grouping   480
  Microplate method   482
  Causes of discrepancies   482
  Differentiation of group A_1 from A_2 484
Rh (D) grouping   484
  Emergency   485
  Rh phenotyping   486
  Antenatal grouping   486
Antibody screening   487
Cross-matching   488
Emergency blood issue   489

Special compatibility testing   489
  In the newborn   489
  Intra-uterine transfusion   490
  Repeated transfusions   490
  In auto-immune haemolytic anaemia   490
Investigation of a transfusion reaction   491
Haemolytic disease of newborn (HDN)   493
  Antenatal serology   493
  Tests at delivery   494
  Anti-D prophylaxis   494
  ABO haemolytic disease of newborn   495

Safe and efficient blood transfusion practice depends on accurate documentation and the elimination of clerical errors (see British Committee for Standards in Haematology (BCSH) *Guidelines on Hospital Blood Bank Documentation and Procedures*[10a] and BCSH *Guidelines on Hospital Blood Bank Computing*[10b]; consideration of the patient's clinical history, particularly with respect to previous transfusions, pregnancy and drugs; constant attention to the reliability of reagents and techniques; a satisfactory pre-transfusion testing procedure to ensure donor-recipient compatibility; and a fail-safe procedure agreed with hospital clinicians and nursing staff to ensure that compatible blood is transfused to the right patient.[25,37]

This chapter is primarily concerned with pre-transfusion compatibility testing and follows the BCSH *Guidelines for Compatibility Testing in Hospital Blood Banks.*[10c] It also includes sections on antenatal antibody screening and the investigation of allo-immune haemolytic disease of the newborn (HDN).

Pre-transfusion compatibility testing

A satisfactory compatibility procedure should include:

1. ABO and Rh(D) grouping of the patient
2. Antibody screening of the patient to detect the presence of clinically significant antibodies and assist the selection of compatible blood
3. Cross-matching to confirm donor-recipient compatibility.

To cross-match or not to cross-match?

The BCSH *Guidelines for Compatibility Testing in Hospital Blood Banks*[10c] and the AABB *Standards for Blood Banks and Transfusion Services*[1] emphasize the importance of the donor-recipient cross-match as the ultimate check of ABO compatibility. Some authorities have advocated abbreviation of the cross-match by omission of the indirect antiglobulin test (IAT) from the compatibility procedure for patients with a negative antibody screen.[17] The technical competence of personnel is a most important factor to be considered when deciding on the compatibility procedure to meet the needs of the hospital, and a continuing unacceptable level of antibody detection failures in external proficiency trials dictates a cautious approach. However, the consultant in charge of the blood bank may, after due consideration of the technical competence of the laboratory staff, decide to delete the antiglobulin phase of the cross-match for patients who have a negative antibody screen and no previous record of irregular antibodies. This decision should be based on periodic assessment of individual staff competence and regular monitoring of cell washing centrifuges as outlined in the BCSH *Guidelines for Compatibility Testing in Hospital Blood Banks.*[10c]

Documentation

The safety of blood transfusion depends on accurate patient and sample identification at all stages, starting with taking the blood sample from the patient for compatibility testing and ending with the transfusion of compatible blood.

The use of computers in the laboratory also helps to eliminate errors.[10b]

Blood samples

Immediately on receipt, laboratory staff should confirm that the blood sample is appropriately labelled and that the information on the sample and request form is identical.

Great care must be taken to identify and label correctly any serum or plasma separated from the patient's original blood sample; the serum or plasma should be stored at or below −20°C.

ABO and Rh (D) grouping

These must be performed by an approved technique with appropriate controls. Before use, all new batches of grouping reagents should be checked for reliability by the techniques used in the laboratory. Grouping reagents should be stored according to the manufacturer's instructions.

ABO GROUPING

Correct interpretation of the patient's ABO group requires confirmation, whenever possible, by tests on the patient's serum or plasma (except for newborn infants up to 4 months of age in whom naturally occurring anti-A and anti-B are normally absent). Ideally, cell and serum or plasma grouping should be carried out by different workers who then check each other's results.

Reagents

Anti-A, anti-B and anti-A,B reagents are used for cell grouping tests. The anti-A,B reagent (group O serum) acts as an additional check on red cells which are agglutinated by anti-A or anti-B, and it should also detect weaker A or B antigens which might otherwise be missed. Conventional polyclonal reagents have been replaced by superior anti-A and anti-B monoclonal reagents,[33] each prepared from blends of two antibodies to optimize the intensity of agglutination for slide tests and their ability to detect the weaker sub-groups of A (e.g. Ax) by tube techniques. Blended monoclonal anti-A,B reagents to optimize anti-A and anti-B reactions are also available. However, the superior performance of specific anti-A and anti-B monoclonal reagents questions the need for the continued use of anti-A,B reagents in ABO grouping.

The monoclonal reagents should contain EDTA (0.1 mol/1 pH 7.1–7.3) to prevent haemolysis should they be used in the presence of fresh patient's serum, as these potent IgM antibodies are strong haemolysins in the presence of complement.

METHODS

ABO grouping may be carried out by tube or slide methods or in microplates. The reader is referred to the BCSH *Guidelines on Microplate Technology*[10d] for the current state of the art in this rapidly changing area of serology.

Tube methods

Spin-tube methods have replaced sedimentation tube methods.

Spin-tube tests may be performed in 75 × 10 or 12 mm glass or plastic tubes. Immediate spin tests may be used in an emergency, whereas routine tests are usually left for 15 min at room temperature (*c* 20°C) before centrifugation. For details of spin force (RCF) and time see p. 460.

Using a commercial reagent dropper or a Pasteur pipette, add 1 drop of each grouping reagent to 3 tubes labelled anti-A, anti-B and anti-A,B respectively, followed by 1 drop of a 2% suspension in phosphate buffered saline of the test red cells. In addition, add 1 volume of patient's serum or plasma to 4 tubes labelled A_1 cells, B cells, O cells and 'auto-agglutination control' respectively. Then add 1 volume of 2% suspensions of the control A_1, B and O cells, and of the test red cells to the appropriate tubes. The layout for tests and controls is shown in Fig. 26.1.

Mix the suspensions by tapping the tubes and leave them undisturbed for 15 min. Agglutination should be read as described in Chapter 24, p. 455.

It is essential to confirm the result of the red cell grouping by examining the patient's serum for the corresponding antibodies (reverse grouping) (Fig. 26.1). Any discrepancy between the results of the red cell grouping and the reverse grouping should be investigated further.

Reverse grouping is not carried out for infants under 4 months of age as the corresponding antibodies are normally absent. The practice of including adult group AB serum as a control to detect possible polyagglutination is not necessary when monoclonal ABO grouping reagents are used, as they lack the contaminating antibody responsible for polyagglutination (p. 483).

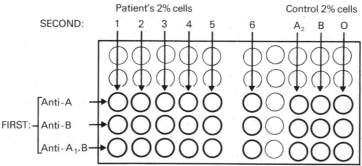

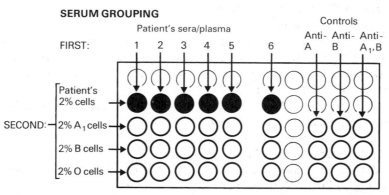

Fig. 26.1 Lay-out for tube grouping tests. The order of adding serum or plasma (first) and cells (second) is indicated. The black circles are 'auto' controls.

Controls

Each grouping test (or series of tests) must be controlled by parallel tests set up exactly as described above, using cells of known group in place of the test (patient's) cells. Group-A_2 and -B cells are used to test the potency of the grouping sera; group-O cells, which should not be agglutinated, are also included to guard against the possibility of false-positive reactions. In addition, the A_1, B and O cells used in the reverse grouping test are checked against standard anti-A, anti-B and anti-A,B grouping sera, during the course of the cell grouping test.

An auto-control should also be included. Any agglutination of the A_1, B or O cells by the test subject's serum cannot be interpreted unless the auto-agglutination control gives a negative result. The possible causes of a positive auto-agglutination test are considered below.

Slide method

In an emergency, ABO grouping may be carried out rapidly on slides or tiles. The method is satisfactory if potent grouping reagents are used (see p. 455). An immediate spin tube test is preferable.

Microplate method

ABO and Rh(D) grouping may be carried out on one U well plate if monoclonal reagents are used. The layout of the plate is as shown in Fig. 26.2.

Using a commercial reagent dropper or Pasteur pipette, add 1 vol of antiserum to each well of the appropriate row (D-H).

Add 1 volume of 2% patient's cells in phosphate buffered saline (PBS) to these rows and the auto control row (C).

Add 1 volume of patient's serum or plasma to the A and B cell rows and the auto control (C) row, followed by 1 volume of 2% A and B cells in PBS.

Add the control cells as indicated. Anti-D controls (p. 485) are incorporated in the ABO control cells, e.g. Arr, Brr and OR$_1$r.

Mix on a microplate shaker. Leave the microplate at room temperature (20°C) for 15 min, then centrifuge at 700 rpm for 1 min.

The plate can be read by one of two methods—streaming (microplate set at an angle) or agitation. Automated microplate readers may also be used.[38]

CAUSES OF DISCREPANCIES IN ABO GROUPING

Before any tests are read the controls must show that the reagents are working correctly.

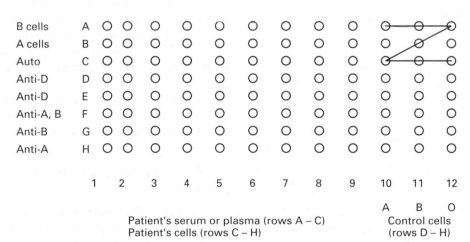

Fig. 26.2 Microplate layout for ABO and Rh(D) grouping. The patient's serum or plasma is added to rows A–C for ABO reverse grouping and the auto control (C). The patient's cells are added to rows C–H for ABO and Rh(D) cell grouping and the auto control (C). The ABO control cells (rows D–H) incorporate controls for the two anti-D reagents, e.g. Arr, Brr, OR$_1$r.

(a) False positive results

(i) Rouleaux formation

Marked rouleaux formation can simulate true agglutination (Figs. 26.3 and 26.4). In reverse grouping the two can be distinguished by repeating the test using the serum diluted 1 in 2 or 1 in 4 in saline. Rouleaux should disappear; agglutination will hardly be affected. If rouleaux are apparent in red cell grouping tests, the tests should be repeated after washing the patient's red cells thoroughly.

(ii) Auto-immune haemolytic anaemia

Cold agglutinins will cause auto-agglutination and apparent panagglutination, if active at room temperature. If this is suspected, the reverse grouping test should be repeated at 37°C, at which temperature the auto-agglutination control should be negative. Any anti-A and/or anti-B present in the patient's serum will, however, still react. The patient's red cells should be washed several times in warm (37°C) saline and the cell grouping repeated. It is advisable, too, to set up an additional test of the patient's cells in group-AB serum containing no antibodies (see below). No agglutination should result.

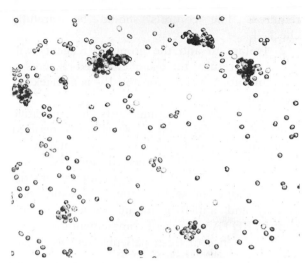

Fig. 26.4   Photomicrograph of a suspension of red cells in serum, showing weak agglutination. ×300. The small agglutinates are more irregularly distributed than the rouleaux and vary more in size. There are also more free cells.

There is no problem with warm IgG auto-antibodies when monoclonal reagents are used.

(iii) Bacterial contamination

Infection of a red-cell suspension by certain bacteria may cause the cells to become agglutinable by normal adult human sera. In vivo, this is thought to be the main cause of the rare phenomenon of polyagglutinability. Bacterial enzymes expose the T-receptor on red cells and polyagglutination is due to the presence of anti-T in most human sera except those of young infants. This problem does not occur with monoclonal grouping reagents which are free of anti-T.

Bacterial contamination of grouping reagents, due to improper storage or handling, may also cause false-positive agglutination.

(b) False-negative reactions in ABO grouping

1. Failure of agglutination or weak reactions are usually due to impotent sera. Loss of potency results if sera are carelessly left at room temperature or stored frozen in large volumes so that repeated freezings and thawings are

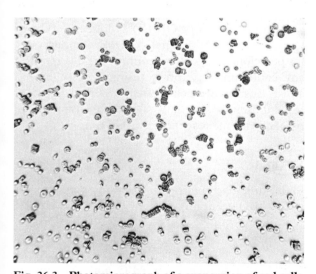

Fig. 26.3   Photomicrograph of a suspension of red cells in serum, showing a minor degree of rouleaux formation. ×300. The numerous small rouleaux are characteristically relatively evenly spaced throughout the field and do not vary greatly in size.

required. The controls should be carefully checked.

2. Failure to add the grouping reagents will cause false results; the use of coloured reagents—blue for anti-A, yellow for anti-B—is a check for this error.

3. In reverse grouping tests false-negative results may be recorded if lysis is not recognized as a positive result. All reverse grouping tubes should be carefully inspected for lysis and its presence recorded before attempting microscopic reading of agglutination. To avoid lysis, anti-A, and anti-B grouping reagents should contain EDTA to prevent complement activation in the presence of fresh patients' sera as in tile grouping.

(c) Mixed-field reactions

These may be due to:

1. The previous transfusion of group O cells to group A or B recipients.
2. An earlier incompatible transfusion.
3. An ABO incompatible bone-marrow transplantation.
4. A permanent dual population of cells, which may be the first indication of blood-group chimerism.

DIFFERENTIATION OF GROUP A_1 FROM GROUP A_2

Group-A_1 and -A_2 cells can be differentiated by using a monoclonal anti-A_1 reagent. The lectin *Dolichos biflorus* extract may also be used for subtyping cells carrying the A antigen.[4,35]

Rh (D) GROUPING

This is usually performed at the same time as ABO grouping to minimize clerical errors that may arise through repeated handling of patients' samples. At least two different anti-D reagents should be used as a double check against errors, as there is no counterpart of 'reverse grouping', as in ABO grouping.

Reagents

The availability of high titre monoclonal IgM anti-D reagents[33] has made it possible to use the same techniques as for ABO grouping. These reagents work equally well at room temperature (*c* 20°C) and at 37°C and are reliable for emergency D grouping by immediate spin tube techniques as described for ABO grouping.

Monoclonal reagents should be used in preference to 'enhanced' anti-D reagents made from polyclonal IgG anti-D which does not cause agglutination in saline unless the IgG antibody has been chemically modified or potentiating substances (e.g. albumin or protease enzymes) have been added to the diluent. These 'enhanced' IgG

anti-D reagents usually require 37°C incubation and must be used strictly according to the manufacturer's instructions.

All anti-D grouping reagents should be checked by the method used in the laboratory for specificity with *positive* (OR_1r or OR_1R_2) and *negative* (Orr or Or'r) controls. Additional controls are necessary for polyclonal reagents to confirm the *absorption* of any contaminating anti-A (using A_1rr cells) and anti-B (using Brr cells). Before a new batch of reagent is introduced, it should be evaluated in parallel with the reagent in current use.

Methods

Slide, tube and microplate methods may be used as for ABO grouping.

Tube method

Working in sequence for ABO and D grouping provides for efficient batch testing (p. 481).

Add 1 volume of anti-D to each tube of the anti-D row of each rack.

Then add 1 volume of the 2% red cell suspension to each tube.

The tests are mixed, incubated and read as described for ABO tests.

Microplate method

ABO and RhD grouping are usually carried out in one microplate using monoclonal reagents (p. 482, Fig. 26.2).

Controls

Controls and tests should be set up in one operation. Each batch of tests should include *positive* (R_1r or R_1R_2) and *negative* (rr) controls. Each test sample must have an *auto*-control (own cells and own serum).

In tests with enhanced IgG anti-D reagents, the auto-control should also be performed with the addition of the enhancing agent, as specified by the manufacturer (*diluent* control). The diluent control is essential to demonstrate that the diluent itself does not promote agglutination of the patient's cells, as might occur with red cells already coated with immunoglobulin due to in-vivo sensitization.

EMERGENCY Rh (D) GROUPING

Spin tube method

For emergency D grouping, use the spin tube method and centrifuge the tubes at $150g$ for 1 min either immediately or after incubation, depending on the time available.

Slide method

Monoclonal anti-D reagents are available that agglutinate D-positive cells within a few minutes. The manufacturer's instructions must be followed (see also p. 455).

For both methods it is essential to use potent anti-D reagents and to include positive and negative controls.

False-positive results in Rh (D) grouping

Misclassification of a D-negative patient as D-positive could lead to the transfusion of D-positive blood. Resultant anti-D sensitization could have potentially harmful clinical consequences, especially for D-negative women of child bearing age (see also p. 486).

False positive results may occur for the following main reasons:

1. Red cells may already be coated with immunoglobulin due to in-vivo sensitization. For this reason antiglobulin and enzyme techniques should not be used for routine D grouping. Furthermore, direct agglutination tests with enhanced anti-D reagents should include an appropriate diluent control to exclude false-positive results.

2. The anti-D grouping reagent may contain a contaminating antibody which has not been adequately absorbed e.g. contaminating anti-A or anti-B, or anti-C (leading to a false-positive result in a D-negative C-positive patient). This type of false positive result may occur when reagents have not been adequately controlled for the method in use or when the reagent manufacturer's instructions have not been followed.

3. Bacterial contamination of reagents may also cause false-positive agglutination.

These problems do not occur when monoclonal reagents are used.

Clinical significance of weak D phenotype (D^u) Discrepant results in D grouping with different anti-D reagents may indicate a serious reagent fault (e.g. contaminating antibody as discussed above), but are usually caused by weak D phenotypes which have fewer D antigen sites than normal (called D^u).[33] The incidence of weak D is c 0.7%, if selected by an IgM monoclonal anti-D at suitable dilution, e.g. MAD-2.

In clinical practice, if the serological reactions with standard methods are equivocal, the patient should be grouped as Rh (D) negative. This 'error' will be of no clinical consequence, since the transfusion of D-negative blood will be compatible with respect to the D antigen. Similarly, a weak D pregnant woman, misclassified as D-negative, will not be harmed by prophylactic IgG anti-D. Nothing is to be gained by further testing of D-negative patients by other techniques, e.g.

antiglobulin or enzyme methods, to detect possible weak D; a more important consideration is the risk of false-positive results with such methods, as indicated above.

In the routine grouping of blood donors at transfusion centres, only some weak D samples will be misclassified as D-negative; the incidence varies, but can be reduced to as low as 0.23% by the sensitive automated methods now being used.[24a] The clinical consequences will not be serious since weak D red cells are thought to be unlikely to undergo accelerated destruction if transfused to an immunized patient; moreover, weak D red cells are thought to be poorly immunogenic and unlikely to provoke a primary immune response in a D-negative recipient.[24a]

In addition to weak D antigens (D[u]), there are rare D-positive individuals who lack some of the epitopes of the complex D antigen (D variants). Most anti-D reagents react with the whole D antigen, but some reagents may be more specific and give negative results with D variant red cells if the antibody is directed against the missing epitopes. If such people require transfusion, they should be regarded as D-negative because they may make antibody against the epitopes which they lack if transfused with the normal (whole) D antigen. Similarly, a D variant mother may be immunized by a normal fetal D antigen, and this could cause Rh (D) haemolytic disease of the newborn.

For blood donors it is therefore important to identify D variants and classify them as D-positive, as they may immunize D-negative recipients against some of the D epitopes. All donor D-negative grouping tests should be confirmed with reagents known to detect D variants (for further details, see Mollison et al[24b]).

Rh PHENOTYPING

Reagents for determining the Rh phenotype are available commercially. It is essential to follow the manufacturer's instructions in doing the tests. The following specificities are required: anti-D, anti-C + C[w], anti-E, anti-c and anti-e.

It is essential to use a panel of cells of known genotypes as controls (see Table 26.1). Cells that are heterozygous for the antigen under test are

Table 26.1   Genotypes of the red cells to use as controls for Rh grouping sera

Antiserum	Negative control	Positive control	Absorption control
Anti-D	*Cde/cde*	*CDe/cde*	A$_1$ B *cde/cde*
Anti-C	*cDE/cDE*	*CDe/cDE*	A$_1$ B *cde/cde*
Anti-E	*cDe/cde*	*CDe/cDE*	A$_1$ B *cde/cde*
Anti-c	*CDe/CDe*	*CDe/cDE*	A$_1$ B *CDe/CDe* or A$_1$ + B, both *CDe/CDe*
Anti-e	*cDE/cDE*	*cDE/cde*	A$_1$ B *cDE/cDE* or A$_1$ + B, both *cDE/cDE*

used as positive controls; cells that do not have the antigen under test (but would be agglutinated by the most common contaminants of the antibody) are used as negative controls. Absorption and appropriate patient 'auto' and reagent 'diluent' controls should be set up as previously described, if monoclonal reagents are not used.

GROUPING IN ANTENATAL WORK

Pregnant women must be grouped for ABO and D and this should be done early in pregnancy as a routine.

Accuracy in D grouping of antenatal samples is particularly important as D-negative women erroneously grouped as D-positive carry the risk of:

1. Being transfused with D-positive blood and consequently being sensitized to the D antigen which could result in severe HDN in subsequent pregnancies.

2. Not receiving prophylactic anti-D immunoglobulin, with the same potential consequences as (1).

3. Being screened serologically less frequently during pregnancy which could result in delayed detection of significant antibodies that could compromise the management of HDN.

Ideally, all pregnant women, whether D-negative or D-positive, should be screened for antibodies other than anti-D. Although HDN due to anti-D is by far the most severe form of the disease, HDN can occur, although less commonly, as the result of the formation of anti-c or anti-E in D-positive mothers. Moreover, HDN has been

Table 26.2 Probability of Rh D-positive genotypes in terms of homozygosity (D/D) or heterozygosity (D/d) in an English population

D	C	c	E	e	Probable genotype	% of total giving these results	Next most probable	% of total giving these results	Relative frequency of heterozygous:homozygous amongst samples giving these results
+	+	+	−		R^1r(D/d)	94	R^1R^0(D/D)	6	15:1
+	+	−	−		R^1R^1(D/D)	96	R^1r(D/d)	4	1:21
+	+	+	+		R^1R^2(D/D)	88	R^1r''(D/d)	8	1:8
+	−	+	+	+	R^2r(D/d)	93	R^2R^0(D/D)	6	15:1
+	−	+	+	−	R^2R^2(D/D)	86	R^2r''(D/d)	14	1:6
+	−	+	−		R^0r(D/d)	97	R^0R^0(D/D)	3	30:1
+	+	−	+		R^1R^2(D/D)	97	R^2r'(D/d)	2	1:41

described, albeit very rarely, as the result of incompatibilities in most of the other major blood-group systems; of these, immunization against the Kell antigen (K) is the commonest.[8] It is best, therefore, not to confine antenatal screening to Rh(D)-negative mothers, but to screen all patients. A schedule for antenatal antibody screening is given on p. 493.

The paternal blood group phenotype should be determined in all cases where the mother has an allo-antibody. If the paternal red cells lack the corresponding antigen, the baby is not at risk. However, caution is advised, as the assumed parent may not be the biological father of the fetus!

It is useful to predict whether the partner of a D-negative woman with anti-D is homozygous or heterozygous for the D antigen. This is essential to forecast the chances of the couple having children affected by Rh (D) haemolytic disease of the newborn (HDN).

No antisera against the 'd' antigen are available as the 'd' antigen is amorphic. Because of the lack of an 'anti-d' serum, the zygosity of the D antigen is usually predicted from the results of tests with anti-C, anti-c, anti-E and anti-e sera, and from

tables of the likelihood of the homo- or heterozygous association of D with the other Rh antigens. These tables have been compiled for different racial groups. It is important, therefore, to tell the specialist laboratory the racial origin of the patient.

Table 26.2 gives the results of testing samples of D-positive red cells from an English population with anti-D and four other anti-Rh antisera, and the interpretation of the data in terms of D homozygosity and heterozygosity for the common and not so common genotypes. The relative frequencies in the last column apply to a random population. They are applicable to D-positive partners of D-negative women in general, but D-positive fathers of children who have had Rh(D) HDN are a selected rather than a random population. The chances of such a father provisionally called 'heterozygous' being in reality homozygous for the D antigen becomes more likely with every child that is affected. It may be helpful to Rh phenotype all his children and his parents.

Now that gene sequence data are available, the PCR method can be used to detect the Rh(D) gene and to measure directly the Rh(D) gene zygosity of a particular individual.[39]

ANTIBODY SCREENING

In parallel with determining the ABO and D groups, all patients should be screened for unexpected allo-antibodies, i.e. other than anti-A and anti-B. This facilitates the selection of suitable blood for a patient requiring transfusion.

The patient's serum or plasma should be tested against at least two red cell suspensions, used

separately and *not* pooled. The screening cells must be group O and should encompass the common antigens of the ethnic population. In the UK the screening cells should express, as a minimum, the following antigens: C,c, D, E, e, M, N, S, s, P_1, K, k, Le^a, Le^b, Fy^a, Fy^b, Jk^a, Jk^b; cells with C^w should also be included if available. At least one cell must have the stronger D antigen combination R_2. It is also desirable, although not always possible, to have antigens in the homozygous state; particularly for Jk^a, Jk^b, S, C, Fy^a, Fy^b, because heterozygous red cells may fail to detect antibodies that would react positively with homozygous cells. Such antibodies have proved to be of clinical importance.

Screening cells are available commercially or from Blood Transfusion Centres.

The antibody screening procedure is designed to detect antibodies of clinical significance. No single test will detect all blood-group antibodies, but an effective compromise is as follows:

1. Direct agglutination test in normal (NISS) or low ionic strength solutions (LISS)—recommended temperature 37°C to avoid detection of insignificant cold antibodies.

2. Indirect antiglobulin test (IAT) after incubation in NISS or LISS (p. 459).

3. Two-stage enzyme tests (p. 454) are considered useful supportive techniques, especially for Rh antibodies, although they may fail to detect some antibodies reactive in a spin-tube antiglobulin test.

New techniques, e.g. the gel test and solid phase, which have a simpler reading phase than standard agglutination tests, are being introduced for routine antibody screening (p. 460).

A positive result in the antibody screen should be followed by antibody identification. The serum or plasma under investigation is normally tested against a panel of eight or more group O red cell samples of known antigen composition, using all the test methods with which the antibody was initially detected. The specificity of a single alloantibody is usually apparent from the pattern of reactivity. Additional antibodies may be present in a serum which displays a reaction pattern indicating a single specificity. Therefore, it is necessary to test the serum against additional red cell samples negative for the apparent specificity. It is also important to know the phenotype of the autologous red cells to predict the specificities of additional antibodies that might be present. The immuno-chemical properties of an antibody assist in the resolution of mixtures of antibodies. If the antibody is clearly cold-reacting and causing direct agglutination in saline at 20°C or 25°C, but is inactive at 37°C, it is not likely to be anti-D; but it might well be anti-P_1 or anti-Le^a. IgG antibodies are usually not active in saline tests and are best detected in enzyme or indirect antiglobulin tests (exceptions are anti-A, anti-B, anti-M and anti-N because the reactive red cells have a very high antigen density). Also, as papain destroys M, N, S and Fy^a antigens, the inclusion of an enzyme test helps to sort out these antibody specificities.

CROSS-MATCHING

The function of the cross-match is to prevent incompatibility. This is most serious when there is ABO incompatibility and, in particular, when A or B cells are transfused into a group-O person with a high titre anti-A/anti-B.

There are two approaches:

1. Follow a 'group, antibody screen and save' policy; or
2. Cross-match all patients who may need a transfusion.

Group, antibody screen and save procedure

This is ideal for operative procedures where blood is often not required, but where it has been customary to have compatible blood on standby. This may be co-ordinated with a maximum blood ordering schedule for planned surgical operations.[10e] The patient's blood is ABO and D grouped and screened for unexpected antibodies; if the antibody screen is negative the patient's sample (serum or plasma and cells) is retained but no blood is cross-matched. When patients with a negative antibody screen require blood urgently, blood of the same ABO and D group can be given, subject only to an immediate spin cross-match to exclude ABO incompatibility. Incubate (c 20°C) equal volumes of a 2% donor cell suspension and the patient's serum or plasma for 2–5 min.

Centrifuge at 100*g* for 1 min (see p. 460) and inspect for agglutination.

If the antibody screen is positive, antigen negative donor units are cross-matched by the routine procedure.

ROUTINE CROSS-MATCHING

Select donor units for cross-matching on the basis of ABO and Rh (D) grouping and antibody identification.

Test the patient's serum or plasma against donor red cells by:

1. Direct agglutination test in NISS or LISS. Inspect for agglutination and haemolysis. The test can be read in the tube after gentle agitation over a × 5 or × 6 magnification illuminated mirror, and incorporated with (2) as one-tube procedure.

2. Indirect antiglobulin test using a minimum incubation 15-min LISS test or a 45-min NISS test. The incubation temperature should be 37°C using a water-bath or warmed block (air incubators are less reliable).

Spin-tube or microplate techniques may be used.

EMERGENCY BLOOD ISSUE (WHERE TIME DOES NOT PERMIT FULL COMPATIBILITY TESTING)

A blood sample should be obtained from the patient before the administration of intravenous colloids, such as Dextran and hydroxethyl-starch (HES), which may cause troublesome red cell aggregation in serological testing.

Laboratories that use LISS for routine work are well placed to meet urgent compatibility requests. However, where laboratories use NISS routinely, it is not recommended that they change to LISS tests for emergency techniques.

Patients should be ABO and D grouped by rapid techniques and group-compatible blood issued. Exclude ABO incompatibility by an immediate spin cross-match and/or by group-checking the blood units before issue.

If this procedure is followed, it should seldom be necessary to have to resort to group-O D-negative blood. Should this need arise, only pre-viously group-checked units should be issued. Furthermore, this should be changed to blood of the patient's own group as soon as possible to avoid subsequent confusion over ABO grouping.

After the emergency has been dealt with, retrospective cross-matching should be undertaken with the pre-transfusion sample.

If a massive transfusion has been given in which the number of units transfused in 24 h exceeds the recipient's blood volume, compatibility testing may be reduced to checking the ABO/D groups of the transfused units or an immediate spin cross-match.

Donor units that have not been tested, or not fully tested, against the patient's serum should be clearly labelled, e.g. 'Selected for patient. . . , but *not* cross-matched'.

SPECIAL TRANSFUSION SITUATIONS

There are some situations where the provision of compatible blood requires special consideration.

Compatibility tests in newborn infants

For infants under 4 months, both baby and maternal blood samples should be ABO and D grouped, the maternal serum screened for unexpected antibodies, and a direct antiglobulin test done on the baby's cells.

If a maternal antibody screen is negative and the baby's direct antiglobulin test is negative, blood of the same ABO and D group as the infant may be issued without cross-matching, even after repeated small volume transfusions, provided the ABO and D groups of the donor units are checked before issue. Recent studies indicate that infants under the age of 4 months do not make red cell allo-antibodies even after multiple small volume transfusions.[23]

If the infant is suffering from haemolytic disease of the newborn (HDN), or if unexpected antibodies are detected in the maternal serum, it is important to use the maternal serum for compatibility testing. This may dictate the use of group-O blood, and if the infant is not group O, care should be taken to ensure that donor units have low titre anti-A and anti-B (i.e. <32). If ABO HDN is suspected, group-O blood of low titre anti-A and anti-B should be used. An alternative to low titre group-O blood is O cells reconstituted in one-third volume of AB plasma. It should be noted that compatible red cells from adult group-A or -B donors should not be used, as adult red cells will almost certainly have more A and B antigen sites than the infant's own red cells and are likely to undergo more rapid destruction by the residual maternal anti-A or anti-B. In the event of an exchange transfusion, plasma-reduced CMV negative blood is indicated.

Compatibility tests for intra-uterine transfusion

Blood for an intra-uterine transfusion should be tested for compatibility with the mother's serum. It should be group O and D-negative (except, for example, when the mother is D-positive and has made antibodies other than anti-D or anti-D mixtures). Kell (K)-negative blood should also be used.[8,18] Compatibility tests for subsequent transfusions must be repeated every time using fresh maternal serum, for the manipulations of intrauterine transfusions are not uncommonly followed by the escape of donor cells into the maternal circulation which could lead to the formation of antibodies of a new specificity. It is essential to test the mother's serum against a phenotyped panel of red cells between each intra-uterine transfusion to identify any new allo-antibodies formed.

Blood for intra-uterine transfusion should, preferably, be less than 24 h old. It should be CMV negative and γ-irradiated (minimum 15 Gy)[2] to avoid graft-versus-host disease. Plasma-reduced blood or washed red cells suspended in saline should be used.

Compatibility tests in patients receiving transfusions at close intervals

Allo-antibodies may develop quickly following a transfusion early in a series. It is important, therefore, to obtain a fresh sample of serum from the recipient before each transfusion if they are separated by an interval of 3 days or longer; while if the patient is receiving daily transfusions, only blood that is likely to be used in the 3 days following the collection of the serum should be matched. It is advisable to do a DAT on the patient's red cells each time, as antibodies that have formed may be adsorbed to incompatible cells and not be present in the serum.

Compatibility tests in auto-immune haemolytic anaemia (AIHA)

(a) Warm-type AIHA

ABO grouping is usually straightforward, but antibody coating on the patient's red cells can cause false-positive D grouping results (p. 485). Saline-reacting monoclonal IgM anti-D reagents will give reliable grouping results.

The problem here is that the auto-antibody almost always reacts with all donor blood samples, so that no cross-match compatible blood can be found. In this situation it is essential to exclude any incompatibility due to the simultaneous presence of allo-antibodies stimulated by previous transfusion or pregnancy. Recent reports indicate that allo-antibodies may be present in up to 40% of cases, the most frequent being anti-C and anti-K.[21,36] It is therefore helpful to determine the patient's Rh phenotype and K type (at least) before transfusions are started, so that donor compatible blood can be selected. Monoclonal reagents should be used when phenotyping the patient's red cells to avoid false-positive reactions due to cell-bound auto-antibody.

Useful advice on the detection of allo-antibodies in the presence of an auto-antibody, which can be quite difficult, has been given by Petz and Garratty[29] (see also p. 512).

(b) Cold-type AIHA

Cold agglutinins cause blood grouping and antibody screening problems (p. 483). Even if agglutination is avoided by performing these tests strictly at 37°C, complement binding may cause false positive results in the antiglobulin test during antibody screening and cross-matching. Useful advice on compatibility testing in the presence of cold agglutinins is given by Petz and Garratty.[29]

INVESTIGATION OF A HAEMOLYTIC TRANSFUSION REACTION

The serologist is particularly concerned with the potential immunological consequences of blood transfusion.[13] These can be considered under two broad headings: allo-immunization and incompatibility (Table 26.3).

Donor-recipient compatibility is essential to ensure normal survival of transfused red cells and to avoid the harmful effects of a haemolytic transfusion reaction. The mechanism of haemolysis depends on the Ig class of the antibody and its ability to fix complement (p. 450). This also determines the site of haemolysis. Haemolytic transfusion reactions (HTR) may be acute (intravascular or extravascular) or delayed (mainly extravascular).

(A) ACUTE INTRAVASCULAR HAEMOLYSIS

Acute intravascular haemolysis is a dreaded complication of blood transfusion. It is usually due to ABO incompatibility resulting from a misidentification error. Although an acute emergency, prompt diagnosis and treatment can be life saving. At the first suspicion of reaction the transfusion must be stopped, as the severity of the clinical consequences depends partly on the volume of red cells transfused to the patient. The laboratory performing the pre-transfusion compatibility testing must be notified immediately.

Diagnosis depends on demonstrating haemolysis in the patient and incompatibility between the donor and the patient (Table 26.4). Patient identification and the donor unit compatibility label should be rechecked at the bedside. As clerical errors involving one patient may involve others cross-matched at the same time, it is essential to check the samples, donor units and documentation of all cross-matches done at that time. Differential diagnosis from other conditions causing a similar clinical presentation is also

Table 26.3 Classification of immunological consequences of blood transfusion

Allo-immunization
i.e. the development of antibodies against:
  (i) Red cell, leucocyte and platelet antigens
  (ii) Plasma protein antigens

Incompatibility
(a) *Red cell incompatibility*
  (i) Intravascular haemolysis
    e.g. ABO incompatibility
  (ii) Extravascular haemolysis
    e.g. Rh incompatibility
    —Immediate
    —Delayed

(b) *Leucocyte and platelet incompatibility*
  (i) Febrile reaction (granulocytes, monocytes)
  (ii) Pulmonary reaction (granulocytes)
  (iii) Post-transfusion purpura (platelets)
  (iv) Poor survival of tranfused platelets and granulocytes
  (v) Graft-versus-host reaction (lymphocytes)

(c) *Plasma protein incompatibility*
Urticarial and anaphylactic reactions

Table 26.4 Investigation of a haemolytic transfusion reaction

I. **Check for haemolysis**
    (i) Examine patient's plasma and urine for haemoglobin
    (ii) Blood film may show spherocytosis

II. **Check for incompatibility**
    (a) *Clerical causes*
        An identification error will indicate the type of incompatibility

    (b) *Serological causes*
    (i) Repeat ABO and D group of patient (pre- and post-transfusion) and donor units
    (ii) Screen for red cell antibodies
    (iii) Repeat cross-match with pre- and post-transfusion serum
    (iv) Direct antiglobulin test (pre- and post-transfusion samples)

III. **Check for DIC**
    (i) Blood film (red cell fragmentation)
    (ii) Platelet count
    (iii) Coagulation screen

IV. **Check for bacterial infection**
    Gram stain and culture donor blood

Table 26.5   Differential diagnosis of acute haemolytic transfusion reaction

---

Red cell incompatibility

Transfusion of infected blood

Other causes of haemolysis
   (i) Post-operative infection (e.g. clostridial septicaemia)
   (ii) Infusion of hypotonic solutions (including hypotonic dialysis)
   (iii) Haemolytic anaemia (e.g. PNH)

Transfusion of lysed red cells
   (i) Thermal damage (pre-transfusion heating or freezing)
   (ii) Mechanical damage (e.g. extracorporeal machines, excessive infusion pressure and/or small bore needle)

---

important, the most serious being the transfusion of infected blood (Table 26.5).

Serological investigations

Specimens required:

1. Pre-transfusion serum and red cells of the patient.
2. Post-transfusion serum and red cells of the patient.
3. The donor unit involved, together with the giving set and any other donor units transfused.
4. Urine from the patient for the first 24 h after the reaction. This will be dark due to the presence of haemoglobin in the case of intravascular haemolysis.

Serological tests

1. Confirm the ABO and D groups of the patient's pre- and post-transfusion samples and the donor units.
2. Perform a DAT on the patient's pre- and post-transfusion washed red cells: a negative DAT post-transfusion does not exclude a severe haemolytic reaction.
3. Repeat the cross-match tests of donor's red cells with patient's serum, using pre- and post-transfusion samples.
4. Screen the donor plasma and the patient's pre- and post-transfusion serum samples for unexpected antibodies.
5. If the donor was group O and the patient group A or B, then titre the anti-A and anti-B levels in the donor plasma, as high titres (>64) are found in 'dangerous group-O donors'.

Haematological tests

1. Blood count—including platelet and reticulocyte counts.
2. Blood film—spherocytosis, red cell fragmentation.
3. Coagulation screen.

Disseminated intravascular coagulation (DIC) is a feature of intravascular HTR and the transfusion of infected blood; severe DIC is a bad prognostic sign.

Bacteriological tests

Inspect the donor unit(s) for any obvious haemolysis. The donor blood unit(s) and giving set should be tested by culturing the remaining blood at 4°C, 20°C and 37°C and by Gram stain and smear examination.

Biochemical tests

The patient's post-transfusion serum should be inspected for haemolysis, tested for free haemoglobin and bilirubin estimated, and the results compared with those of the pre-transfusion sample.

If the above testing does not indicate a haemolytic transfusion reaction or infected blood, other possible causes of an adverse immunological reaction, e.g. leucocyte antibodies, allergic reactions to plasma proteins (Table 26.3), should be taken into consideration when selecting blood for further transfusions.

(B) ACUTE EXTRAVASCULAR HAEMOLYSIS

Acute extravascular haemolysis is a feature of IgG antibodies that do not cause complement lysis, e.g. anti-D. This is a less severe haemolytic reaction. The main clinical features are fever, sometimes with rigors, and an inadequate haemoglobin response to the transfusion that cannot be explained by blood loss; jaundice may occur, but haemoglobinuria is not common. These reactions are not commonly seen due to improved pre-transfusion antibody screening and cross-matching procedures. Diagnosis should follow the procedure set out in Table 26.4.

(C) DELAYED HAEMOLYTIC REACTIONS

Delayed haemolytic reactions may occur in patients allo-immunized by previous pregnancy or transfusion. The antibody titre is too low to be detected in the pre-transfusion compatibility testing, but after re-exposure to the incompatible antigen, a secondary (anamnestic) immune response occurs. IgG antibodies are made and the transfused red cells are destroyed; anti-Jk[a] is such an antibody (p. 449).

Haemolysis is usually extravascular, and typically the patient develops anaemia, fever, jaundice and sometimes haemoglobinuria about 1 week after transfusion. The clinical picture may resemble an auto-immune or drug-induced immune haemolytic anaemia with a positive direct antiglobulin test (in this case due to allo-antibody on the donor cells), spherocytosis and reticulocytosis. However, the history of a preceding transfusion should suggest the correct diagnosis, which should be confirmed as in Table 26.4. There is usually no need for further action in most cases as the process is self-limiting. Many delayed haemolytic transfusion reactions of this type almost certainly go undetected.

HAEMOLYTIC DISEASE OF THE NEWBORN (HDN)

HDN is an immune haemolytic anaemia affecting the fetus and newborn infant. It occurs when maternal allo-antibody to fetal red cell antigens crosses the placenta and causes haemolysis of fetal red cells. As IgG is the only immunoglobulin transferred across the placenta, only red cell antibodies of this class are a potential cause of HDN. Anti-D causes the most severe form of HDN. However, the success of anti-D prophylaxis has reduced the number of cases of Rh (D) HDN; consequently the relative proportion of cases due to other antibodies has increased, notably anti-c, anti-E and anti-K, but almost every other red cell IgG antibody has been reported as a cause of HDN. ABO-HDN is considered separately as a number of special factors combine to protect the fetus from the effects of ABO incompatibility. For a more detailed discussion of HDN the reader is referred to the review by Bowman et al[9] and the textbook by Mollison et al.[24c]

ANTENATAL SEROLOGY

Maternal ABO and D grouping and antibody screening (p. 486) are the basis of any system for the prediction and management of HDN. Protocols for antenatal screening vary in detail, but depend on the maternal D group, antibody status, transfusion history, and obstetric history of HDN. It is important to screen both D-positive and D-negative women; the D-positive woman, particularly if she has been transfused, may develop allo-antibodies that are dangerous for the fetus. A satisfactory testing schedule can be summarized as follows.[3]

Without antibodies

	Test at
D-negative and previously transfused women	Booking
	24–28 weeks
	34–36 weeks
	Delivery
Other D-positive women	Booking
	34–36 weeks

With antibodies

Mothers with antibodies or a history of HDN should be tested more frequently, e.g. monthly until 28 weeks, then at shorter intervals, e.g. every 2 weeks.

Antibody screening should be carried out as previously described (p. 487); in addition it is recommended that ABO and D grouping be repeated on each occasion to minimize the risk of error.

Antenatal assessment of severity of Rh (D) HDN

The role of the serologist is to carry out serial antibody measurements on sensitized women to determine the titre or concentration (µg/ml plasma) of anti-D. Manual titrations are less sensitive than quantitative automated assays for detecting changes in antibody levels; a two-fold change in antibody concentration must occur before the titre is affected. Nevertheless, titration of maternal anti-D plays an important part in identifying pregnancies at risk. Individual laboratories working with local obstetricians generally establish the clinical significance of their own titration results, e.g. antiglobulin titres of the order of 8–32 suggest the need for further intervention to assess the severity of HDN.

Automated measurement of the amount of anti-D (IU or µg/ml) may define the fetal risk more accurately,[5,16] as also may the antibody-dependent cell-mediated cytotoxicity (ADCC) assay used as a model of in-vivo haemolysis in the fetus.[15,20,31] However, further essential information regarding management depends on amniotic fluid spectro-photometry[22] and on direct fetal blood sampling by ultrasound-guided cordocentesis.[14] The last pro-cedure provides not only direct diagnostic information,[26,27] but also a new approach to fetal therapy by direct fetal intravascular transfusion.[19,28]

The declining incidence of severe Rh (D) HDN and the increasingly specialized management of severely affected pregnancies has meant that these women are now being referred to specialist centres dealing with this condition.

TESTS ON MATERNAL AND CORD BLOOD AT DELIVERY

It should be standard practice to collect an adequate sample (e.g. 20 ml) of cord blood (both EDTA and clotted specimens) for serological studies, as subsequent (small) samples from the baby may not be enough for all the necessary tests to be carried out. There should be an agreed local procedure for labelling mother's and baby's samples to avoid misidentification errors.

The following tests should be carried out on all D-negative mothers and their babies:

(a) Tests on cord blood

1. ABO and D grouping.
2. DAT (if positive, test the mother's serum

against a cell panel to identify the antibody).
3. Haemoglobin.
4. Bilirubin (D-positive babies).

(b) Tests on maternal blood

1. Repeat ABO and D grouping.
2. Repeat antibody screen (in case anti-D sensitization has occurred in a previously unsensitized woman).
3. Kleihauer test for feto-maternal red cell leakage (p. 137) if the baby is shown to be D-positive; this determines the prophylactic dose of anti-D immunoglobulin to be given to the mother to prevent sensitization (see below).

The above tests should also be carried out on the cord blood of all babies born to mothers with antibodies other than anti-D. Ideally, a DAT should be done on all cord blood samples, as this offers the opportunity of detecting unsuspected ABO HDN (p. 495), and other antibodies against rare or private (paternal) antigens which may affect subsequent pregnancies. Attractive as this proposal is on clinical grounds, it seems unlikely that it could be generally applied on economic grounds.

ANTI-D PROPHYLAXIS

The dose of anti-D for D-negative women at risk depends on the size of the feto-maternal red cell leakage, as determined by the Kleihauer acid elution technique (p. 137). The method depends on the Hb F of fetal red cells resisting acid elution to a greater extent than the Hb A of maternal red cells. When a treated maternal blood film is stained with eosin the fetal cells stain dark pink and the maternal cells appear as pale 'ghosts'.

Using a ×40 objective and ×10 eyepieces (i.e. low power), count the darkly staining fetal red cells in a single low power field (LPF). The dose of anti-D is calculated as follows:

Kleihauer count	Dose of anti-D immunoglobulin
Up to 200 cells per 50 LPFs	500 IU
For every 100 cells in excess of 200 per 50 LPFs	*Extra* 500 IU

e.g. for a Kleihauer count of 500 cells per 50 LPF the dose of anti-D would be 2000 IU. The dose of anti-D can also be expressed in µg (1 µg = 5 IU).

The administration of an adequate dose of anti-D to prevent maternal sensitization is the responsibility of the clinician in charge of the patient. The following guidelines for preventing D immunization by pregnancy are based on the recommendations set out in Mollison et al.[24d]

1. Minimize the risk of misclassifying D-negative women as D-positive by D grouping on at least two separate occasions, i.e. (a) during pregnancy, and (b) at delivery. This presupposes accurate and unique patient identification throughout pregnancy.

2. An adequate dose of anti-D immunoglobulin should be given to *all as yet unimmunized D-negative women*. The following procedure is recommended:

(a) After delivery

1. To avoid the situation where anti-D is sometimes withheld because a report on the baby's D group has not been received, all Rh(D)-negative women should be given a *standard* intramuscular dose of anti-D (500 IU) within 72 h of delivery, unless the baby is known to be D-negative.

2. On the basis of the Kleihauer test, *extra* anti-D may be indicated to cover a larger fetomaternal leakage of red cells.

(b) During pregnancy

1. For abortion before 20 weeks a standard dose of 250 IU should be given; after 20 weeks give 500 IU or more based on the Kleihauer count.

2. Following obstetric manipulations (e.g. amniocentesis, version) and antepartum haemorrhage (APH) give 500 IU of anti-D or more, based on the Kleihauer count.

Prophylactic anti-D is also given routinely in the third trimester in some countries,[7] but this is not current standard practice in the UK.

ABO HAEMOLYTIC DISEASE OF THE NEWBORN

This is considered separately, as a number of special factors combine to protect the fetus from the effects of ABO incompatibility. For practical purposes, only group-O individuals make high titres of IgG anti-A and anti-B. Therefore only A and B infants of group-O mothers are at risk from ABO-HDN. Although 15% of births are susceptible, only about 1% are affected; even then the condition is usually mild and very rarely severe enough to need exchange transfusion. Two mechanisms protect the fetus against anti-A and anti-B: one is the relative weakness of A and B antigens on fetal red cells; the other is the widespread distribution of A and B glycoproteins in fetal fluids and tissues, which diverts much of the maternal IgG antibody away from the fetal red cell 'target'.

ABO-HDN may be seen in the first incompatible pregnancy. This is unlike anti-D HDN, where immunization usually takes place at the end of the first pregnancy, the first child thus being unaffected.

Serological investigation

ABO haemolytic disease is difficult to diagnose, especially in Caucasians, as the DAT may be negative or weak even in a case of severe haemolytic disease. Furthermore, anti-A or anti-B is normally present in the mother's serum and special tests are needed to demonstrate a high titre of IgG anti-A or anti-B in the presence of IgM anti-A or anti-B.

In cases of suspected ABO HDN the main features are.[34]

1. It is almost always confined to infants of group-O mothers as there is more IgG anti-A and anti-B in group-O than in group-B or group-A mothers.

2. As anti-A and anti-B are always present in group-O mothers, evidence for ABO-HDN depends on demonstrating a high titre of IgG anti-A or anti-B, e.g. by treating the mother's serum with 2-mercapto-ethanol (2-ME) or dithiothreitol (DTT) to distinguish between IgG and IgM antibodies (for method, see p. 524).

3. The DAT on cord blood is often weak or negative; the latter at least excludes any other serological incompatibility. This probably reflects

the low A and B antigen density on the red cells of newborn infants.

4. The simplest evidence for the occurrence of ABO haemolytic disease is obtained by testing the serum of the cord blood sample for incompatible anti-A or anti-B by the antiglobulin method with adult A_1, B and O cells. If the baby is group A the important test is with the A_1 cells which will be positive in ABO HDN. A strong reaction with B cells will always occur with a group-A baby. The test with O cells should be negative, but if positive, it indicates the presence of a further antibody as a possible contributory or major cause of the disease, especially if the DAT is strongly positive. Similarly, if the baby is group-B the critical test is with adult B cells; a strong reaction will also be found with A_1 cells, but this will not harm the baby's B cells.

Note: If the blood sample from the baby is not taken until the time of crisis of the disease, usually about 2–3 days after delivery, the serological tests may be negative because most, if not all, of the maternal anti-A or anti-B will have been absorbed in the destruction of the baby's red cells.

5. The best diagnostic test of ABO HDN is to prepare a heat eluate from the baby's red cells (from the cord blood sample), and test it (together with the last wash supernatant as a control) by the antiglobulin method with adult A_1, B and O cells. In some cases reactions occur with both A_1 and B cells due to anti-A,B cross-reacting antibodies, but most severe cases of ABO HDN involve separate specific anti-A or anti-B anti-bodies.[32] The tests with O cells and the last wash control should be negative.

Antenatal prediction

Antenatal prediction of ABO HDN is not essential for medical management, as there is time to observe the baby after birth and to treat according to the severity of the condition. Nevertheless, a baby is likely to be more severely affected if the maternal IgG anti-A (-B) titre is greater than 128.[6]

A recent study using an ADCC assay, in which monocytes from normal donors were incubated with normal red cells sensitized with maternal anti-A or anti-B serum, suggests that a strongly positive result with this assay correlates with severe HDN.[11,12] The most severe haemolysis was associated with a maternal antibody of IgG3 subclass and a high antigen density on the fetal red cells. While the ADCC assay is not advocated as a routine screening test in group-O mothers at risk, it could be used selectively to predict the outcome of a pregnancy when there has been a previously severely affected infant.

ACKNOWLEDGEMENTS

The author wishes to thank Mrs Judith Chapman, FIMLS, and Dr. D. Voak for advice in the preparation of this chapter and, with great respect, to pay tribute to the late Eleanor Lloyd, FIMLS, who was his co-author in the previous edition.

REFERENCES

1 AABB (1993). *Standards for Blood Banks and Transfusion Services*, 15th edn. Ed. F. Widmann. American Association of Blood Banks, Bethesda, MD.
2 ANDERSON, K. C., GOODNOUGH, L. T., SAYERS, M., PISCIOTTO, P. T., KURTZ S. R., LANE T. A., ANDERSON, C. S. and SIBERSTEIN, L. E. (1991). Variation in blood component irradiation practice: implications for prevention of transfusion associated graft-versus-host disease. *Blood*, 77, 2096.
3 ANONYMOUS (1986) Prenatal screening for irregular blood group antibodies. *Lancet*, ii, 1369.
4 BIRD, G. W. G. (1988) Lectins in haematology and blood banking. *Methods in Haematology*, 17, 125.
5 BOWELL, P. J., WAINSCOAT, J. S., PETO, T. E. A. and GUNSON, H. H. (1982). Maternal anti-D concentrations and outcome in rhesus haemolytic disease of the newborn.

British Medical Journal, 285, 327.
6 BOWLEY, C. C. and VOAK, D. (1971). What is the optimal serological analysis of haemolytic disease of the newborn due to ABO incompatibility? International Forum. *Vox Sanguinis*, 20, 183.
7 BOWMAN, J. M. (1985). Controversies in Rh prophylaxis: who needs Rh immune globulin and when should it be given? *American Journal of Obstetrics and Gynecology*, 151, 289.
8 BOWMAN, J. M. (1990). Treatment options for the fetus with alloimmune hemolytic disease. *Transfusion Medicine Reviews*, 4, 191.
9 BOWMAN, J. M., POLLOCK, J. M. and BIGGINS, K. R. (1988). Antenatal studies and the management of hemolytic disease of the newborn. *Methods in Hematology*, 17, 163.

[10] BRITISH COMMITTEE FOR STANDARDS IN HAEMATOLOGY (1991). *Standard Haematology Practice*. Ed. Roberts, B., (a) p. 128, (b) p. 139, (c) p. 150, (d) p. 164, (e) p. 189. Blackwell Scientific Publications, Oxford.

[11] BROUWERS, H. A. A., OVERBEEKE, M. A. M., van ERTBRUGGEN, I. et al (1988). What is the best prediction of the severity of ABO-haemolytic disease of the newborn? *Lancet*, **ii,** 641.

[12] BROUWERS, H. A. A., OVERBEEKE, M. A. M., VAN ERTBRUGGEN, I., VAN LEEUWEN, E. F., STOOP, J. W. and ENGELFRIET, C. P. (1988). Maternal antibodies against fetal blood-group antigens A or B; lytic activity of IgG subclasses in monocyte-driven cytotoxicity and correlation with ABO-haemolytic disease of the newborn. *British Journal of Haematology*, **70,** 465.

[13] CONTRERAS, M. and MOLLISON, P. L. (1992). Immunological complications of transfusion. In *ABC of Transfusion*, 2nd edn. Ed. Contreras, M., p. 41. British Medical Journal, London.

[14] DAFFOS, F., CAPELLA-PAVLOVSKY, M. and FORESTIER, F. (1985). Fetal blood sampling during pregnancy with use of a needle guided by ultrasound; a study of 606 consecutive cases. *American Journal of Obstetrics and Gynaecology*, **153,** 655.

[15] ENGELFRIET, C. P. and OUWEHAND, W. H. (1990). ADCC and other cellular bioassays for predicting the clinical significance of red cell alloantibodies. *Baillière's Clinical Haematology*, **3,** 321.

[16] FRASER, I. D. and TOVEY, G. H. (1976). Observations on Rh iso-immunization: past, present and future. *Clinics in Haematology*, **5,** 149.

[17] GARRATTY, G. (1982). The role of compatibility tests. *Transfusion*, **22,** 169.

[18] GIBLETT, E. R. (1977). Blood group alloantibodies: an assessment of some laboratory practices. *Transfusion*, **17,** 299.

[19] GRANNUM, P. A., COPEL, J. A., PLAXE, S. C., SCIOSCIA, A. L. and HOBBINS, J. C. (1986). In utero exchange transfusion by direct intravascular injection in severe erythroblastosis fetalis. *New England Journal of Medicine*, **314,** 1431.

[20] HADLEY, A. G. GARNER, S. F. and TAVERNER, J. M. (1993). Autoanalyzer quantification, monocyte-mediated cytotoxicity and chemiluminescence assays for predicting the severity of haemolytic disease of the newborn. *Transfusion Medicine*, **3,** 195.

[21] LAINE, M. L. and BEATTIE, K. M. (1985). Frequency of alloantibodies accompanying autoantibodies. *Transfusion*, **25,** 545.

[22] LILEY, A. W. (1961). Liquor amnii analysis in management of pregnancy complicated by rhesus immunization. *American Journal of Obstetrics and Gynecology*, **82,** 1359.

[23] LUDVIGSEN, C. W. Jr, SWANSON, J. L., THOMPSON, T. R. and McCULLOUGH, J. (1987). The failure of neonates to form red blood cell alloantibodies in response to multiple transfusions. *American Journal of Clinical Pathology*, **87,** 250.

[24] MOLLISON, P. L., ENGELFRIET, C. P. and CONTRERAS, M. (1993). *Blood Transfusion in Clinical Medicine*, 9th edn., (a) p. 211, (b) p. 212, (c) p. 543, (d) p. 579. Blackwell Scientific Publications, Oxford.

[25] MOORE, P. B. L. (1986). Good laboratory practice before and after blood transfusion. *Haematologia*, **19,** 241.

[26] NICOLAIDES, K. H., RODECK, C. H., MILLAR, D. S. and MIBASHAN, R. S. (1985). Fetal haematology in rhesus isoimmunization. *British Medical Journal*, **290,** 661.

[27] NICOLAIDES, K. H., RODECK, C. H., MIBASHAN, R. S. and KEMP, J. R. (1986). Have Liley charts outlived their usefulness? *American Journal of Obstetrics and Gynecology*, **155,** 90.

[28] NICOLAIDES, K. H., SOOTHILL, P. W., RODECK, C. H. and CLEWELL, W. (1986). Rh disease: intravascular fetal blood transfusion by cordocentesis. *Fetal Therapy*, **1,** 185.

[29] PETZ, L. D. and GARRATTY, G. (1980). *Acquired Immune Hemolytic Anemias*, (a) p. 365, (b) p. 376. Churchill Livingstone, New York.

[30] SZYMANSKI, I. O. and ARASZKIEWICZ, P. (1989). Quantitative studies on the D antigen of red cells with the D^u phenotype. *Transfusion*, **29,** 103.

[31] URBANIAK, S. J., AYOUB GREISS, M., CRAWFORD, R. J. and FERGUSON, M. J. C. (1984). Prediction of the outcome of Rhesus haemolytic disease of the newborn; additional information using an ADCC assay. *Vox Sanguinis*, **46,** 323.

[32] VOAK, D. (1968). The serological specificity of the sensitising antibodies in ABO hetero-specific pregnancy of the group-O mother. *Vox Sanguinis*, **14,** 271.

[33] VOAK, D. (1990). Monoclonal antibodies as blood grouping reagents. *Baillière's Clinical Haematology*, **3,** 219.

[34] VOAK, D. and BOWLEY, C. C. (1969). A detailed serological study on the prediction and diagnosis of ABO haemolytic disease of the newborn (ABO HD). *Vox Sanguinis*, **17,** 321.

[35] VOAK, D., LODGE, T. W. and REED, J. V. (1969). The enhancement of *Ulex europaeus* anti-H activity by human serum. *Vox Sanguinis*, **17,** 134.

[36] WALLHERMFECHTEL, M. A., POLK, B. A. and CHAPLAIN, H. (1984). Alloimmunisation in patients with warm autoantibodies. A retrospective study employing three donor alloabsorptions to aid antibody detection. *Transfusion*, **24,** 482.

[37] WATERS, A. H. and DAVIDSON, J. F. (1988). Clinical interface of blood transfusion. *Journal of Clinical Pathology*, **41,** 601.

[38] WHITROW, W. and ROSS, D. W. (1990). Automation in blood grouping: impact of microplate technology. *Baillière's Clinical Haematology*, **3,** 255.

[39] WOLTER, L. C. and HYLAND, C. A. (1993). Rhesus D genotyping using polymerase chain reaction. *Blood*, **82,** 1682.

27. Serological investigation of the auto-immune and drug-induced immune haemolytic anaemias

Revised by A. H. Waters

Types of auto-antibody   500
  Warm auto-antibodies   500
  Cold auto-antibodies   501
Methods of investigation   502
  Collection of samples of blood and serum   502
  Storage of samples   502
Scheme for the serological investigation of a patient suspected of suffering from a haemolytic anaemia of immunological origin   503
Detection of incomplete antibodies by means of the direct antiglobulin test (DAT)   505
  Qualitative direct antiglobulin test   506
  Quantitative direct antiglobulin test   506
Reactions with antiglobulin sera against IgG subclasses   507
Significance of a positive direct antiglobulin test   508
  Positive DATs in normal subjects   509
  Positive DATs in hospital patients   509
False-negative antiglobulin tests   510
DAT-negative AIHA   510
  Preparation of and testing a concentrated ether eluate   510
  Manual direct Polybrene test   511
Determination of the blood groups of a patient with AIHA   511

Demonstration of free antibodies in serum   512
Identification by absorption techniques of co-existing allo-antibodies in AIHA   513
Elution of antibodies from red cells   517
  Landsteiner and Miller's method   517
  Rubin's method   517
Determination of the specificity of warm auto-antibodies   518
Demonstration of lysis by warm auto-antibodies   518
Titration of cold agglutinins   519
Specificity of cold antibodies   519
Determination of thermal range of cold agglutinins   520
Lysis by cold antibodies   520
Donath-Landsteiner (D-L) antibody   522
  Direct Donath-Landsteiner test   522
Treatment of serum with 2-mercapto-ethanol and dithiothreitol   524
Drug-induced haemolytic anaemias of immunological origin   524
  Drug-dependent immune haemolytic anaemias   524
  Drug-dependent auto-immune haemolytic anaemias   525
  Detection of anti-penicillin antibodies   525
  Detection of antibodies against drugs other than penicillin   526

In many cases of acquired haemolytic anaemia the increased haemolysis is brought about by the production of auto-antibodies directed against the patient's own red cells. These are known as the auto-immune haemolytic anaemias (AIHA). They exist as disorders of obscure origin — the 'idiopathic' type — and secondary or symptomatic types, which are mainly associated with malignant diseases of the lympho-reticular system or other auto-immune diseases, particularly systemic lupus erythematosus (SLE), or may follow atypical (Mycoplasma) pneumonia, infectious mononucleosis, or other virus infections. Paroxysmal cold haemoglobinuria (PCH) also belongs to this group of disorders.

Occasionally, drugs may give rise to a haemolytic anaemia of immunological origin which closely mimics clinically and serologically idiopathic AIHA. Thus the red cells of about 20% of patients on long-term α-methyldopa (Aldomet) treatment give a positive direct antiglobulin test (DAT) and may have auto-antibodies in their serum which will react with normal red cells, even though they often show no evidence of increased red cell destruction. Other drugs such as penicillin, phenacetin, quinidine, quinine, the sodium salt of p-aminosalicylic acid and salicylazosulphapyridine (see p. 524) can also in rare cases cause haemolytic anaemia by immunological mechanisms. With these drugs (with the exception of Aldomet) the antibody is directed primarily against the drug and only secondarily involves the red cells.

TYPES OF AUTO-ANTIBODY

The diagnosis of an auto-immune haemolytic anaemia (AIHA) depends primarily upon the demonstration of auto-antibodies attached to the patient's red cells. This can be achieved by showing that the red cells are agglutinated by an anti-human globulin (AHG) serum (see p. 457).

Auto-antibodies can often be demonstrated free in the serum of a patient suffering from an AIHA. The ease with which the antibodies can be detected depends on how much antibody is being produced, its affinity for the corresponding antigen on the red cell surface and the effect that temperature has on the adsorption of the antibody, as well as on the technique used to detect it. The auto-antibodies associated with AIHA can be separated into two broad categories depending on how their interaction with antigen is affected by temperature; i.e. into warm antibodies which are able to combine with their corresponding red cell antigen readily at 37°C, and cold antibodies which cannot combine with antigen at 37°C, but form an increasingly stable combination with antigen as the temperature falls from 30–32°C to 2–4°C.

Cases of AIHA can similarly be separated into two broad categories according to the temperature characteristics of the associated auto-antibodies, i.e. into warm-type AIHA and cold-type AIHA. The relative frequency of the two categories is illustrated in Table 27.1.

WARM AUTO-ANTIBODIES

The commonest type of warm auto-antibody is an IgG immunoglobulin which behaves in vitro very similarly to an anti-Rh allo-antibody; indeed many IgG auto-antibodies have Rh specificity. IgA and IgM warm auto-antibodies are much less common, and when present they are usually formed in addition to an IgG auto-antibody (Table 27.2).

Quite frequently, patients with warm-type AIHA have complement adsorbed to their red cells, i.e. the cells are agglutinated by antisera specific for complement or a complement component, e.g. C3d (Table 27.2). In these cases

the complement is probably not being bound by an IgG antibody but is on the cell surface as the result of the action of small and otherwise undetected amounts of IgM auto-antibody. (IgA auto-antibodies are thought not to cause the binding on of complement.)

Table 27.1 Relative incidence of different types of auto-immune haemolytic anaemia[*]

	Males	Females	Total
Warm antibodies			
'Idiopathic'	46	65	111
Associated with drugs (mostly α-methyldopa)	1	10	11
Secondary			
Associated with:			
Lymphomas	14	23	37
SLE	1	15	16
Other possible or probable auto-immune disorders	8	13	21
Infections and miscellaneous	9	4	13
Ovarian teratoma	0	1	1
Totals	79	131	210
Cold antibodies			
'Idiopathic' (CHAD)	16	22	38
Secondary			
Associated with:			
Atypical or mycoplasma pneumonia	5	18	23
Infectious mononucleosis	1	1	2
Lymphomas	3	4	7
Paroxysmal cold haemoglobinuria			
'Idiopathic'	7	1	8
Secondary	4	3	7
Totals	36	49	85

[*]From Dacie and Worlledge.[6]

Table 27.2 Direct antiglobulin test in warm-antibody auto-immune haemolytic anaemia: incidence of different reactions to specific antiglobulin sera[5]

Anti-IgG	Anti-IgA	Anti-IgM	Anti-C	No. of patients	%
+	−	−	−	43	36
−	+	−	−	3	2
+	+	−	−	4	3
+	−	−	+	52	43
+	−	+	+	6	5
−	−	−	+	13	11
				121	100

Sometimes patients with warm-type AIHA appear to have only complement on the red cell surface. This is more difficult to interpret, as weak reactions of this type are not uncommon in patients with a variety of disorders in whom there is little evidence of increased red cell destruction. In some patients this may be due to the binding to the red cells of circulating immune complexes.

Warm auto-antibodies free in the patient's serum are best detected by means of the indirect antiglobulin test (IAT) or by the use of enzyme-treated, e.g. trypsinized or papainized, red cells. (Antibodies that agglutinate unmodified cells directly are seldom present.) Not infrequently, antibodies that agglutinate enzyme-treated cells, sometimes at high titres, are present in the sera of patients in whom the IAT using unmodified cells is negative (Table 27.3). Occasionally, too, they are present in the sera of patients in whom the DAT is negative.

Antibodies in serum that can be shown to lyse unmodified red cells at 37°C in the presence of complement (warm haemolysins) are rarely demonstrable.[4a] If present, the patient is likely to suffer from extremely severe haemolysis. Antibodies in serum that lyse as well as agglutinate enzyme-treated cells but do not affect unmodified cells are, on the other hand, quite commonly met with. Their specificity is uncertain — they are not anti-Rh — and their presence is not necessarily associated with increased haemolysis.

COLD AUTO-ANTIBODIES

Cold auto-antibodies are nearly always IgM in type. In vivo, the antibodies can cause chronic intravascular haemolysis, the intensity of which is characteristically influenced by the ambient temperature. The resultant clinical picture is generally referred to as the cold-haemagglutinin syndrome or disease (CHAD). Haemolysis is due to destruction of the red cells by complement which is bound to the red cell surface by the antigen-antibody reaction which takes place in the blood vessels of the exposed skin where the temperature is 28–32°C or less.

The red cells of patients suffering from CHAD characteristically give positive antiglobulin reactions only with anti-complement (anti-C) sera. This is due to the presence of red cells which have irreversibly adsorbed sublytic amounts of complement; it is a sign, therefore, of an antigen-antibody reaction which has taken place at a temperature below 37°C. The complement component responsible for the reaction with anti-C sera is the C3dg derivative of C3 (see p. 450).

In vitro, a cold-type auto-antibody will often lyse normal red cells at 20–30°C in the presence of fresh human complement, especially if the cell-serum mixture is acidified to pH 6.5–7.0; it will usually lyse enzyme-treated red cells readily in unacidified serum, and agglutination and lysis of these cells may still be present at 37°C. Most of

Table 27.3 Results of testing for free auto-antibodies in the sera of 210 patients with warm-antibody auto-immune haemolytic anaemia*

Indirect antiglobulin test	Agglutination at 37°C of enzyme-treated red cells	Lysis at 37°C of enzyme-treated red cells	Agglutination at 20°C of normal red cells	No. and percentage of patients in group	
+	+	+	+	4	
+	+	+	−	16	
+	+	−	−	64	41%
+	−	−	−	2	
+	−	−	+	1	
−	+	+	+	16	
−	+	+	−	31	
−	+	−	−	29	40%
−	+	−	+	7	
−	−	−	−	39	19%

*From Dacie and Worlledge.[6]

Notes: 1. In 41% of the patients the IAT was positive and in 80% of the patients the tests with enzyme-treated cells were positive + (in half of these patients the IAT was negative).

2. In 19% of the patients both tests were negative.

3. In 13% of the patients normal red cells were agglutinated at 20°C, probably by cold agglutinins.

Table 27.4 Main characteristics of IgG, IgM and IgA auto-antibodies

	IgG	IgM	IgA
Mol wt (daltons)	146 000	970 000	160 000
Sedimentation constant (s)	7	19	7
No. of heavy-chain sub-classes	4	1	2
Cross placenta	Yes	No	No
Cause activation of complement	Yes	Yes	No
Cause monocyte/macrophage attachment	Yes	No	No
No. of antigen binding sites	2	5 or 10	2
Types of AIHA produced	Warm; PCH	Usually cold	Warm

these cold-type auto-antibodies have anti-I specificity; i.e. they react strongly with the vast majority of adult red cells and only weakly with cord-blood red cells. A minority are anti-i and react strongly with cord-blood cells and weakly with adult red cells.[25] Rarely, the antibodies have anti-Pr or anti-M specificity and react with antigens on the red cell surface that are destroyed by enzyme treatment.

Another quite distinct, but rarely met with, type of cold antibody is the Donath-Landsteiner (D-L) antibody. This is an IgG globulin and has anti-P specificity. The clinical syndrome the antibody produces is referred to as paroxymal cold haemoglobinuria (PCH).

Some of the characteristics of IgG, IgM and IgA antibodies are illustrated in Table 27.4.

The clinical, haematological and serological aspects of the auto-immune haemolytic anaemias have by now an extensive literature. Relatively recent reviews include those of Pirofsky,[30] Petz and Garratty,[29] Sokol, Hewitt and Stamps,[39] Issitt,[18] Sokol and Hewitt[37] and Dacie.[4]

METHODS OF INVESTIGATION

Many of the methods used in the investigation of a patient suspected of suffering from AIHA have already been described in Chapter 24. Detailed description is given here of precautions to be taken when collecting blood samples from the patient and of methods of particular value in his or her investigation.

Collection of samples of blood and serum

It is convenient in dealing with a patient suspected of having AIHA to collect venous blood using a syringe and needle already warmed to 37°C and to deliver the blood (a) into a defibrinating container warmed in a water-bath at 37°C and (b) into ACD or CPD solution (1 ml of ACD or 0.5 ml of CPD is sufficient for 4 ml of whole blood).

Defibrination has an advantage over allowing blood to clot undisturbed in that large volumes of red cells are obtained as well as serum. In the first examination of a patient, it is desirable to carry out defibrination at 37°C rather than at room temperature, so as to prevent adsorption of a cold auto-antibody should one be present.

When defibrination is complete, the blood should be centrifuged to separate the serum at 37°C, e.g. in an ordinary centrifuge into the buckets of which water warmed to 37–40°C has been placed.

The red cells are available for antibody elution and the serum can be examined for free antibody or other abnormalities. The ACD or CPD sample is used for the DAT and other tests involving the patient's red cells. If the auto-antibody in a particular case is known to be warm in type, the blood may be defibrinated and separated at room temperature; otherwise, as already indicated, this should be carried out at 37°C. When samples are sent by post, it is best to send separately: (a) serum (separated at 37°C) and (b) whole blood added to ACD or CPD solution. Sterility must be maintained.

Storage of samples

Samples of patient's blood, while keeping quite well in ACD or CPD at 4°C, are more difficult to preserve than normal red cells. In particular, if marked spherocytosis is present considerable lysis develops on storage. However, satisfactory eluates can be made from washed red cells frozen at −20°C for weeks or months.

The patient's serum should be stored at −20°C or below in small (1–2 ml) volumes. If complement is to be titrated, the serum should be frozen as soon as practicable at −70° or below if the titration is not performed immediately.

SCHEME FOR THE SEROLOGICAL INVESTIGATION OF A PATIENT SUSPECTED OF SUFFERING FROM A HAEMOLYTIC ANAEMIA OF IMMUNOLOGICAL ORIGIN

The problem arises as to which are the most profitable tests to carry out and the order in which they should be done. A suggested scheme covering the more important tests follows, it has been set out in the form of answers (right-hand side) to questions (left-hand side).

Question

1. Are the patient's red cells 'coated' by immunoglobulins or complement (indicating antigen-antibody reaction)? [If the DAT is negative, the diagnosis is unlikely to be an auto-immune haemolytic anaemia (AIHA), although not impossible. See DAT-negative AIHA (p. 510).]

2. If the DAT is positive, are immunoglobulins or complement adsorbed to the red cells?

3. If immunoglobulins are present on the red cells, are they auto-antibodies?

4. What is the patient's blood group?

Answer

Direct antiglobulin tests (DAT) using a potent 'broad-spectrum' reagent at suitable dilutions (p. 457).

Repeat the DAT using serial dilutions of polyspecific and monospecific sera (p. 457). i.e. broad-spectrum, anti-IgG, anti-IgM, anti-IgA and anti-C.

Prepare eluates from the patient's red cells. Test these later (see 6a).

Determine the patient's ABO and Rh (D) and other blood-group antigens as far as possible. The Rh phenotype is particularly important in warm-type AIHA; other antigens must be determined if allo-antibodies are to be differentiated from auto-antibodies (see p.516).

Question	Answer

Question

5. Is there free antibody in the serum? How does it react, at what temperatures and by what methods can it be demonstrated?

6. If there is a warm antibody:

(a) What is the specificity of the antibody adsorbed to the red cells?

(b) What is the specificity of any irregular (unexpected) antibody detected in the serum? Is it an auto- or allo-antibody?

(c) What is the agglutinin titre of the antibody?

(d) If the antibody is lytic, what is the lysis titre?

7. If there is a cold antibody:

(a) Has the antibody any specificity? Is it an auto-antibody or an allo-antibody? What is its titre?

(b) What is the thermal range of the antibody?

(c) Has the antibody any lytic activity?

Answer

(i) Screen the serum with two or three samples of adult enzyme-treated red cells for agglutination and lysis at 20°C and 37°C and by the IAT (p. 512). The red cells chosen must be ABO-compatible and bear between them the antigens of all the common blood-group systems. If these are not available, use group-O, R_1R_2 (CDe/cDE) cells.
(ii) Determine the agglutinin titre at 4°C with ABO-compatible adult red cells, cord-blood cells and adult enzyme-treated cells. (p. 519).

These tests will show whether cold or warm antibodies are present in the serum or a mixture of the two.

Test the eluate with a selected ABO-compatible panel of red cells of known blood groups by the IAT and by using enzyme-treated red cells (p. 518).

Titrate the serum by the methods that have given positive results in the screening test using the same panel of red cells (5i).

Titrate in saline and/or in albumin using normal and enzyme-treated cells and by the IAT.

Determine the lysis titre with enzyme-treated red cells (or PNH red cells) at 37°C, or with normal cells if these have been lysed in the screening test (5i).

Titrate at 4°C with ABO-compatible adult (I) cells, cord-blood (i) cells, the patient's cells, adult (i) cells (if possible) and enzyme-treated adult (I) cells (p. 519).
(i) Determine the highest temperature at which auto-agglutination of the patient's whole blood takes place (p. 520).
(ii) Titrate the patient's serum at 20°C and 30°C with the panel of cells listed under 5(i). If there was any agglutination or lysis at 37°C in the screening test (5i), titrate with the appropriate cells at this temperature.
(i) Titrate the antibody in fresh normal ABO-compatible serum with normal ABO-compatible I (or i) red cells and enzyme-treated I (or i) red cells at 20°C and (if necessary) at 37°C (p. 520).

Paroxysmal noctural haemoglubinuria (PNH) red cells, if available, can be used as a valuable and sensitive reagent for detecting lytic activity by both warm and cold antibodies.

Question	Answer
7. (c) Cont.	(ii) If PCH is suspected, carry out the direct and indirect Donath-Landsteiner tests (p. 522).
8. Is a drug suspected as the cause of the haemolytic anaemia?	(i) If a penicillin is suspected, test for antibodies using cells pre-incubated with the appropriate drug (p. 525). (ii) If other drugs are suspected, add the drug in solution to a mixture of the patient's serum, normal cells and fresh normal serum (p. 526). Look for agglutination of normal and enzyme-treated cells and use the IAT
9. Are there any other serological abnormalities?	Consider carrying out the following tests: quantitative estimation of serum proteins; electrophoresis and quantitative estimation of immunoglobulins; estimation of complement; tests for LE cells; tests for anti-nuclear factor (ANF); titration of heterophile (anti-sheep red cell) antibodies; Wassermann and Kahn reactions; test for mycoplasma antibodies.

The above scheme summarizes what may be done by way of serological investigation of a patient suspected of having AIHA. It is not suggested that every patient has to be investigated in such depth. However, there are other considerations than scientific interest and curiosity. For instance, not infrequently clinical diagnosis and prognosis depend on accurate investigation; and an exact knowledge of the specificity of an antibody may be of great importance in relation to blood transfusion. In some patients, too, quantitative measurements of antibody activity or immunoglobulin may provide valuable evidence of the efficacy of treatment. As in all spheres of laboratory medicine, a close collaboration between clinician and laboratory helps in deciding what tests should be done in any particular case.

DETECTION OF INCOMPLETE ANTIBODIES BY MEANS OF THE DIRECT ANTIGLOBULIN (COOMBS) TEST (DAT)

Principle. As already described, the DAT involves testing the patient's cells without prior exposure to antibody in vitro. For the investigation of cases of AIHA, antiglobulin reagents specific for IgG, IgM and IgA should be used. These reagents are available from commercial sources. Monoclonal antibodies specific for the complement component C3d can also be obtained.

Precautions

Certain precautions are necessary when investi-

gating a patient with possible AIHA. The patient's red cells should be washed four times in a large volume of saline* warmed to 37°C. The warm saline is used as a routine in order to wash off cold antibodies and obtain a smooth suspension of cells — there is no risk of washing off adsorbed complement components. However, the washing process should be accomplished as quickly as

---

*Throughout this Chapter 'saline' refers to 9g/l NaCl buffered to pH 7.0 (see p. 579).

possible and the test should be set up immediately afterwards, for, occasionally, bound warm-antibody elutes off the cells when they are washed and false-negative results may be obtained. If for any reason the washing process has to be interrupted once it has begun, the cell suspension should be placed at 4°C to slow down the dissociation of the antibody. A tile method is particularly useful in the investigation of AIHA since it enables an estimation of the speed of agglutination as well as the final strength of the reaction.

QUALITATIVE DIRECT ANTIGLOBULIN TEST

A spin tube technique, as described on p. 459, is recommended.

Make a 2–5% suspension of washed red cells in saline. Add 1 volume (drop) of the cell suspension to 2 volumes (drops) of antiglobulin reagent at its recommended dilution. Centrifuge for 10–60 s (see p. 460).

Examine for agglutination after gently re-suspending the button of cells. A concave mirror helps in macroscopic readings. If the result appears to be negative, confirm this microscopically.

Each DAT or batch of tests should be carefully controlled as previously described (p. 458).

Check negative results with the anti-IgG and anti-C reagents by the addition of IgG-sensitized cells and complement-coated cells.

If the qualitative DAT is positive, quantitative tests may be undertaken. The results with such tests reflect the degree to which the patient's red cells are coated with IgG and/or complement. For comparative purposes, the same antiglobulin reagent must be used throughout.

QUANTITATIVE DIRECT ANTIGLOBULIN TEST

A convenient method utilizing four-fold dilutions of antiglobulin and allowing the antiglobulin and cell suspension to interact on a translucent opal tile is described below. Alternatively, the reactions can be allowed to take place in 75 × 10 or 12 mm glass tubes using 2–5% suspensions of red cells, and the results read macroscopically or microscopi-

cally after the cell suspensions have spontaneously sedimented at the end of 1 h at room temperature.

Wash the cells as already described. Make four-fold dilutions of broad-spectrum, anti-IgG and anti-C reagents, ranging normally from a 1 in 4 dilution to 1 in 4096. Place 6 drops of saline in each of the master tubes to be used for preparing dilutions and add 2 drops of the appropriate undiluted antiglobulin to the first tube (1 in 4 dilution) (see Fig. 27.1), dry the pipette, mix the diluted antiglobulin serum, place 1 drop on the tile and 2 drops in the next tube, and so on. The final layout is shown in Fig. 27.1. Care must be taken to minimize the carry-over of more concentrated antiglobulin into the tubes destined to contain highly diluted antiglobulin. A simple way to minimize this is to wipe the sides and tip of the pipette with absorbent tissue between each dilution. For greater accuracy (not required for routine purposes) separate pipettes should be used for each dilution. The effect of carry-over is illustrated in Table 27.5.

Anti-IgM and anti-IgA reagents should also be used if they have given a positive reaction in the qualitative test.

As soon as possible after the dilutions of antiglobulin have been placed on the tile, add 1 drop of a 20% suspension of the patient's washed

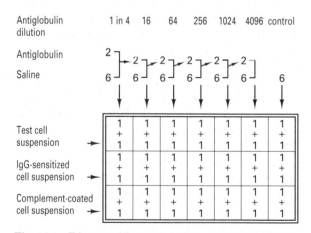

Fig. 27.1 Diagram illustrating the quantitative DAT. The top half of the diagram indicates how the antiglobulin dilutions are made (in tubes). The figures represent drops. One drop of the antiglobulin dilution and one drop of the appropriate red cell suspension are mixed in a square on the tile (or in a tube). A pattern of reactions is shown in Fig. 27.2.

Table 27.5 Comparison of titration end-points of a high-titre cold agglutinin using conventional doubling dilution techniques with those obtained by making dilutions with separate pipettes

Final serum dilution		1 in 1024	1 in 4096	1 in 16 000	1 in 64 000	1 in 256 000	1 in 1 000 000	Control (saline)
1. Doubling dilutions using Pasteur pipette								
(a) no mixing in stem	macro	+	+	+	[+]	−	−	−
	micro	+	+	+	+	+	[+]	−
(b) with mixing in stem	macro	+	+	+	weak*	−	−	−
	micro	+	+	+	+	+	[+]	−
2. Doubling dilutions using glass automatic	macro	+	+	+	[+]	(?)	−	−
pipette	micro	+	+	+	+	+	[+]	−
3. Dilutions prepared using a separate	macro	+	+	[+]	(?)	−	−	−
pipette for each dilution	micro	+	+	+	[+]	−	−	−

*The titre read macroscopically was recorded as 32 000.

Only the results of readings made on the last seven alternate tubes of the titrations are recorded. The doubling dilutions were prepared commencing with undiluted serum, and the separate dilutions (Series 3) were prepared from an initial serum dilution of 1 in 256.

The titrations were carried out at room temperature (18°C) and the end-points of the titrations were determined macroscopically (macro) using a concave mirror, and also microscopically (micro). The end-points are indicated thus [+].

The end-points determined *macroscopically* using the conventional doubling-dilution techniques give results which closely approximate to the truth, assuming that the correct titration figure is obtained when dilutions of serum are prepared using a separate pipette for each dilution and the result is read microscopically.

cells to each drop of diluted antiglobulin, mix using a wooden swab-stick, starting with the saline control and finishing with the highest concentration of antiglobulin. Use a separate swab-stick for each series of dilutions. Rock gently and observe at 1 min intervals, assessing the results at the end of a predetermined time (e.g. 5 min) and scoring as illustrated in Table 24.6 (p. 456).

Normal (unsensitized) cells and normal sensitized (control) cells should be used to check the specificity and sensitivity of the antiglobulin reagent.

Typical results illustrating different types of quantitative DATs are shown in Table 27.6. The appearance of positive tests with cells coated with complement and IgG, respectively, are shown in Fig. 27.2.

Antiglobulin test titration scores give a good indication of the degree of sensitization of the red cells with IgG and complement without the necessity of performing sophisticated quantitative measurements. However, whilst a high titre (> 1000) with anti-IgG is likely to be associated with increased haemolysis, titration scores cannot be used to determine whether or not increased haemolysis is occurring. Titres are, however, of value in the follow-up of an individual patient:

e.g. a fall in titre is often associated with remission and a rising titre with relapse. In warm-type AIHA the presence of complement on the red cell surface as well as IgG is more frequently associated with secondary than with 'idiopathic' AIHA. However, IgG without complement is typical of an α-methyldopa-induced positive DAT.

REACTIONS WITH IgG SUBCLASS ANTIGLOBULIN REAGENTS

When the DAT is positive with anti-IgG, it is of interest to determine the subclass of IgG. The majority of IgG red cell auto-antibodies are IgG1, sometimes in combination with IgG2 or IgG3. The formation of IgG3 (either alone or with IgG1) appears to be associated with active disease and marked haemolysis. Patients with IgG1 only on the red cell surface may or may not have marked haemolysis, whilst IgG2 and IgG4 do not appear to be associated with any increased haemolysis.[7] Thus it is of value to know whether IgG3 is present since its presence indicates the likelihood of aggressive disease. The reactions with subclass reagents can be ascertained using four-fold dilutions of the specific reagents exactly

Table 27.6   Patterns of agglutination in the direct antiglobulin test using broad-spectrum and specific antiglobulin reagents

IgG type

Reagent	Dilutions of antiglobulin							
	1 in 1	4	16	64	256	1024	4096	Saline
Broad-spectrum	1 +	2 +	3 +	4 +	4 +	3 +	2 +	0
Anti-IgG	1 +	2 +	3 +	4 +	4 +	3 +	2 +	0
Anti-C	0	0	0	0	0	0	0	0

IgG + C type

Reagent	Dilutions of antiglobulin							
	1 in 1	4	16	64	256	1024	4096	Saline
Broad-spectrum	3 +	3 +	3 +	2 +	2 +	1 +	0	0
Anti-IgG	0	1 +	1 +	2 +	2 +	1 +	0	0
Anti-C	3 +	3 +	2 +	1 +	0	0	0	0

C only type

Reagent	Dilutions of antiglobulin							
	1 in 1	4	16	64	256	1024	4096	Saline
Broad-spectrum	3 +	3 +	2 +	1 +	0	0	0	0
Anti-IgG	0	0	0	0	0	0	0	0
Anti-C	3 +	3 +	2 +	1 +	0	0	0	0

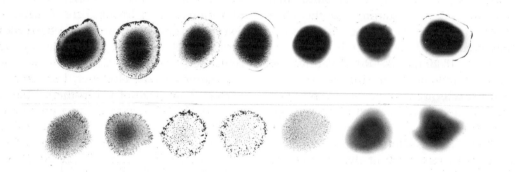

Fig. 27.2   Antiglobulin reactions carried out on a tile using various dilutions of an antiglobulin reagent.
Upper series: red cells coated by complement. *Lower series*: red cells sensitized with an IgG antibody. The dilutions of antiglobulin reagent ranged from 1 in 4 to 1 in 4096. The red cell suspension on the extreme right is the control with 9 g/l NaCl substituted for the antiglobulin reagent.

as has already been described. The sub-class reagents are available commercially*.

SIGNIFICANCE OF POSITIVE DIRECT ANTIGLOBULIN TEST[46]

A positive DAT does not necessarily mean that the patient has auto-immune haemolytic anaemia.[6] However, it certainly calls attention to this possibility. The causes of a positive test include

the following:

1. An auto-antibody on the red cell surface with or without haemolytic anaemia.

2. An allo-antibody on the red cell surface, as for example in haemolytic disease of the newborn or after an incompatible transfusion.

*e.g. from the Central Laboratory of the Netherlands Red Cross Blood Transfusion Service, Amsterdam.

3. Antibodies provoked by drugs adsorbed to the red cell (p. 524).

4. Normal globulins adsorbed to the red cell surface as the result of damage by drugs, e.g. cephalothin.

5. Interaction between the antiglobulin sera and anti-T, as with polyagglutinable red cells.

6. Anti-albumin and anti-transferrin antibodies in antiglobulin sera giving rise to false-positive reaction.

7. Adsorption of immune complexes to the red cell surface. This may be the mechanism of the (usually weak) reactions that are found in approximately 8% of hospital patients suffering from a wide variety of disorders (see below).

8. Sensitization in vitro. If, for instance, clotted or defibrinated normal blood is allowed to stand in a refrigerator at 4°C, or even at room temperature, and the antiglobulin test is subsequently carried out, the reaction may be positive due to the adsorption of incomplete cold antibodies and complement from normal sera.[4e] Samples of blood taken into EDTA or ACD and subsequently chilled do not give this type of false-positive result as the anticoagulant inhibits the complement reaction.

9. It is not unknown for the DAT to be positive with the blood of apparently perfectly healthy individuals, e.g. blood donors. Such occurrences are rare and have not been satisfactorily explained (see below). The possibility that α-methyldopa is being taken as an antihypertensive drug must not be overlooked: up to 20% of such patients on long-term therapy develop positive DATs — most show no signs of overtly increased haemolysis.

In connection with positive reactions given by normal cells, it should be pointed out that slowly developing weak agglutination, occurring even in well diluted antiglobulin serum, is not uncommon. With suspensions on an opalescent tile, this is not, as a rule, evident to the naked eye under at least 5 min. However, this agglutination is probably real and appears to represent an interaction between globulins normally adsorbed to the red cell surface and the antiglobulin serum (see below). Tests should normally be read before this type of false-positive agglutination occurs.

Stratton and Renton[41] emphasized yet another possible cause of false-positive agglutination. This is due to a silica gel derived from glass, and it is most commonly produced by using sodium citrate solutions autoclaved in glass bottles or in the case of tests carried out on glass tiles by scraping the surface of the tile in the course of mixing cells and serum with a corner of a microscope slide or glass rod.

Positive DATs in normal subjects

The occurrence of a clearly positive DAT in an apparently healthy subject is a rare but well-known phenomenon. Worlledge[46] had reported an incidence in blood donors of approximately 1 in 9000. In a more recent report, Gorst et al[11] estimated that the incidence was approximately 1 in 14 000. 65 positive tests had been encountered in blood donors: of 59 samples that had been tested with anti-complement (anti-C) sera as well as with anti-IgG sera, 23 had been positive with anti-IgG sera alone, 28 by anti-C sera alone and eight by both anti-IgG and anti-C sera. 32 of the donors giving positive tests had been recalled for further study; none presented any abnormal clinical findings and all were fit and well. All except one (see below) remained healthy subsequently (for up to 18 years). The exception was a donor who, having had a positive DAT for 2 years, subsequently developed typical AIHA. It is interesting to note that the data of Gorst et al indicated an increasing likelihood of a positive test with increasing age. Their report, and other subsequent reports,[1,40] certainly suggests that the finding of a positive DAT, using an anti-IgG serum, in an apparently healthy person is usually of little clinical significance and that overt AIHA, although it may develop, hardly ever does. In some patients, too, the DAT eventually becomes negative!

Positive DATs in hospital patients

In contrast to the rarity of positive DATs in strictly healthy people, positive tests are much more frequent in hospital patients. Worlledge[46] reported that the red cells of 40 out of 489 blood samples (8.9%) submitted for routine tests had been agglutinated by anti-complement (anti-C sera). Only one sample was agglutinated by an anti-IgG serum and this had been obtained from a patient being treated with α-methyldopa. Freedman[8] reported a similar incidence — 7.8% positive tests with anti-C sera. Lau et al[23] had used anti-IgG sera only. The tests were seldom positive (0.9% positive out of 4664 tests). The probable explanation for the relatively high incidence of positive tests with anti-C sera is that the reaction is between anti-complement antibodies and immune complexes adsorbed to the red cells.

Hypergammaglobulinaemia

Another possible explanation for positive DATs in hospital patients is hypergammaglobulinaemia. Symanski et al[42] employed an AutoAnalyser and used Ficoll and PVP to enhance agglutination by an anti-IgG serum highly diluted (usually to 1 in 5000) in 0.5% bovine serum albumin. In this sensitive system the strength of agglutination was clearly positively correlated with the serum γ-globulin concentration, being subnormal in hypogammaglobulinaemia and supranormal in hypergammaglobulinaemia.

It is typical to find in hypergammaglobulinaemic patients in whom the DAT is positive that attempts to demonstrate antibodies in eluates fail i.e., that eluates are non-reactive.[14,17]

FALSE-NEGATIVE ANTIGLOBULIN TESTS

There are several causes:

1. Failure to wash the red cells properly—the antisera may then be neutralized by immuno-globulins or complement in the surrounding serum or plasma (p. 459).

2. Excessive agitation at the reading stage may break up agglutinates leading to a false-negative result.

3. The use of impotent antisera so that weakly sensitized cells are not detected.

4. The use of incorrect dilutions of the antisera.

5. The use of antisera lacking the antibody corresponding to the subclass of immunoglobulin responsible for the red cell sensitization.

6. The antibody being readily dissociable and eluted in the washing process.

DAT-NEGATIVE AIHA

In approximately 2–6% of patients who present with the clinical and haematological features of AIHA the DAT is negative on repeated testing.[3,46,47]

In some of these patients auto-antibodies are being formed but they are of such a nature or present in such small amounts that routine testing fails to detect them. In such patients evidence for auto-antibody formation can often be obtained by careful screening of a concentrated ether eluate made from the patient's red cells or by the manual Polybrene test.

More complex techniques have, too, been used successfully to demonstrate low levels of immuno-globulin on the red cell surface in patients with a provisional diagnosis of DAT-negative AIHA. These methods include radio-immunoassay,[36] the use of the agglutination enhancers Polybrene and PVP in automated tests,[15,21] the complement-fixing antibody consumption (CFAC) test[10] and enzyme-linked immunosorbent assays (ELISA) and enzyme-linked antiglobulin tests (ELAT).[2,38]

PREPARATION AND TESTING A CONCENTRATED ETHER ELUATE

This technique concentrates low levels of immunoglobulin present on the red cell surface so that antibody may then be detected by screening the eluate with enzyme-treated normal group-O red cells and by the IAT.

Method

1. Prepare a concentrated eluate by adding 1 volume of saline to 7 volumes of washed, packed red cells. After this initial step the eluate is prepared by Rubin's method,[32] as described on p. 517.

2. Screen the eluate for the presence of antibody with the group-O red cells of three

donors, using enzyme-treated cells and the IAT, as described on p. 518

MANUAL DIRECT POLYBRENE TEST

The following method[26] is modified from that described by Petz and Branch[27] who based their technique on that of Lalezari and Jiang.[20] Polybrene is a polyvalent cationic molecule, hexadimethrine bromide, which can overcome the electrostatic repulsive forces between adjacent red cells, bringing the cells closer together. When low levels of IgG are present on the red cell surface antibody linkage of adjacent red cells is enhanced. The Polybrene is then neutralized using a negatively charged molecule such as trisodium citrate. Sensitized red cells remain agglutinated after neutralization of the Polybrene. Unsensitized red cells will disaggregate after neutralization.

Reagents

Polybrene stock. 10% Polybrene in 9 g/l NaCl, pH 6.9 (saline).

Working Polybrene solution. Dilute the stock Polybrene solution 1 in 250 in saline.

Resuspending solution. 60 ml of 0.2 mol/l trisodium citrate added to 40 ml of 50 g/l dextrose.

Washing solution. 50 ml of 0.2 mol/l trisodium citrate in 950 ml of saline.

Low ionic medium (LIM). 50 g/l dextrose containing 2 g/l disodium ethylenediamine tetraacetate. Adjust the pH of half the batch to 6.4. Store the remainder at the original pH (approx. 4.9); use this to repeat tests that are negative using LIM at pH 6.4.

Method

Ensure all reagents are at room temperature.

Positive control

Dilute an IgG anti-D in normal group-AB serum. Find a dilution which gives a positive result with papainized cells but is negative by the IAT on standard testing with group-O, D-positive red cells (a dilution of 1 in 10 000 is often suitable).

Negative control

Normal group-AB serum which fails to agglutinate papainized group-O, D-positive red cells.

1. Wash the cells four times in saline and make 3–5% suspensions of test and normal group-O Rh (D) red cells in saline.

2. Set up three 75×10 mm tubes as shown in Table 27.7. Leave at room temperature for 1 min.

3. Add 1 drop of working Polybrene solution to each tube and mix gently. Leave for 15 s at room temperature.

4. Centrifuge for 10 s at 1000g. Decant, taking care to remove all the supernatant.

5. Leave for 3–5 min at room temperature before adding 2 drops of resuspending solution and mixing gently. Within 10 s aggregates will dissociate leaving true agglutination in the positive tubes.

6. Read macroscopically after 10–60 s. Check all negative results microscopically and compare with the negative control.

7. Repeat negative tests using LIM at the lower pH (approx. 4.9).

If the direct Polybrene test is negative, a supplementary antiglobulin test may be performed by washing the cells twice in the washing solution, and testing with an anti-IgG antiglobulin reagent.

DETERMINATION OF THE BLOOD GROUP OF A PATIENT WITH AIHA

ABO grouping

No difficulty should be encountered in ABO

Table 27.7 Setting up a direct manual Polybrene test

	Test	Positive control	Negative control
AB serum*	2	0	2
Dilute anti-D in AB serum*	0	2	0
2–3% test cells*	1	0	0
2–5% normal O Rh (D) cells*	0	1	1
LIM	0.6 ml	0.6 ml	0.6 ml

*Drops.

grouping patients with warm-type AIHA, but the presence of cold agglutinins may well cause difficulties. The cells should in all cases be washed in warm (37°C) saline. They should then be groupable without trouble; the reactions must, however, be controlled with normal AB serum. Reverse grouping should be performed strictly at 37°C or, in an emergency, on a warmed tile. Warm the known A_1, B and O cells to 37°C before adding them to the patient's serum at 37°C. Read the results on microscope slides warmed to 37°C (p. 483).

Rh (D) grouping

When the DAT is positive monoclonal anti-D reagents should be used, as the cells will spontaneously agglutinate in the presence of albumin or other enhancing medium. Appropriate controls should be included. (See p. 485.)

DEMONSTRATION OF FREE ANTIBODIES IN SERUM

The sera of patients suffering from AIHA often contain free auto-antibodies. This is the rule in cold-haemagglutinin disease, but in the warm-antibody type of disease IgG antibodies detectable by the indirect antiglobulin test (IAT) are usually only found free in the serum of patients who are suffering from a moderate or marked degree of haemolysis. Free warm antibodies detectable by the use of enzyme-treated cells are, on the other hand, not infrequently found and they may often be detected in patients in clinical and haematological remission. In investigating a patient's serum for auto-antibodies a comprehensive screening procedure should be followed. If positive results are obtained, a more detailed quantitative assessment should be undertaken. If the results are negative, no further tests need to be carried out.

ROUTINE SCREENING TESTS FOR AUTO- (AND ALLO-) ANTIBODIES IN SERUM

The patient's serum is tested under optimal conditions for agglutination and lysis and by the IAT using two or three samples of group-O adult red cells (chosen to possess between them all the common red cell antigens) and the same cells enzyme-treated, e.g. pre-papainized.

The serum is tested undiluted and diluted 1 in 2 with fresh normal human ABO-compatible serum, both at the normal pH of the serum (pH 7.5–8.0) and acidified so that the pH of the cell-serum mixture is c 6.8. The pH of the serum should be checked before the cells are added; a pH of 6.0–6.5 is required. Fresh serum is added because the sera of some patients with AIHA may be deficient in complement. Acid is added because the pH optimum for the lytic activity of some types of antibodies is 6.5–6.8. Tests are carried out strictly at 37°C and at 20°C, the cells and serum being allowed to come to the chosen temperature before they are mixed and being centrifuged subsequently at that temperature. In tests at 37°C the tubes should be centrifuged at that temperature, e.g. in a centrifuge the buckets of which are surrounded by water warmed to 37°–40°C. For the IAT the cells should be washed in saline at the appropriate temperature. The fresh normal serum used as complement must be tested against the same samples of test cells to ensure that it is free from antibody. Such sera should be separated immediately after collection and stored at –40°C or below.

Method

Set up a series of 30 tubes (75 × 10 mm), as illustrated in Fig. 27.3, the back row acting as master tubes. The master tubes contain the mixtures indicated A–F.

Pipette 9-drop samples from the master tubes A–F into each of four tubes. Incubate the first and third rows of tubes at 37°C, and leave the second and fourth rows of tubes at 20°C, as shown in the figure. Add 1 volume of 50% group-O normal cells to the first two rows of tubes,

Tube No.	A	B	C	D	E	F
Patient's serum	40	36	20	20	0	0
Fresh normal serum (complement)	0	0	20	16	40	36
0.2 mol/l HCl	0	4	0	4	0	4

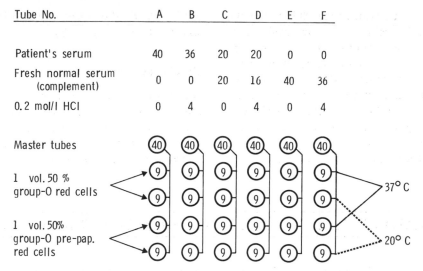

Master tubes

1 vol. 50% group-O red cells

1 vol. 50% group-O pre-pap. red cells

37° C

20° C

Fig. 27.3   Suggested procedure for setting up a serum screening test for auto-immune haemolytic anaemia. The top row of circles represents the large master tubes in which the primary dilutions are made; the lower four rows of circles represent the tubes in which the tests are carried out. The figures represent drops or volumes.

and 1 volume of 50% group-O pre-papainized cells to the other two rows. Mix and allow to stand for 1–1½ h. Inspect all the tubes macroscopically for agglutination over a diffuse light source and then centrifuge at the temperature of the test and read for lysis by eye.

Wash the cells in the first row in warm saline at 37°C four times and carry out an IAT using anti-IgG and anti-C sera at their optimal dilutions. If the DAT had been positive with an anti-IgM or anti-IgA serum the cells should also be set up against the optimal dilution of the appropriate antiglobulin reagent.

Wash the cells in the second row at room temperature and carry out an IAT as described above.

By using this technique the serum has been screened to see whether:

1. Free antibody is present which agglutinates normal group-O red cells at 37°C (first row) or at 20°C (second row).

2. Free antibody is present which agglutinates enzyme-treated group-O red cells at 37°C (third row) or at 20°C (fourth row).

3. Free antibody is present which reacts in the IAT with normal group-O cells.

4. The group-O normal or enzyme-treated cells are lysed and whether this shows pH dependence.

5. There is evidence of a lack of complement, lysis taking place in the presence of fresh normal serum but not without it (tubes 3 and 4, columns B and C).

If the screening test is positive, further tests are necessary to confirm the finding and demonstrate the antibody specificity.

Allo-antibodies will be detected by the screening procedure and will have to be carefully distinguished from auto-antibodies (see below). Representative examples of results of the screening tests in the different types of AIHA are shown in Table 27.8.

IDENTIFICATION BY ABSORPTION TECHNIQUES OF CO-EXISTING ALLO-ANTIBODIES IN THE PRESENCE OF WARM AUTO-ANTIBODIES

Absorption techniques for the detection of allo-antibodies present in the sera or eluates of patients with suspected or proved AIHA can be helpful in the following situations:

1. In screening for co-existing serum allo-antibodies in patients with AIHA who have been pregnant or previously transfused and are found to have significant titres (>8) of a pan-reactive antibody in their serum.

Table 27.8(1)　Antibody screening test: typical result with IgG antibody (direct antiglobulin test positive with anti-IgG only)

Method		Red cells	Temp. (°C)	S	AS	S + C	AS + C	C	AC
Indirect antiglobulin test	anti-IgG	N	37	3 +	4 +	2 +	3 +	–	–
	anti-C	N	37	–	–	–	–	–	–
	anti-IgG	N	20	2 +	3 +	1 +	2	–	–
	anti-C	N	20	–	–	–	–	–	–
Agglutination		N	37	–	–	–	–	–	–
		N	20	–	–	–	–	–	–
Lysis		N	37	–	–	–	–	–	–
		N	20	–	–	–	–	–	–
Agglutination		EN	37	3 +	3 +	3 +	3 +	–	–
		EN	20	2 +	2 +	2 +	2 +	–	–
Lysis		EN	37	–	–	–	–	–	–
		EN	20	–	–	–	–	–	–

Table 27.8(2)　Antibody screening test: typical result with antibody(ies) giving positive direct antiglobulin tests with anti-IgG and anti-C

Method		Red cells	Temp. (°C)	S	AS	S + C	AS + C	C	AC
Indirect antiglobulin test	anti-IgG	N	37	1 +	2 +	1/2 +	1 +	–	–
	anti-C	N	37	1 +	2 +	3 +	3 +	–	–
	anti-IgG	N	20	1/2 +	–	–	–	–	–
	anti-C	N	20	1 +	2 +	2 +	3 +	–	–
Agglutination		N	37	–	–	–	–	–	–
		N	20	1 +	1 +	–	–	–	–
Lysis		N	37	–	–	–	–	–	–
		N	20	–	–	–	–	–	–
Agglutination		EN	37	1 +	1 +	–	–	–	–
		EN	20	2 +	2 +	1 +	1 +	–	–
Lysis		EN	37	1 +	2 +	3 +	4 +	–	–
		EN	20	–	–	1 +	2 +	–	–

Table 27.8(3)　Antibody screening test: typical result with antibody giving positive direct antiglobulin tests with anti-C only

Method		Red cells	Temp. (°C)	S	AS	S + C	AS + C	C	AC
Indirect antiglobulin test	anti-IgG	N	37	–	–	–	–	–	–
	anti-C	N	37	2 +	3 +	2 +	2 +	–	–
	anti-IgG	N	20	–	–	–	–	–	–
	anti-C	N	20	2 +	3 +	1 +	2 +	–	–
Agglutination		N	37	–	–	–	–	–	–
		N	20	–	–	–	–	–	–
Lysis		N	37	–	–	–	–	–	–
		N	20	–	–	–	–	–	–
Agglutination		EN	37	–	–	1 +	1 +	–	–
		EN	20	1 +	1 +	2 +	2 +	–	–
Lysis		EN	37	3 +	4 +	1 +	2 +	–	–
		EN	20	1 +	2 +	–	–	–	–

Table 27.8(4) Antibody screening test: typical result in the cold-haemagglutinin disease (direct antiglobulin test positive with anti-C only)

Method		Red cells	Temp. (°C)	S	AS	S + C	AS + C	C	C
Indirect antiglobulin test	⎰ anti-IgG	N	37	–	–	–	–	–	–
	⎱ anti-C	N	37	–	–	–	–	–	–
	anti-IgG	N	20						
	anti-C	N	20	⎱ Cells too agglutinated to test					
Agglutination		N	37	–	–	–	–	–	–
		N	20	4 +	4 +	4 +	2 +	–	+
Lysis		N	37	–	–	–	–	–	–
		N	20	–	–	–	2 +	–	–
Agglutination		EN	37	2 +	2 +	2 +	1 +	–	–
		EN	20	4 +	4 +	2 +	1 +	–	–
Lysis		EN	37	–	–	2 +	3 +	–	–
		EN	20	–	–	2 +	3 +	–	–

N, pooled normal adult group O red cells; EN, the same cells pre-treated with the enzyme papain; S, patient's undiluted serum; AS, patient's undiluted serum acidified to pH 6.0–6.5; C (complement), fresh normal human compatible serum; AC, fresh normal human compatible serum acidified to pH 6.0–6.5; S + C, equal volumes of patient's serum and complement.

2. In differentiating between auto- and allo-antibodies in the eluate of recently transfused patients with AIHA.

3. In investigating haemolytic transfusion reactions due to red cell allo-antibodies in patients with AIHA.

In some cases of AIHA an underlying allo-antibody may be detected by titrating the patient's serum and eluate against a panel of phenotyped red cells from normal donors. However, a high-titre auto-antibody may mask the allo-antibody; hence the need for absorption techniques, especially in the situations outlined above. The techniques described are based on those of Petz and Branch.[27]

USE OF ZZAP REAGENT FOR USE IN AUTO-ABSORPTION TECHNIQUES

'ZZAP' reagent[27] is a mixture of dithiothreitol and papain. It dissociates an auto-antibody already coating the patient's red cells and enzyme-treats them, thus increasing the amount of auto-antibody that can subsequently be adsorbed onto the patient's cells in vitro.

Reagents

Dithiothreitol (DTT), 0.2 mol/l.
Papain, 1%.

Phosphate buffered saline (PBS), pH 6.8–7.2.

Prepare a suitable volume of ZZAP by making up the reagents in the following ratio: 0.2 mol/l DTT 5 volumes; 1% papain 1 volume.

Check the pH and adjust to pH 6.0–6.5 using one drop at a time of 0.2 mol/l HCl or 0.2 mol/l NaOH.

METHOD FOR AUTO-ABSORPTION USING ZZAP

1. Add 2 volumes of ZZAP to 1 volume of four-times-washed packed red cells. Incubate at 37°C for 30 min mixing occasionally.

2. After incubation, wash the cells four times in saline, packing hard after the last wash.

3. Divide the cells into two equal volumes. To one volume add an equal volume of the serum to be absorbed. Incubate at 37°C for 1 h.

4. Centrifuge at 1000*g*. Remove the serum and add to the remaining volume of cells.

5. Repeat the absorption procedure.

6. Remove the absorbed serum and store at −20% or below for allo-antibody screening or cross-matching, which may be performed by standard techniques.

Notes

The auto-absorption techniques should only be used in the following circumstances:

1. When the patient has not been transfused in the previous 6 weeks, as the presence of transfused red cells may allow the absorption of allo-antibody as well as auto-antibody.

2. When at least 2–3 ml of packed red cells are available from the patient.

3. When the auto-antibodies present react well with enzyme-treated red cells.

If they do not, heat elution should be substituted for ZZAP treatment. Heat elution may be performed by shaking the washed cells for 5 min in a 56°C water-bath and then washing the cells.

ALLO-ABSORPTION USING PAPAINIZED R_1R_1, R_2R_2 AND rr CELLS

This method may be used when auto-absorption is not appropriate — for instance when the patient has been transfused in the previous 6 weeks or when at least 2–3 ml of patient's red cells are not available.

1. Select three normal group-O red cell samples, which individually lack some of the blood-group antigens which commonly stimulate the production of clinically significant antibodies, e.g. C, E, K, Fy^a, Fy^b, Jk^a, Jk^b, S, s (Table 27.9).

2. Papainize 2 ml of packed cells from each sample after washing the cells in saline 4 times.

3. Add to 1 ml of each sample of washed, packed, papainized cells 1 ml of the patient's serum. Incubate for 1 h at 37°C.

4. Centrifuge to pack the cells. Remove the supernatant serum and add it to the second 1 ml volume of papainized cells. Incubate for 1 h at 37°C.

5. Centrifuge again to pack the cells. Remove the supernatant and store at −20°C or below for further testing, e.g. allo-antibody screening and cross-matching.

Method for testing allo-absorbed sera

Allo-antibody screening. Each absorbed serum is tested against a panel of phenotyped red cells by the IAT, using undiluted serum and by a short titration, 1 in 2 to 1 in 16, against papainized cells.

Cross-matching. Each absorbed serum must be tested separately against the donor red cells by the IAT, using undiluted serum.

Example of allo-antibody detection using the allo-absorption technique in a recently transfused patient with AIHA

The patient's serum when first tested against a panel of group-O phenotyped red cells revealed only pan-reactive antibodies. In contrast, three absorbed sera, A, B and C, obtained by absorbing the patient's serum with three selected phenotyped samples of group-O cells, were shown to contain anti-E and anti-Jk^a when tested against a panel of phenotyped group-O cells using the IAT. The results of testing the

Table 27.9   Testing an allo-absorbed serum against a phenotyped panel of red cells

	Red cell phenotypes															Results of IAT		
No.	Rh	M	N	S	s	P_1	Lu^a	Le^a	Le^b	K	Kp^a	Fy^a	Fy^b	Jk^a	Jk^b	Serum A	Serum B	Serum C
1.	R_1R_1	+	+	+	+	+	−	−	−	+	−	+	+	+	+	1 +	1 +	−
2.	R_1R_1	+	−	−	+	−	+	−	+	−	−	+	+	+	+	1 +	3 +	−
3.	R_2R_2	+	+	+	+	+	+	+	−	−	−	−	+	−	+	1 +	−	3 +
4.	R_1R_2	+	+	+	−	+	−	−	+	−	−	−	+	+	−	1 +	4 +	1 +
5.	r'r	+	−	+	+	+	−	−	+	−	−	+	+	−	+	−	−	−
6.	r"r	+	+	+	−	+	−	−	+	−	−	+	−	+	+	2 +	2 +	2 +
7.	rr	+	+	−	+	+	−	−	−	+	−	+	+	+	−	2 +	2 +	−
8.	rr	+	−	+	+	+	−	+	−	−	−	+	−	+	−	1 +	2 +	(+)
9.	rr	−	+	−	+	+	−	+	−	−	+	+	+	+	+	2 +	2 +	−
10.	R_1R_2	−	+	+	+	−	−	−	+	+	−	−	+	+	−	1 +	3 +	2 +

Phenotype of cells selected for absorption of serum   Absorbed serum
1. R_1R_1, C^w +,   K −,   Fy (a + b −),   Jk(a −b +),   M +, N −, s −   Serum A
2. R_2R_2, C^w −,   K−   Fy (a − b +),   Jk(a − b +),   M +, N +, s +   Serum B
3. rr, C^w K+   Fy (a + b −),   Jk(a + b −),   M +, N −, s −   Serum C

absorbed sera, A, B and C, are shown in Table 27.9. The patient's red cell phenotype was R_1r, Jk(a– b–).

Explanation of the results of testing allo-absorbed sera, A, B and C

1. As the R_1R_1-absorbing cells were negative for the E and Jk^a antigens, absorbed serum A could contain anti-E and anti-Jk^a. Testing the absorbed serum A against the panel of cells suggested that this was so.

2. As the R_2R_2-absorbing cells were positive for the E antigen but negative for the Jk^a antigen, absorbed serum B could contain anti-Jk^a but not anti-E. Testing absorbed serum B against the panel of cells confirmed the presence of anti-Jk^a.

3. As the rr-absorbing cells were negative for the E antigen but positive for the Jk^a antigen, absorbed serum C could contain anti-E but not anti-Jk^a. Testing absorbed serum C against the panel of cells confirmed the presence of anti-E.

4. As the phenotype of the patient's own red cells was R_1r, Jk (a– b–), the anti-E and anti-Jk^a detected in the allo-absorbed sera must be allo-antibodies. Blood for transfusion should be E-negative, Jk^a-negative.

Additional notes on absorption techniques

1. If the patient's serum contains a haemolytic antibody, EDTA should be added to prevent the uptake of complement and subsequent lysis of the cells used for absorption.

Add 1 volume of neutral EDTA (potassium salt) (see p. 576) to 9 volumes of serum.

2. It is often useful to allo-absorb both serum and eluate to differentiate between auto- and allo-antibodies, particularly if the auto-antibody is the mimicking type described by Issitt.[18]

3. If the auto-antibody does not react with papainized cells, do *not* papainize the cells for absorption.

ELUTION OF ANTIBODIES FROM RED CELLS

The preparation of potent antibody-containing eluates from the red cells of patients with AIHA is essential in determining the specificity of the antibody.

Several methods are available for the preparation of eluates; each has advantages and disadvantages. The first step is to wash the red cells at least four times in a large volume of saline. At the last washing, centrifuge for 10 min at 1200–1500g and save the supernatant. Ideally, 2–5 ml of packed red cells should be left at the end of this washing.

Landsteiner and Miller's method[22]

To the washed, packed cells add a suitable volume of saline containing 1% of human serum albumin or AB serum (see below). If the DAT gives a strong reaction (i.e. + + or + + +), add a volume of saline equal to the volume of the cells; if the reaction is a weak one (i.e. ± or +), add only half the volume. Mix and agitate continuously in a water-bath at 56°C for 5 min. Centrifuge rapidly while still hot and remove the cherry-red supernatant at once — this is the eluate.

Eluates made into saline must be tested at once; those made into albumin-saline or AB serum will keep quite well at –20°C, but the AB serum must be known to be free of any antibody.

Rubin's modification[32] of Vos and Kelsall's method[44]

To washed packed red cells in a glass tube add a suitable volume of saline (see above); then add a volume of ether twice that of the packed red cells. Stopper loosely, allowing release of vapour frequently and shake vigorously for 1 min. Place at 37°C for 30 min, mixing frequently; centrifuge at 1200–1500g at 37°C for 10 min, after which, three layers will be found. The top layer is ether — this is discarded. The bottom haemoglobin-stained layer is the eluate. Collect this with a pipette passed through the middle layer of red cell stroma. Free the eluate of residual ether by leaving it at 37°C for 30–60 min. The smell of ether should have vanished before the eluate is tested or frozen for testing at a later date. Eluates prepared by Rubin's method into saline keep well if stored at –20°C.

Hughes-Jones, Gardner and Telford[16] estimated that if the elution process is carried out as described above, 70% of antibody will be recovered, while Landsteiner and Miller's method[22] yields only a third as much antibody from the same volume of cells. For this reason, and because of the ease with which eluates can be prepared by Rubin's method, this is the method we recommend for use in the investigation of cases of AIHA.

SCREENING ELUATES

The eluate and the saline of the last wash (control) are first screened against two or three samples of washed normal group-O cells to see if they contain any antibodies:

   1. *By titration against enzyme-treated group-O cells.* Prepare doubling dilutions of eluate and control in saline to give dilutions of 1 in 1 to 1 in 32. To 1 drop of eluate or dilution add 1 drop of 2% enzyme-treated cells. Incubate at 37°C for 1–1½ h and read microscopically.
   2. *By the indirect antiglobulin test (IAT).* To 10 drops of eluate or control add 1 drop of a 50% suspension of group-O cells. Incubate for 1–1½ h at 37°C. Wash four times and, using optimal dilutions of anti-IgG (and of anti-IgM and anti-IgA if these sera gave positive reactions in the DAT), carry out the IAT by either the tile or tube method.

   If the control preparation (the supernatant saline from the last washing) gives positive reactions, the possibility that any eluate contains serum antibody has to be considered.

Determination of the specificity of warm auto-antibodies in eluates and sera

When tested against a phenotyped panel, about two-thirds of auto-antibodies appear to have Rh specificity and in about half these cases specificity against a particular antigen can be demonstrated.[6,18,29]

The other one-third of auto-antibodies may show specificity against other very high incidence antigens, for example, Wr[b] and En[a], and rarely other blood-group specificities are involved. It is essential to differentiate between auto- and allo-antibodies, especially if transfusion is being considered. The presence of allo-antibodies in addition to auto-antibodies is suggested by any discrepancy between the serum and eluate results.

The ascertainment of specificity is not difficult but it is essential to have available a panel of normal red cells, the blood groups of which have been determined as completely as possible. Access to a source of –D– / –D– or Rh[null] cells is a great advantage. Within the Rh system anti-e is the commonest specificity. This will be shown by R_2R_2 cells reacting much more weakly than do cells of the other common Rh genotypes. So-called 'Rh specificity' is demonstrated by Rh[null] cells reacting very weakly or failing to react while all the other cells on the panel react strongly.

As already mentioned, the presence of allo-antibodies in a serum complicates the determination of the specificity of an auto-antibody, and it can be argued that it would be better to test only the eluted auto-antibody and to leave the serum strictly alone. However, only a small volume of an eluate may be available, especially in anaemic patients, and it is generally wise to test both serum and eluate. The procedure is the same for both.

Titration of antibodies in eluates or sera

The methods used have already been described in Chapter 24, p. 461. The exact technique chosen, and the red cells used, should be those which have given the clearest results in the screening tests.

DEMONSTRATION OF LYSIS BY WARM AUTO-ANTIBODIES

As referred to on p. 500, auto-antibodies in serum capable of bringing about lysis in vitro of normal red cells at 37°C ('warm haemolysins') have rarely been demonstrated in cases of AIHA.[4a] In contrast, it is not rare for warm antibodies — presumably of the IgM variety — to bring about lysis, in the presence of complement, of enzyme-treated cells at 37°C, and it is significant that patients whose sera lyse these modified cells, but *not* normal cells, do not necessarily suffer from a serious degree of haemolysis.[43] PNH red cells, too, can be used, if available, as sensitive reagents for demonstrating the lytic potentiality of the antibodies[4b] (see p. 291).

Red cells which have been stored for several days at 4°C may occasionally undergo agglutination (or lysis) in certain pathological sera.[19] When this occurs at 37°C in the screening test, the preparation should be set up again with the same cells taken freshly from the donor. Not infrequently, lysis will not occur with perfectly fresh red cells even though sublytic amounts of complement may be bound. In all lysis tests using normal red cells the pH of the cell-serum mixtures should be adjusted to about 6.8, as this the optimum pH for lysis. Adjustment of pH is less critical using enzyme-treated or PNH cells than when normal unmodified cells are used.

TITRATION OF COLD AGGLUTININS

While setting up screening procedures using serum, as described above, it is convenient to set up titrations for cold agglutinins in order to screen for their presence, and if present to obtain an indication of their specificity.

Prepare doubling dilutions of the serum in saline ranging from 1 in 1 to 1 in 512 and add 1 drop of each serum dilution into three series of small (e.g. 38 × 6.4 mm) glass tubes so that three replicate titrations can be made. Add 1 drop of a 2% suspension of saline-washed adult group-O (I) cells to the first row, 1 drop of enzyme-treated adult group-O cells to the second row and 1 drop of cord-blood group-O (i) cells to the third row. Mix and leave overnight at 4°C. Before reading place pipettes and a tray of slides at 4°C. Read microscopically at room temperature using the chilled slides.

Normal range. Using sera from normal adult Caucasians and normal adult I red cells, the cold-agglutinin titre at 4°C is from 1 to 32; using enzyme-treated I red cells the titre is from 1 to 64 and with cord-blood (i) cells 0 to 8. In cold-haemagglutinin disease (CHAD) the end-point may not have been reached at a dilution of 1 in 512; if so, further dilutions should be prepared and tested.

If a cold agglutinin is present at a raised titre, the presence of a cold allo-antibody has to be excluded. In this case the patient's own red cells will be found to react *much* less strongly than do normal adult I red cells. It should be noted that in CHAD the patient's cells commonly react rather less strongly than do normal adult I cells (see Table 27.10).

SPECIFICITY OF COLD ANTIBODIES

High-titre cold auto-antibodies have a well defined blood-group specificity which is almost invariably within the I/i system.[18,31,45] Since the I antigen is poorly developed in cord-blood red cells, whilst the i antigen is well developed, group-O cord-blood red cells should be included in the panel used to test for I/i specificity. Adult cells almost always have the I antigen well expressed but the strength of the antigen varies and it is of considerable advantage to have available adult cells known to possess strong I antigen. (The rare adult i cells, if available, are also a useful reagent.)

Table 27.10 Agglutination titres using various types of cold auto-antibodies and normal adult and normal cord red cells, the patient's red cells and enzyme-treated (papainized) normal adult red cells

Patient	Agglutination titre (4°C)			Papainized adult (I) cells
	Adult (I) cells	Cord (i) cells	Patient's cells	
A. G.	4000	512	2000	8000
F. B.	512	32000	128	8000
A. R.	2000	2000	2000	16

A. G. This patient had the cold-haemagglutinin disease. The antibody was of the common anti-I type.
F. B. This patient had a terminal haemolytic anaemia associated with a lymphoma. The antibody was of the anti-i type.
A. R. This patient had the cold-haemagglutinin disease. The antibody was of the rare anti-Pr type.

Cold agglutinin titration patterns

The presence of high-titre cold agglutinins in a patient's serum will be indicated by the screening procedure described above. To demonstrate that the agglutinins are auto-antibodies, it is necessary to show that the patient's own cells are also agglutinated. It is interesting to note that the titre using the patient's cells is usually less (one-half or one-quarter) than that of control normal adult red cells (Table 27.10).

In cold-haemagglutinin disease, whether 'idiopathic' or secondary to mycoplasma pneumonia or lymphoma, the auto-antibodies usually have anti-I specificity (Patient A.G. in Table 27.10).

In rare cases of haemolytic anaemia associated with infectious mononucleosis an auto-antibody of anti-i specificity has been demonstrated (Patient F.B. in Table 27.10), and this specificity, too, has been found in certain patients with lymphoma. Rarely, in chronic CHAD, the antibody has been shown to have anti-Pr or anti-M specificity; in either type of case the antigen is destroyed by enzyme treatment (Patient A.R. in Table 27.10).

DETERMINATION OF THE THERMAL RANGE OF COLD AGGLUTININS

From a series of master doubling dilutions of serum in saline place 1 drop of serum or serum dilution into four rows of small (38 × 6.4 mm) agglutinin tubes. Set them up at 30°C, 25°C and 20°C and to each tube add 1 drop of a 2% saline suspension of the following cells:

1. Pooled normal adult group-O (I) red cells.
2. Pooled enzyme-treated (e.g. pre-papainized) normal adult group-O (I) red cells.
3. Pooled cord-blood group-O (i) red cells.
4. Patient's red cells.

Titration should also be carried out at 37°C, if there had been agglutination at this temperature in the screening tests. After incubation at the appropriate temperature for 1½–2 h, determine the presence or absence of agglutination macroscopically, using a concave mirror, as described on p. 456. It is hardly practical to read agglutination microscopically on slides warmed or cooled to the appropriate temperatures.

Alternatively, the thermal range of an antibody may be determine in the following simple way. Place three tubes each containing 10 drops of the patient's serum at 37°C. To each tube add 1 drop of a 50% saline suspension of pre-warmed red cells: to the first, normal adult group-O (I) red cells; to the second, normal cord-blood group-O (i) red cells, and to the third, the patient's own red cells. Mix the contents of each tube and allow the red cells to sediment for about 1 h in a water-bath at 37°C. After this time, transfer the tubes to a beaker containing water at 37°C which is allowed to cool slowly and in which a thermometer records the fall in temperature. Inspect the three tubes visually for agglutination at 37°C by tipping them gently and watching the behaviour of the red cells, and re-inspect each time the temperature falls by 1°C until agglutination is unmistakeable. Results typical of a case of chronic cold-haemagglutinin disease are given in Table 27.11.

LYSIS BY COLD ANTIBODIES

If lysis is detected in the serum screening tests, the lysis titre and the thermal range for lysis should be determined and also the specificity of the antibody, e.g. anti-I, anti-i or anti-Pr. To estimate the titre, dilutions of the patient's serum are made in fresh normal serum to provide a source of complement. Typically, although not

Table 27.11   Macroscopic agglutination at different temperatures of various red cell samples by the serum of a patient suffering from chronic cold-haemagglutinin disease

Cells	Temperature (°C)										
	30	29	28	27	26	25	24	23	22	21	20
Patient (I)	−	−	½ +	1 +	2 +	2 +	3 +	3 +	3 +	3 +	3 +
Normal adult (I)	−	½ +	1 +	1 +	2 +	3 +	3 +	3 +	3 +	3 +	3 +
Normal cord (i)	−	−	−	−	−	−	−	−	−	?	½ +

invariably, more lysis takes places if the mixture of serum and complement is acidified.[4c]

Method

Prepare suitable dilutions of the patient's serum in fresh normal serum acidified to a pH of 6.0–6.5 (see p. 289). A series of master doubling dilutions should be set up initially. If a high lysis titre is anticipated, it is convenient to prepare a 1 in 10 dilution initially and then set up doubling dilutions (1 in 10, 1 in 20, etc., to a dilution of 1 in 640.

To 5 drops of each dilution add 1 drop of a 25% saline suspension of red cells. The cells used in the test should be:

1. Adult group-O cells known to possess a strong I antigen.
2. The same cells after treatment with papain.
3. Group-O (i) cord-blood cells.

Each test should be set up at 20°C, 30°C and 37°C, and it is most important that the cells and serum are brought to the correct temperature before they are mixed.

Optimum temperature for demonstrating lysis by a high-titre cold antibody

A temperature of 25°C is about optimum for the demonstration of lysis by high-titre (anti-I) antibodies. Below 15°C lysis will not take place because some complement components will not bind at a low temperature; above 30°C, depending on the thermal range of the antibody, lysis is prevented because antibody is not adsorbed. Lysis taking place in one phase at normal bench temperature without preliminary chilling has been referred to as monophasic (Fig. 27.4). This contrasts with lysis brought by the Donath-Landsteiner (D-L) antibody which is typically described as biphasic. Preliminary chilling below normal bench temperature is usually necessary to bring about binding of the antibody, followed by warming for lysis to occur (see p. 522). It should be noted that high-titre anti-I antibodies will often, too, bring about lysis when the red cell-serum suspension is treated biphasically, i.e. give a type of positive D-L antibody test. Conversely, but rarely, genuine D-L antibodies, if active at a

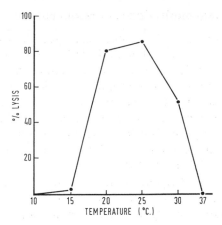

Fig. 27.4 Effect of temperature on lysis by a high-titre cold auto-antibody (anti-I). Chronic cold haemagglutinin disease. Normal group O (I) red cells in patient's serum. The serum was diluted with an equal volume of fresh normal serum and acidified by the addition of a one-tenth volume of 0.2 mol/l HCl. Incubation was carried out for 10 min at each temperature.

sufficiently high temperature, cal also give rise to lysis monophasically, e.g. at 20°C. Anti-I antibodies can be distinguished from D-L antibodies by virtue of their remarkable agglutinating properties at low temperatures and in other ways even if they give a positive D-L test.

It is particularly important that the concentrated cell suspension be delivered directly into the serum dilution without running down the side of the tube, for tightly agglutinated cells lyse extremely easily under these conditions, even in the absence of complement. Lysis is usually read visually after the red cells have sedimented for 2 h or, if practicable, after remixing and centrifuging at the appropriate temperature.

Enzyme-treated cells are typically much more sensitive to lysis by high-titre anti-I and anti-i antibodies than are normal red cells (Table 27.12), and they may even be lysed at 37°C. PNH cells are particularly easily lysed because of their remarkable sensitivity to complement[4d] (Table 27.12), and the lysis titre with these cells at 30°C is usually as great as or may exceed the agglutination titre. PNH cells can be used as a sensitive and reliable tool for the demonstration of the lytic potential of any antibody which fixes complement. However, when using PNH cells the serum must not be acidified, and the control tube, containing fresh normal serum but no patient's serum, must be carefully examined for lysis.

To ensure that lysis is easily visible a stronger cell-serum suspension should be used than that used for agglutination tests. A final concentration of about 5% is suitable and this is attained by the method described above. The lysis titre is given by the reciprocal of the highest serum dilution causing (+) lysis. It is convenient to score complete lysis as C; (+) represents definite but weak lysis compared with the colour of the supernatant of the control, while +, + + and + + + represent intermediate degrees of lysis.

Typical results obtained in a patient with chronic cold-haemagglutinin disease due to anti-I antibody are shown in Table 27.12.

Table 27.12 Relative sensitivity of red cells to lysis by a high-titre cold antibody at 20°C

Type of cell	pH	Dilution of serum								Control (normal serum diluent)
		1 in 1	1 in 4	1 in 16	1 in 64	1 in 256	1 in 1024	1 in 4096	1 in 16 000	
Normal (I)	8.0	–	Trace	–	–	–	–	–	–	–
Normal (I)	6.5	Trace	+	(+)	Trace	–	–	–	–	–
Trypsinized normal (I)	8.0	+	+ + +	+ +	+	(+)	–	–	–	–
PNH	8.0	+ + +	+ + +	+ + +	+ + +	+ + +	+ +	+ +	+	–

+ + + denotes lysis; + +, + and (+) denote lesser but definite degrees of lysis; – denotes no lysis.

DETECTION AND TITRATION OF THE DONATH-LANDSTEINER (D-L) ANTIBODY

The Donath-Landsteiner (D-L) antibody of paroxysmal cold haemoglobinuria differs from the high-titre cold antibodies referred to previously in that it is an IgG antibody and has a quite different specificity. It is, too, far more lytic to normal cells in relation to its titre than are anti-I or anti-i antibodies. Thus the lysis titre of a D-L antibody may be the same or greater than its agglutination titre. Almost maximal lysis develops in unacidified serum.

DIRECT DONATH-LANDSTEINER TEST

Collect two samples of venous blood into glass tubes containing no anticoagulant, previously warmed at 37°C. Incubate the first sample at 37°C for 1½ h. Put the second sample in a beaker packed with ice and allow to stand for 1 h; then place the tube at 37°C for a further 20 min. Centrifuge both tubes at 37°C and examine the supernatant serum for lysis. A positive test is indicated by lysis in the sample which had been chilled.

INDIRECT DONATH-LANDSTEINER TEST

Serum obtained from the patient's blood which has been allowed to clot at 37°C is used for this test.

Add 1 volume of a 50% suspension of washed normal group-O, P-positive red cells to 9 volumes of patient's unacidified serum in a glass tube.

Chill the suspension in crushed ice at 0°C for 1 h, then place the tube at 37°C for 30 min.

Centrifuge at 37°C and examine for lysis. Three controls should be set up at the same time:

1. A duplicate of the test cell-serum suspension, but kept strictly at 37°C for the duration of the test.

2. A duplicate of the test cell-serum suspension, except that an equal volume of ABO-compatible fresh normal serum is first added to the patient's

serum as a source of complement. The same cells are added and the suspension is chilled and subsequently warmed in the same way as the test suspension. (This control excludes false-negative results due to the patient's serum being deficient in complement.)

3. A duplicate of the test cell-serum suspension, except that fresh normal serum is used in place of the patient's serum. This control, too, is chilled and subsequently warmed.

A positive test will be indicated by lysis in the test suspension and in control No. 2. If ABO compatible *pp* cells are available they should be used in a duplicate set of tubes. No lysis will develop — confirming the P specificity of the antibody.

Titration of a Donath-Landsteiner antibody

Prepare doubling or four-fold dilutions of the patient's serum in fresh normal human serum. To each tube add a one-tenth volume of a 50% suspension of washed group-O P-positive red cells and immerse each of the tubes in crushed ice at 0°C. After 1 h place at 37°C and incubate for a further 30 min. Then centrifuge and inspect for lysis.

Detection of a Donath-Landsteiner antibody by the indirect antiglobulin test

Since the D-L antibody is an IgG antibody, it can be detected by the indirect antiglobulin test (IAT) using an anti-IgG serum if the cells which have been exposed to the antibody in the cold are washed in cold (4°C) saline. At this temperature the antibody will not be eluted during washing. It should be noted, however, that exposing normal red cells at 4°C to many fresh normal sera results in a positive IAT with broad-spectrum antiglobulin sera because of the adsorption of incomplete anti-H (a normally-occurring cold antibody) on to the red cells. At a low temperature, complement is bound, too, and it is its adsorption which gives rise to the positive tests with broad-spectrum sera. The adsorption of complement can be prevented by adding an anticoagulant such as EDTA to the serum.

Method

Add a one-tenth volume of EDTA, buffered to pH 7.0 (see p. 576) to the patient's serum. Prepare doubling dilutions in saline from 1 in 1 to 1 in 28.

Add 1 volume (drop) of a 50% suspension of group-O, P-positive red cells to 10 volumes (drops) of each dilution. Mix and chill at 4°C (preferably in a cold room).

After 1 h wash the red cells four times in a large volume of cold (4°C) saline. Then carry out an antiglobulin test using an anti-IgG reagent, as described on p. 459, but keeping the red cell-antiglobulin serum suspension at 4°C.

As controls, set up a series of tests using a serum known to contain a D-L antibody and a normal serum, respectively.

This technique is the most sensitive way of detecting, especially in stored sera, the D-L antibody present in an amount insufficient to bring about actual lysis.

Thermal range of a Donath-Landsteiner (D-L) antibody

The highest temperature at which D-L antibodies are usually adsorbed to red cells is about 18°C. Hence little or no lysis can be expected unless the cell-serum suspension is cooled below this temperature. Chilling in crushed ice results in maximum adsorption of the antibody and leads to the binding of complement which brings about lysis when the cell suspension is subsequently warmed at 37°C. Hence the 'cold-warm' biphasic procedure necessary for lysis to be demonstrated by a typical D-L antibody.

Specificity of the Donath-Landsteiner antibody

The D-L antibody appears to have a well-defined specificity within the P blood-group system, namely, anti-P. However, in practice, almost all samples of red cells are acted upon, for the cells that will not react (P^k and *pp*) are extremely rare.[24,48] Cord-blood cells are lysed to about the same extent as are adult P_1 and P_2 cells.

TREATMENT OF SERUM WITH 2-MERCAPTO-ETHANOL (2-ME) OR DITHIOTHREITOL (DTT)

Weak solutions of 2-ME or DTT destroy the inter-chain sulphydryl bonds of gamma globulins. IgM antibodies treated in this way lose their ability to agglutinate red cells while IgG antibodies do not.[9,18] IgA antibodies may or may not be inhibited depending upon whether or not they are made up of polymers of IgA. Since almost all auto-antibodies are either IgM or IgG, treatment of serum or an eluate with 2-ME or DTT gives a reliable indication of the Ig class of auto-antibody under investigation.[9,18]

Method

(a) 2-Mercapto-ethanol (2-ME)

To 1 volume of undiluted serum add 1 volume of 0.1 mol/l 2-mercapto-ethanol in phosphate buffer, pH 7.2 (see p. 578).

As a control, add a volume of the serum to the phosphate buffer alone. Incubate both at 37°C for 2 h.

Then titrate the treated serum and its control with the appropriate red cells.

If IgG antibody is present, the antibody titration in the control serum will be the same as that of the treated serum. However, if the antibody is IgM, the treated serum will fail to agglutinate the test cells or agglutinate them to a much lower titre compared with the control untreated serum.

The control must remain active to show that the absence of agglutination is due to reduction of IgM antibody and not due to dilution.

(b) Dithiothreitol (DTT)

0.01 mol/l DTT can be used in place of 0.1 mol/l 2-ME in the above method.

DRUG-INDUCED HAEMOLYTIC ANAEMIAS OF IMMUNOLOGICAL ORIGIN

As already mentioned (p. 499), acquired haemolytic anaemias may develop as the result of immunological reactions consequent on the administration of certain drugs.[13,28,29] Clinically, they often closely mimic AIHA of 'idiopathic' origin and for this reason a careful enquiry into the taking of drugs is a necessary part of the interrogation of any patient suspected of having an acquired haemolytic anaemia.

Two immunological mechanisms leading to a drug-induced haemolytic anaemia are recognized. These mechanisms are commonly referred to as 'drug-dependent immune' and 'drug-dependent auto-immune'. Both types of antibody may be present in some patients.[12,33,34] In a unifying concept, the target orientation of these antibodies covers a spectrum in which the primary immune response is initiated by an interaction between the drug or its metabolites and a component of the blood cell membrane to create a neoantigen.[35] Drug-dependent antibodies bind to both the drug and the cell membrane, but not to either separately. If the drug is withdrawn, the immune reaction subsides. In the case of the auto-antibodies, the greater part of the neoantigen is sufficiently similar to the normal cell membrane to allow binding without the drug being present. Similar mechanisms have been described for drug-induced immune thrombocytopenia and neutropenia of immunological origin (p. 467).

DRUG-DEPENDENT IMMUNE HAEMOLYTIC ANAEMIAS

In these cases the drug is required in the in-vitro system for the antibodies to be detected. The red cells become damaged by one of two mechanisms:

1. *Complement lysis.* A typical history is for haemolysis, which may be severe and intravascular, to follow the re-administration of a drug with which the patient has previously been treated,

and for the haemolysis to subside when the offending drug has been identified and withdrawn. The DAT is likely to become strongly positive during the haemolytic phase, the patient's red cells being agglutinated by anti-C and sometimes by anti-IgG.

Drugs which have been shown to cause haemolysis by the above mechanism include quinine, quinidine and rifampicin, as well as chlorpropamide, hydrochlorothiazide, nomifensine, phenacetin, salicylazosulphapyridine, the sodium salt of p-aminosalicylic acid and stibophen. Petz and Branch[28] listed 25 drugs reported to have brought about haemolysis by this mechanism.

2. *Extravascular haemolysis*. This is brought about by IgG antibodies that usually do not activate complement, or if they do, not beyond C3. The DAT will be positive with anti-IgG, and sometimes also with anti-C.

The haemolytic anaemia associated with prolonged high-dose penicillin therapy is caused by the above mechanism, and other penicillin derivatives, as well as cephalosporins and tetracycline may cause haemolysis in a similar fashion. Haemolysis ceases when the offending drug has been identified and withdrawn.

Cephalosporins, in addition to causing the formation of specific antibodies, may alter the red cell surface so as to cause non-specific adherence of complement and immunoglobulins. This may lead to a positive DAT but is seldom associated with increased haemolysis.

DRUG-DEPENDENT AUTO-IMMUNE HAEMOLYTIC ANAEMIAS

In these cases the antibody reacts with the red cell in the absence of the drug. The anti-red cell auto-antibodies seem to be serologically identical to those of 'idiopathic' warm-type AIHA. The great majority of cases have followed the use of the anti-hypertension drug α-methyldopa (Aldomet). The red cells are coated with IgG and the serum contains auto-antibodies which characteristically have Rh specificity.

Other drugs that have been reported to act in a similar fashion to α-methyldopa include chlordiazepoxide (Librium), mefenamic acid (Ponstam), flufenamic acid and indomethicine.[6]

Typical serological features of the different types of drug-induced haemolytic anaemia of immunological origin are summarized in Table 27.13.

DETECTION OF ANTI-PENICILLIN ANTIBODIES

The characteristic features of penicillin-induced haemolytic anaemia are:

1. Haemolysis occurs only in patients receiving large doses of a penicillin for long periods (e.g. weeks).

2. The DAT is strongly positive with anti-IgG reagents.

3. The patient's serum and antibody eluted from the patient's red cells react *only* with penicillin-treated red cells — they do not react with normal untreated red cells.

Reagents

Barbitone buffer. 0.14 mol/l, pH 9.5 (see p. 577).
Penicillin solution. 0.4 g of penicillin G dissolved in 6 ml of barbitone buffer.

Penicillin-coated normal red cells

Wash group-O normal red cells three times in

Table 27.13 Serological features of the different types of drug-induced haemolytic anaemia of immunological origin

Mechanism	Prototype drug	DAT	IAT No drug	IAT	
				Serum + drug	Eluate + drug
Drug-dependent antibody:					
(a) C-activation	Quin(id)ine	C*	Neg	C*	Neg
(b) No C-activation	Penicillin	IgG	Neg	IgG	IgG
Auto-antibody	α-Methyldopa	IgG	IgG		

*Occasionally also IgG.

saline and make a *c* 15% suspension in saline to which a one-tenth volume of barbitone buffer has been added. Add 2 ml of the red cell suspension to 6 ml of penicillin solution and incubate at 37°C for 1 h. Then wash 4 times in saline and make up 2% (for tube tests) and 20% (for tile tests) red cell suspensions in saline.

Control normal red cells

These should be treated in exactly the same way as the penicillin-coated red cells except that the 6 ml of penicillin solution is replaced by 6 ml of barbitone buffer.

Method

Anti-penicillin antibodies can be detected by the IAT in the usual way using the penicillin-coated red cells in place of normal unmodified cells. However, three extra controls are necessary.

1. Red cells which have not been exposed to penicillin should be added to the patient's serum.
2. Penicillin-treated red cells should be added to two normal sera known not to contain anti-penicillin antibodies (*negative controls*).
3. Penicillin-treated red cells should be added to a serum (if one is available) known to contain anti-penicillin antibodies (*positive control*).

Cephalosporin can be used in a similar way to sensitize red cells. Control (2) is particularly important when penicillin derivatives such as cephalosporin are used, since over-exposure in vitro to these drugs can lead to positive results with normal sera.

High-titre IgG anti-penicillin antibodies often cause direct agglutination of penicillin-treated red cells in low dilutions of serum. The antibodies can be differentiated from IgM-agglutinating antibodies by treatment with 2-ME or DTT (p. 524).

DETECTION OF ANTIBODIES AGAINST DRUGS OTHER THAN PENICILLIN

In a patient with an immune haemolytic anaemia whose serum and red cell eluate does *not* react

Table 27.14   Investigation of a suspected drug-induced haemolytic anaemia

	Tube No.					
	1	2	3	4	5	6
Patient's serum volumes (drops)	10	10	5	5	0	0
Fresh normal serum volumes (drops)	0	0	5	5	10	10
Drug solution volumes (drops)	2	0	2	0	2	0
Saline volumes (drops)	0	2	0	2	0	2
50% normal group-O cells volumes (drops)	1	1	1	1	1	1

with normal red cells and who is receiving a drug or drugs other than penicillin or a penicillin derivative, antibodies which react with red cells only in the presence of the suspect drugs or drugs should be looked for in the following way.

The patient's serum and red cell eluates should be tested with normal and enzyme-treated group-O red cells, carrying out the tests with and without the drug that the patient is receiving. The approach is essentially empirical. A saturated solution of the drug or its metabolite should be prepared in saline and the pH adjusted to 6.5–7.0.

Set up six tubes containing the patient's serum and the drug solution in the proportions shown in Table 27.14 and add one drop of a 50% saline suspension of group-O cells to each tube. Incubate at 37°C for 1 h and examine for agglutination and lysis. Wash the red cells four times in saline and carry out an IAT using anti-IgG and anti-C separately.

Interpretation

Tubes 1 and 2 test the patient's serum (? drug-dependent antibody) and normal red cells in the presence of (Tube 1) and without the drug (Tube 2).

Tubes 3 and 4 test the effect of added complement on the above reactions.

Tubes 5 and 6 without the patient's serum act as controls for Tubes 3 and 4.

REFERENCES

[1] BAREFORD, D., LONGSTER, G., GILKS, L. and TOVEY, L. A. D. (1985). Follow-up of normal individuals with a positive antiglobulin test. *Scandinavian Journal of Haematology*, **35**, 348.

[2] BODENSTEINER, D., BROWN, P., SKIKNE, B. and PLAPP, F. (1983). The enzyme-linked immunosorbent assay: accurate detection of red blood cell antibodies in autoimmune hemolytic anemia. *American Journal of Clinical Pathology*, **79**, 182.

[3] CHAPLIN, H. Jr (1973). Clinical usefulness of specific antiglobulin reagents in autoimmune hemolytic anemia. *Progress in Hematology*, **8**, 25.

[4] DACIE, J. (1992). *The Haemolytic Anaemias*, Vol. 3. *The Auto-Immune Haemolytic Anaemias*, 3rd edn, (a) p. 136, (b) p. 139, (c) p. 275, (d) p. 228, (e) p. 276. Churchill Livingstone, Edinburgh.

[5] DACIE, J. V. (1975). Auto-immune hemolytic anemias. *Archives of Internal Medicine*, **135**, 1293.

[6] DACIE, J. V. WORLLEDGE, S. M. (1969). Auto-immune hemolytic anemias. *Progress in Hematology*, **6**, 82.

[7] ENGELFRIET, C. P., VON DEM BORNE, A. E. G., BECKERS, D. and VAN LOGHEM, J. J. (1974). Auto-immune haemolytic anaemia: serological and immunochemical characteristics of the auto-antibodies: mechanisms of cell destruction. *Series Haematologica*, **VII**, 328.

[8] FREEDMAN, J. (1979). False-positive antiglobulin tests in healthy subjects. *Journal of Clinical Pathology*, **32**, 1014.

[9] FREEDMAN, J., MASTERS, C. A., NEWLANDS, M. and MOLLISON, P. L. (1976). Optimal conditions for the use of sulphydryl compounds is dissociating red cell antibodies. *Vox Sanguinis*, **30**, 231.

[10] GILLILAND, B. C., BAXTER, E. and EVANS, R. S. (1971). Red-cell antibodies in acquired hemolytic anemia with negative antiglobulin serum test. *New England Journal of Medicine*, **285**, 252.

[11] GORST, D. W., RAWLINSON, V. I., MERRY, A. H. and STRATTON, F. (1980). Positive direct antiglobulin test in normal individuals. *Vox Sanguinis*, **38**, 99.

[12] HABIBI, B. (1985). Drug induced red blood cell autoantibodies co-developed with drug specific antibodies causing haemolytic anaemias. *British Journal of Haematology*, **61**, 139.

[13] HABIBI, B. (1987). Drug-induced immune haemolytic anaemias. *Baillières Clinical Immunology and Allergy*, **1**, 343.

[14] HEDDLE, N. M., KELTON, J. G., TURCHYN, K. L. and ALI, M. A. M. (1988). Hypergammaglobulinemia can be associated with a positive direct antiglobulin test, a nonreactive eluate, and no evidence of haemolysis. *Transfusion*, **28**, 29.

[15] HSU, T. C. S., ROSENFIELD, R. E., BURKART, P., WONG, K. Y. and KOCKWA, S. (1974). Instrumental PVP augmented antiglobulin tests. II. Evaluation of acquired hemolytic anemia. *Vox Sanguinis*, **26**, 305.

[16] HUGHES-JONES, N. C., GARDNER, B. and TELFORD, R. (1963). Comparison of various methods of dissociation of anti-D, using ^{131}I-labelled antibody. *Vox Sanguinis*, **8**, 531.

[17] HUH, Y. O., LIU, F. J., ROGGE, K., CHAKRABARTY, L. and LIGHTIGER, B. (1988). Positive direct antiglobulin test and high serum immunoglobulin G levels. *American Journal of Clinical Pathology*, **90**, 197.

[18] ISSITT, P. D. (1985). Serological diagnosis and characterization of the causative autoantibodies. *Methods in Hematology*, **12**, 1.

[19] JENKINS, W. J. and MARSH, W. L. (1961). Autoimmune haemolytic anaemia. Three cases with antibodies specifically active against stored red cells. *Lancet*, **ii**, 16.

[20] LALEZARI, P. and JIANG, A. C. (1980). The manual Polybrene test: a simple and rapid procedure for detection of red cell antibodies. *Transfusion*, **20**, 206.

[21] LALEZARI, P. and OBERHARDT, B. (1971). Temperature gradient dissociation of the red cell antigen-antibody complexes in the Polybrene technique. *British Journal of Haematology*, **21**, 131.

[22] LANDSTEINER, K. and MILLER. C. P. Jnr (1925). Serological studies on the studies of blood of primates. II. The blood groups in anthropoid apes. *Journal of Experimental Medicine*, **42**, 853.

[23] LAU, P., HAESLER, W. E. and WURZEL, H. A. (1976). Positive direct antiglobulin reaction in a patient population. *American Journal of Clinical Pathology*, **65**, 368.

[24] LEVINE, P., CELANO, M. J. and FALKOWSKI, F. (1963). The specificity of the antibody in paroxymal cold hemoglobinuria (P. C. H.). *Transfusion*, **3**, 278.

[25] MARSH, W. L. and JENKINS, W. J. (1960). Anti-i: a new cold antibody. *Nature* (London), **188**, 753.

[26] OWEN, I. and HOWS, J. (1990). Evaluation of the manual Polybrene technique in the investigation of autoimmune haemolytic anaemia. *Transfusion*, **30**, 814.

[27] PETZ, L. D. and BRANCH, D. R. (1983). Serological tests for the diagnosis of immune hemolytic anemias. *Methods in Hematology*, **9**, 12.

[28] PETZ, L. D. and BRANCH, D. R. (1985). Drug-induced immune hemolytic anemias. *Methods in Hematology*, **12**, 47.

[29] PETZ, L. D. and GARRATTY. G. (1980). *Acquired Immune Hemolytic Anemias*. Churchill Livingstone, New York.

[30] PIROFSKY, B. (1969). *Autoimmunization and the Autoimmune Hemolytic Anemias*. Williams & Wilkins, Baltimore.

[31] ROELCKE, D. (1989). Cold agglutination. *Transfusion Medicine Review*, **3**, 140.

[32] RUBIN, H. (1963). Antibody elution from red blood cells. *Journal of Clinical Pathology*, **16**, 70.

[33] SALAMA, A., GÖTTSCHE, B. and MUELLER-ECKHARDT, C. (1991). Autoantibodies and drug- or metabolite-dependent antibodies in patients with diclofenac-induced immune haemolysis. *British Journal of Haematology*, **77**, 546.

[34] SALAMA, A. and MUELLER-ECKHARDT, C. (1987). Cianidanol and its metabolites bind tightly to red cells and are responsible for the production of auto- and/or drug-dependent antibodies against these cells. *British Journal of Haematology*, **66**, 263.

[35] SALAMA, A. and MUELLER-ECKHARDT, C. (1992) Immune-mediated blood dyscrasias related to drugs. *Seminars in Hematology*, **29**, 54.

[36] SCHMITZ, N., DJIBEY, T., KRETSCHMER, V., MAHN, I. and MUELLER-ECKHARDT, C. (1981). Assessment of red cell autoantibodies in autoimmune hemolytic anemia of warm type by radioactive anti-IgG test. *Vox Sanguinis*, **41**, 224.

[37] SOKOL, R. J. and HEWITT, S. (1985). Autoimmune hemolysis: a critical review. *CRC Critical Reviews in Oncology/Hematology*, **4**, 125.

[38] SOKOL, R. J., HEWITT, S., BOOKER, D. J. and STAMPS, R. (1985). Enzyme linked direct antiglobulin tests in patients with autoimmune haemolysis. *Journal of Clinical Pathology*, **38**, 912.

[39] SOKOL, R. J., HEWITT, S. and STAMPS, B. K. (1981). Autoimmune haemolysis: an 18-year study of 865 cases referred to a regional transfusion centre. *British Medical Journal*, **282**, 2023.

[40] STRATTON, F., RAWLINSON, V. I., MERRY, A. H. and THOMSON, E. E. (1983). Positive direct antiglobulin test in normal individuals. *Clinical and Laboratory Haematology*, **5**, 17.

[41] STRATTON, F. and RENTON, P. H. (1955). Effect of crystalloid solutions prepared in glass bottles on human red cells. *Nature (London)*, **175**, 727.

[42] SZYMANSKI, I. O., ODGREN, P. R., FORTIER, N. L. and SNYDER, L. M. (1980). Red blood cell associated IgG in normal and pathologic states. *Blood*, **55**, 48.

[43] VON DEM BORNE, A. E. G. Kr., ENGELFRIET, C. P., BECKERS, D., VAN DER KORT-HENKES, G., VAN DER GIESSEN, M. and VAN LOGHEM, J. J. (1969). Autoimmune haemolytic anaemia. II. Warm haemolysins — serological and immunochemical investigations and ^{51}Cr studies. *Clinical and Experimental Immunology*, **4**, 333.

[44] VOS, G. H. KELSALL, G. A. (1959). A new elution technique for the preparation of specific immune anti-Rh serum. *British Journal of Haematology*, **2**, 342.

[45] WIENER, A. S., UNGER, L. J., COHEN, L. FELDMAN, J. (1956). Type-specific cold auto-antibodies as a cause of acquired hemolytic anemia and hemolytic transfusion reactions: biologic test with bovine red cells. *Annals of Internal Medicine*, **44**, 221.

[46] WORLLEDGE, S. M. (1978). The interpretation of a positive direct antiglobulin test. *British Journal of Haematology*, **39**, 157 (Annotation).

[47] WORLLEDGE, S. M. and BLAJCHMAN, M. A. (1972). The autoimmune haemolytic anemias. *British Journal of Haematology*, **23** (Suppl), 61.

[48] WORLLEDGE, S. M. and ROUSSO, C. (1965). Studies on the serology of paroxysmal cold haemoglubinuria (P. C. H.) with special reference to a relationship with the P blood group system. *Vox Sanguinis*, **10**, 293.

28. DNA techniques in haematology

By T. Vulliamy and J. Kaeda

Introduction to the analysis of DNA   529
Extraction of DNA from peripheral blood   530
Southern blot analysis   530
Diagnosis of α-thalassaemia by Southern blot analysis   532
Southern blot analysis of β-thalassaemia   534
Diagnosis and characterization of lymphoproliferative disorders by Southern blot analysis   534
The polymerase chain reaction (PCR)   538
Analysis of PCR products   539
   Restriction enzyme digestion   539
   Allele-specific oligonucleotide hybridization (ASOH)   539
   Amplification refractory mutation system (ARMS)   540

Investigation of haemoglobinopathies using the PCR   541
G6PD deficiency   543
Diagnosis of genetic disease by linkage analysis   544
   Diagnosis of haemophilia A   544
RNA techniques   546
Appendices: Technical methods   546
   A: Extraction of genomic DNA   546
   B: Southern blot analysis   548
   C: DNA probes   551
   D: PCR 553
   E: Restriction enzyme digestion of PCR products   554
Glossary   555

In the diagnosis of the majority of haematological disorders, conventional procedures are perfectly adequate. But inevitably there are times when a diagnosis is uncertain, ambiguous, or cannot be made at all. There are also instances when these procedures cannot be applied, particularly in early prenatal diagnosis. In some of these cases DNA analysis can be useful, since virtually all haematological disorders have a genetic basis, be it inherited or acquired. Rapid advances over the last decade in the techniques available have made the analysis of DNA possible.[41] It is certain that as more of the relevant genes and mutations are characterized, this analysis will play an increasingly important role in the diagnostic laboratory.

INTRODUCTION TO THE ANALYSIS OF DNA

DNA is the genetic material. Information for the construction of proteins is encoded in its four-letter alphabet. The four letters, A, C, G and T are the initials of the four bases adenine, cytosine, guanine and thymine that lie along the sugar-phosphate backbone of the DNA molecule. Although it is beyond the scope of this chapter to describe the structure of DNA in detail,[40] the points listed below should help in the understanding of the methods described.

1. The DNA found in the nucleus of all eukaryotic cells is a double stranded molecule.

2. The two strands are held together by hydrogen bonds that form specifically between A and T residues and G and C residues.

3. Because of this, the sequence of bases on one strand of the DNA molecule (say TAGGCTAG) has only one possible partner on the other strand (ATCCGATC). These sequences are called complementary.

4. The strands have a polarity; one end is called the 5' end, the other is the 3' end. The two strands are antiparallel as they run in opposite directions.

The ability to manipulate DNA as recombinant molecules followed from the discovery of bacterial DNA modifying enzymes such as restriction enzymes*. These are endonucleases that cut DNA molecules wherever there is a short specific sequence of bases. More than 100 different restriction enzymes are now commercially available. Using these enzymes it is possible to cut up the genetic material found in human nuclei—the human genome—into specific fragments of a manageable size.

With the necessary DNA modifying enzymes, these restriction fragments can be inserted into cloning vectors such as plasmids. Bacteria that host these plasmids can be isolated as colonies and subsequently propagated indefinitely. In this way genes can be isolated as cloned recombinant DNA molecules and their DNA sequence established. They can also be used as gene probes. A recent innovation that has revolutionized many aspects of DNA analysis is the ability to amplify specific DNA fragments from small amounts of starting material by the polymerase chain reaction (PCR).[27] The great advantages of this method of analysis is that it is simple, rapid, relatively inexpensive and does not require the use of radionuclides.

There has been a vast expansion in the application of DNA-based methods in diagnosis, and many alternative protocols have become available. A comprehensive laboratory manual describing the techniques of molecular biology now runs to three volumes.[29] In this chapter the techniques described centre around two main procedures: Southern blot analysis[32] for the detection of large deletions, gene rearrangements and DNA polymorphisms; and amplification by the PCR followed by the appropriate analysis for the detection of small and large deletions, point mutations and DNA polymorphisms.

Here the most relevant examples of their application in a diagnostic haematology laboratory are described. While the emphasis is shifting towards the use of PCR-based techniques, they cannot yet replace Southern blot analysis in all situations.

EXTRACTION OF DNA FROM PERIPHERAL BLOOD

DNA can be extracted from virtually any blood sample. The quality and quantity of the DNA obtained will vary depending on the size, age and white blood cell count of the sample. It is extracted from all nucleated cells and is called genomic DNA as it contains all the genetic information inherited by humans.

In the nucleus, the DNA is tightly associated with many different proteins in a structure called chromatin. It is important to remove these as well as other cellular proteins in order to extract the DNA. This is achieved through the use of organic solvents. An aqueous solution of DNA is obtained from which the DNA can be further purified by ethanol precipitation.

Nuclear DNA has a very high molecular weight. To maintatin its integrity, special procedures must be employed. The method which is described in Appendix A yields DNA that is of sufficiently high quality for all routine analysis.[33]

SOUTHERN BLOT ANALYSIS

This technique is used for the detection of specific sequences among DNA fragments separated by gel electrophoresis.[32] The size of a specific DNA fragment from a particular individual can therefore be determined by its mobility. Among other things, this information can be used to identify deletion mutations, gene rearrangements and genetic polymorphisms. Examples of its application include the diagnosis of α-thalassaemia, lymphoproliferative disorders and haemophilia A. For whatever genetic defect is being anlaysed, the

---

*Restriction enzymes are named after the bacterial strains from which they are isolated. For example, EcoR I is derived from *Escherichia coli* RY 13, BamH I from *Bacillus amyloliuefaciens* H, Hind III from *Haemophilus influenza* Rd, and so on.

method is the same; it is the choice of restriction enzyme, the choice of probe and the interpretation of results that will differ. These aspects will be discussed in the relevant sections.

Principle. The digestion of human genomic DNA with a restriction enzyme that recognizes a six base-pair sequence yields fragments that can be conveniently separated according to size by electrophoresis in an agarose gel. Good resolution is obtained in the size range of about 500 base pairs (bp) to about 20 kilobases (kb). DNA is negatively charged in a neutral buffer; smaller fragments migrate faster towards the anode than larger fragments.

A specific DNA fragment is detected using a labelled probe. The probe is usually a purified DNA fragment which can be labelled to a high specific activity with a radionucleotide. The specificity of DNA-DNA base pairing means that, in the appropriate conditions, the denatured probe will only hybridize to its perfectly complementary sequence among the digested DNA fragments. The location of the signal seen after autoradiography allows the size of the DNA fragment to be determined with reference to a size marker run on the gel.

The agarose gel in which the DNA fragments are resolved is not a suitable matrix for this hybridization. After denaturing the fragments by immersing the gel in alkali, they are transferred to a nylon membrane by capillary action; this is a Southern blot.

Reagents and methods

See Appendix B, p. 548.

DNA probes

Any piece of DNA can be used as a probe, from total genomic DNA to a short oligonucleotide. The only requirements are that there is a sufficient amount (more than 20 ng) and the DNA can be labelled. A probe that is in regular use is typically a DNA fragment, between a few hundred bp and a few kb in length, which has been cloned into a plasmid vector. Many plasmids have been specifically engineered to enable the efficient propagation of these DNA fragments as cloned recombinant molecules in *E. coli*.

It is beyond the scope of this chapter to go into the details of how these clones are produced. Those that are described in this chapter are all freely available from the laboratories in which they were first isolated. With any probe it is important to obtain the following information in order to use it properly: (1) whether the fragment is derived from genomic DNA or cDNA; (2) which vector the fragment has been cloned into; (3) the restriction enzymes that were used in the cloning, and those that can be used to release the DNA fragment (or insert) from the vector; (4) the size of the insert; and (5) a restriction map of the region of DNA from which the probe is derived.

Probes will usually be sent out as plasmid DNA or bacterial strains harbouring the recombinant plasmid. They may also be obtained from commercial companies in a form in which they are ready to use. Protocols for the transformation of competent* *E. coli* with plasmid DNA and the large scale preparation of plasmid DNA from liquid cultures of *E. coli* are to be found in specialist laboratory manuals.[29] The preparation of the insert from plasmid DNA and a recommended method[7] for labelling the insert with $[\alpha^{32}P]dCTP$ are described in Appendix C (p. 551).

Problems and interpretation

The most commonly encountered problem in Southern blot analysis is poor signal quality. As there are so many steps involved in the procedure, it is never easy to identify the problem, especially when no signal is obtained. Two common reasons for failure are: (1) the specific activity of the probe—unless the isotope is relatively fresh, and the incorporation has been good, the probe will not be hot enough to give a good signal; (2) failure to rinse away all the alkali that remains on the filter—it is common to neutralize the gel before transfer, although with the positively-charged nylon membranes that are currently in use this is not necessary and is omitted from our protocol.

E. coli that are made receptive to the uptake of DNA by chemical treatment.

A high background signal can also be a problem. Among other reasons, this may be caused by letting the filter dry before the washes are complete, by a failure to remove all the unincorporated radiolabelled nucleotide from the probe, or by using a poor quality probe.

Because this method permits the detection of pg amounts of target DNA in the digested genomic DNA sample, contamination of the samples with cloned plasmid DNAs (which may be in the laboratory in mg quantities) can be a serious problem. It is usually quite distinctive with a consistent size, and the intensity of hybridization to any contaminant is most often disproportionate compared to the expected signal.

Incomplete digestion of the genomic DNA may also be a problem in that additional fragment sizes will be detected which are artefactual. These can be recognized because they have a consistent size with the same probe and the same enzyme; there may also be some indication of partial digestion from the photograph of the ethidium bromide stained agarose gel.

Finally, and most importantly, comes the problem of interpretation. To recognise a change from the normal situation, it is necessary to know what the expected pattern of restriction fragments is for a given gene, and what changes may be expected. A restriction map and the previous experience of others can supply these. Below, the application of Southern blot analysis to the diagnosis of α- and β-thalassaemia and in the characterization and diagnosis of lymphoproliferative disorders is discussed.

DIAGNOSIS OF α-THALASSAEMIA BY SOUTHERN BLOT ANALYSIS

As described, it is possible to determine the size of a specific gene fragment by Southern blot analysis. The α-thalassaemias, which are mostly caused by gene deletions[15] (Fig. 28.1), can therefore be identified by this procedure. The common α⁺-thalassaemias are caused by deletions which are readily detected using an α globin gene probe. The clinically significant α⁰-thalassaemias are caused by larger deletions that remove both of the α globin genes from one chromosome, and therefore go undetected when an α globin gene probe is used. In the most common of these, the South-East Asian (_ _ᵉᵃ) and Mediterranean (_ _ᵐᵉᵈ) forms, the deletions extend from within the ζ globin genes to the region of the α globin 3′ hypervariable region (HVR). The resulting disruption of the ζ globin genes can be detected by Southern blot analysis using a ζ globin gene probe.

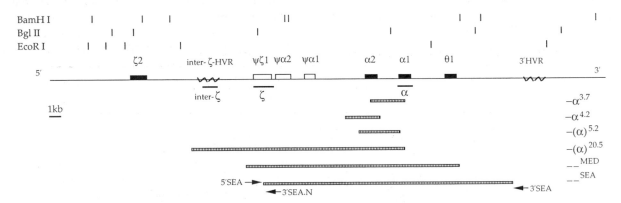

Fig. 28.1 The α globin gene cluster. The location of the genes (black boxes) and pseudogenes (open boxes), restriction sites (vertical bars) and gene probes (horizontal bars) are shown on a sketch of the α globin gene cluster (after ref. 15). The hatched bars below show the extent of the deletions, commonly found in α thalassaemia, that are discussed in the text. The arrows show the position of the PCR primers used in the detection of the _ _ ᴿᴱᴬ deletion. HVR, hypervariable region; SEA, South-East Asian; MED, Mediterranean.

Probes

The α globin gene probe used is a 1.6 kb Pst I α_1 genomic fragment.[22] The extensive homology of the two α genes (α_1 and α_2) means that this probe will hybridize to both of these genes. The same is true for the ζ globin gene probe, which is a 1.8 kb Sac I ζ_1 genomic fragment[22] that will hybridize to both the ζ_1 and ζ_2 genes. The choice of restriction enzymes for the digestion of the genomic DNA for the different probes is shown in Table 28.1. Also shown are the expected fragment sizes seen in the different α globin genotypes.

Interpretation

The identification of α^+-thalassaemia is relatively straightforward: in addition to the normal 14.0 kb fragment, BamH I fragments of 10.3 kb or 9.8 kb are seen with an α globin gene probe in individuals that are heterozygous for the $-\alpha^{3.7}$ and $-\alpha^{4.2}$ deletions, respectively (Table 28.1). The precise genotype is confirmed in Bgl II digests using the ζ globin probe: the 3.7 kb deletion ($-\alpha^{3.7}$) removes the Bgl II site between the two α globin genes, so that the normal 12.6 kb fragment is replaced by a larger 16.0 kb fragment. With the 4.2 kb deletion ($-\alpha^{4.2}$), the α_2 globin gene is lost and the 12.6 kb Bgl II fragment is reduced to 8.4 kb.

When a 10.3 kb BamH I fragment alone is seen by the α globin gene probe, individuals may have either the $\alpha-/\alpha-$ or the $\alpha-/--$ genotype. The latter may be excluded by hybridization with the ζ globin probe, as described below, or simply by the absence of Hb H on haemoglobin electrophoresis.

When a 14.0 kb fragment is seen by the α globin gene probe in BamH I digests, this is in keeping with a normal genotype but does not exclude the non-deletional type of α-thalassaemia or heterozygous α^0-thalassaemia. To detect the α^0 thalassaemias, the ζ globin probe is used. Bgl II digests give fragments of 10.5 kb and 13.9 kb with the $--^{SEA}$ and $--^{MED}$ genotypes, respectively.

However, the interpretation of Bgl II digests is made difficult in such cases by the presence of a hypervariable region between the two ζ globin genes (inter-ζ HVR)[14] which is highly polymorphic in both normal and α-thalassaemic individuals. It is further complicated by a rare Bgl II polymorphic site between the ζ_2 and α_2 globin genes which splits the 12.6 kb fragment into 5.2 kb and 7.4 kb fragments (the latter is not seen by the ζ globin probe). Variation can also be observed resulting from the triplication or the deletion of one of the ζ globin genes.

These problems in the interpretation of Bgl II digests can be overcome by using the ζ globin probe against either EcoR I or BamH I digests which generate abnormal fragments of 17.0 or 20.0 kb, respectively, in individuals with the $--^{SEA}$ deletion. The $--^{MED}$ deletion is not easily detected using these digests, and is only identified with confidence using an inter ζ probe which reveals an abnormal fragment of 7.5 kb in EcoR I digests.

Table 28.1 Restriction enzyme (RE) fragment sizes in different α globin gene deletions

Probe	RE	GENOTYPE				
		$\alpha\alpha$	$-\alpha^{3.7}$	$-\alpha^{4.2}$	$--^{SEA}$	$--^{MED}$
α	BamH I	14.0	10.3	9.8	–	–
	EcoR I	23.0	19.3	18.8	–	–
	Bgl II	12.6; 7.4	16.0	8.4; 7.4	–	–
ζ	BamH I	10.8; 5.7	10.8; 5.7	10.8; 5.7	20.0	5.9
	EcoR I	23.0; 4.8	19.3; 4.8	18.8; 4.8	17.2; 4.8	4.8
	Bgl II	12.6	16.0	8.4	10.5	13.9
		9.5–12.5*	9.5–12.5*	9.5–12.5*	9.5–12.5*	9.5–12.5*
Inter-ζ	BamH I	10.8	10.8	10.8	20.0	7.5

Fragment sizes given in kb. *Range of normal fragment sizes is due to the inter-ζ HVR.

Recently, a PCR based method for detecting these deletions has been devised and is described in the PCR section. A possible strategy to identify α^0-thalassaemia would be to exclude the common deletions using the PCR and then use the appropriate enzymes and probes to exclude the rare deletions such as $_{-\ -}$FIL and $_{-\ -}$THAI.[8]

Comments

Unlike the β-thalassaemias, α-thalassaemias are not easily diagnosed using routine haematological techniques. The diagnosis of α-thalassaemia is often made following exclusion of β-thalassaemia and/or iron deficiency. Since the vast majority of cases of α-thalassaemia are of the clinically benign type (i.e. α^+-thalassaemia), it is debatable whether molecular analysis is justified in order to reach a definitive diagnosis in these individuals.

However, it is essential that individuals with α^0-thalassaemia are identified and, if it is appropriate, are investigated at the molecular level. This is particularly relevant if prenatal diagnosis is to be offered to a couple who are at risk for having a hydrops child, where there is an increased risk for maternal death at delivery. Women of child-bearing age and those attending antenatal clinics who have an MCH less than 24 pg and an MCHC of between 30 and 32 g/dl should be investigated at the molecular level for α-thalassaemia. Women of South-East Asian origin should be investigated for α-thalassaemia irrespective of the MCHC value if the MCH is 24.5 pg or below. It is also advisable to screen for H bodies in individuals who fall into these categories, as in our experience H bodies are always present in α^0-heterozygotes. However, it should be stressed that in all cases where a woman attending an antenatal clinic has thalassaemic indices, her partner should have a peripheral blood count without delay (see also Chapter 14, p. 273).

SOUTHERN BLOT ANALYSIS OF β-THALASSAEMIAS

The majority of the β-thalassaemias, unlike the α-thalassaemias, are due to point mutations,[16,18] which in most cases cannot be detected by Southern blot analysis. However, the 1.35 kb and the 619 bp deletions common in the blacks and the Asian Indians, respectively, can be identified due to the decrease in DNA fragment sizes seen with the β globin gene probe.[37] When digested with Bgl II, the normal 5.2 kb fragment of the β globin gene is reduced to 3.8 kb by the 1.35 kb deletion and to 4.6 kb by the 619 bp deletion.

The δ-β fusion globins, Hb Lepore,[10] are also detected by the β globin gene probe: Xba I digests reveal an abnormal fragment of 3.8 kb instead of the normal 10.8 kb fragment.

Deletions giving rise to δβ-thalassaemia or HPFH need to be analysed by Southern blotting, but in heterozygotes the β globin gene probe will only reveal normal fragments from the normal β globin gene cluster. However, they can be identified using a γ or ψβ globin probe, both of which hybridize to a restriction enzyme fragment that spans the breakpoint of the deleted DNA. The HPFH 1 and 2 deletions are identified by the presence of abnormal 14.0 kb and 16.0 kb BamH I fragments, respectively, replacing the normal 18.0 kb fragment seen with the γ globin probe.[34]

DIAGNOSIS AND CHARACTERIZATION OF LYMPHOPROLIFERATIVE DISORDERS BY SOUTHERN BLOT ANALYSIS

The vast majority of lymphoproliferative disorders can be readily diagnosed using cytochemical and immunological techniques as described in Chapter 9. However, in certain cases where the diagnosis is ambiguous, genetic techniques may be useful.[11,38] Examples include cases of controversial lineage, lymphomas in which the histology is ambiguous and occult lymphomas. DNA analysis may also help in determining whether a lymphocytosis is monoclonal, oligoclonal or polyclonal and in establishing the extent and monitoring the treatment of a known lymphoproliferative disorder.

Principle

This analysis is possible because the immunoglobulin (Ig) and T cell receptor (TCR) genes undergo a rearrangement during the normal differentiation of B and T lymphocytes, but not in other cells. This rearrangement disrupts the DNA around the joining region of these genes, causing a change in the DNA restriction fragment sizes seen. As described above, this can be detected by Southern blot analysis.

However, the rearranged fragments from any one clone are only detected when it represents an abnormally large proportion of the cells in the population being studied, as it will in a clonal lymphoproliferative disorder. In a polyclonal population, each of the many different rearranged fragments that are present, which are derived from the large number of different clones, will be below the level of detection by this method. In this situation only the germ line fragments will be seen.

Probes

The most informative probes used in gene rearrangement studies are the JH probe, for the joining region of the immunoglobulin heavy chain gene, and the Cβ probe, for the constant region of the TCR β chain gene.

The JH probe

The immunoglobulin heavy chain gene rearranges before the light chain genes in almost all B cells, and is therefore the best choice for studying B cell clonality. A suitable probe is a 2.6 kb genomic clone[9] that extends beyond the 3′ joining segments of this gene (Fig. 28.2).

Convenient restriction enzymes to use are Hind III which gives a 10 kb germ line fragment and BgI II which gives a 4 kb germ line fragment. Both cut on each side of the joining region, and so while the 3′ site will be unaffected by any rearrangement, the 5′ site will be deleted out and replaced by another in the incoming variable segment of the gene.

The Cβ probe

The majority of T cells express a receptor that is a heterodimer of α and β chains. While the α gene has many different joining regions spread over a considerable genetic distance, the β chain gene has only two different sites where rearrangement can occur, and is therefore the gene of choice in this procedure. A suitable probe is a cDNA probe[31] that will hybridize to both the $C\beta_1$ and $C\beta_2$ segments, due to their extensive homology (Fig. 28.2). EcoR I digests will detect rearrangements at $J\beta_1$, Hind III digests will detect rearrangements at $J\beta_2$ while BamH I digests should detect all rearrangements, although the fragment sizes involved may be too large to be easily resolved in a normal Southern blot. A routine screen is carried out using these three enzymes. Hind III digests give germ line fragments of 7.3 kb, 5.8 kb and 3.5 kb, EcoR I digests give germ line fragments of 12 kb and 4 kb, and BamH I digests give a germ line fragment of 23 kb.

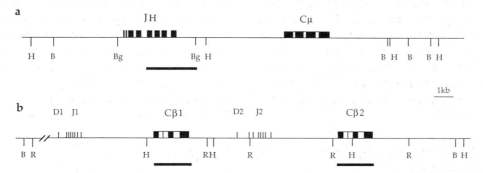

Fig. 28.2   Restriction maps of the Ig JH and TCR Cβ genes. (a) A sketch of the joining region of the immunoglobulin heavy chain gene shows the location of restriction enzyme sites (H, Hind III; R, EcoR I; B, BamH I; Bg, Bgl II), the joining segments (black boxes), the JH probe (black bar) and the constant region of the μ chain, Cμ (after ref. 9). (b) A sketch of the constant region of the T cell receptor β chain gene (after ref. 31). C, constant; D, diversity; J, joining. The black bars show the position of hybridization of the Cβ cDNA probe. Restriction sites are shown as in panel (a).

Other TCR gene probes

The Jγ probe, for the joining region of the TCR γ chain gene, may be informative in the detection of abnormal T cell clones that express a γδ TCR. However, due to the limited number of variable segments of this gene, faint rearranged fragments will be seen in normal samples and so this probe is not useful when the abnormal clone only represents a small proportion of the total cell population. It is preferable therefore to identify these rare T cell clones that express a γδ TCR using probes to the δ TCR gene, which will detect rearrangements in BamH I and Hind III digests. One problem with this analysis is the fact that the δ TCR chain gene is known to be rearranged in a significant proportion of B cell malignancies.

Interpretation

The detection of a rearranged fragment with a TCR or Ig gene probe that is different in size to the germ line fragments, indicates the presence of an abnormal lymphocyte clone. In all cases it is important to corroborate the findings seen with one restriction enzyme by seeing the same pattern with another enzyme.

Some general principles should always apply in the interpretation of these gene rearrangements. If a single rearranged band is seen, then the abnormal clone has a rearranged gene on one chromosome only. The relative intensity of the rearranged band, compared to the intensity of the germ line band, will be the same in different digests. If two rearranged bands are seen, then the abnormal clone has both alleles of the gene rearranged. In this case, the rearranged bands will be of the same intensity. Again, the same pattern should be observed in different digests that detect rearrangements at the same position. In all cases, the intensity of the rearranged band indicates the size of the abnormal clone as a proportion of the total cell population.

Some examples that illustrate these general points, as well as problems encountered in this analysis, are shown in Figs. 28.3 and 28.4. Panel (a), Fig. 28.3, shows the detection of an abnormal B cell clone in a patient with CLL.

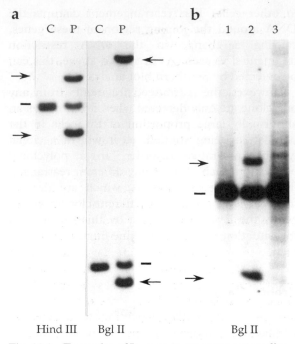

Fig. 28.3   Examples of Ig gene rearrangement studies. The panels show the results of Southern blot analysis using JH probe. Dashes to the left and right of each panel indicate the position of the germ line fragments. The arrows point to the rearranged fragments. C, control sample; P, patient sample. The restriction enzymes used are shown beneath each panel. For explanations, see text.

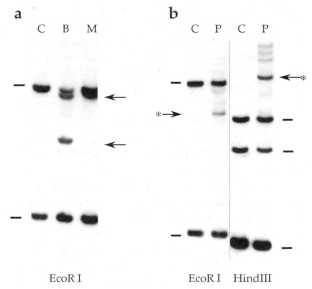

Fig. 28.4   Examples of TCR gene rearrangement studies. The panels show the results of Southern blot analysis using the Cβ probe. Markings are as for Fig. 28.3. *Fragments generated by partial digestion. B, peripheral blood sample; M, bone marrow sample. For explanations, see text.

Using the JH probe to Hind III and Bgl II digests, only a single germ line fragment is seen in the control sample. In the patient, two additional rearranged bands of roughly equal intensity are seen representing two rearranged alleles in the clone. The relative intensity of these bands to the germ line band shows that the clone represents a large proportion of the mononuclear cells in peripheral blood, from where the DNA was extracted.

Panel (b) in Fig. 28.3 shows the hybridization of the JH probe to Bgl II digests of DNA from the peripheral blood of a patient with a lymphocytosis (lane 1), CLL (lane 2) and cold agglutinins (lane 3). In lane 1, only a germ line fragment is seen, demonstrating that the lymphocytosis is not due to a clonal expansion of B cells. In lane 2, two rearranged alleles from the abnormal B cell clone are detected. In lane 3 there are clearly a number of faint rearranged bands detected in addition to the germ line fragment. The significance of this pattern is not altogether clear and it has been called an oligoclonal expansion of B cell clones.

In panel (a) in Fig. 28.4, the two expected germ line fragments are seen with the Cβ probe in an EcoR I digest of DNA extracted from a control sample. Two rearranged bands are seen in DNA extracted from peripheral blood mononuclear cells and a bone-marrow aspirate of a patient with pure red cell aplasia. These bands are strong in the blood sample, indicating the presence of a relatively large abnormal T cell clone, but much weaker in the bone marrow aspirate where the clone represents a much smaller proportion of the total cell population. Two rearranged bands in EcoR I digests indicate that the clone has rearranged both alleles at $J\beta_1$. Two rearranged bands were also seen in BamH I digests with the Cβ probe, but in Hind III digests only germ line fragments were seen. This is to be expected since the $J\beta_2$ region remains in its germ line configuration when $J\beta_1$ rearranges. If a rearrangement is seen in Hind III digests with the Cβ probe, only germ line fragments will be seen in EcoR I digests from the same allele, as $C\beta_1$ will be deleted. Accordingly, the 12 kb EcoR I fragment may be visibly reduced in intensity if the clone is large.

In panel (b), Fig. 28.4, additional bands are seen with the Cβ probe in the same patient in both Hind III and EcoR I digests. In this case, however, it is very likely that these bands do not represent gene rearrangement, but partial digestion. The Hind III and EcoR I sites at $C\beta_2$ are particularly resistant to digestion in sub-optimal conditions. This results in additional fragments of 13 kb in Hind III digests and 8 kb in EcoR I digests. Additional larger faint bands are also seen in this patient, which is again indicative of incomplete digestion. These partial fragments will be the same size in all the different samples in which they are seen, while genuine rearranged fragments will almost invariably be of a different size in different patients. Partial digestion is a problem encountered with the JH probe as well, but again the fragments generated are of a consistent size.

Problems

Two of the major problems in this analysis are poor film quality and partial digestion. The second of these, which has been illustrated, is at least relatively easy to identify. Poor film quality is the more frustrating, as the sensitivity of this technique depends on obtaining good signals against a low background. At their best, these gene rearrangement studies can detect clones that represent as little as 1% of the total cell population.

Misinterpretation of a band that is an artefact is another major pitfall. In looking for very minor bands the technique is open to this possibility, for example if a tiny contaminant is present at any stage. This may even occur if there is the slightest crossover from probe to probe through aerosols on the base of the micropipette. The best guard against this problem is always to corroborate findings in different digests and if necessary in different experiments.

As with all Southern blot analysis, a reasonable amount (at least 30 μg) of high quality DNA is required. Although this is not usually a problem with blood or marrow samples, it can be a major problem in dealing with small tissue biopsies. There is no real way around this problem, and it is one of the principal reasons for attempting to develop PCR based methods for the study of gene rearrangements.[3,30]

Finally, there are other problems intrinsic to the method itself. These include the time taken to perform the analysis, the experience required to obtain consistently high quality autoradiographs and the use of a radionuclide, which is still the only way to obtain the strength of signal required in this procedure.

THE POLYMERASE CHAIN REACTION (PCR)

The invention of the polymerase chain reaction[27] (PCR) has had a dramatic impact on the study and analysis of nucleic acids. Not more than 6 yr ago, the analysis of DNA involved the basic techniques of Southern blotting and gene cloning. Only specialist centres could carry these out with any degree of success. Now, with the PCR, many more laboratories have a simple method allowing access to the analysis of DNA.

Through the use of a thermostable DNA polymerase, PCR results in the amplification of a specific DNA fragment such that it can be visualized by ethidium bromide staining on an agarose gel. The procedure takes only a few hours, does not require the use of radionucleotides, and requires only a very small amount of starting material. These advantages have resulted in the PCR being applied in a wide variety of research and diagnostic procedures.

Principle. A DNA polymerase will synthesize the complementary strand of a DNA template in vitro. A stretch of double-stranded DNA is required for the synthesis to be initiated. This double-stranded sequence can be generated by annealing an oligonucleotide (oligo), which is a short single stranded DNA molecule usually between 17 to 22 bases in length, to a single-stranded DNA template. These oligos, which are synthesized in vitro, will prime the DNA synthesis and are therefore referred to as primers.

In the PCR two oligos are used. One primes the synthesis of DNA in the forward direction, or along the coding strand of the DNA, while the other primes DNA synthesis in the reverse direction, or along the non-coding strand. The other components of the reaction are the DNA template from which the DNA fragment will be amplified, the four deoxynucleotide triphosphates (dATP, dTTP, dCTP and dGTP) required as the building blocks of the DNA that is to be synthesized, the necessary buffer and the thermostable DNA polymerase, or *Taq** polymerase.

The first step of the reaction is to denature the template DNA by heating the reaction mixture to 95°C. The reaction is then cooled to a temperature, usually between 50°C and 60°C, that permits the annealing of the oligos to the DNA template, but only at their specific complementary sequences. The temperature is then raised to 72°C at which the *Taq* polymerase efficiently synthesizes DNA, extending from the oligo in a 5′ to 3′ direction. Cyclical repetition of the denaturing, annealing and extension steps, by simply changing the temperature of the reaction in an automated heating block, results in exponential amplification of the DNA that lies between the two oligos.

The specificity of the DNA fragment that is amplified is therefore determined by the sequences of the oligos used. A sequence of 17 bp is theoretically unique in the human genome and so oligos of this length and above will anneal at only one specific place on a template of genomic DNA. One general requirement of the PCR is therefore some knowledge of the DNA sequence of the gene that is to be amplified. The relative positioning of the two oligos is another important consideration. They must prime DNA synthesis in opposite directions, but pointing towards one another. There is also an upper limit to the distance apart that the oligos can be placed; fragments of several kb in length can be amplified, but the process is most efficient for fragments of several hundred bp.

---

*This DNA polymerase is named after the bacterium it is isolated from, *Thermus aquaticus*.

Reagents and methods

See Appendix D, p. 553.

Problems and Interpretation

If the amplification has been successful a discrete fragment of the expected size is seen in an ethidium-bromide-stained agarose gel in all samples, except where a blank control is loaded. If a product is seen in the blank control, then one of the solutions has been contaminated. In this case, the experiment and all the working solutions should be discarded, and the micropipettes cleaned.

The absence of a fragment in all tracks indicates that the PCR has failed. This could be due to a number of reasons, the most obvious being the poor quality or omission of one of the essential reagents. The reaction may also fail if the magnesium concentration is too low, or the annealing temperature is too high. If one particular DNA sample repeatedly fails to amplify, then the sample should be re-extracted with phenol and chloroform, and re-precipitated in 1/10 volume of 5 mol/l ammonium acetate and 2.5 volumes of ethanol (see DNA extraction protocol). Another problem is the presence of non-specific fragments or just a smear of amplified product. This can occur if the magnesium concentration is too high, or the annealing temperature is too low.

Products of the PCR may be analysed in a variety of different ways. The identification of point mutations that create or destroy restriction enzyme sites can be achieved through the appropriate digestion. Allele-specific oligo-nucleotide hybridization can also be used in the detection of point mutations. The presence of an amplified fragment may in itself be informative, e.g. in the analysis of deletion mutations and in the use of allele-specific primers. These methods, which are described in the next section, may be applied to any genetic disorder where the sequence and mutations of the relevant gene are known. Examples of their application in the diagnosis of the haemoglobinopathies are given below.

ANALYSIS OF PCR PRODUCTS

RESTRICTION ENZYME DIGESTION

Principle. A single base substitution, or point mutation, that creates or destroys the recognition sequence of a particular restriction enzyme can be identified due to the change in DNA fragment sizes that will result from digestion by that enzyme. This change in a restriction fragment size can be detected by Southern blot analysis, but is more simply achieved through the analysis of the appropriate PCR product.

Method

See Appendix E, p. 554.

Interpretation

A difference in the size of the restriction fragments seen in normal and mutant samples can be predicted from a restriction map of the amplified fragment and the site of the mutation that changes a restriction site. The observed fragments should be consistent with either the mutant or the normal pattern. An example is shown below in the diagnosis of the sickle-cell mutation.

ALLELE-SPECIFIC OLIGONUCLEOTIDE HYBRIDIZATION (ASOH)

Principle. The long DNA probes described for the Southern blot analysis are not able to detect single base changes (point mutations) or small insertions or deletions. However, under appropriate conditions, short oligonucleotide probes will hybridize to their exact complementary sequence, but not to a sequence where there is even a single base mismatch.[39] A pair of oligos are therefore used to test for the presence of a point mutation: a mutant oligo complemetary to the mutant sequence and a normal oligo complementary to the normal sequence, with the sequence difference placed near the centre of the oligo.

The stability of the duplex formed between the oligo and the target DNA being tested (the product of a PCR reaction) depends on the temperature, the base composition and length of the oligo, and the ionic strength of the washing solution. For allele-specific oligonucleotide hybridization (ASOH) studies, an empirical formula has been derived for the dissociation temperature (Td), the temperature at which half of the duplexes are dissociated. This value is used as a guideline; the exact temperature at which only perfect base pairing is maintained is usually found by trial and error. The method is described in other specialized laboratory manuals.[29]

Interpretation

The oligos should hybridize to their exact complementary DNA sequence, such that the mutant oligo gives a signal with a homozygous mutant control but not with a normal control. When this is the case, the interpretation of the result is straightforward; a positive signal from a particular oligo indicates the presence of that allele in the test sample. Heterozygotes and homozygotes are distinguished by using the mutant and normal oligos in tandem.

If there is no significant difference in the intensity of the radioactive signal seen in the control samples, then a further wash of the filters at a higher temperature (e.g. Td + 2°C) may be necessary. A problem with the method is that it is relatively time consuming, and care has to be taken in establishing the correct washing condition for each oligo. Non-radioactive probes, with detection systems involving horse-radish peroxidase, are now quite widely used in this procedure.[28]

AMPLIFICATION REFRACTORY MUTATION SYSTEM (ARMS)

Principle. Point mutations and small insertions or deletions can be identified directly by PCR amplification using allele-specific primers.[20,25] As in ASOH, two different oligos are used that differ only at the site of the mutation (the ARMS primers). In this case, however, the mismatch is at the 3′ end of the oligo rather than in its centre. In a PCR, an oligo with a mismatch at its 3′ end will fail to prime the extension step of the reaction. Each test sample is amplified in two separate reactions containing either a mutant ARMS primer or a normal ARMS primer. The mutant primer will prime amplification from DNA with this mutation, but not from a normal DNA. A normal primer will do the opposite. To increase the instability of the 3′ end mismatch, and so ensure the failure of the amplification, it is sometimes necessary to introduce a second nucleotide mismatch three or four bases from the 3′ end of both oligos. A second pair of unrelated primers at distance from the ARMS primers is included in each reaction as internal control, to demonstrate that efficient amplification has occurred. This is essential because a failure of the ARMS primer to amplify is interpreted as a significant result and must not be due to sub-optimal reaction conditions.

Method

The amplification of DNA with ARMS primers is carried out in exactly the same way as a standard PCR, except for the fact that each PCR mixture includes two pairs of primers, instead of one pair. Each ARMS primer (either the mutant or the normal oligo) requires another common primer to yield an amplified product. A second pair of primers, which will amplify a nearby but irrelevant fragment, are included as internal controls for the PCR mixture.

A 25 µl reaction is sufficient for this analysis, with the buffer, nucleotide and primer concentrations being adjusted accordingly. The volume of the water is reduced to allow for the presence of the four primers included in each reaction. It may be convenient to prepare a pre-mix for a set of both normal and mutant oligo reactions, as described in Appendix D.

Interpretation

In all the samples, apart from the blank control, the fragment produced by amplification with the internal control primers must be seen. If this is the case, then the presence or absence of a mutation is simply determined by the presence or absence of the expected fragment produced by amplification with the mutant ARMS primer and the common primer. The presence or absence of the normal allele is determined in the same way in the reaction that includes the normal ARMS primer. In this way, heterozygous, homozygous normal, and homozygous mutant individuals can be distinguished. An example of this in the diagnosis of a β-thalassaemia mutation is given below.

INVESTIGATION OF HAEMOGLOBINOPATHIES USING THE PCR

SICKLE-CELL DISEASE

The presence of a sickle-cell gene can be determined by haemoglobin cellulose acetate electropheresis or a sickling test. However, there are occasions when it is beneficial to make this diagnosis by DNA analysis: examples of this are in prenatal diagnosis, which can be performed at 10 weeks of pregnancy, or when HbS β-thalassaemia is suspected, or in confirming the diagnosis of sickle-cell anaemia in a neonate. For the type of specimens collected for prenatal diagnosis, refer to Chapter 14, p. 284.

The identification of the sickle-cell mutation was initally carried out by indirect linkage analysis.[17] It is now possible to detect the mutation directly by restriction enzyme analysis of a DNA fragment generated by the PCR. This is possible because the sickle cell mutation in codon 6 of the β globin gene (GAG → GTG) results in a loss of a Bsu36 I (or Mst II, Sau I,

Oxa NI, or Dde I) restriction enzyme site that is present in the normal gene[26] (Fig. 28.5).

A pair of primers are used to amplify exons 1 and 2 of the β globin gene, and the products of the PCR are digested with Bsu36 I. The loss of a Bsu36 I site in the sickle cell gene gives rise to an abnormally large restriction fragment that is not seen in normal individuals (Fig. 28.5).

Even though the Hb C mutation is also within codon 6 of the β globin gene (GAG → AAG), this does not result in the loss of the Bsu36 I restriction site, and so a Hb S/C patient will give the same pattern as a Hb A/S individual. The Hb C mutation may be detected by ASOH or ARMS.

Other haemoglobin variants that can be detected by restriction enzyme analysis include the Hbs D, O-Arab and E. The first two both abolish an EcoR I site in exon 3 of the β globin gene while Hb E abolishes an Mnl I site in exon 1.

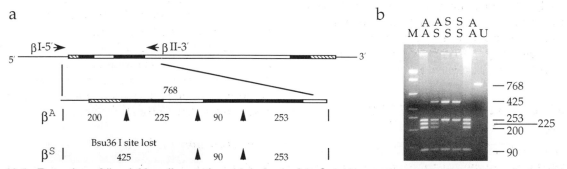

Fig. 28.5   Detection of the sickle cell mutation. (a) A sketch of the β globin gene shows the position of the primers used to amplify a 768 bp fragment in a PCR. The sequence of β I-5′ is 5′TAAGCCAGTGCCAGAAAGAGCC3′ and that of β II-3′ is 5′CATTCGTCTGTTTCCCATTCTA3′. Maps of the Bsu36 I restriction sites and the fragment sizes from βA and βS genes are shown below. (b) An ethidium-bromide-stained minigel illustrates the fragment sizes generated by Bsu36 I digestion of the PCR product from normal (A/A), sickle-cell trait (A/S) and sickle-cell anaemia (S/S) individuals, along with the undigested amplified fragment (U) and the molecular size marker (M).

β-THALASSAEMIA

The ethnic groups with the highest incidence of β-thalassaemia are the Mediterranean, Asian Indians, Chinese and Africans. Although over 100 β-thalassaemia mutations are known,[16,18] each of these groups has its own sub-set of mutations, so that only five different mutations may account for more than 90% of the affected individuals in any one population. This makes the direct detection of β-thalassaemia mutations a reasonable possibility and it has become the method of choice where it is most important—in pre-natal diagnosis.[4]

A significant proportion of the mutations either abolish or create a restriction enzyme site. These mutations can therefore be identified in the same way as described for the sickle-cell mutation, i.e. by amplifiying a region of the β globin gene around the mutation, and then digesting the fragment obtained with the appropriate restriction enzyme.

If a restriction enzyme digestion is not applicable, then ASOH or allele-specific amplification, using the ARMS, may be used for the detection of point mutations. Larger deletions can be identified directly from the size of the amplified product. If the mutation is not known, or has not been identified by using ASOH, ARMS or restriction enzyme analysis, then the mutation may only be identified by sequence analysis, which is beyond the scope of this chapter.

Example 1: the 619 bp deletion

Using primers that flank this common deletion mutation, the size of the product of the PCR is directly informative (Fig. 28.6). A small fragment of 224 bp is seen when the deletion is present, compared to the 843 bp fragment derived from the normal chromosome. This pair of primers can be used as internal controls for the PCR when using ARMS primers, as described below.

Example 2: the 41/42 frameshift mutation

In this diagnosis, the presence or absence of the product generated by the ARMS oligos and the common primer determine the genotype of the test individual. An example of this is shown in Fig. 28.7. All individuals have amplified with the control primers (upper band) and the normal primer (lower band, lanes 6–9). Two have also amplified with the mutant primer (lanes 3 and 4): these two individuals are therefore heterozygous for the 41/42 frameshift mutation.

α-THALASSAEMIA

A PCR-based strategy to detect the common forms of α⁰-thalassaemia has recently been described.[1] The primers are designed and positioned adjacent to the 5′ and 3′ breakpoints of each deletion and an internal primer is included, such that a PCR product is observed whether the deletion is present or not. The presence of an α⁺ deletion on the other

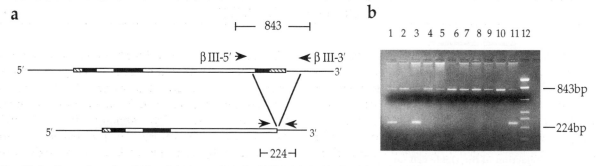

Fig. 28.6   Detection of a 619 bp deletion using the PCR. (a) A sketch of the normal β globin gene and the deleted gene shows the location of the primers (arrows) used to amplify across this deletion. The sequence of β III-5′ is 5′A CAGTGATAAT TTCTGGGTT 3′ and that of β III-3′ is 5′TAAGCAAGAGAACTGAGTGG3′. (b) A minigel shows the expected 843 bp fragment yielded by the two primers from a normal β globin gene in all lanes, and the 224 bp fragment derived from a deleted gene in individuals who are heterozygous for the mutation in lanes 1, 3, and 11.

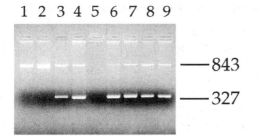

1 2 3 4 5 6 7 8 9

——843

——327

Fig. 28.7 Diagnosis of the 41/42 (-TTCT) frameshift mutation using ARMS. The gel shows the 843 bp fragment generated by the internal control primers (β III-5′ and β III-3′) in all lanes, except lane 5 which is the blank control. Four DNA samples are tested with the mutant ARMS primer (5′GTCTACCCTTGGACCCAGAGGTTGA3′) in combination with the common primer (5′CATTCGTCTGTTTCCCATTCTA -3′) in lanes 1–4, and with the normal ARMS primer (5′GTCTACCCTTGGACCCAGAGGTTCTT3′) in combination with the common primer in lanes 6–9. The presence of a 327 bp product in lanes 3 and 4 and lanes 6–9 indicates that the individuals in lanes 3 and 4 are heterozygous for the 41/42 frameshift mutation, while individuals 1 and 2 are normal with respect to this mutation.

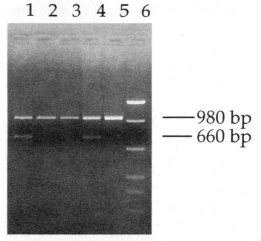

1 2 3 4 5 6

——980 bp
——660 bp

Fig. 28.8 Detection of South-East Asian α⁰-thalassaemia (_ _ ^{SEA}) by the PCR. The location of the primers 5′SEA (5′CTCTGTGTTCTCAGTATTGGAG3′), 3′SEA. N (5′TGAAGAGCCTGCAGGACCAGTCA3′) and 3′SEA (5′ATATATGGGTCTGGAAGTGTATC3′) are shown in Fig. 28.1. A normal fragment of 980 bp is generated by the primers 5′ SEA and 3′ SEA.N in all lanes, except lane 6 which is a molecular weight marker. The primers 5′SEA and 3′ SEA generate a smaller fragment of 66 0 bp, which is seen in lanes 1 and 4; these individuals are heterozygous for the deletion.

chromosome does not affect the identification of the α⁰ delelion.

The PCR is set up with the following modifications: PCR buffer II is used instead of PCR buffer I, and DMSO is added to a final concentration of 10% (see Appendix D, p. 552). Three primers are included in each reaction. The location of the primers used for the detection of the _ _^{SEA} deletion is shown in Fig. 28.1. The fragment generated by these primers across the

deletion breakpoint is different in size to the fragment generated from the normal chromosome. The primers that flank the deletion breakpoint are too far apart to generate a fragment from the normal chromosome in the PCR. Only when these are brought closer together as a result of the deletion, can a fragment be produced (Fig 28.8).

G6PD DEFICIENCY

Glucose-6-phosphate dehydrogenase (G6PD) deficiency, the most common human enzymopathy, may be responsible for acute and sometimes chronic haemolytic anaemia. It is essential that G6PD deficiency is excluded in patients with unexplained haemolysis. Most of the polymorphic variants that are associated with acute haemolysis have been defined at the molecular level and it may be important to distinguish these from a G6PD-deficient variant that is the cause of chronic haemolysis. Since it is an X-linked

disorder, it may be difficult to identify heterozygous females, in whom levels of enzyme activity may vary from reduced to normal levels. This is particularily important in female relatives of men with chronic haemolytic anaemia due to G6PD deficiency. Furthermore, G6PD deficiency can be masked by reticulocytosis in individuals with acute haemolysis and in neonates.

In such cases it may be beneficial to test for a G6PD-deficient variant by DNA analysis. Although more than 50 G6PD mutations have now been described,[36] some of the most common deficient variants are readily diagnosed by restriction enzyme digestion of the appropriate PCR products. For example, the G6PD Mediterranean mutation creates an Mbo II site in exon 6, and the two mutations found in G6PD A– create an Nla III site in exon 4 and a Fok I site in exon 5 of the G6PD gene.

DIAGNOSIS OF GENETIC DISEASE BY LINKAGE ANALYSIS

In the preceding sections we have described the diagnosis of inherited haematological disorders for which the molecular basis is known. In these cases, the direct detection of a specific mutation is possible. However, there are still a large number of inherited diseases for which the mutations remain uncharacterized. This is true of a large proportion of the hereditary red cell membrane disorders as well as many disorders of coagulation. Although great effort has led to the identification of a large number of mutations in the factor IX gene,[12] the majority of mutations in the factor VIII gene that cause haemophilia A are yet to be identified.[35] Two reasons for this are the extraordinarily large size of the gene, and the high rate of sporadic new mutations that give rise to this disorder.

Using haemophilia A as an example, this section will describe how prenatal diagnosis can be performed and carrier status determined for unknown mutations through genetic linkage analysis.

Principle

Genetic loci that lie close to one another on a chromosome are linked. The chances of a recombination event occurring between them during meiosis is dependent on the distance that they are apart. Closely linked loci are likely to be inherited together without crossing over. A silent or anonymous marker locus that is tightly linked to a mutation that causes disease can therefore be used to track the mutation in families, even if the mutation itself is unknown.

Restriction fragment length polymorphisms (RFLPs) have proved to be very useful genetic markers.[2,23] These are usually silent base substitutions occurring at random throughout the genome that cause the recognition sequence for a particular restriction enzyme to be either lost or gained. They must have a polymorphic frequency in the general population to be informative. The presence or absence of the restriction site can easily be determined by Southern blot analysis or by PCR followed by restriction enzyme digestion. More recently, a large number of highly polymorphic markers that are due to simple sequence repeats (or a variable number of tandem repeats, VNTRs) have been described that can be readily genotyped by the PCR.[42,43]

In a family with an affected individual, the linkage of one allele of a marker RFLP or VNTR to the disease-causing mutation can be established. Following this allele through the family, where the appropriate members are heterozygous for the marker and therefore informative, allows carrier status to be established and prenatal diagnosis to be offered.

THE DIAGNOSIS OF HAEMOPHILIA A

The factor VIII gene is X-linked. Female carriers of mutations in this gene will express intermediate levels of factor VIII. However, it is often not possible to determine without doubt the carrier status of a woman based on factor VIII levels due to the range of values seen in normal and heterozygous individuals. It is therefore desirable to use a genetic test in order to determine whether or not a woman, who is related to a haemophiliac, is a carrier. If a carrier is identified, or a woman is an obligate carrier, genetic analysis can also be employed to determine through prenatal diagnosis whether or not a fetus is affected.

Within the factor VIII gene there are several polymorphic restriction enzyme sites of which two are particularily informative: an Xba I site in intron 22 and a Bcl I site in intron 18 for which the frequencies of the minor alleles are 0.41 and 0.30, respectively.

The Xba I polymorphism is detected using the probe p482.6.[44] Genomic DNA is digested with the enzymes Kpn I and Xba I together to resolve a cross-hybridizing constant fragment from the two polymorphic fragments. When Xba I does not cut, a fragment of 6.1 kb is detected in addition to the constant band of 6.8 kb. When the Xba I site is present, the 6.1 kb fragment is lost and a 4.8 kb fragment is detected. The Bcl I polymorphism is seen with the probe p114.2[13] Alleles of approximately 1.3 kb or 1.0 kb are detected.

Both of these polymorphisms can also be analysed through PCR amplification and subsequent restriction enzyme digestion,[19] as described above for the sickle cell mutation. The sequences of the oligos used to prime the amplification of a DNA fragment of 142 bp that includes the polymorphic Bcl I site are: 5′TTCGAATTCTGAAATTATCTTGTT3′ and 5′TAAAAGCTTTAAATGGTCTAGGC3′. Bcl I digestion, which is carried out at 50°C, will yield fragments of 99 bp and 43 bp if the site is present, or leave the 142 bp fragment intact if the site is absent. The polymorphic Xba I site can be analysed in the same way using the primers 5′CTGCAGGGGGGGGGGGACA3′ and 5′CGAGCTCTCCATCTGAACAT3′ which generate a fragment of 88 bp which is cut into fragments of 68 bp and 20 bp by Xba I when the site is present.

Southern blot analysis of the segregation of the Xba I polymorphism in a family is shown in Fig. 28.9. The boy with haemophilia A has the 6.1 kb allele of this Xba I polymorphism; this allele is therefore linked to the mutation in this family. The mother is heterozygous, with the affected 6.1 kb allele and an unaffected 4.8 kb allele, and so the polymorphism is informative in this family. The father has a normal 6.1 kb allele, and the question is whether or not the sister is a carrier of haemophilia A. Because she must have inherited the normal 6.1 kb allele from her father, she has inherited the 4.8 kb allele from her mother and is therefore not a carrier.

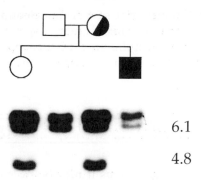

Fig. 28.9   Carrier status of haemophilia A. A family tree is drawn over the appropriate lanes of an autoradiograph showing the hybridization of the factor VIII probe, p482.6, to Xba I + Kpn I restriction digests. The sizes of the two alleles of the Xba I polymorphism are indicated. The daughter is not a carrier of haemophilia A (see text).

Problems

The example described above is a simple one: the mother is an obligate carrier as she has an affected brother as well as an affected son and she is heterozygous for the intragenic Xba I polymorphism. However, these two requirements are often not fulfilled. Because a significant proportion of cases of haemophilia A arise through new mutation, female relatives may or may not be affected, even if they carry the same marker allele as the affected boy. The study of RFLPs can exclude carrier status for some of these women, but in other cases the results are unhelpful.

When women are homozygous at each of the different intragenic RFLPs, genetic analysis will not distinguish the affected and unaffected chromosomes even if they are obligate carriers. One possible way around this problem is to use other genetic markers that are linked to the factor VIII gene, but lie at some distance from it. A highly polymorphic marker called st14,[24] has been used in this way. The problem with this is that there is a 5% chance that a recombination event will occur between this marker and the mutation in the factor VIII gene. When this happens, an incorrect diagnosis will be made.

More recently, an informative repeat polymorphism (VNTR) has been identified within the factor VIII gene.[21] This consists of between

16 and 24 copies of a of CA dinucleotide, and the chances that a woman is heterozygous for the number of copies of this repeat is estimated to be 0.91. The polymorphism is detected by PCR amplification of a small DNA fragment around this $(CA)_n$ repeat, followed by polyacrylamide gel electrophoresis to resolve the different sizes of the various alleles.

RNA TECHNIQUES

For some diagnostic tests it may be necessary to analyze the messenger RNA (mRNA) of a particular gene of interest. Because these tests are rarely employed, only some general points will be mentioned here. The main difference that must be appreciated in the handling of RNA when compared with handling DNA is the relative stability of the two molecules. In contrast to DNA, RNA is highly susceptible to degradation. It is therefore important to work on freshly obtained blood samples in sterile containers with solutions that have been autoclaved. RNase inhibitors are often used during extraction procedures, and the purified RNA should be stored frozen at a low temperature, ideally at −80°C. The amount of each RNA species will vary, sometimes greatly, between different cell types. It is therefore necessary to consider an appropriate cell separation prior to RNA extraction.

A number of useful and quick extraction procedures have been described.[5,29] RNA is analysed by Northern blotting and the use of a specific gene probe, or through reverse transcription of the RNA to create an RNA/DNA double stranded molecule followed by PCR amplification.

The analysis of RNA may be necessary in the detection of mutations in genes that have their coding sequences spread over very large genomic regions, for example the spectrin genes, band 4.1 and factor VIII. The identification of fusion transcripts resulting from chromosomal translocations may also require the analysis of RNA rather than DNA. An example is the detection of the bcr-abl fusion message that is specific to Philadelphia chromosome positive cells of CML. The power of amplification by the PCR can be employed here in the detection of minimal residual disease.[6]

APPENDICES: TECHNICAL METHODS

APPENDIX A: EXTRACTION OF GENOMIC DNA

Reagents

General note: *for all the buffers and solutions described in this chapter it is recommended that reagents of the highest grade available and double distilled deionized water are used throughout.*

Stock solutions

NaCl 5 mol/l. Weigh 146.1 g of NaCl into a beaker and make up the volume to 500 ml with water; stir until dissolved.

Tris-HCl, 1 mol/l, pH 8.5. Dissolve 60.5 g of Trizma base (tris(hydroxy)methylaminomethane) in 350 ml water; add concentrated HCl until the pH falls to 8.5; make up to 500 ml with water.

Tris-HCl, 1 mol/l pH 7.4. Prepare as for above but reduce the pH to 7.4 with HCl.

NaOH, 5 mol/l. Add 200 g of NaOH to 800 ml water and stir until dissolved; make up to 1 litre with water.

Ethylenediamine tetra-acetic acid (EDTA), 0.5 mol/l, pH 8.0. Weigh 93 g of EDTA disodium salt (dihydrate) and add to 400 ml of water; stir until most of it has dissolved. Add 0.5 mol/l NaOH until the pH rises to 8.0, when the rest of the solid should go into solution. Make up to 500 ml with water.

Phosphate-buffered saline (PBS), pH 7.3. See p. 579 for preparation.

Nonidet P-40 (NP40), 10%. Add 10 ml of NP40 to 90 ml water and mix well.

Sodium dodecyl sulphate (SDS, lauryl sulphate), 20%. Weigh 100 g of SDS and add to 350 ml of water. *Caution*: SDS is a respiratory irritant: wear a face mask; stir and heat to 65°C until it is in solution and top up to 500 ml with water.

Working solutions

PBS + 0.1% NP40. Add 5 ml of 10% NP40 to 495 ml of PBS.

Ten times concentrated (10 ×) lysis buffer. Mix 60 ml of 5 mol/l NaCl, 20 ml of 0.5 mol/l EDTA, 10 ml of 1 mol/l Tris pH 7.4 and 10 ml of water to give 100 ml of 3 mol/l NaCl, 100 mmol/l EDTA, 100 mmol/l Tris.

Lysis solution. Prepare an appropriate amount of this solution fresh every time; for 50 ml weigh 21 g of urea (7 mol/l), add 5 ml of × 10 lysis buffer and make up to a final volume of 50 ml with water.

Chloroform/isoamyl alcohol (24:1). Add 20 ml of isoamyl alcohol to 480 ml of chloroform.

Ethanol 70%. Add 30 ml of water to 70 ml of absolute ethanol.

TE (10 mmol/l Tris, 1 mmol/l EDTA). Add 5 ml of 1 mol/l Tris pH 7.4 and 1 ml of 0.5 mol/l Na$_2$EDTA to 494 ml water.

TE equilibrated phenol. The condition of the phenol is crucial to the quality of the DNA obtained. DNA is soluble in acidic water-saturated phenol, and so it is necessary to equilibrate it to a neutral pH. Take 500 ml of water-saturated phenol. Prepare 500 ml of 0.5 mol/l Tris pH 8.5, add 150 ml of this to the phenol and mix by inversion for 2–3 min. Leave to stand until the aqueous and organic phases have separated. Remove and discard the upper aqueous layer. Add another 125 ml of 0.5 mol/l Tris, mix, stand and remove the aqueous layer as before and then repeat. To the remaining 100 ml of 0.5 mol/l Tris, add 400 ml of water to give 500 ml of 0.1 mol/l Tris. Add 150 ml of this to the phenol, and then mix, stand and remove as above. Repeat two more times. To the remaining 50 ml of 0.1 mol/l Tris add 449 ml of water and 1 ml of 0.5 mol/l EDTA to give 500 ml of TE. Add, mix, stand and remove this in three stages as before. The phenol will have reduced in volume during this procedure, but is now TE equilibrated and ready for use.

Method

1. Freeze an anticoagulated blood sample at –20°C. EDTA, ACD or preservative-free heparin are all suitable anticoagulants. It is convenient to collect the blood in a tube that can be centrifuged, such as a disposable plastic 30 ml universal container. Any sample size from 2 to 20 ml will be satisfactory.

2. Thaw the blood and centrifuge at 700*g* for 15 min. Carefully pour off the supernatant. The pellet is hard to see at this stage, and may be quite loose.

3. Resuspend the pellet in 1–2 ml of PBS + 0.1% NP40 by mixing up and down in a wide bore standard plastic transfer pipette. Top up the suspension to the original volume with PBS + 0.1% NP40.

4. Centrifuge again at 700*g* for 15 min and pour off the supernatant. If necessary, repeat until the pellet has lost most of its red colour.

5. Add 2–3 drops of lysis solution. Break up the pellet into this solution using a non-wettable sterile stick (for example a plastic disposable bacterial inoculating loop) or a clean siliconized glass rod. The solution will become viscous. Make it as homogeneous as possible.

6. Add successive 0.5 ml volumes of the lysis solution, mixing each time, until the viscosity is such that the solution can be pipetted up and down without difficulty. The final volume will depend on the size, nature and quality of the blood sample. For 10 ml of freshly frozen normal blood use 2–3 ml of lysis solution.

7. Add 1/10 volume of 20% SDS. Mix gently with a transfer pipette and incubate at 37°C for a minimum of 15 min. The samples can be left overnight at this stage.

8. Transfer the sample to a polypropylene tube. Add an equal volume of chloroform/isoamyl alcohol and an equal volume of phenol. Mix gently by inversion for 5 min. Centrifuge at 1300*g* for 15 min.

9. Transfer the upper aqueous phase to a new tube. Leave behind the white protein interface and the organic phase. This may be difficult if the solution is too viscous, in which case further dilution with lysis solution is necessary.

10. Repeat steps 8 and 9 at least once more and continue until the interface is clear. Add an equal volume of chloroform/isoamyl alcohol and mix gently by inversion for five min. Centrifuge as before and again transfer the aqueous phase to a new tube.

11. Add 2.5 volumes of absolute ethanol. Mix the solution by inverting the tube several times. The DNA should precipitate as a 'cotton wool' ball. Using a micropipette tip, transfer the DNA to a microcentrifuge tube containing 1 ml of 70% ethanol.

12. Centrifuge in a microcentrifuge at 12 000g for 5 min. Pour off the 70% ethanol. Centrifuge again for a few seconds to bring down the residual ethanol, and remove all of this with a micropipette.

13. Leave to dry on the bench for 10 min.

14. Add 50–500 µl of TE depending on the size of the pellet. Aim to have a DNA concentration of approximately 0.5 mg/ml. Leave to resuspend for at least one night. Mix gently by flicking the tube; never vortex. The DNA can be stored for long periods at 4°C or frozen at –20°C.

DNA extraction kits

A number of systems are now available that reduce the amount of time required for DNA extraction, and bypass the use of organic solvents, some of which are hazardous and may be difficult to obtain. One such procedure involves sodium perchlorate extraction followed by the use of a protein-binding silica suspension. The DNA can then be recovered after a single centrifugation.

Extraction of DNA from other sources

For the analysis of immunoglobulin and T cell receptor gene rearrangements it is necessary to enrich a peripheral blood sample for lymphocytes prior to DNA extraction. This is achieved through the separation of mononuclear cells on Ficoll/Hypaque (or Lymphoprep). After washing the cell pellet in PBS, lysis and DNA extraction can proceed as from step 5 above.

DNA is extracted from bone marrow aspirates in the same way as from peripheral blood, except that before freezing they are diluted in at least 5 volumes of PBS.

Tissue biopsies vary greatly in nature, size and cell content and, as a result, so does the quality and quantity of DNA obtained from them. To obtain sufficient quantities of high molecular weight DNA for Southern blot analysis the biopsy must be several mm^3 in size and fresh frozen. After thawing in a small Petri dish, it is mechanically disrupted into PBS firstly by chopping finely with a clean blade and then broken up with the blunt end of a 5 ml syringe plunger. The suspension is centrifuged to obtain a pellet, from which DNA is extracted as above (from step 5).

Determining the DNA concentration

Take 5 µl of the DNA solution and dilute into 245 µl of water. Mix well by vortexing. (This DNA is to be discarded and can therefore be treated in this way.) Read the absorbance (A) in a spectrophotometer at 260 nm against a water blank. An A of 1.0 is obtained from a solution of DNA at a concentration of 50 µg/ml. Therefore, multiply the A reading obtained by 2500 to get the concentration of the original DNA solution in µg/ml. The ratio of the A_{260} to the A_{280} gives an indication as to the purity of the DNA solution. This ratio should be in the range 1.7–2.0.

APPENDIX B: SOUTHERN BLOT ANALYSIS

Reagents

Restriction enzymes

A number of different companies now supply a comprehensive list of restriction enzymes, but they may vary greatly in their cost. Those that are in regular use are generally quite cheap compared with the more specialized enzymes that are used only occasionally and may be 10–100 times more expensive.

Restriction enzyme buffers

These are now almost always supplied with each restriction enzyme. Buffer compositions are always given, and will vary from enzyme to enzyme. The commonly used restriction enzymes all cut perfectly well in a single universal buffer. This is prepared using the following stock solutions:

Tris-acetate, 2 mol/l, pH 7.5. Dissolve 24.2 g of Trizma base in 60 ml of water, adjust the pH to 7.5 with glacial acetic acid and make up to 100 ml.

Potassium acetate, 2 mol/l. Weigh out 19.62 g, make up to 100 ml with water and dissolve.

Magnesium acetate, 2 mol/l. Weigh out 42.89 g, make up to 100 ml with water and dissolve.

BSA fraction V (molecular biology grade), 20 mg/ml.

Dithiothreitol (DTT), 0.5 mol/l. Weigh out 0.771 g, make up to 10 ml with water, dissolve and store at –20°C.

Spermidine (*N*-(3-aminopropyl)-1, 4-butanediamine), 1 mol/l. Weigh out 1.273 g, make up to 10 ml with water, dissolve and store at –20°C.

10 × RE buffer. For a 10-times concentrated buffer prepare a solution that is 300 mmol/l Tris-acetate pH 7.5, 660 mmol/l potassium acetate, 100 mmol/l magnesium acetate, 1 mg/ml BSA, 10 mmol/l DTT and 30 mmol/l spermidine; aliquot into microcentrifuge tubes and store at –20°C.

Other reagents

40 × Tris-acetate-EDTA (TAE) buffer. To 1600 ml water add 387.2 g of Trizma base, 29.6 g of EDTA and 92 ml of glacial acetic acid. Stir to dissolve and bring the pH to 7.4 with acetic acid. Top up the solution to 2 l with water. Dilute 1 in 40 for use.

Ethidium bromide, 10 mg/ml. Dissolve 1 g of ethidium bromide in 100 ml of water, and keep in brown or foil-wrapped bottle. **Caution**: ethidium bromide is a known teratogen; wear a face mask and handle with double gloves.

Tracking dye. Weigh 25 g of Ficoll (type 400), 0.25 g of bromophenol blue and 0.25 g of xylene cyanol. Make up to 100 ml with water, cover and mix by inversion; it will take quite a considerable amount of mixing to get the solution homogeneous. Dispense into aliquots.

Denaturation solution, 1.5 mol/l NaCl, 0.5 mol/l NaOH. Prepare this solution fresh every time by weighing 44 g of NaCl, making up to 450 ml with water and adding 50 ml of 5 mol/l NaOH.

20 × Standard sodium citrate (SSC). Add 351 g of NaCl and 176.5 g of sodium citrate (trisodium salt) to 1600 ml of water and stir to dissolve. Bring the pH to 7.0 with a very small amount of citric acid (anydrous free acid), and make up to 2 l.

100 × Denhardt's solution. Weigh 10 g of Ficoll (type 400), 10 g of polyvinylpyrrolidone and 10 g of BSA (fraction V, 96–99% purity) and make up to 500 ml with water. Dissolve and freeze at –20°C in 50 ml aliquots.

Carrier DNA, 10 mg/ml. Dissolve 1 g of salmon sperm DNA in 100 ml of water by heating to 65°C and leaving for several hours. Aliquot into 20 ml fractions and sonicate until the viscosity is reduced such that the solution can be pipetted with ease. Boil for 20 min and freeze at –20°C.

20% SDS. See DNA extraction procedure, (p. 546).

Hybridization solution, 6 × SSC, 2 × Denhardt's solution, 0.1 mg/ml carrier DNA and 1% SDS. For 100 ml, take 62 ml of water and add 30 ml of 20 × SSC, 2 ml of 100 × Denhardt's solution, 1 ml of 10mg/ml carrier DNA and 5 ml of 20% SDS.

Agarose. Type II medium electro-endosmosis.

Whatman paper. Large sheets of 17 mm and 3 mm paper.

Nylon membrane or filter. A selection of different hybridization membranes are commercially available. Always check the manufacturers' recommendations for their use.

Methods

Restriction enzyme digestion

For the digestion of genomic DNA it is necessary to take into account the following points: 5–10 µg of DNA are required to obtain a good signal from a Southern blot. Restriction enzymes are usually sold at a concentration of around 10 u/µl. The unit is defined as the amount of enzyme that will cut 1 µg of cloned DNA in 1 h at the appropriate temperature. A 4–6 fold excess of enzyme is used to ensure the complete digestion of genomic DNA, and the digestion is allowed to continue for at least 6 h. The volume of enzyme added must be less than 10% of the final reaction volume, in order to avoid non-specific digestion. Finally, attempt to keep the reaction volume below that of the well in the agarose gel (see below) into which the digested DNA solution will be loaded.

A typical reaction mixture is set up in a 1.5 ml microcentrifuge tube as follows:

10× RE buffer	7 μl
Water	38 μl
Genomic DNA (0.5 μg/μl)	20 μl
Restriction enzyme (10 u/μl)	5 μl

The components are added in the order they are listed above. The suspension is mixed by a flicking of the tube, the contents are centrifuged to the bottom by a pulse centrifugation, and incubated at 37°C.

Agarose gel electrophoresis

A large horizontal-bed electrophoresis tank is required, with the appropriate gel casting tray and combs. Good resolution of DNA fragments from 20 samples can be obtained in a gel that is 20 × 24 cm. The % agarose of the gel depends on the size of the DNA fragments to be resolved; for most purposes described in this chapter a 0.8% gel is suitable.

1. Add 3.2 g of agarose to 400 ml of 1 × TAE buffer in a 1 litre flask. Melt the agarose by boiling either in a microwave oven or in a saucepan of water over a Bunsen burner. Ensure the agarose is fully dissolved and well mixed in.

2. Cool to 55°C in a water-bath, add 40 μl of 10 mg/ml ethidium bromide, mix and pour on to the casting tray that has been taped up appropriately and has a comb to form wells in place. Remove any bubbles, and allow to set at room temperature.

3. To the completed restriction enzyme digests, add 1/10 volume of tracking dye and load into the gel, with the wells nearest the cathode so that the DNA runs towards the anode. Include a track with a size marker: 2.5 μg of λ bacteriophage DNA cut with the restriction enzyme Hind III in 40 μl of water with 4 μl of tracking dye is the standard marker used, and gives fragments of approximately 23, 9.6, 6.4, 4.5, 2.3, 2.0 and 0.56 kb.

4. Run the electrophoresis overnight, or until the bromophenol blue dye reaches the end of the gel.

Southern transfer

1. Remove the gel from the tank on its support into a tray containing TAE buffer. Photograph the gel on a transilluminator under UV illumination. Cut off the bottom right-hand corner of the gel for orientation.

2. Pour off the TAE and add 500 ml of denaturation solution. Leave for 40 min, preferably on a gently rocking platform.

3. Cut 3 pieces of 3 mm Whatman paper and one sheet of nylon hybridization transfer membrane to the size of the gel.

4. According to the instructions of the manufacturer of the nylon membrane it may be necessary to neutralize the gel prior to transfer. This is done by immersing the gel in 500 ml of 1.0 mol/l Tris pH 8.0, 1.5 mol/l NaCl for 40 min.

5. Prepare the transfer apparatus as follows: pour 500 ml of 20 × SSC into a tray. Place a glass plate over the tray to act as a bridge; this plate should be larger than the size of the gel. Cut a piece of 17 mm Whatman paper to cover the plate and pass down into the 20 × SSC to act as a wick. Wet it with the 20 × SSC by first passing it under the bridge.

6. Place the gel on to the wick. Carefully lay on the nylon membrane (or filter). Cover the rest of the platform, all around the gel, with cling film. Do not leave any air bubbles between wick and gel or gel and filter.

7. One at a time, wet the three pieces of 3 mm Whatman paper in the denaturing solution and lay them on to the nylon filter. Roll out any bubbles that may be trapped using a graduated pipette.

8. Lay on a stack of paper towels about 10 cm high, unfolded to the size of the gel for the first 1 cm. Then place over the paper stack a glass

plate and a weight (about 200 ml of water in a 500 ml bottle is convenient) so that good contact is maintained between the different layers of the blot. Leave overnight.

9. Remove the weight, the paper towels and Whatman papers. Mark the origins on the nylon filter with a pen and cut the corner for orientation.

10. Remove the filter and rinse in two changes of 200 ml of 3 × SSC to remove traces of alkali and reduce the salt concentration. Dry the filter to dampness on a piece of Whatman paper.

11. Bake the filter in an oven at 80°C for 2 h to fix the DNA to the filter.

Hybridization and autoradiography

1. Prepare 50 ml of the hybridization solution and prewarm it at 65°C.

2. Wet the filter by floating it on 3 × SSC, place it in a thick polythene bag and seal close to the filter around three edges.

3. Pour in 40 ml of the hybridization solution. Remove all the air bubbles from the bag by rolling a pipette along the outside of it, taking care not to lose the solution, and seal the bag at a distance of about 10 cm from the fourth edge of the filter.

4. Leave at 65°C for 4 h for prehybridization.

5. Label the probe DNA with $[\alpha^{32}P]dCTP$ as described below. Boil it for 5–10 min in 0.5 ml carrier DNA and place immediately into ice.

6. Cut open the bag, leaving a gap between the filter and the opening and pour off the prehybridization solution. Pour in 5–10 ml of the hybridization solution, depending on the size of the filter; 10 ml is sufficient for a filter of 20 × 22 cm; for smaller filters the volume should be reduced accordingly.

7. Add the probe to the hybridization solution and push out most of the air. Seal at the edge of the bag. Roll the radioactive air bubbles into the space between the filter and the edge using a pipette as before, leaving the hybridization solution around the filter, and seal close to the filter.

8. Leave overnight at 65°C.

9. Pre-warm the following washing solutions at 65°C: 500 ml of 3 × SSC + 0.1% SDS (made from 422.5 ml of water, 75 ml of 20 × SSC and

2.5 ml of 20% SDS); 1 litre 2 × SSC + 0.1% SDS (895 ml of water, 100 ml of 20 × SSC and 5 ml of 20% SDS); 1 litre of 0.2 × SSC + 0.01% SDS (prepared by diluting the previous solution 1:10 with water).

10. Cut open the hybridization bag and pour off the solution. *Caution*: carefully dispose of the radioactivity according to local regulations. Remove the filter and immediately plunge it into the 3× SSC. Leave for about 5 min to rinse away most of the radioactivity.

11. Pour off the 3 × SSC and pour on 500 ml of the 2 × SSC solution. Leave at 65°C for 20 min.

12. Repeat this wash in 2 × SSC and then do two further 20 min washes in the 0.2 × SSC solution, all at 65°C.

13. Remove the filter and dry to dampness on Whatman paper.

14. Wrap the filter in cling film with a fluorescent orientation marker, and expose to X-ray film for at least one night at –80°C in a cassette with intensifying screens.

15. Develop the film, mark the position of the origins and orientation of the filter, and examine the position of the hybridizing signal with reference to the photograph taken of the gel. The size of the bands seen can be estimated by comparison with the λ Hind III marker on the gel: on semi-log paper, plot the distance travelled by the marker fragments on the linear scale against their size on the log scale to give a standard curve.

APPENDIX C: DNA PROBES

Plasmid insert purification

The DNA fragment to be labelled can be purified away from the vector DNA, in which it is cloned, by size separation on an agarose gel and subsequent elution of the insert from the agarose.

Reagents

Plasmid DNA. 10 × RE buffer and restriction enzyme(s). See protocol for Southern blot analysis (p. 548).

Tris-borate-EDTA (TBE) buffer. This can be

used as an alternative to TAE as an electrophoresis buffer. $10 \times$ TBE: add 216 g of Trizma base, 18.6 g of EDTA and 110 g of orthoboric acid to 1600 ml water, dissolve and top up to 2 l; dilute 1 in 20 for use as $0.5 \times$ TBE buffer.

Ultrapure (low melting) agarose.

Sodium acetate, 3 mol/l, pH 5.2. Dissolve 40.8 g of sodium acetate. $3H_2O$ in 80 ml of water, and adjust the pH to 5.2 with glacial acetic acid. Make up the volume to 100 ml with water.

Dialysis tubing. Boil strips of tubing in 2% sodium bicarbonate, 1 mmol/l EDTA for 10 min. Rinse well with water and then boil for 10 min in water. Store at 4°C.

Sephadex G50. Swell the Sephadex G50 powder in an excess volume of water overnight; take off the water that is above the beads and replace with TE (see p. 547). Mix up the beads, allow them to settle, remove the TE; repeat twice.

Method

1. Digest 5–10 µg of the plasmid with 20–40 U of the appropriate restriction enzyme in RE buffer and sufficient water such that the volume of enzyme is less than 10% of the final volume.

2. Pour a medium sized 1% agarose gel in $0.5 \times$ TBE buffer, and load the digested DNA into a wide (3 cm) well. Carry out electrophoresis until the insert resolves from the vector DNA fragment.

3. On a UV transilluminator, cut out a gel slice containing the insert.

4. Put the gel slice lengthways into a strip of dialysis tubing that has been rinsed well with water, clipped at one end and filled with $0.5 \times$ TBE buffer. Empty out most of the TBE buffer, leaving only enough to cover the gel slice, and clip the other end of the tubing without leaving any air bubbles.

5. Replace into the electrophoresis tank and continue the current for another 2–4 h with the gel slice toward the negative terminal.

6. Reverse the current for 30 s.

7. Open the dialysis bag and transfer the buffer in 400 µl aliquots into 1.5 ml microcentrifuge tubes, add 40 µl of 3 mol/l sodium acetate and 1 ml of absolute ethanol and freeze on dry ice for 30 min or at −20°C overnight.

8. Centrifuge at 12 000g in a microcentrifuge

for 5 min, pour off the supernatant, centrifuge again for a few seconds, remove all the remaining ethanol with a micropipette and allow to dry on the bench with the cap open.

9. Resuspend in a total of 50 µl of water, pool and load onto a G50 spinning column as described below.

G50 spin column

1. Plug an empty 1 ml syringe with a pinch of polymer wool; fill completely with TE equilibrated G50 Sephadex and allow the beads to settle.

2. Place the syringe in a 10 ml centrifuge tube so that the wings of the syringe hold it on to the rim of the tube and there is a void space between the end of the syringe and the bottom of the tube.

3. Centrifuge for 30 s at 400g; the beads will pack down to about 0.9 ml. Fill the tube to the top with TE and centrifuge again for 30 s at 400g.

4. Pour away the TE if this has risen above the bottom of the syringe, add two drops of TE to the top of the column and centrifuge for 4 min at 400g.

5. Take out the column, pour the TE out of the centrifuge tube and drop a 0.5 ml microcentrifuge tube without its cap into the 10 ml tube.

6. Replace the column and if necessary support the microcentrifuge tube so that the end of the syringe sits inside it. Load the DNA solution on to the top of the G50 column and centrifuge for 4 min at 400g; collect the eluate from the column from the microcentrifuge tube.

7. To assess the amount of insert DNA recovered, load a small aliquot (2 µl) on to an agarose minigel and compare the intensity of ethidium bromide staining against a known standard.

LABELLING A DNA FRAGMENT WITH [32]P

There are several different ways of labelling a DNA fragment. The one that is preferred for generating probes of high specific activity for use in Southern blotting is called random priming.[7]

Principle

The DNA fragment to be labelled is denatured in the presence of short random oligonucleotides (6 or 9 bp in length), made of all the possible sequence combinations. As the DNA cools, these oligos anneal to the DNA along its length and act as primers for DNA synthesis by the Klenow fragment of DNA polymerase using the DNA fragment as a template and the four deoxy-nucleotide triphosphates (dNTPs) as building blocks. This synthesis is carried out in the presence of a radiolabelled nucleotide (usually $[\alpha^{32}P]dCTP$) so that the copies of the DNA fragment are made radioactive. Unincorporated nucleotides are removed from the DNA, which is then boiled again before use as a probe so that the labelled single stranded DNA molecules can hybridize to their complementary sequences in the target DNA.

Method

To obtain efficient incorporation of the labelled nucleotide and generate probes with a sufficiently high specific activity for use in genomic Southern hybridization experiments, it is recommended to use a labelling kit. The Megaprime labelling system from Amersham can consistently yield probes with a specific activity greater than 5×10^8 cpm/µg DNA. The method is clearly described in a booklet that accompanies the kit.

Non-radioactive labelling

A number of non-radioactive labelling systems are now available. The advantages of working without hazardous radioisotopes are obvious, and probes can be obtained that will detect single copy genes in a standard Southern blot analysis. An additional advantage is that labelled probes can be stored at −20°C for significant periods of time (at least 3 months), while ^{32}P-labelled probes decay rapidly and need to be freshly prepared each time they are used. However, it is still the case that the sensitivity of a ^{32}P-labelled probe, exposed to X-ray film for 10–14 days, is greater than any non-radioactive method.

The principle of these non-radioactive labelling systems is the same as described above in that random priming is used to generate a labelled DNA fragment. The difference is that instead of a ^{32}P-labelled nucleotide, other labels are utilized such as fluorescein-dUTP. Detection of the hybridization involves horse-radish peroxidase conjugated antibodies and colour or luminescent visualization of bound antibody.

APPENDIX D: PCR

Reagents

PCR buffer I

Take 0.5 ml of 2 mol/l Tris-HCl pH 8.3, 2.5 ml of 2 mol/l KCl, 0.15 ml of 1 mol/l MgCl$_2$, 0.1 ml of 10% gelatin, 0.5 ml of 10% Nonidet P40 and 0.5 ml of 10% Tween 20 and make up the volume to 10 ml with water. Dispense into microcentrifuge tubes and store at −20°C. This is a $10 \times$ concentrated PCR buffer. The final reaction concentration will be 10 mmol/l Tris, 50 mmol/l KCl, 1.5 mmol/l MgCl$_2$, 0.01% gelatin, 0.05% NP40 and 0.05% Tween 20.

PCR buffer II

Take 3.35 ml of 2 mol/l Tris-HCl pH 8.8, 1.66 ml of 1 mol/l (NH$_4$)$_2$SO$_4$, 0.125 ml of 2 mol/l MgCl$_2$, 13.4 µl of 0.5 mol/l Na$_2$EDTA, 80 µl of 20 mg/ml BSA (molecular biology grade) and 70 µl of 14.3 mol/l β-mercapto-ethanol and make up to 10 ml with water. Again, this is a $10 \times$ buffer, the final concentration of which is 670 mmol/l Tris, 166 mmol/l (NH$_4$)$_2$SO$_4$, 25 mmol/l MgCl$_2$, 670 µmol/l Na$_2$EDTA, 160 µg/ml BSA and 100 mmol/l β-mercapto-ethanol. This buffer is used in conjunction with 10% DMSO in the final reaction mixture.

Other reagents

dNTP, 10 mmol/l.
Dimethylsulphoxide (DMSO).
Taq polymerase. See p. 538. This can be purchased from a variety of different companies and may be diluted on arrival with glycerol (final concentration of 50%) and $1 \times$ PCR buffer I (without the MgCl$_2$) to give an enzyme concentration of 1 u/µl. The oligonucleotide primers can be obtained from several commercial companies and they are usually 18–22 bases in length.

Method

The method was first described by Saiki et al[27] in

1988 using PCR buffer I. PCR buffer II, in combination with 10% DMSO, may give better amplification of genes with a high GC content. The magnesium chloride concentration may need to be altered for some primers, with the optimal concentration being derived empirically.

The PCR reaction is set up in a final volume of 25–100 µl; in most cases a 50 µl volume is sufficient to check whether the amplification has been successful and to perform at least one subsequent manipulation. A blank control should always be included (i.e. a reaction without any template) in order to check for contamination. A DNA sample that is known to amplify can also be included and this sample may then be used as a normal or positive control.

Precautions that can greatly reduce the risk of contamination include the use of plugged micropipette tips and an area of the laboratory dedicated to setting up these reactions, away from the area in which they are analysed. In preparing a group of reactions, pipetting errors can be minimized by making a pre-mix solution which can be dispensed into microcentrifuge tubes to which the DNA sample is added last.

1. Prepare a PCR mixture for four reactions (with a final volume of 50 µl for each DNA sample) as follows:

Stock solution	Vol (µl)	Final concentration
10 × PCR buffer	20	1×
10 mmol/l dNTP	4	0.2 mmol/l
Primer (1) 20 pmol/µl	4	0.4 pmol/µl
Primer (2) 20 pmol/µl	4	0.4 pmol/µl
Taq polymerase 1 u/µl	2	0.01 u/µl
Water	162	–
Final volume	196	–

2. Aliquot into four microcentrifuge tubes (i.e. 49 µl into each tube). Add 1 µl of DNA at approximately 0.5 µg/µl into three of the tubes and 1 µl of double distilled water into the fourth tube. Mix well and centrifuge for 5 s in a microcentrifuge.

3. Overlay the mixture with 75 µl of light paraffin oil and place the tubes in a PCR machine, programmed for the following conditions: an initial step of 5 min at 94°C and then 30 cycles of 56°C for 1 min, 72°C for 1 min and 94°C for 1 min in sequence followed by a final extension step at 72°C for 10 min. These conditions are suitable for the majority of primers although some may require a different annealing temperature, or longer extension time.

4. While the PCR program is running, a 1.5% agarose mini-gel (approximately 100 × 76 mm) is prepared: add 0.75 g of agarose to 50 ml of 0.5 × TBE buffer and heat until completely dissolved. Add 5 µl of ethidium bromide (10 mg/ml), allow the agarose to cool slightly and pour with the appropriate comb in position.

5. To check if the amplification has been successful, add 1 µl of tracking dye to a 10 µl aliquot of the PCR reaction mixture, being careful not to pipette the mineral oil overlaying the PCR reaction.

6. Load the gel and run at a constant voltage of 100 V for 1 h in 0.5 × TBE buffer. A molecular size marker should be included to establish the size of the amplified fragment; these are commercially available. The marker used in this chapter is the plasmid pEMBL 8 digested with Taq I and Pvu II to yield fragments of 1443, 1008, 613, 357, 278, 193 and 108 bp.

7. Visualize the DNA on a UV transilluminator and, if required, take a photograph.

APPENDIX E: RESTRICTION ENZYME DIGESTION OF PCR PRODUCTS

The restriction enzyme digest is set up as described below in a final volume of 40 µl using 1–5 units of the restriction enzyme. In many cases the universal restriction enzyme buffer (see Appendix A) is suitable, but it is important to check with the enzyme manufacturer's instructions for the precise conditions. For example, the enzyme Mae I, which detects the common β^0-thalassaemia mutation in codon 39 of the β globin gene, fails to cut in the universal buffer.

1. Transfer 30 µl of the amplified product to a new microcentrifuge tube, being careful not to transfer any of the mineral oil. Add 4 µl of 10 × restriction enzyme buffer, 4.5 µl of double distilled water and 2–5 units of the appropriate restriction enzyme (usually 0.5 µl), giving a final volume of 40 µl.

2. Incubate at 37°C (or other appropriate temperature) for a minimum of 4 h. In preparing

more than one digestion with the same restriction enzyme, sufficient buffer, enzyme and water can be pre-mixed and dispensed into micro-centrifuge tubes before adding 30 µl of the PCR product.

3. While the tubes are incubating, a 3.0% agarose mini gel is poured. The gel is made up of 1:1 mixture of type II medium electroendosmosis agarose and Nusieve agarose (from FMC Bioproducts), i.e. 0.75 g of agarose and 0.75 g of Nusieve agarose in 50 ml of half-strength (0.5 ×) TBE buffer (see Appendix C).

4. After the incubation period, add 4 µl of tracking dye to the digests and load the samples on to the gel. The electrophoresis is continued until a clear separation of all the expected fragments is achieved, which may be checked at intervals by placing the gel on a UV trans-illuminator.

GLOSSARY (Courtesy of Professor Lucio Luzzatto)

Alleles. Alternate forms of a gene found at a particular locus, e.g. β^A, β^S and β^{thal}. There may be many different alleles in a population, but two at the most in one individual.

Base pair (bp). A single pairing of the nucleotides A with T or G with C in a DNA double helix (in RNA, A pairs with U).

cDNA. A DNA molecule complementary to an RNA molecule, usually synthesized in vitro by the enzyme reverse transcriptase.

Clone, cellular. The progeny of a single cell. Cells belonging to the same clone are referred to as a monoclonal cell population.

Clone, molecular. A large number of identical DNA molecules, usually obtained by propagation of a single plasmid or bacteriophage molecule in bacteria.

Codon. A triplet of nucleotides that codes for an amino acid or termination signal.

Deletion. A mutation caused by the removal of a sequence of DNA, with the regions on either side being joined together.

Exon. A segment of a gene that codes for protein.

Gene. The unit of inheritance. In biochemical terms a gene specifies the structure of a protein, which is the gene product. In molecular terms, a gene is a stretch of DNA that is transcribed in one block, a transcription unit.

Genomic clone. A molecular clone consisting of a portion of cellular DNA.

Genotype. The genetic constitution of an individual

Heterozygote. An individual with two different alleles on the homologous chromosomes at a particular locus.

Hybridization. The pairing of complementary RNA or DNA strands to give an RNA-DNA hybrid or a DNA duplex.

Intron. A segment of a gene that is transcribed but is removed in the mature messenger RNA and therefore does not code for protein.

Linkage. The co-inheritance of genes as a result of their neighbouring location on the same chromosome.

Locus. The position on a chromosome where a particular gene is located.

Mutation. A particular change in the sequence of genomic DNA.

Northern blotting. A technique for transfering RNA from an agarose gel to a nitrocellulose or nylon filter on which it can be recognized by a suitable probe.

Oligonucleotide (Oligo). A short single stranded DNA molecule, usually synthesized in vitro.

Phenotype. The appearance of an individual person or cell. In relation to a particular genetic character, the phenotype reflects the genotype conferring that character plus the effects of the environment.

Plasmid. An autonomously replicating extra-chromosomal circular DNA molecule, e.g. pBR322 and pUC19.

Point mutation. A change of a single base pair in DNA.

Polymerase chain reaction (PCR). A technique for amplifying an individual DNA sequence in vitro. The reaction is primed by using specific oligonucleotides.

Primers. Oligonucleotides use to initiate DNA synthesis in vitro by the enzyme DNA polymerase.

Probe. A fragment of DNA that can be used to hybridize to a specific DNA sequence or RNA molecule.

Recombinant DNA. Any DNA molecule constructed artificially by bringing together DNA segments of different origin.

Restriction enzymes. Enzymes that recognize short DNA sequences (usually 4 or 6 base pairs) and cut the DNA wherever those sequences are found (e.g. BamH I, Bgl II, EcoR I, Hind III, Pst I and Sac I). These sequences are called restriction sites.

Southern blotting. The procedure for transfering denatured DNA from an agarose gel to a nitrocellulose or nylon filter, where it can be recognized by an appropriate probe.

Vector. A DNA molecule capable of replication and specifically engineered to facilitate the cloning of another DNA molecule of interest.

LIST OF ABBREVIATIONS

ARMS	Amplification refractory mutation system
ASOH	Allele specific oligonucleotide hybridization
bp	Base pair
CTP	Cytosine triphosphate
DNA	Deoxyribonucleic acid
Ig	Immunoglobulin
kb	Kilobase pairs
PCR	Polymerase chain reaction
RE	Restriction enzyme
RFLP	Restriction fragment length polymorphism
RNA	Ribonucleic acid
SDS	Sodium dodecyl sulphate
SSC	Standard sodium citrate
TAE	Tris acetate EDTA buffer
TBE	Tris borate EDTA buffer
TCR	T cell receptor
TE	Tris EDTA buffer
VNTR	Variable number tandem repeat

REFERENCES

[1] BOWDEN, D. K., VICKERS, M. A. and HIGGS D. R. (1992). A PCR-based strategy to detect the common severe determinants of α thalassaemia. *British Journal of Haematology*, **81**, 104.

[2] BOTSTEIN, D., WHITE, R. L., SKOLNICK, M. and DAVIES, R. W. (1980). Construction of a genetic linkage map in man using restriction fragment length polymorphisms. *American Journal of Human Genetics*, **32**, 314.

[3] BOURGUIN, A., TUNG, R., GALILI, N. and SKLAR, J. (1990). Rapid, nonradioactive detection of clonal T-cell receptor gene rearrangements in lymphoid neoplasms. *Proceedings of the National Academy of Sciences, U.S.A*, **87**, 8536.

[4] CAO, A. and ROSATELLI, R. (1993). Screening and prenatal diagnosis of the haemoglobinopathies. *Balliére's Clinical Haematology*, **6**, 263.

[5] CHOMCZYNSKI, P. and SACCHI, I. (1987). Single step method of RNA isolation by acid guanidinium thiocyanate phenol chloroform extraction. *Annals of Biochemistry*, **162**, 156.

[6] CROSS, N. C. P., HUGHES, T. P., FENG, L., O'SHEA, P., BUNGEY, J., MARKS, D. I., FERRANT, A., MARTIAT, P. and GOLDMAN, J. M. (1993). Minimal residual disease after allogeneic bone marrow transplantation for chronic myeloid leukaemia in first chronic phase: correlation with acute graft versus host disease and relapse. *British Journal of Haematology*, **84**, 67.

[7] FEINBERG, A. P. and VOGELSTEIN, B. (1984). A technique for radiolabelling DNA restriction endonuclease fragments to high specific activity. *Annals of Biochemistry*, **137**, 266

[8] FISCHEL-GHODSIAN, N., VICKERS, M. A., SEIP, M., WINICHAGOON, P. and HIGGS, D. R. (1988). Characterization of two deletions that remove the entire human ζ-α globin gene compex (--THAI and --FIL). *British Journal of Haematology*, **70**, 2338.

[9] FLANAGAN, J. C. and RABBITTS, T. H. (1982). Arrangement of human immunoglobulin heavy chain constant region genes implies evolutionary duplication of a segment containing γ, ε and α genes. *Nature*, **300**, 709.

[10] FLAVELL, R. A., KOOTER, J. W. Q. and DE BOER, E. (1978). Analysis of the β globin gene in normal and Hb Lepore DNA. Direct determination of gene linkage and intergene distance. *Cell*, **15**, 25.

[11] FORONI, L., MASON, P. and LUZZATTO, L. (1991). Immunoglobulin and T-cell receptor gene analysis for the investigation of lymphoproliferative disorders. In *The Leukemic Cell*. Ed. D. Catovsky, pp. 339–391. Churchill Livingstone, Edinburgh.

[12] GIANNELLI, F., GREEN, P. M., HIGH, K. A., SOMMER, S., LILLICRAP, D. P., LUDWIG, M., OLEK, K., REITSMA, P. H., GOOSENS, M., YOSHIOKA, A. and BROWNLEE, G. G. (1992). Haemophilia B: database of point mutations and short additions and deletions—third edition, 1992. *Nucleic Acids Research*, **20**, 2027.

[13] GITSCHIER, J., DRAYNA, D., TUDDENHAM, E. G. D., WHITE, R. L. and LAWN, R. M. (1985). Genetic mapping and diagnosis of haemophilia A achieved through a Bcl I polymorphism in the factor VIII gene. *Nature*, **314**, 738.

[14] GOODBOURN, S. E. Y., HIGGS, D. R., CLEGG, J. B. and WEATHERALL, D. J. (1983). Molecular basis of length polymorphism in the human ζ globin gene complex. *Proceedings of the National Academy of Sciences, U.S.A*, **80**, 5022.

[15] HIGGS, D. R., VICKERS, M. A., WILKIE, A. O. M., PRETORIUS, I.-M., JARMAN, A. P. and WEATHERALL, D. J. (1989). A review of the molecular genetics of the human α-globin gene cluster. *Blood*, **73**, 1081.

[16] HUISMAN, T. H. J. (1992). The β- and δ-thalassaemia repository. *Haemoglobin*, **16**, 237.

[17] KAN, Y. W. and DOZY, A. M. (1978). Antenatal diagnosis of sickle-cell anaemia by DNA analysis of amniotic-fluid cells. *Lancet*, **ii**, 910.

[18] KAZAZIAN, H. H. (1990). The thalassaemic syndromes: molecular basis and prenatal diagnosis in 1990. *Seminars in Haematology*, **27**, 209.

[19] KOGAN, S. C., DOHERTY, M. and GITSCHIER, J. (1987). An improved method for prenatal diagnosis of genetic diseases by analysis of amplified DNA sequences: application to hemophilia A. *New England Journal of Medicine*, **317**, 985.

[20] NEWTON, C. R., GRAHAM, A., HEPTINSTALL, L. E., POWELL, S. J., SUMMERS, C., KALSHEKAR, N. and SMITH, J. C. (1989). Analysis of any point mutation in DNA. The amplification refractory mutation system (ARMS). *Nucleic Acids Research*, **17**, 2503.

[21] LALLOZ, M. R., MCVEY, J., PATTINSON, J. and TUDDENHAM, E. G. D (1991). Haemophilia A diagnosis by analysis of a hypervariable dinucleotide repeat within the factor VIII gene. *Lancet*, **338**, 207.

[22] NICHOLLS, R. D., FISCHEL-GHODSIAN, N. and HIGGS, D. R. (1987). Recombination at the human α globin gene cluster: sequence features and topological constraints. *Cell*, **49**, 369.

[23] NIH/CEPH COLLABORATIVE MAPPING GROUP (1992). A comprehensive genetic linkage map of the human genome. *Science*, **258**, 67.

[24] OBERLE, I., CAMERINO, G., HELIG, R., GRUNEBAUM, L., CAZENAVE, J.-P., CRAPANZANO, C., MANNUCCI, P. M. and MANDEL, J.-L. (1985). Genetic screening for hemophilia A (classic hemophilia) with a polymorphic DNA probe. *New England Journal of Medicine*, **312**, 682.

[25] OLD, J. M., VARAWALLA, N. Y. and WEATHERALL, D. J. (1990). Rapid detection and prenatal diagnosis of β-thalassaemia: studies in Indian and Cypriot populations in the U.K. *Lancet*, **336**, 834.

[26] ORKIN, S. H., LITTLE, K. P. F. R., KAZAZIAN, H. H. and BOEHM, C. D. (1982). Improved detection of the sickle mutation by DNA analysis. *New England Journal of Medicine*, **307**, 30.

[27] SAIKI, R., GELFAND, D. H., STOFFEL, B., SCHARF, S. J., HIGUCHI, R., HORN, G. T., MULLIS, K. B. and ERLICH, H. A. (1988). Primer-directed enzymatic amplification of DNA with a thermostable DNA polymerase. *Science*, **239**, 487.

[28] SAIKI, R. K., CHANG, C. A., LEVENSON, C. H., WARREN, B. A., BOEHM, C. D., KAZAZIAN, H. H. and ERLICH, H. A. (1988). Diagnosis of sickle cell anemia and beta-thalassemia with enzymatically amplified DNA and non-radioactive allele specific oligonucleotide probes. *New England Journal of Medicine*, **319**, 537.

[29] SAMBROOK, J., FRITSCH, E. F. and MANIATIS, T. (1989). *Molecular Cloning. A Laboratory Manual*, 2nd edn. Cold Spring Harbor Laboratory Press, Cold Spring Harbor.

[30] SEGAL, G. H., WITTWER, C. T., FISHLEDER, A. J., STOLER, M. H., TUBBS, R. R. and KJELDSBERG, C. R. (1992). Identification of monoclonal B-cell populations by rapid cycle polymerase chain reaction. *American Journal of Pathology*, **141**, 1291.

[31] SIMMS, J. E., TUNNACLIFFE, A., SMITH, W. J. and RABBITTS, T. H. (1984). Complexity of human T-cell antigen receptor β chain constant and variable region genes. *Nature*, **312**, 541.

[32] SOUTHERN, E. (1975). Detection of specific sequences using DNA fragments separated by gel electrophoresis. *Journal of Molecular Biology*, **98**, 503.

[33] SYKES, B. C. (1983). DNA in heritable disease. *Lancet*, **ii,**. 787.

[34] TUAN, D., MURNANE, M. J., DE RIEL, J. K. and FORGET, B. G. (1980). Heterogeneity in the molecular basis of hereditary persistence of fetal haemoglobin. *Nature*, **285**, 335.

[35] TUDDENHAM, E. G. D., COOPER, D. N., GITSCHIER, J., HIGUCHI, M., HOYER, L. M., YOSHIOKA, A., PEAKE, I. R., SCHWABB, R., OLEK, K., KAZAZIAN, H. H., LAVERGNE, J.-M., GIANELLI, F. and ANTONARAKIS, S. E. (1991). Haemophilia A—database of nucleotide substitutions, deletions, insertions and rearrangements of the factor VIII gene. *Nucleic Acids Research*, **19**, 4821.

[36] VULLIAMY, T. J., BEUTLER, E. and LUZZATTO, L. (1993). Variants of glucose-6-phosphate dehydrogenase are due to missense mutations spread throughout the coding region of the gene. *Human Mutation*, **2**, 159.

[37] WAINSCOAT, J. S., OLD, J, M., WOOD, W. G., TRENT, R. J. and WEATHERALL, D. J. (1984). Characterization of an Indian (δβ)° thalassaemia. *British Journal of Haematology*, **58**, 353.

[38] WALDMANN, T. A. (1987). The arrangement of immunoglobulin and T cell receptor genes in human lymphoproliferative disorders. *Advances in Immunology*, **40**, 247.

[39] WALLACE, R. B., SHAFFER, J., MURPHY, R. F., BONNER, J., HIROSE, T. and IKATURA, K. (1979). Hybridization of synthetic oligodeoxyribonucleotides to PhiX174 DNA: the effect of single base pair mismatch. *Nucleic Acids Research*, **6**, 3543.

[40] WATSON, J. D., GILMAN, M., WITKOWSKI, J. and ZOLLER, M. (1992). *Recombinant DNA*, 2nd edn. Scientific American Books, Freeman & Company, New York.

[41] WEATHERALL, D. J. (1991). *The New Genetics and Clinical Practice*, 3rd edn. Oxford University Press, Oxford.

[42] WEBER J. L. and MAY, P. E. (1989). Abundant class of human DNA polymorphisms which can be typed using the polymerase chain reaction. *American Journal of Human Genetics*, **44**, 388.

[43] WEISSENBACH, J., GYPAY, G., DIB, C., VIGNAL, A., MORISETTE, J., MILLASSEAU, P., VAYSSEIX, G. and LATHROP, M. (1992). A second generation linkage map of the human genome. *Nature*, **359**, 794.

[44] WION, K-L., TUDDENHAM, E. G. D. and LAWN, R. (1986). A new polymorphism in the factor VIII gene for prenatal diagnosis of haemophilia A. *Nucleic Acids Research*, **14**, 4535.

29. Miscellaneous tests

Tests for the acute phase response 559
Erythrocyte sedimentation rate (ESR) 559
  Westergren method 559
  Modified methods 560
Plasma viscosity 563
Whole-blood viscosity 563

Tests for infectious mononucleosis 564
  Slide screening test 564
  Paul Bunnell test 565
Demonstration of antinuclear factors 568
Demonstration of LE cells 569
Erythropoietin 571

TESTS FOR THE ACUTE PHASE RESPONSE

Inflammatory response to tissue injury (the acute phase response) includes alteration in serum protein concentration, especially increases in fibrinogen and C-reactive protein and decrease in albumin. The changes occur in both acute inflammation and during active phases of chronic inflammation.

Measurement of the acute phase response is a helpful indicator of the presence and extent of inflammation and its response to treatment. Useful tests include estimation of C-reactive protein, fibrinogen and measurement of the erythrocyte sedimentation rate and plasma viscosity.

THE ERYTHROCYTE SEDIMENTATION RATE (ESR)

The erythrocyte sedimentation rate is influenced both by the proteins of the acute phase response and by anaemia which may be present in inflammatory disease, whereas plasma viscosity reflects only the protein component. The method for measuring the ESR which has been recommended by the International Council for Standardization in Haematology[43,47] and also by various national authorities[11,62] is based on that of Westergren.[80] In this, diluted blood is sedimented in an open-ended glass tube of 30 cm length mounted vertically on a stand. To make the test more reproducible a standardized method has been proposed in which EDTA blood is used and its PCV is adjusted to 0.35. This is, however, too laborious for routine use. Because of the biohazard risk of blood contamination inherent in using open-ended tubes, it is now recommended that, where possible, a closed system be used in routine practice.[78] Several automated closed systems are now available, e.g. Sediscan (Becton Dickinson) and Starrsed (R & R Mechatronics). These use either blood collected in special evacuated tubes containing citrate or EDTA blood which is taken up through a piercable cap and then automatically diluted in the system.

Westergren method

The recommended tube is a straight glass tube 30 cm in length and not less than 2.55 mm in diameter. The bore must be uniform to within 5% throughout. A scale graduated in mm extends over the lower 20 cm. The tube must be clean and dry and kept free from dust.

After use it should be thoroughly washed in tap

water, then rinsed with acetone and allowed to dry before being reused. Specially made racks with adjustable levelling screws are available for holding the sedimentation tubes firmly in an exactly vertical position. The rack must be constructed so that there will be no leakage of the blood from the tube. It is conventional to set up sedimentation-rate tests at room temperature (18–25°C). Sedimentation is normally accelerated as the temperature rises[58] and if the test is to be carried out at a higher ambient temperature, a normal range should be established for that temperature. Exceptionally, when high-thermal-amplitude cold agglutinins are present, sedimentation becomes noticeably less rapid as the temperature is raised towards 37°C.

109 mmol/l trisodium citrate (32 g/l $Na_3Ca_6H_5O_7.2H_2O$) is used as the anticoagulant diluent solution. It is filtered through a micropore filter (0.22 μm) into a sterile bottle. It can be stored for several months at 4°C but must be discarded if it becomes turbid through the growth of moulds. The test is performed on venous blood diluted accurately in the proportion of 1 volume of citrate to 4 volumes of blood. The usual practice is to collect the blood directly into the citrate solution. The test, however, can be carried out equally well with blood anticoagulated with EDTA, provided that 1 volume of 109 mmol/l (32 g/l) trisodium citrate is added to 4 volumes of blood immediately before the test is performed. The sedimentation rate is reduced in stored blood; the test should thus be carried out within 4 h of collecting the blood, although a delay of up to 6 h is permissible provided that the blood is kept at 4°C.

Mix the blood sample thoroughly and then draw it up into the Westergren tube to the 200 mm mark by means of a teat or a mechanical device; mouth suction should never be used. Place the tube exactly vertical and leave undisturbed for 60 min, free from vibrations and draughts, and not exposed to direct sunlight. Then read to the nearest 1 mm the height of the clear plasma above the upper limit of the column of sedimenting cells. The result is expressed as ESR = X mm in 1 h. This is not strictly a 'rate'; some procedures give readings after a shorter period, but these results should then be

'normalized' to the values which would be expected at 1 h. A poor delineation of the upper layer of red cells, so called 'stratified sedimentation', has been attributed to the presence of many reticulocytes.[75]

Range in health

The mean values and the upper limit for 95% of normal adults are given in Table 29.1. There is a progressive increase with age, but above 70 years it is difficult to define a strictly healthy population for determining normal values.

In the newborn the ESR is usually low. In childhood and adolescence it is the same as for normal men with no differences between boys and girls.

Modified methods

A number of variations have been developed, especially for automated methods and closed systems. Whenever a different method is planned, a preliminary test should be carried out in order to compare results with those obtained by the standardized method described below.

Length of tube. The overall length of the tube is not a critical dimension for the test provided that it fits firmly in an appropriate holding device. The tube must, however, be long enough to ensure that packing of the cells does not start before the test has been completed.

Plastic tubes. A number of plastic materials—for example, polypropylene and polycarbonate—are possible substitutes for glass in Westergren tubes.[72] Nevertheless, not all plastics have similar pro-

Table 29.1   ESR ranges in health

Age (years)	95% upper limit
Men	
17–50	10
51–60	12
61–70	14
>70	c 30
Women	
17–50	12
51–60	19
61–70	20
>70	c 35

perties and it must be demonstrated that the results with the chosen tubes are reproducible and comparable with those obtained with the standard method.

Disposable glass tubes. These should be supplied clean and dry and ready for use. It is necessary to show that neither the tube material nor the manufacturer's cleaning process affects the ESR.

Capillary method. Short tubes of narrower bore than in the standard tube are available mainly for tests on infants. Sedimentation is slower in these tubes and it is necessary to establish normal ranges or a correction factor to convert results to the equivalent ESR by the standard Westergren method.

ICSH STANDARDIZED METHOD[47]

This is carried out on EDTA blood not diluted in citrate, using Westergren tubes as described above. The PCV should be 0.35 or less; if necessary, adjust the PCV by centrifuging the specimen, remove an appropriate amount of plasma or red cells and then resuspend the cells by thorough mixing.

Immediately before filling the ESR tube, mix the specimen by at least eight complete inversions. Measure the ESR on each specimen (undiluted) by the standardized Westergren method.

Correct the reading for lack of dilution as follows:

Corrected ESR (mm in 1 h) =
(undiluted ESR × 0.86) – 12.

Verification of a method[47]

Select 10 EDTA blood specimens the ESR of which by the routine method is in the range 15–105 mm in 1 h and PCV is 0.30–0.35. Fill the tubes as described above for the standardized method. At the same time carry out the ESR by the method which is to be verified on aliquots of the same specimens (after appropriate dilution) or on blood collected separately from the same subjects in accordance with specified requirements, e.g. directly into tubes containing citrate.

The routine method is satisfactory if 95% of results are within the limits given in Table 29.2.

Quality control[78]

Perform a quality control check whenever routine ESR tests are performed. Select one blood sample with a PCV between 0.30 and 0.36 and perform the ESR by the routine method and by the undiluted Westergren ESR method as described above. Apply the formula to obtain the corrected ESR for the undiluted sample.

The test is satisfactorily controlled if the results by the routine method do not differ from those obtained by the ICSH standardized method by more than the limits shown in Table 29.2.

Mechanism of erythrocyte sedimentation

The phenomenon of erythrocyte sedimentation has been investigated exhaustively.[10,34,46,81]

The rate of fall of the red cells is influenced by a number of inter-reacting factors. Basically, it depends upon the difference in specific gravity between red cells and plasma, but it is influenced very greatly by the extent to which the red cells form rouleaux, which sediment more rapidly than single cells. Other factors which affect sedimentation include the ratio of red cells to plasma, i.e. the PCV, the plasma viscosity, the verticality or otherwise of the sedimentation tube, the bore of the tube and the dilution, if any, of the blood.

The all-important rouleaux formation and red-cell clumping are mainly controlled by the concentrations of fibrinogen and other acute-phase proteins, e.g. haptoglobin, ceruloplasmin, α_1 acid-glycoprotein, α_1 antitrypsin and c-reactive protein. Rouleaux formation is also enhanced by the immunoglobulins. It is retarded by albumin. Defibrinated blood normally sediments extremely slowly, not more than 1 mm in 1 h, unless the serum-globulin concentration is raised or there is an unusually high globulin:albumin ratio.

Anaemia, by altering the ratio of red cells to plasma, encourages rouleaux formation and accelerates sedimentation. In anaemia, too, cellular factors may affect sedimentation. Thus in iron-deficiency anaemia a reduction in the intrinsic ability of the red cells to sediment may compensate for the accelerating effect of an increased proportion of plasma.[68]

Sedimentation can be observed to take place in three stages: a preliminary stage of at least a few

Table 29.2 ESR values (mm) for verification of comparability of working (routine) method with ICSH standardized method

Standardized method*	Working method limits**	Standardized method*	Working method limits**	Standardized method*	Working method limits**
15	3–13	45	18–37	75	40–68
16	4–14	46	18–38	76	40–69
17	4–15	47	19–38	77	41–70
18	4–15	48	20–39	78	42–71
19	5–16	49	20–40	79	43–72
20	5–17	50	21–41	80	44–73
21	6–17	51	22–42	81	45–74
22	6–18	52	22–43	82	45–76
23	6–19	53	23–44	83	46–77
24	7–19	54	24–45	84	47–78
25	7–20	55	24–46	85	48–79
26	8–21	56	25–47	86	49–80
27	8–21	57	26–48	87	50–82
28	9–22	58	26–49	88	51–83
29	9–23	59	27–50	89	52–84
30	10–24	60	28–51	90	53–85
31	10–25	61	29–52	91	53–86
32	11–25	62	29–53	92	54–88
33	11–26	63	30–54	93	55–89
34	12–27	64	31–56	94	56–90
35	12–28	65	32–57	95	57–91
36	13–29	66	32–58	96	58–93
37	13–30	67	33–59	97	59–94
38	14–30	68	34–60	98	60–95
39	14–31	69	35–61	99	61–96
40	15–32	70	35–62	100	62–98
41	15–33	71	36–63	101	63–99
42	16–34	72	37–64	102	64–100
43	17–35	73	38–65	103	65–101
44	17–36	74	39–66	104	66–103
				105	67–104

*Standardized method: EDTA anticoagulated but undiluted whole blood of haematocrit of 0.35 or less.
**Working method: 4 volumes EDTA blood plus 1 volume citrate diluent.
The values incorporate a correction for dilution of blood by citrate in the working method. Proposed working method valid if 95% of results are within indicated limits.
Reproduced with permission from the *Journal of Clinical Pathology*.[47]

minutes during which time rouleaux occur and aggregations form; then a period in which the sinking of the aggregates takes place at approximately a constant speed, and finally a phase during which the rate of sedimentation slows as the aggregated cells pack at the bottom of the tube. It is obvious that the longer the tube used the longer the second period can last and the greater the sedimentation rate may appear to be. This is an advantage of the Westergren tube. With a shorter tube, e.g. a Wintrobe tube, packing may start before an hour has elapsed.

Significance of the measurement of the erythrocyte sedimentation rate in clinical medicine

Although the ESR is a non-specific phenomenon, its measurement is clinically useful in disorders associated with an increased production of acute-phase proteins. In rheumatoid arthritis or tuberculosis it provides an index of progress of the disease, and it is also useful as a screening test in the routine examination of patients. An elevated ESR occurs as an early feature in myocardial infarction.[32] Although a normal ESR cannot be taken to exclude the presence of organic disease, the fact remains that the vast majority of acute or chronic infections and most neoplastic and degenerative diseases are associated with changes in the plasma proteins which lead to an acceleration of sedimentation. The ESR is higher in women than in men, and correlates with sex differences in fibrinogen levels.[6] An increase in fibrinogen occurs in normal pregnancy, resulting in increased red cell aggregation and elevated sedimentation.[42] The ESR is influenced by age, stage of the menstrual cycle and drugs (e.g. corticosteroids, contraceptive pills); it is especially low (0–1 mm) in polycythaemia, hypofibrinogenaemia and congestive cardiac failure, and when there are abnormalities of the red cells such as poikilocytosis, spherocytosis or sickle cells.

PLASMA VISCOSITY

The ESR and plasma viscosity in general increase in parallel. Plasma viscosity is, however, primarily dependent on the concentration of plasma proteins, especially fibrinogen, and it is not affected by anaemia. Change in viscosity seems to reflect the clinical severity of disease more closely than does the ESR.[24,35] Also, changes in the ESR may lag behind changes in plasma viscosity by 24–48 h.[24]

There are several types of viscometer; these are based on three principles.[35,46]

1. The rotational viscometer in which shear stress is determined at different shear rates.
2. The rolling ball viscometer in which the rate of rolling of a metal ball is measured in a tilted tube filled with plasma and calibrated with fluids of known viscosity.
3. The capillary viscometer in which comparison is made of the flow rate of plasma and distilled water under equal pressure and constant temperature through capillary tubes of equal bore and length. The results are expressed as viscosity of plasma relative to that of water.

Most reports of clinical studies have been based on the capillary viscometer. It requires only 0.3–0.5 ml of plasma, obtained from EDTA blood. Results are highly reproducible (CV 1%);

they are, however, very sensitive to changes in temperature. The test is usually performed at 25°C although some workers recommend 37°C;[44,65] in either case the temperature should be closely controlled, with a variation of less than ±0.5°C.

Precision is also affected by the way the plasma sample has been obtained and prepared; the formation of a fibrin clot will invalidate the test. Venous blood should be collected with minimum stasis into EDTA (1.2 mg/ml) and, as soon as possible, centrifuged in a stoppered tube at 3000g for 5 min to obtain clear plasma. After separation, the plasma, if sterile, can be stored in a stoppered tube at room temperature (not in a refrigerator) for up to 1 week without change to its viscosity.

The actual test should be carried out as described in the instruction manual for the particular instrument used.

Reference values[44,46]

Normal plasma has a viscosity of 1.16–1.33 (mean 1.24) mPa/s* at 37°C; 1.50–1.72 (mean 1.60) mPa/s at 25°C. Plasma viscosity is lower in the newborn (0.98–1.25 mPa/s at 37°C), rising to adult values by the third year; it is slightly higher in old age. There are no significant differences in plasma viscosity between men and women, or in pregnancy. It is remarkably constant in health, with little or no diurnal variation, and it is not affected by exercise. A change of only 0.03–0.05 mPa/s is thus likely to be clinically significant.

WHOLE-BLOOD VISCOSITY

The viscosity of blood reflects its rheological properties; it is influenced by PCV, plasma viscosity, red cell aggregation and red cell deformability. It is especially sensitive to PCV, with which it is closely correlated. Its measurement has, however, limited clinical value as it does not take account of the interaction of the red cells with blood vessels which greatly influences

---

*Previously measured in 'poise' (P); 1 cP = 1 mPa/s.

blood flow in vivo. Guidelines for measuring blood viscosity and red cell deformability by standardized methods have been published.[44,45]

Rotational and capillary viscometers are suitable for measuring blood viscosity. Deformability can be measured by recording the rate at which red cells in suspension pass through a filter with pores 3–5 μm in diameter.

TESTS FOR HETEROPHILE ANTIBODIES IN HUMAN SERUM: THE PAUL-BUNNELL TEST FOR THE DIAGNOSIS OF INFECTIOUS MONONUCLEOSIS

The presence of anti-sheep-cell haemagglutinins at unusually high titres in the sera of patients suffering from infectious mononucleosis (glandular fever) was described in 1932 by Paul and Bunnell.[63] These (Paul-Bunnell) antibodies are immunologically related to but distinct from the type of anti-sheep red cell antibodies which may develop in serum sickness (see p. 566). The Paul-Bunnell antibodies are, however, not specific for sheep red cells. Thus, they react with horse red cells and ox red cells also; but they do not react with human red cells. They are known to be IgM (19S) globulins.[12,13]

For the diagnosis of infectious mononucleosis, it is necessary to demonstrate that the antibody present has the characters of the Paul-Bunnell antibody, i.e. it is absorbed by ox red cells but not by guinea-pig kidney. This is the basis of the absorption tests for infectious mononucleosis. Although sheep red cells have been widely used to demonstrate the Paul-Bunnell antibody, horse red cells give even better results.[54] Either type of cell, preserved by formalin, can be used in screening tests,[38] however, the preserved cells are less able to detect low-titre antibodies than are fresh horse cells.[53,74]

A SLIDE SCREENING TEST FOR INFECTIOUS MONONUCLEOSIS

Reagents

Sera. Patient's serum (fresh or inactivated by heating at 56°C for 30 min), and positive and negative control sera.

Red cell suspension. 20% suspension of horse blood in 109 mmol/l (32 g/l) trisodium citrate. Before use the suspension must be well mixed by repeated inversion. For the screening test it is unnecessary to wash the cells.

Guinea-pig kidney emulsion. See p. 567.

10% autoclaved ox red suspension. See p. 568.

Method[53]

Place 1 large drop (approximately 30 μl) of guinea-pig kidney emulsion and 1 large drop of ox-cell suspension on two adjacent squares on an opal glass tile. Add 1 drop of test serum adjacent to each. Deliver 10 μl of horse-blood suspension to the corner of each square, by means of a micropipette avoiding contact with the drops in the squares. With a wooden applicator stick, mix the reagents (guinea-pig kidney emulsion or ox-cell suspension, serum and horse-blood suspension) and then examine with the naked eye for agglutination, using oblique light at an angle over a dark background. Negative and positive serum controls should always be set up at the same time. The appearances are shown in Fig. 29.1.

Interpretation

Positive. Agglutination is stronger in the square containing guinea-pig kidney emulsion than in the square containing ox red cell suspension.

Negative. Agglutination is absent in both squares.

In one study on 500 students the test was shown to have a sensitivity of 86% and specificity of 99%[31] where the diagnosis was established by the presence of EBV-specific antibody. False

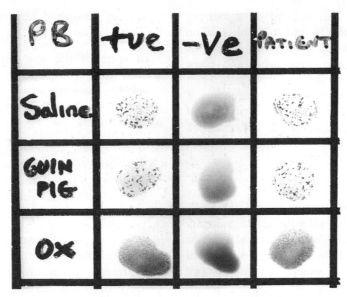

Fig. 29.1 Slide screening test for infectious mononucleosis. Upper: guinea pig kidney. Lower: ox cell suspension.

positives have been reported in malignant lymphomas,[59] malaria,[69] rubella[63] and other diseases, and also occasionally without any apparent underlying disease.[40] A false negative is likely to occur with plasma from EDTA blood.

The reagents for the screening test are available commercially as diagnostic kits (e.g. Monospot (Ortho) and Serascan (Biostat). As different kits have been reported to vary in their performance,[71] positive and negative controls should always be used. Infectious mononucleosis is caused by the Epstein-Barr virus (EBV). Infection gives rise to specific antibody reactions to the nuclear antigen-1 (anti-EBNA-1).[77] Immunofluorescent tests have been developed which are designed to demonstrate the presence of these antibodies and to distinguish IgM antibody which occurs at high titre in the early phase of infection, diminishing during convalescence, from IgG antibody which persists at high titre for years after infection.[26,37]

Screening tests are available based on enzyme-linked immunosorbent assay (ELISA) (e.g. Monalert (Ortho)) and on immunochromatographic assay (Cards Mono kit, Pacific Biotech (Biostat)). These tests are more elaborate than the slide screening test described above, but they are said to be more sensitive and specific.

QUANTITATIVE PAUL-BUNNELL TEST

When the screening test is positive or doubtful a quantitative test with differential absorption should be carried out. The technique described below is based upon that of Barrett[7] and uses sheep red cells, but horse red cells, as recommended by Lee, Davidson and Slaby[54] can equally well be used.

Reagents

Patient's serum and positive control serum. 1 ml, previously inactivated by heating at 56°C for 30 min.

Guinea-pig kidney emulsion. See p. 567.

10% autoclaved ox red cell suspension. See p. 568.

Sheep red cells. 0.4% suspension in 9 g/l NaCl (saline). The sheep blood should preferably be not more than 7 days old. If stored red cells are used instead, they should be washed three times in saline immediately before the test.

Absorption of serum

Deliver three 0.25 ml volumes of patient's inactivated serum into three small glass or plastic tubes, A, B and C. Add 1.0 ml of saline to Tube

A, 0.75 ml of saline and 0.3 ml of guinea-pig kidney emulsion to Tube B, and 0.75 ml of saline and 0.25 ml of 10% ox-cell suspension to Tube C. Mix the contents of the three tubes and place them at 4°C for at least 2 h or overnight. Then centrifuge the tubes and retain the supernatants. 1 in 5 dilutions in saline of unabsorbed serum and of the serum absorbed with guinea-pig kidney and ox red cells, respectively, are thus obtained.

Method

Make serial dilutions of the sera from Tubes A, B and C in saline; 0.15–0.2 ml volumes are suitable. Nine 75 × 8 mm tubes and a control tube to contain saline are usually sufficient. Add equal volumes of the 0.4% sheep (or horse) cell suspension to each tube, giving final serum dilutions of from 1 in 10 (Tube 1) to 1 in 2560 (Tube 9). After mixing their contents, incubate the tubes for 2 h at 37°C before reading the results. A standardized method of reading the end-point should be adopted. Macroscopic reading using a concave mirror is recommended (p. 456). A serum known to contain Paul-Bunnell antibody provides a control for the potency of the absorbents and the agglutinability of the red cells.

Interpretation

The following figures are given as examples of typical results with sheep cells:

1. Unabsorbed serum, end-point Tube 7; titre 640. Guinea-pig kidney absorbed serum, end-point Tube 7; titre 640.
   Ox-cell absorbed serum, end-point Tube 4; titre 80.

Such a result would be positive for infectious mononucleosis, the antibody being not absorbed by guinea-pig kidney and significantly absorbed by ox cells. Naturally occurring antibody is absorbed by guinea-pig kidney, but not by ox cells, and that of serum sickness is absorbed by both reagents.

2. Unabsorbed serum, end-point Tube 3; titre 40. Guinea-pig kidney absorbed serum, end-point Tube 3, titre 40.

Ox-cell absorbed serum, no agglutination in Tube 1.

In spite of the low titre in the unabsorbed serum, this result would also be positive for infectious mononucleosis, the antibody being not absorbed by the guinea-pig kidney but absorbed by the ox cells.

3. Unabsorbed serum, end-point Tube 3; titre 40. Guinea-pig kidney absorbed serum, no agglutination in Tube 1.
   Ox-cell absorbed serum, end-point Tube 3; titre 40.

This is a normal result, and the screening test would have been negative. Caution is needed in interpreting the results when they are weakly positive or when there is only partial absorption by guinea-pig kidney.

Lack of complete absorption with guinea-pig kidney is not in itself diagnostic of infectious mononucleosis, as this may occasionally be observed with normal serum.[7] A positive test requires at least a two-tube difference in titre before and after absorption with ox cells.

The antibodies normally present in human sera which agglutinate sheep red cells are of the Forssman type, i.e. they react against an antigen widely spread in animal tissues. Antibodies of this type are formed by rabbits injected with an emulsion of guinea-pig kidney. The antibodies react with dog, cat and mouse tissues as well as with sheep and horse red cells, but not with the tissues of man, ox or rat.[83] The antibody formed in infectious mononucleosis is of a different nature and is not absorbed by red cells or tissues containing the Forssman antigen; hence the use, as absorbing agents, of guinea-pig kidney, rich in the antigen, and ox red cells, deficient in the antigen but capable of absorbing the Paul-Bunnell antibody.

The antibodies are lytic as well as agglutinating, and it is possible to read the results by recording lysis, if titrations are carried out in the presence of complement. Fresh ox red cells may be used instead of an autoclaved suspension, although less conveniently. Leyton suggested that an ox red cell lytic test might prove to be a satisfactory substitute for the orthodox Paul-Bunnell agglutination test.[57] He stated that lysins for ox red cells develop sooner and persist longer than do agglutinins for sheep red cells. Other workers have subsequently advocated the lytic test using ox red cells on the grounds of its greater sensitivity.[28,61] The use of horse kidney instead of guinea-pig kidney as an absorbing agent has also been recommended because of the ease with which a large amount of a standard stable reagent can be prepared.[21]

Davidsohn and Lee compared several serological tests and concluded that the differential absorption, enzyme and ox red-cell lysin tests were all equally valuable in the diagnosis of infectious mononucleosis.[22]

An immune-adherence haemagglutination test has been developed for assay of heterophile antibody. It has been reported to be as specific as other tests but to be more sensitive and to remain positive for a longer time.[30]

Technical factors affecting results

Temperature. The Paul-Bunnell antibody of infectious mononucleosis reacts well at 37°C; but agglutination is enhanced at lower temperatures and higher titres are obtained if the tests are carried out at 4°C. At this temperature, however, the test is less specific.[86] A cold agglutinin, anti-i, may appear transiently during the immunological response to infectious mononucleosis,[48,73] but as the antibody does not agglutinate sheep cells its presence does not affect the Paul-Bunnell test. It is usually present in a low titre but it may on rare occasions cause haemolytic anaemia if present at high titre.

Varying sensitivity of sheep red cells. A cause of difficulty in serial studies is the comparatively wide variation in sensitivity between one sample of sheep red cells and the next. Zarofonetis and Oster tested 24 sera with the red cells from 24 different sheep.[85] They found the titres given by the most sensitive cells to be from 4 to 16 times those given by the least sensitive cells. Comparable studies do not seem to have been carried out with horse red cells.

Clinical value of the Paul-Bunnell test

Infectious mononucleosis is caused by the Epstein-Barr virus (EBV). Specific tests have been developed to demonstrate the IgG EBNA-1 (see above). However, tests for the heterophile antibody were developed before the EB virus was identified and they remain a useful aid to the diagnosis of the disease. The Paul-Bunnell test is not infallible. Most authors have reported 80–90% of positive results in patients thought to be suffering from infectious mononucleosis.[9,23,49] Antibodies are often present as early as the fourth to sixth day of the disease and are almost always found by the 21st day. They disappear as a rule within 4–5 months. There is no unanimity as to how frequently negative reactions are found in 'true' infectious mononucleosis. Occasionally, the characteristic antibodies develop very late in the course of the disease, perhaps weeks or even months after the patient becomes ill, and it is also known that a positive reaction may be transient and that the antibodies may be present at such low titres that they may be missed or may produce anomalous agglutination reactions when associated with the naturally occurring antibody at similar titres. For all the above reasons it is difficult to state categorically that any particular patient has not or will not produce antibodies. EBV-specific antibody has been demonstrated in the serum of 86% of patients with clinical and/or haematological features of infectious mononucleosis.[30]

As far as false-positive reactions are concerned, there is no substantial evidence that sera containing agglutinins in high concentration giving the typical reactions of infectious mononucleosis are ever found in other diseases uncomplicated by infectious mononucleosis. In particular, the heterophile-antibody titres in the lymphomas are similar to those found in unselected patients not suffering from infectious mononucleosis.[33] In virus hepatitis, although one-fifth of the patients in one series had antibody titres greater than normal, in only one patient did the result of absorption tests suggest the presence of the Paul-Bunnell antibody.[55]

Preparation of guinea-pig kidney suspension and heated ox red cell suspension (after Barrett[7])

Guinea-pig kidney suspension

Strip the capsules and perirenal fat from at least

two pairs of kidneys. Then wash them well in running water. Homogenize the tissue in 9 g/l NaCl (saline) in a blender for 2 min, sterilize it at 121°C (by autoclaving at 15 lb pressure for 20 min) and blend it again so as to obtain a fine suspension. Then centrifuge the suspension in saline and wash the deposit in two changes of saline. Finally, add to the deposit about four times its volume of 5 g/l phenol in saline. After resuspension, centrifuge the sample in a haematocrit tube in order to estimate its concentration. Then add sufficient phenol-saline to the remainder to produce a 1 in 6 suspension. Use it without further dilution. Its absorbing power must be tested with known positive and negative sera.

The reagent will remain potent for at least 1 yr if stored at 4°C.

Ox red cell suspension

Wash ox cells in several changes of 9 g/l NaCl (saline) and make a 30% suspension. Then sterilize it at 121°C (by autoclaving at 15 lb pressure for 20 min). When cool, adjust the PCV to 0.20 with saline and add an equal volume of 10 g/l phenol-saline to give a 10% suspension.

The ability of the suspension to absorb the infectious mononucleosis antibody must be tested with known positive sera. It should remain potent for several years if stored at 4°C.

DEMONSTRATION OF ANTINUCLEAR FACTORS

Antinuclear antibodies, or antinuclear factors (ANF), occur in the serum in a wide range of auto-immune disorders, including systemic lupus erythematosus (SLE), Sjögren's syndrome, rheumatoid arthritis, chronic hepatitis, thyroiditis, myasthenia gravis, pernicious anaemia, ulcerative colitis, red cell aplasia; they may be present, too, in cases of drug reactions. The antibodies may be specific for DNA, soluble nucleoprotein or an extract of cell nuclei (Sm antigen). There are also antibodies which react with cytoplasmic antigens (Ro antigen), and mixed nuclear and cytoplasmic antigens (La antigen). Several techniques for demonstrating the antibodies in patients with SLE and other disorders have been described.[70]

Some antibodies react with animal tissue antigens. Immunofluorescence provides a sensitive method for detecting this reaction. The serum under investigation is added to a section of tissue (e.g. rat liver). Uptake of antinuclear factor (ANF) will be shown by fluorescence of cell nuclei when fluorescein-labelled rabbit anti-human-γ-globulin serum is subsequently added (indirect test).[39] A characteristic of SLE is the presence of 7S IgG antibodies to double-stranded DNA (ds-DNA);[41] they can be detected and measured quantitatively by indirect immunofluorescence.[66]

Radio-immunoassay also provides a sensitive and specific method for the detection of anti-DNA antibodies. Antigen labelled with a radionuclide (e.g. [125]I) is added to the serum under test and the resultant mixture is then treated with 50%-saturated ammonium sulphate in order to precipitate immunoglobulins; the precipitate will contain radioactivity only if an antigen-antibody reaction has occurred, and the amount of antibody can be estimated from the radioactivity in the antigen-antibody complex.[84]

A rapid and simple qualitative method for detecting the presence of antinuclear antibodies is based on the ability of the serum to aggregate polystyrene latex particles coated with the appropriate nuclear components. Thus, the antinuclear antibody can be demonstrated fairly reliably and rapidly with a reagent comprising latex-bound desoxyribonucleoprotein. This is available as a kit from commercial suppliers (e.g. Lorne Laboratories and Biostat Diagnostics).

Antinuclear antibodies can also be detected by the LE-cell test (see below). They have the property of causing in-vitro lysis of the nuclei of neutrophil polymorphonuclears and subsequent phagocytosis of the lysed nuclei by other neutrophils. The test requires four components: antinuclear antibody (the 'LE-cell' factor); nuclear protein material; complement, and actively phago-cytic neutrophils. To provide access to the nuclear protein material the cell membranes must first be damaged by mechanical or chemical means.

Although more laborious than the tests described above, it is a useful method as the facilities to carry it out are readily available in any haematology laboratory.

DEMONSTRATION OF LE CELLS

In Romanowsky-stained preparations the LE cell appears as a neutrophil in the cytoplasm of which is a large spherical body (the LE body) which stains shades of pale purple. The nucleus of the ingesting leucocyte is usually displaced to one side and typically its lobes appear to be wrapped around the ingested material (Fig. 29.2). The LE body, although derived from nuclear material, usually shows no evidence of nuclear structure and appears as an opaque homogenous mass. The ingesting leucocyte is almost invariably and characteristically a neutrophil polymorphonuclear, very rarely a monocyte or eosinophil.

The 'Tart'* cell is a monocyte—rarely a neutrophil—which has phagocytosed another cell or the nucleus of another cell. The phagocytosed material most often resembles a lymphocyte nucleus, in which case a definite nuclear pattern can be seen (Fig. 29.3); a common alternative form is a pyknotic nucleus smaller than an LE body and staining far more intensely (Fig. 29.4). Tart cells are often associated with leuco-agglutinins and may occasionally occur in patients on drug therapy.[50] Such reactions have to be distinguished from the drug-induced lupus syndrome in which genuine LE cells occur.[25]

Many methods of demonstrating LE cells have been described. It seems clear that some degree of trauma to leucocytes is necessary for a successful preparation, for the LE factor does not appear to be capable of acting upon healthy living leucocytes. A good method of achieving the necessary degree of trauma is to rotate whole blood to which glass beads have been added before concentrating the leucocytes by centri-fugation. The method described in the following section is based on that of Zinkham and Conley.[87]

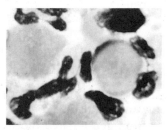

Fig. 29.2   Typical LE cells. The rounded amorphous LE body is well shown to the right of the picture with the segments of a neutrophil nucleus wrapped around it. Below and to the left is shown more amorphous nuclear material, but this is less obviously phagocytosed. ×1000.

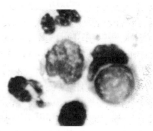

Fig. 29.3   'Tart' cell. A lymphocyte, with intact nuclear structure, has been engulfed by a monocyte, the nucleus of which has been compressed. ×1000.

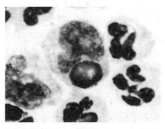

Fig. 29.4   'Tart' cell. A pyknotic lymphocyte nucleus has been phagocytosed by a monocyte. ×100.

*'Tart' apparently refers to the name of the patient in whom cells of this type were first seen.

I. METHOD USING THE PATIENT'S BLOOD

Blood to which the minimum amount of heparin has been added should be used. Transfer 1 ml of the blood into a 75 × 12 mm glass test-tube; add four glass beads and seal the tube with a tightly fitting rubber bung. Rotate the preparation at c 33 rpm at c 20°C for 30 min; place it at 37°C for 10–15 min, and then transfer the contents of the tube to a Wintrobe haematocrit tube. Make buffy coat films after centrifuging for 10 min at 150–200g. Allow the films to dry in the air, fix them in methanol and stain by a Romanowsky method in the usual way.

II. METHOD USING THE PATIENT'S SERUM AND NORMAL LEUCOCYTES

Patient's serum. Obtain this from blood allowed to clot undisturbed at room temperature or at 37°C or from defibrinated blood. It should be stored frozen at –20°C until used.

Normal leucocyte suspension. Deliver 5 ml of freshly drawn group-O blood into a container in which 1 mg of heparin has been dried. After mixing, centrifuge the blood at 1200–1500g for 15 min. Remove the lower half of the column of packed red cells with a Pasteur pipette and discard it; remix the remaining red cells and the supernatant plasma, place in a tube of about 10 mm diameter and allow to sediment at 37°C. The removal of some of the red cells increases the rate of sedimentation.

Allow the blood to sediment until 1–2 ml of plasma are available. This usually takes 30–60 min. Place the supernatant plasma, which contains leucocytes, platelets and a small number of red cells, in a 75 × 12 mm tube and wash once in 9 g/l NaCl (saline). It is important to centrifuge the leucocyte suspension at a slow speed (150–200g) and for no longer than 5 min. Before the saline is added, it is essential to resuspend, by tapping the tube, the button of leucocytes in the small volume of fluid that remains after the supernatant fluid has been poured off. After washing, remove the supernatant by pipette as completely as possible. Resuspend the leucocyte button in the fluid remaining in the tube; it is then ready for use.

Technique of test

Mix equal volumes (5–10 drops) of leucocyte suspension and patient's serum in a 75 × 12 mm tube and add three small glass beads. Fit the tube with a rubber bung and rotate it at c 33 rpm for 30 min at c 20°C, after which transfer its contents to a Wintrobe haematocrit tube. Make films of the deposited leucocytes after centrifuging at 150–200g for 10 min. Dry them in the air, fix in methanol and stain by a Romanowsky method.

Examination of films

Slides should be examined for at least 10 min before a negative report is given. With practice it is possible to recognize LE cells using a 10 × objective. In addition to intracellular LE bodies, extracellular material may also be seen. This consists of basophilic aggregations, either amorphous or in the form of round bodies. Extracellular material may be seen in SLE, but it may also be found in rheumatoid arthritis, discoid LE, cirrhosis of the liver, myelomatosis and possibly even in normal subjects.[5] The material should not be considered of significance unless the characteristic LE cells are also seen.

Interpretation

The number of LE cells found in cases of SLE varies within wide limits. Occasionally, large numbers are present; infrequently, particularly in patients who have received corticosteroid therapy, scattered cells are found only after a prolonged search. If sufficiently numerous, they may be reported as the number present per 1000 neutrophils. 'Tart' cells can usually be clearly differentiated from LE cells, but they are occasionally a source of difficulty, and, when LE cells are outnumbered by Tart cells, SLE should not be diagnosed.

Both the techniques described above are sensitive. That using the patient's whole blood is the simplest and should be used first, as positive results are more likely to be obtained in most instances than by the use of patient's serum. The chief value of the indirect method is in the retrospective assessment of the effect of treatment on the LE-cell-forming activity of a sample of the patient's serum, when a stored sample of the patient's serum can be used as a control.

The LE-cell phenomenon, its relationship to SLE and other auto-immune disorders, and methods for its demonstration, have a large literature.[60] A positive LE-cell test is very suggestive of SLE and LE-cell demonstration is a useful diagnostic test. However, the test is positive in only c 75% of patients with SLE,[41] and conversely, 'false' positive results have sometimes been found when immunofluorescence has failed to demonstrate antinuclear factor.[50] Moreover, clearly positive reactions have been reported in lupoid hepatitis, and in patients on drug therapy.[14,25] Positive tests, too, have been found in 3.6% of patients with rheumatoid arthritis, especially when the disease is severe and highly active.[56]

ERYTHROPOIETIN

Erythropoietin is a heat-stable glycoprotein which regulates red cell production. It is produced mainly in the kidney. Only a small quantity is demonstrable in normal plasma or urine.

The original method for measuring plasma eryhtropoietin was an in-vivo biological assay, based on the uptake of ^{59}Fe by laboratory animals (usually rats) following the injection of test plasma or extract.[16,79] This was a fairly laborious procedure which has been replaced in clinical practice by in-vitro methods using mouse spleen cell culture[51] and by radioimmune assay (RIA).[15,18] The mouse spleen method is sensitive but it is influenced by other serum factors, especially when erythropoietin is low. RIA has also been shown, in some cases, to give anomalous results,[8] but the recent availability of a pure form of human erythropoietin from recombinant DNA (r-HuEPO) has led to a more reliable specific RIA.[8,27,52] Commercial kits are now available for this test.

Results are expressed in international units by reference to an international (WHO) standard. This was originally a urinary extract,[17] and a preparation of urinary erythropoietin is now available with a potency of 10 IU per ampoule.[4] A standard has also been established for r-HuEPO with a potency of 86 IU per ampoule.[76]

Normal range

The normal range in plasma or serum has varied considerably according to the method of assay. By radioimmune assay the range has been reported as 18–35 (mean 25) mIU/ml;[20] or as 11–23 (mean 16) mIU/ml.[36] In normal children the levels are the same as in adults, except for infants under 2 months when the level is low.[36]

There is a diurnal variation, with the highest values at night.[82] A sex difference has also been reported,[1,2] and in pregnancy erythropoietin concentration increases with gestation.[19]

Significance

Increased levels of erythropoietin are found in the plasma in various anaemias and there is normally an inverse relationship between haemoglobin and erythropoietin.[67] In renal disease there is a progressive decline in the erythropoietin response to anaemia, and in end-stage renal failure the concentration is normal or even lower than normal despite increasing anaemia. Some impairment of production of erythropoietin may also occur in the anaemias of neoplastic and chronic inflammatory diseases.[67]

Raised concentrations of erythropoietin occur in secondary polycythaemia due to respiratory and cardiac disease, in the presence of abnormal haemoglobins with high oxygen affinity, in association with hypernephroma and erythopoietin secreting tumours such as hepatoma, uterine fibroma, ovarian carcinoma and some other rare tumours.[3]

In primary proliferative polycythaemia ('polycythaemia vera') the plasma levels are often lower than nomal but in some cases they may be within the normal range.[20,29] In secondary polycythaemia the level of erythropoietin is never suppressed below normal. Assay is particularly useful in patients with erythrocytosis of undetermined cause. However, in such cases there may be an intermittent increase in erythropoietin secretion. Thus, determining the erythropoietin level in a single sample of plasma may be misleading.[20]

REFERENCES

[1] ADAMSON, J. W., ALEXANIAN, R., MARTINEZ, C. and FINCH, C. A. (1966). Erythropoietin excretion in normal man. *Blood*, **28**, 354.

[2] ALEXANIAN, R. (1966). Urinary excretion of erythropoietin in normal men and women. *Blood*, **28**, 344.

[3] ALEXANIAN, R. (1977). Increased erythropoietin production in man. In *Kidney Hormones, Vol. II: Erythropoietin.* Ed. J.W. Fisher, p. 531. Academic Press, London.

[4] ANNABLE, L., COTES, P. M. and MUSSETT, M. V. (1972). The second international reference preparation of erythropoietin, human, urinary, for bioassay. *Bulletin of the World Health Organization*, **47**, 99.

[5] ARTERBERRY, J. D., DREXLER, E. and DUBOIS, E. L. (1964). Significance of hematoxylin bodies in lupus erythematosus cell preparations. *Journal of American Medical Association*, **187**, 389.

[6] BAIN, B. J. (1983). Some influences on the ESR and the fibrinogen level in healthy subjects. *Clinical and Laboratory Haematology*, **5**, 45.

[7] BARRETT, A. M. (1941). The serological diagnosis of glandular fever (infectious mononucleosis): a new technique. *Journal of Hygiene (Cambridge)*, **41**, 330.

[8] BECHENSTEEN, A. G., LAPPIN, T. R. J., MARSDEN, J., MUGGLESTON, D. and COTES, P. M. (1993). Unreliability in immunoassays of erythropoietin: anomalous estimates with an assay kit. *British Journal of Haematology*, **83**, 663.

[9] BERNSTEIN, A. (1940). Infectious mononucleosis. *Medicine (Baltimore)*, **19**, 85.

[10] BULL, B. S. (1981). Clinical and laboratory implications of present ESR methodology. *Clinical and Laboratory Haematology*, **3**, 283.

[11] BRITISH STANDARDS INSTITUTION (1987). *Specification for Westergren Tube and Support for the Measurement of Erythrocyte Sedimentation Rate.* BS 1554. BSI, London.

[12] CARTER, R. L. (1966). Antibody formation in infectious mononucleosis. I. Some immunochemical properties of the Paul-Bunnell antibody. *British Journal of Haematology*, **12**, 259.

[13] CARTER, R. L. (1966). Antibody formation in infectious mononucleosis. II. Other 19 S antibodies and false-positive serology. *British Journal of Haematology*, **12**, 268

[14] CONDEMI, J. J., BLOMGREN, S. E. and VAUGHAN, J. H. (1970). The procainamide induced lupus syndrome. *Bulletin on Rheumatic Diseases*, **20**, 604.

[15] COTES, P. M. (1982). Immunoreactive erythropoietin in serum. I. Evidence for the validity of the assay method and the physiological relevance of estimates. *British Journal of Haematology*, **50**, 427.

[16] COTES, P. M. and BANGHAM, D. R. (1961). Bio-assay of erythropoietin in mice made polycythaemic by exposure to air at reduced pressure. *Nature (London)*, **191**, 1065.

[17] COTES, P. M. and BANGHAM, D. R. (1966). The international reference preparation of erythropoietin. *Bulletin of the World Health Organization*, **35**, 751.

[18] COTES, P. M., CANNING, C. E. and GAINES DAS, R. E. (1983). Modification of a radioimmunoassay for human serum erythropoietin to provide increased sensitivity and investigate non-specific serum responses. In *Immunoassays for Clinical Chemistry.* Eds. W. M. Hunter and J. E. T. Corrie, p. 106. Churchill Livingstone, Edinburgh.

[19] COTES, P. M., CANNING, C. E and LIND, T. (1983). Changes in serum immunoreactive erythropoietin during the menstrual cycle and normal pregnancy. *British Journal of Obstetrics and Gynaecology*, **90**, 304.

[20] COTES, P. M., DORÉ, C. J., LIU YIN, J. A., LEWIS, S. M., MESSINEZY, M., PEARSON, T. C. and REID, C. (1986). Determination of serum immunoreactive erythropoietin in the investigation of erythrocytosis. *New England Journal of Medicine*, **315**, 283.

[21] DAVIDSOHN, I. and GOLDIN, M. (1955). The use of horse kidney in the differential test of infectious mononucleosis. *Journal of Laboratory and Clinical Medicine*, **45**, 561.

[22] DAVIDSOHN, I. and LEE, C. L. (1964). Serologic diagnosis of infectious mononucleosis. A comparative study of five tests. *American Journal of Clinical Pathology*, **24**, 115.

[23] DAVIDSOHN, I., STERN, K. and KASHIWAGI, C. (1951) The differential test for infectious mononucleosis. *American Journal of Clinical Pathology*, **21**, 1101.

[24] DINTENFASS, L. (1976). *Rheology of Blood in Diagnostic and Preventive Medicine.* Butterworth, London.

[25] DUBOIS, E. L. (1975). Serological abnormalities in spontaneous and drug-induced systemic lupus erythematosus. *Journal of Rheumatology*, **2**, 204.

[26] EDWARDS, J. M. B. and McSWIGGEN, D. A. (1974). Studies on the diagnostic value of an immunofluorescence test for EB virus-specific IgM. *Journal of Clinical Pathology*, **27**, 647.

[27] EGRIE, J. C., COTES, P. M., LANE, J., GAINES DAS, R. E. and TAM, R. C. (1987). Development of radioimmunoassays for human erythropoietin using recombinant erythropoietin as tracer and immunogen. *Journal of Immunological Methods*, **9**, 235.

[28] ERICSON, C. (1960). Sheep cell agglutinin and ox cell hemolysin in the serological diagnosis of mononucleosis infectiosa. *Acta Medica Scandinavica*, **166**, 225.

[29] ERSLEY, A. J., CARO, J., KANSU, E., MILLER, O. and COBBS, E. (1979). Plasma erythropoietin in polycythemia. *American Journal of Medicine*, **66**, 243.

[30] EVANS, A. S. and NIEDERMAN, J. C. (1982). EBV-IgA and new heterophile antibody tests in diagnosis of infectious mononucleosis. *American Journal of Clinical Pathology*, **77**, 555.

[31] FLEISHER, G. R., COLLINS, M. and FARGER, S. (1983). Limitations of available tests for diagnosis of infectious mononucleosis. *Journal of Clinical Microbiology*, **17**, 619.

[32] FROOM, P., MARGALIOT, S., CAINE, Y. and BENBASSAT, J.

(1984). Significance of erythrocyte sedimentation rate in young adults. *American Journal of Clinical Pathology*, **82**, 198.

33 GOLDMAN, R., FISHKIN, B. G. and PETERSON, E. T. (1950). The value of the heterophile antibody reaction in the lymphomatous diseases. *Journal of Laboratory and Clinical Medicine*, **35**, 681.

34 HARDWICKE, J. and SQUIRE, J. R. (1952). The basis of the erythrocyte sedimentation rate. *Clinical Science*, **11**, 333.

35 HARKNESS, J. (1971). The viscosity of human plasma; its measurement in health and disease. *Biorheology*, **8**, 171.

36 HELLEBOSTAD, M., HAGA, P. and COTES, M. P. (1988). Serum immunoreactive erythropoietin in healthy normal children. *British Journal of Haematology*, **70**, 247.

37 HENLE, W., HENLE, G. E. and HORWITZ, C. A. (1974). Epstein-Barr virus specific diagnostic tests in infectious mononucleosis. *Human Pathology*, **5**, 551.

38 HOFF, G. and BAUER, S. (1965). A new rapid slide test for infectious mononucleosis. *Journal of the American Medical Association*, **194**, 351.

39 HOLBOROW, E. J., WEIR, D. M. and JOHNSON, G. D. (1957). A serum factor in lupus erythematosus with affinity for tissue nuclei. *British Medical Journal*, **ii**, 732.

40 HORWITZ, C. A., HENLE, W., HENLE, G., PENN, G., HOFFMAN, N. and WARD, P. C. J. (1979). Persistent falsely positive rapid tests for infectious mononucleosis. Report of five cases with four–six year follow-up data. *American Journal of Clinical Pathology*, **72**, 807.

41 HUGHES, G. R. V. (1973). The diagnosis of systemic lupus erythematosus (Annotation). *British Journal of Haematology*, **25**, 409.

42 HUISMAN, A., AARNOUDSE, J. G., KRANS, M., HUISJES, H. J., FIDLER, V. and ZIJLSTRA, W. G. (1988). Red cell aggregation during normal pregnancy. *British Journal of Haematology*, **68**, 121.

43 INTERNATIONAL COMMITTEE FOR STANDARDIZATION IN HAEMATOLOGY (1977). Recommendation for measurement of erythrocyte sedimentation rate of human blood. *American Journal of Clinical Pathology*, **68**, 505.

44 INTERNATIONAL COMMITTEE FOR STANDARDIZATION IN HAEMATOLOGY (1984). Recommendation for selected method for the measurement of plasma viscosity. *Journal of Clinical Pathology*, **37**, 1147.

45 INTERNATIONAL COMMITTEE FOR STANDARDIZATION IN HAEMATOLOGY (1986). Guidelines for measurement of blood viscosity and erythrocyte deformability. *Clinical Hemorheology*, **6**, 439.

46 INTERNATIONAL COMMITTEE FOR STANDARDIZATION IN HAEMATOLOGY (1988). Guidelines on the selection of laboratory tests for monitoring the acute-phase response. *Journal of Clinical Pathology*, **41**, 1203.

47 INTERNATIONAL COUNCIL FOR STANDARDIZATION IN HAEMATOLOGY (1993). ICSH recommendations for measurement of erythrocyte sedimentation rate. *Journal of Clinical Pathology*, **46**, 198.

48 JENKINS, W. J., KOSTER, H. G., MARSH, W. L. and CARTER, R. L. (1965). Infectious mononucleosis: an unsuspected source of anti-i. *British Journal of Haematology*, **11**, 480.

49 KAUFMAN, R. E. (1944). Heterophile antibody in infectious mononucleosis. *Annals of Internal Medicine*, **21**, 230.

50 KOLLER, S. R., JOHNSTON, C. L., MONCURE, C. W. and WALLER, M. V. (1976). Lupus erythematosus cell preparation-antinuclear factor incongruity. A review of diagnostic tests for systemic lupus erythematosus. *American*

51 KRYSTAL, G. (1983). A simple microassay for erythropoietin based on ^{3}H-thymidine incorporation into spleen cells from phenylhydrazine treated mice. *Experimental Hematology*, **11**, 649.

52 LAPPIN, T. R. J., ELDER, G. E., TAYLOR, T., McMULLIN, M. F. and BRIDGES, J. M. (1988). Comparison of the mouse spleen assay and a radioimmunoassay for the measurement of serum erythropoietin. *British Journal of Haematology*, **70**, 117.

53 LEE, C. L., DAVIDSOHN, I. and PANCZYSZYN, O. (1968). Horse agglutinins in infectious mononucleosis, II. The spot test. *American Journal of Clinical Pathology*, **49**, 12.

54 LEE, C. L., DAVIDSOHN, I. and SLABY, R. (1968). Horse agglutinins in infectious mononucleosis. *American Journal of Clinical Pathology*, **49**, 3.

55 LEIBOWITZ, S.(1951). Heterophile antibody in normal adults and in patients with virus hepatitis. *American Journal of Clinical Pathology*, **21**, 201.

56 LENOCH, F. and VOJTISEK O. (1967). The prevalence of LE cells in 1000 consecutive patients with active rheumatoid arthritis. *Acta Rheumatologica Scandinavica*, **13**, 313.

57 LEYTON, G. B. (1952). Ox-cell haemolysins in human serum. *Journal of Clinical Pathology*, **5**, 324.

58 MANLEY, R. W. (1957). The effect of room temperature on erythrocyte sedimentation rate and its correction. *Journal of Clinical Pathology*, **10**, 354.

59 MERRILL, R. H. and BARRETT, O. (1976). Positive mono-spot test in histiocytic medullary reticulosis. *American Journal of Clinical Pathology*, **65**, 407.

60 MIESCHER, P. W. and REITHMÜLLER, D. (1965). Diagnosis and treatment of systemic lupus erythematosus. *Seminars in Hematology*, **2**, 1.

61 MIKKELSEN, W., TUPPER, C. J. and MURRAY, J. (1958). The ox cell hemolysin test as a diagnostic procedure in infectious mononucleosis. *Journal of Laboratory and Clinical Medicine*, **52**, 648.

62 NATIONAL COMMITTEE FOR CLINICAL LABORATORY STANDARDS (1977). *Standardized Methods for the Human Erythrocyte Sedimentation Rate (ESR) Test (ASH-2)*. NCCLS, Villanova, PA.

63 PAUL, J. R. and BUNNELL, W. W. (1932). The presence of heterophile antibodies in infectious mononucleosis. *American Journal of Medical Sciences*, **183**, 90.

64 PHILLIPS, G. M. (1972). False-positive monospot test in rubella. *Journal of American Medical Association*, **222**, 585.

65 PHILLIPS, M J. and HARKNESS, J. (1981). A study of plasma viscosity-temperature relationships. *Bibliotheca Anatomica*, **20**, 215.

66 PINCUS, T., SCHUR, P. H. and TALAL, N. (1968). A diagnostic test for systemic lupus erythematosus using a DNA binding assay. *Arthritis and Rheumatism*, **11**, 837.

67 PIPPARD, M. J., HUGHES, R. T. and COTES, P. M. (1992). Erythropoietin. In *Recent Advances in Haematology; No. 6*. Eds. A. V. Hoffbrand and M. K. Brenner, p. 1. Churchill Livingstone, Edinburgh.

68 POOLE, J. C. F. and SUMMERS, G. A. C. (1952). Correction of E.S.R. in anaemia. Experimental study based on interchange of cells and plasma between normal and anaemic subjects. *British Medical Journal*, **i**. 353.

69 REED, R. E. (1974). False-positive monospot tests in malaria. *American Journal of Clinical Pathology*, **61**, 173.

70 REICHLIN, M. (1981). Current perspectives on serological reactions in SLE patients. *Clinical and Experimental*

Immunology, **44**, 1.

[71] RIPPEY, J. H. and BOWMAN, H. E. (1979). Infectious mononucleosis test performance in CAP survey specimens. *American Journal of Clinical Pathology*, **72**, 363.

[72] RODDIE, A. M. S. and POLLOCK, A. (1987). Plastic ESR tubes: does static electricity affect the results? *Clinical and Laboratory Haematology*, **9**, 175.

[73] ROSENFELD, R. E., SCHMIDT, P. J., CALVO, R. C. and McGINNISS, M. H. (1965). Anti-i, a frequent cold agglutinin in infectious mononucleosis. *Vox Sanguinis*, **10**, 631.

[74] SCOTT, G. L. and PRIEST, C. J. (1972). An evaluation of the Monosticon rapid slide test diagnosis of infectious mononucleosis. *Journal of Clinical Pathology*, **25**, 783.

[75] STEPHENS, J. G. (1938). Stratified blood sedimentation—isolation of immature red cells. *Nature (London)*, **141**, 1058.

[76] STORRING, P. L. and GAINES DAS, R. E. (1992). The international standard for recombinant DNA-derived erythropoietin: collaborative study of four recombinant DNA-derived erythropoietins and two highly purified human erythropoietins. *Journal of Endocrinology*, **134**, 459.

[77] STRNAD, B. C., SCHUSTER, T. C., HOPKINS, R. F., NEUBAUER, R. H. and RABIN, H. (1981). Identification of an Epstein-Barr virus nuclear antigen by fluoro-immunoelectrophoresis and radioimmuno-electrophoresis. *Journal of Virology*, **38**, 996.

[78] STUART, J. and LEWIS, S. M. (1993). Recommendations for standardization, safety and quality control of erythrocyte sedimentation rate. *WHO Document LBS / 93.1*. World Health Organization, Geneva.

[79] WEINTRAUB, A. H., GORDON, A. S. and CAMISCOLI, J. F. (1963). Use of the hypoxia-induced polycythemic mouse in the assay and standardization of erythropoietin. *Journal of Laboratory and Clinical Medicine*, **62**, 743.

[80] WESTERGREN, A. (1921). Studies of the suspension stability of the blood in pulmonary tuberculosis. *Acta Medica Scandinavica*, **54**, 247.

[81] WHICHER, J. T. and DIEPPE, P. A. (1985). Acute phase proteins. *Clinics in Immunology and Allergy*, **5**, 425.

[82] WIDE, L., BENGTSSON, C. and BIRGEGARD, G. (1988). Circadian rhythm of erythropoietin in human serum. *British Journal of Haematology*, **72**, 85.

[83] WILSON, C. S. and MILES, A. A. (1964). In *Topley and Wilson's Principles of Bacteriology and Immunity*, 5th edn., p. 1330. Arnold, London.

[84] WOLD, R. T., YOUNG, F. E., TAN, E. M. and FARR, R. S. (1968). Desoxyribonucleic acid antibody: a method to detect its primary interaction with desoxyribonucleic acid. *Science*, **161**, 806.

[85] ZAROFONETIS, C. J. D. and OSTER, H. L. (1950). Heterophile agglutination variability of erythrocytes from different sheep. *Journal of Laboratory and Clinical Medicine*, **36**, 283.

[86] ZAROFONETIS, C. J. D., OSTER, H. L. and COLVILLE, V. F. (1953). Cold agglutination of sheep erythrocytes as a factor in false positive heterophile agglutination tests. *Journal of Laboratory and Clinical Medicine*, **41**, 906.

[87] ZINKHAM, W. H. and CONLEY, C. L. (1956). Some factors influencing the formation of L.E. cells. A method for enhancing L.E. cell production. *Bulletin of the Johns Hopkins Hospital*, **98**, 102.

30. Appendices

Preparation of reagents, anticoagulants and preservative
   solutions   575
Buffers   577
Preparation of glassware   580
   Flask for defibrination of blood   580
   Siliconized glassware   580
Methods of cleaning slides and apparatus   580
Sizes of tubes   581
Speed of centrifuging   581
Units of weight and measurement   581

Microscopic magnification   583
Atomic weights and molecular concentrations   583
Statistical procedures   584
   Analysis of difference by t-test   584
   Analysis of variance by F-test   585
Microscope maintenance   588
Rabbit brain thromboplastin   589
PTT Phospholipid reagent   589
Reference reagents and standards   590

1. PREPARATION OF CERTAIN REAGENTS, ANTICOAGULANTS AND PRESERVATIVE SOLUTIONS

Acid-citrate-dextrose (ACD) solution—'NIH-A'

Trisodium citrate, dihydrate (75 mmol/l)	22 g
Citric acid, monohydrate (42 mmol/l)	8 g
Dextrose (139 mmol/l)	25 g
Water	to 1 litre

Sterilize the solution by autoclaving at 121°C for 15 min. Its pH is 5.4. For use, add 10 volumes of blood to 1.5 volumes of solution.

Alsever's solution[3]

Dextrose (114 mmol/l)	20.5 g
Trisodium citrate, dihydrate (27 mmol/l)	8.0 g
Sodium chloride (72 mmol/l)	4.2 g
Water	to 1 litre

Adjust the pH to 6.1 with citric acid (c 0.5 g) and then sterilize the solution by micropore filtration (0.22 μm) or by autoclaving at 121°C for 15 min.

For use, add 4 volumes of blood to 1 volume of solution. For use in red cell survival studies see p. 405.

Citrate-phosphate-dextrose (CPD) solution, pH 6.9

Trisodium citrate, dihydrate (102 mmol/l)	30 g
Sodium dihydrogen phosphate, monohydrate (1.08 mmol/l)	0.15 g
Dextrose (11 mmol/l)	2 g
Water	to 1 litre

Sterilize the solution by autoclaving at 121°C for 15 min. After cooling to c 20°C, it should have a brown tinge and its pH should be 6.9.

575

Citrate-phosphate-dextrose (CPD) solution, pH 5.6–5.8

Trisodium citrate, dihydrate (89 mmol/l)	26.30 g
Citric acid, monohydrate (17 mmol/l)	3.27 g
Sodium dihydrogen phosphate, monohydrate (16 mmol/l)	2.22 g
Dextrose (142 mmol/l)	25.50 g
Water	to 1 litre

Sterilize the solution by autoclaving at 121°C for 15 min. For use as an anticoagulant-preservative, add 7 volumes of blood to 1 volume of solution.

Citrate-phosphate-dextrose-adenine (CPD-A) solution, pH 5.6–5.8

Trisodium citrate, dihydrate (89 mmol/l)	26.30 g
Citric acid, monohydrate (17 mmol/l)	3.27 g
Sodium dihydrogen phosphate, monohydrate (16 mmol/l)	2.22 g
Dextrose (177 mmol/l)	31.8 g
Adenine (2.04 mmol/l)	0.275 g
Water	to 1 litre

Sterilize the solution by autoclaving at 121°C for 15 min. For use as an anticoagulant-preservative, add 7 volumes of blood to 1 volume of solution.

Low ionic strength solution[3]

Sodium chloride (NaCl) (30.8 mmol/l)	1.8 g
Disodium hydrogen phosphate (Na_2HPO_4) (1.5 mmol/l)	0.21 g
Sodium dihydrogen phosphate (NaH_2PO_4) (1.5 mmol/l)	0.18 g
Glycine (NH_2CH_2COOH) (240 mmol/l)	18.0 g
Water	to 1 litre

Dissolve the sodium chloride and the two phosphate salts in c 400 ml of water; dissolve the glycine separately in c 400 ml of water; adjust the pH of each solution to 6.7 with 1 mol/l NaOH. Add the two solutions together and make up to 1 litre.

Sterilize by Seitz filtration or autoclaving. The pH should be within the range of 6.65–6.85, the osmolality 270–285 mmol, and conductivity 3.5–3.8 mS/cm at 23°C.

EDTA

Ethylenediamine tetra-acetic acid, dipotassium or disodium salt	100 g
Water	to 1 litre

Allow appropriate volumes to dry in bottles at c 20°C so as to give a concentration of 1.5 ± 0.25 mg/ml of blood.

Neutral EDTA, pH 7.0, 110 mmol/l

Ethylenediamine tetra-acetic acid, dipotassium salt	44.5 g
or disodium salt	41.0 g
1 mmol/l NaOH	75 ml
Water	to 1 litre

Neutral buffered EDTA, pH 7.0

Ethylenediamine tetra-acetic acid, disodium salt (9 mmol/l)	3.35 g
Disodium hydrogen phosphate (Na_2HPO_4) (26.4 mmol/l)	3.75 g
Sodium chloride (NaCl) (140 mmol/l)	8.18 g
Water	to 1 litre

Saline

Sodium chloride (NaCl) (154 mmol/l)	9.0 g
Water	to 1 litre

Trisodium citrate

($Na_3C_6H_5O_7.2H_2O$), 109 mmol/l

Dissolve 32 g* in 1 litre of water. Distribute convenient volumes (e.g. 10 ml) into small bottles and sterilize by autoclaving at 121°C for 15 min.

---

*or 38 g of $2Na_3 C_6H_5O_7. 11H_2O$.

Heparin

Powdered heparin (lithium salt) is available with an activity of c 160 IU/mg. Dissolve it in water at a concentration of 4 mg/ml. Sodium heparin is available in 5 ml ampoules with an activity of 1000 IU/ml. Add appropriate volumes of either solution to a series of containers and allow to dry at c 20°C so as to give a concentration not exceeding 15–20 IU/ml of blood.

Gibson and Harrison's artificial haemoglobin standard

Chromium potassium sulphate	
($CrK (SO_4)_2.12H_2O$)	11.61 g
Cobaltous sulphate (anhydrous)	
($CoSO_4$)	13.1 g
Potassium dichromate ($K_2Cr_2O_7$)	0.69 g
Water	to 500 ml

Add 1.8 ml of 1 mol/l sulphuric acid to the dissolved salts and heat the mixture to boiling. After boiling for 1 min, cool the solution and make up the volume to 1 litre with water. The chromium potassium sulphate crystals must be free from any signs of whitening due to efflorescence. The cobaltous sulphate must be anhydrous. Heat c 30 g of $CoSO_4.7H_2O$ for c 2 h in a small porcelain dish placed in an oven at a temperature just below its melting point (96°C). Then heat the coarser particles overnight in an electric muffle furnace kept at 400°C. The product should be a uniform lilac powder. Transfer while still hot to a stoppered bottle. As soon as it has cooled, weigh out 13.1 g and dissolve in 80 ml of water with the aid of heat. As the anhydrous salt is hygroscopic, seal in glass tubes immediately after preparation.

The undiluted standard is equivalent to 160 ± 2 g Hb per l (based on iron determinations) when used as described on p. 53.

Water

For most purposes still-prepared distilled water or deionized water is equally suitable. Throughout this text this is implied when 'water' is referred to. When doubly-distilled or glass-distilled water is required this has been specially indicated, and when tap-water is satisfactory or indicated, this, too, has been stated.

---

2. BUFFERS*

Barbitone buffer, pH 7.4

Sodium diethyl barbiturate	
($C_8H_{11}O_3N_2Na$) (57 mmol/l)	11.74 g
Hydrochloric acid (HCl)	
(100 mmol/l)	430 ml

Barbitone buffered saline, pH 7.4

NaCl	5.67 g
Barbitone buffer, pH 7.4	1 litre

Before use, dilute with an equal volume of 9 g/l NaCl.

Barbitone-buffered saline, pH 9.5

Sodium diethyl barbiturate	
($C_8H_{11}O_3N_2Na$) (98 mmol/l)	20.2 g
Hydrochloric acid (HCl)	
(100 mmol/l)	20 ml
NaCl	5.67 g

Before use, dilute the buffer with an equal volume of 9 g/l NaCl.

---

*Other buffers which are used for specific purposes are described under the appropriate tests.

Barbitone-bovine serum albumin (BSA) buffer, pH 9.8

Sodium diethyl barbiturate
  ($C_8H_{11}O_3N_2Na$) (54 mmol/l)   10.3 g
NaCl (102 mmol/l)   6.0 g
Sodium azide (31 mmol/l)   2.0 g
Bovine serum albumin (e.g. Sigma)   5.0 g
Water   to 1 litre

Dissolve the reagents in *c* 900 ml of water. Adjust the pH to 9.8 with 5 mol/l HCl. Make up the volume to 1 litre with water. Store at 4°C.

Citrate-saline buffer

Trisodium citrate ($Na_3C_6H_5O_7.2H_2O$)
  (5 mmol/l)   1.5 g
NaCl (96 mmol/l)   5.6 g
Barbitone buffer, pH 7.4   200 ml
Water   800 ml

Glycine buffer, pH 3.0

Glycine (NH_2CH_2COOH)
  (82 mmol/l)   6.15 g
NaCl (82 mmol/l)   4.80 g
Water   820 ml
0.1 mol/l HCl   180 ml

HEPES buffer, pH 6.6

4-(2-Hydroxyethyl)-1-piperazineethane
  sulphonic acid (100 mmol/l)   23.83 g

Dissolve in *c* 100 ml of water. Add a sufficient volume of 1 mol/l NaOH (*c* 1 ml) to adjust the pH to 6.6. If the buffer is intended for use with Romanowsky staining (p. 87), then add 25 ml of dimethyl sulphoxide (DMSO). Make up the volume to 1 litre with water.

HEPES-saline buffer, pH 7.6

HEPES (4-(2-Hydroxyethyl)-1-piperazine-
  ethane sulphonic acid (20 mmol/l)   4.76 g
NaCl   8.0 g

Dissolve in *c* 100 ml of water. Add a sufficient volume of 1 mol/l NaOH to adjust the pH to 7.6. Make up volume to 1 litre with water.

Imidazole-buffered saline, pH 7.4

Imidazole (50 mmol/l)   3.4 g
NaCl (100 mmol/l)   5.85 g

Dissolve in *c* 500 ml of water. Add 18.6 ml of 1 mol/l HCl and make up the volume to 1 litre with water. Store at room temperature (18–25°C).

Phosphate buffer, iso-osmotic

(A) $NaH_2PO_4.2H_2O$ (150 mmol/l)   23.4 g/l
(B) Na_2HPO_4 (150 mmol/l)   21.3 g/l

pH	Solution A	Solution B
5.8	87 ml	13 ml
6.0	83 ml	17 ml
6.2	75 ml	25 ml
6.4	66 ml	34 ml
6.6	56 ml	44 ml
6.8	46 ml	54 ml
7.0	32 ml	68 ml
7.2	24 ml	76 ml
7.4	18 ml	82 ml
7.6	13 ml	87 ml
7.7	9.5 ml	90.5 ml

Normal human serum has an osmolality of 289 ± 4 mmol. Hendry[2] recommended slightly different concentrations of the stock solution, namely, 25.05 g/l $NaH_2PO_4.2H_2O$ and 17.92 g/l Na_2HPO_4 for an iso-osmotic buffer.

Phosphate-buffered saline

Equal volumes of iso-osmotic phosphate buffer
and 9 g/l NaCl.

Phosphate buffer, Sörensen's

66 mmol/l stock solutions:
- (A) KH_2PO_4 9.1 g/l
- (B) Na_2HPO_4 9.5 g/l or
-     $Na_2HPO_4.2H_2O$ 11.9 g/l

100 mml/l and 150 mmol/l stock solutions may
be similarly prepared. To obtain a solution of the
required pH, add A and B in the indicated
proportions:

pH	A	B
5.4	97.0	3.0
5.6	95.0	5.0
5.8	92.2	7.8
6.0	88.0	12.0
6.2	81.0	19.0
6.4	73.0	27.0
6.6	63.0	37.0
6.8	50.8	49.2
7.0	38.9	61.1
7.2	28.0	72.0
7.4	19.2	80.8
7.6	13.0	87.0
7.8	8.5	91.5
8.0	5.5	94.5

This buffer is not iso-osmotic with normal
plasma (see above).

Tris-HCl buffer (200 mmol/l)

Tris(Hydroxymethyl)aminomethane
(24.23 g/l)   250 ml

To obtain a solution of the required pH add
the appropriate volume of 1 mol/l HCl and then
make up the volume to 1 litre with water:

pH	Volume
7.2	44.5 ml
7.4	42.0 ml
7.6	39.0 ml
7.8	33.5 ml
8.0	28.0 ml
8.2	23.0 ml
8.4	17.5 ml
8.6	13.0 ml
8.8	9.0 ml
9.0	5.0 ml

100 mml/l, 150 mmol/l, 300 mmol/l and
750 mmol/l stock solutions may be similarly
prepared with an appropriate weight of Tris and
volume of acid.

Tris-HCl bovine serum albumin (BSA) buffer, pH 7.6, 20 mmol/l

Tris (hydroxymethyl) aminomethane
(20 mmol/l)   2.42 g
EDTA, disodium salt (10 mmol/l)   3.72 g
NaCl (100 mmol/l)   5.85 g
Sodium azide (3 mmol/l)   0.2 g

Dissolve the reagents in c 800 ml of water. Adjust
the pH to 7.6 with 10 mol/l HCl. Add 10 g of
bovine serum albumin and make up to 1 litre with
water.

3. PREPARATION OF GLASSWARE

FLASK FOR THE DEFIBRINATION OF BLOOD

Provide a 100 ml conical flask with a central glass rod to the bottom end of which are fused pieces of glass capillary (Fig. 1.1, p. 3). The rod is kept in position with a cotton-wool plug. Deliver 10–50 ml of blood into the flask and, after re-inserting the central rod, hold the flask by the neck and rotate it by hand. The blood is usually successfully defibrinated within 5 min, the fibrin forming on the glass rod, usually in one piece. Little or no lysis is caused, and the blood is as a rule completely free from small clots.

SILICONIZED GLASSWARE

Use c 2% solution of silicone (dimethyldichloro-silane) in solvent. This is available commercially*. Immerse the clean glassware or syringes to be coated in the fluid and allow to drain dry. (It is advisable to wear rubber gloves and to prepare the apparatus in a fume cupboard provided with an exhaust fan). Then rinse the coated glassware thoroughly in water, and allow to dry in an oven at 100°C for 10 min or overnight in an incubator.

4. METHODS OF CLEANING SLIDES AND APPARATUS

New slides

Place them in 3 mol/l HCl for at least 48 h. Wash the treated slides well in running tap-water, rinse in water and store in 95% ethanol until used. Dry with a clean linen cloth and carefully wipe free from dust before they are used.

Dirty slides

When discarded, place in a detergent solution, heat to 60°C for 20 min and then wash in hot running tap-water. Finally, rinse in water before being dried with a clean linen cloth.

Chemical apparatus and glassware

Wash in running tap-water and then boil in a detergent solution, rinse in acid and wash in hot running tap-water, as described above. Alternatively, the apparatus can be soaked in 3 mol/l HCl.

For the removal of deposits of protein and other organic matter, 'biodegradable' detergents are recommended. Decon 90 (Decon Laboratories Ltd., Hove BN3 3LY, UK) is suitable but a number of similar preparations are also available.

Iron-free glassware

Wash in a detergent solution, then soak in 3 mol/l HCl for 24 h and finally rinse in de-ionized, double-distilled water.

---

*e.g. BDH Silicone solution (Merck); Sigmacote (Sigma).

5. SIZES OF TUBES

The sizes of tubes recommended in the text have been chosen as being appropriate for the tests described. The dimensions given are the length and external diameter (in mm). The equivalent in inches, as given in some catalogues, and certain corresponding internal diameters, are as follows:

75 × 10 mm (internal
diameter 8 mm)   = 3 × $\frac{3}{8}$ "

75 × 12 mm (internal
diameter 10 mm)   = 3 × $\frac{1}{2}$ "

65 × 10 mm   = $2\frac{1}{2}$ × $\frac{3}{8}$ "

38 × 6.4 mm   = $1\frac{1}{2}$ × $\frac{1}{4}$ " ('precipitin
tubes')

100 × 12 mm   = 4 × $\frac{1}{2}$ "

150 × 16 mm   = 6 × $\frac{5}{8}$ "

150 × 19 mm   = 6 × $\frac{3}{4}$ "

6. SPEED OF CENTRIFUGING

Throughout the book the unit given is the relative centrifugal force (**g**). Conversion of this figure to rpm depends upon the radius of the centrifuge; it can be calculated by reference to the nomogram illustrated in Fig. 30.1 (see p. 582), or from the formula for relative centrifugal force:

$$RCF = 118 \times 10^{-7} \times r \times N^2$$

where r = radius (cm) and N = speed of rotation (rpm).

The following centrifugal forces are recommended:

'Low-spun' platelet-
rich plasma   150–200 **g** (for 10–15 min).
'High-spun' plasma   1200–1500 **g** (for 15 min).
Packing of red cells   2000–2300 **g** (for 30 min).

7. UNITS OF WEIGHT AND MEASUREMENT IN COMMON USE IN HAEMATOLOGY

Throughout the book measurements have been expressed in SI units, in accordance with international recommendations.[4] These units are derived from the metric system. The base units are shown below and the abbreviated forms are indicated alongside.

Weight—unit: gram (g)
  × 10^3 = kilogram (kg)
  × 10^{-3} = milligram (mg)
  × 10^{-6} = microgram (µg) (formerly γ)
  × 10^{-9} = nanogram (ng) (formerly µmg)
  × 10^{-12} = picogram (pg) (formerly µµg)

Length—unit: metre (m)
  × 10^{-1} = decimetre (dm)
  × 10^{-2} = centimetre (cm)
  × 10^{-3} = millimetre (mm)
  × 10^{-6} = micrometre (µm) (formerly µ)
  × 10^{-9} = nanometre (nm) (formerly mµ)

Volume—unit: litre (l or L) = dm^3
  × 10^{-1} = decilitre (dl) (formerly 100 ml)
  × 10^{-3} = millilitre (ml) = cm^3 (formerly cc)
  × 10^{-6} = microlitre (µl) = mm^3
  × 10^{-9} = nanolitre (nl)
  × 10^{-12} = picolitre (pl) (formerly µµl)
  × 10^{-15} = femtolitre (fl) = µm^3

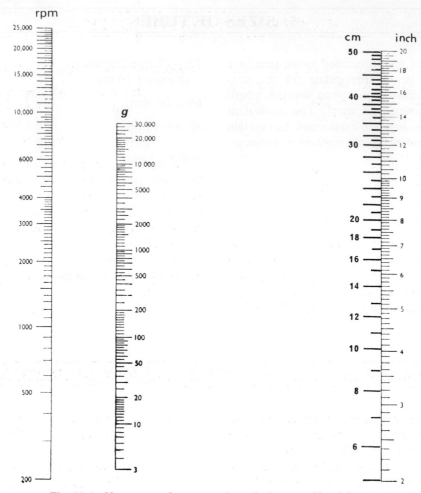

Fig. 30.1 Nomogram for computing relative centrifugal forces.

Amount of substance—unit: mole (mol)
  $\times 10^{-3}$ = millimole (mmol)
  $\times 10^{-6}$ = micromole (μmol)

Substance concentration—unit: moles per litre (mol/l)
(formerly M) see p. 583.
  $\times 10^{-3}$ = millimole per litre (mmol/l)
  $\times 10^{-6}$ = micromole per litre (μmol/l)

Mass concentration—unit: gram per litre (g/l)
  $\times 10^{-3}$ = milligram per litre (mg/l)
  $\times 10^{-6}$ = microgram per litre (μg/l)

When preparing a small amount of a reagent, it is more appropriate to express its concentration per ml or dl.

To convert a measurement from mass concentration to molar concentration, divide by the molecular mass. Thus, for example, if Hb = 160 g/l, as the molecular mass of haemoglobin is 16 125 (see p. 51), then Hb = 160 ÷ 16 125 = 0.0099 mol/l = 9.9 mmol/l.

8. MICROSCOPE MAGNIFICATION

It has become customary for the objective lenses of microscopes to be marked with their magnifying power rather than their focal length. The approximate equivalents are as follows:

Focal length (mm)	Magnification
2	× 100
4	× 40
16	× 10
40	× 4

The working distance of the objective is the distance between the objective and the object to be visualized. The greater the magnifying power of the objective, the smaller the working distance. If the cover-glass is too thick it will not be possible to focus at high magnification.

Objective	Working distance
×10	5–6 mm
×40	0.5–1.5 mm
×100	0.15–0.20 mm

Thus, the cover-glass should be no more than 0.15 mm thick for examination of covered preparations by the ×100 oil-immersion lens. Obviously, preparations which are not covered can be examined under oil immersion without this problem.

If the glass slide is too thick, this may prevent correct focus of the light path through condenser to the object.

9. ATOMIC WEIGHTS AND MOLECULAR CONCENTRATIONS

The concentration of a substance in solution can be expressed either in g/l or in mol/l.* The molecular weight or relative molecular mass (RMM) of the substance (including water of crystallization if present in the chemical form) expressed as g/l is equivalent to 1 mole (or 1000 mmol/l). Thus, e.g.

RMM of NaCl	= 58.5	
∴ 1 mol/l	= 58.5 g/l	
9 g/l	= 9 ÷ 58.5	= 0.154 mol/l
		= 154 mmol/l

The atomic weights of some chemicals which are commonly used in preparation of reagents are as follows:

Calcium	40
Carbon	12
Chlorine	35
Chromium	52
Hydrogen	1
Iron	56
Magnesium	24
Nitrogen	14
Oxygen	16
Phosphorus	31
Potassium	39
Sodium	23
Sulphur	32

*In earlier editions of this book, and in a few places in the present edition, molarity has been expressed by the symbol M rather than as concentration in mol/l. Thus, for example, 0.1M HCl is equivalent to 0.1 mol/l.

10. STATISTICAL PROCEDURES

Mean ($\bar{x}$) is the sum of all the measurements (Σ) divided by the number of measurements (n).

Median (m) is the point on the scale that has an equal number of observations above and below.

Mode is the most frequently occurring result.

Gaussian distribution describes events or data which occur symetrically about the mean (see Fig. 2.1); with this type of distribution mean, median and mode will be approximately equal. The extent of spread of measurements about the mean is expressed as the standard deviation (SD). Its calculation is described below. 68% of all the measurements will be within the ±1 SD range, 95% within ±2 SD and 99% within ±3 SD.

Log normal distribution describes events which are asymetrical (skewed) with a larger number of observations towards one end. The mean will thus be nearer that end; the mean, median and mode may differ from each other. To calculate geometric mean and SD the data are first converted to their logarithms and after calculating the mean and SD of the logarithms, the results are reconverted to the antilog.

Poisson distribution describes events which are random in their occurrence. This will be the case, for example, when blood cells are counted in a diluted suspension. The number of cells which are counted in a given volume will vary on each occasion; this count variation (σ) is 0.92 $\sqrt{\lambda}$, where λ = the total number of cells counted (see p. 56). It is an estimate of the standard deviation of the entire population whereas SD denotes the standard deviation of the items that were actually measured.

Coefficient of variation (CV) is another way of indicating standard deviation, related to the actual measurement so that variation at different levels can be compared. It is expressed as a percentage.

Standard error of mean (SEM) is a measure of dispersion of the mean of a set of measurements. It is used to compare means of two sets of data.

CALCULATIONS

Variance $(s^2) = \dfrac{\Sigma(x - \bar{x})^2}{n - 1}$

Standard deviation (SD) = $\sqrt{s^2}$

Coefficient of variation (CV) = $\dfrac{SD}{\bar{x}} \times 100\%$

Standard error of mean (SEM) = $\dfrac{SD}{\sqrt{n}}$

Standard deviation of paired (duplicate) results =

$$\sqrt{\frac{\Sigma d^2}{2n}}$$

Where d = difference between duplicates,
     n = number of duplicate measurements.

Standard deviation of median =
$$\frac{\text{Central 50\% of results}^\star}{1.35}$$

(*i.e. between 25% and 75%)

ANALYSIS OF DIFFERENCES BY t-TEST

This is a method for comparing two sets of data, e.g. to assess the accuracy of a new method against a reference method.

Calculation

(1) Variance $(s^2) = \dfrac{\Sigma(d - \bar{d})^2}{n - 1}$

  where d = differences between paired
       measurements
    $\bar{d}$ = mean of the differences
    n = number of paired measurements

(2) $t = \bar{d} \div \sqrt{\dfrac{s^2}{n}}$

From the t-test chart (Table 30.1 p. 585) read the value of t for the appropriate degree of freedom (i.e. n – 1). Express results as the level of probability (p) that there is *no* significant difference between the sets of data that are being compared.

Table 30.1   Critical values of t-test

df	50 (0.5)	40 (0.4)	30 (0.3)	20 (0.2)	10 (0.1)	5 (0.05)	1 (0.01)
			% Probability level				
1	1.000	1.376	1.963	3.078	6.314	12.706	63.657
2	0.816	1.061	1.386	1.886	2.920	4.303	9.925
3	0.765	0.978	1.250	1.638	2.353	3.182	5.841
4	0.741	0.941	1.190	1.533	2.132	2.776	4.604
5	0.727	0.920	1.156	1.476	2.015	2.571	4.032
6	0.718	0.906	1.134	1.440	1.943	2.447	3.707
7	0.711	0.896	1.119	1.415	1.895	2.365	3.499
8	0.706	0.889	1.108	1.397	1.860	2.306	3.355
9	0.703	0.883	1.100	1.383	1.833	2.262	3.250
10	0.700	0.879	1.093	1.372	1.812	2.228	3.169
11	0.697	0.876	1.088	1.363	1.796	2.201	3.106
12	0.695	0.873	1.083	1.356	1.782	2.179	3.055
13	0.694	0.870	1.079	1.350	1.771	2.160	3.012
14	0.692	0.868	1.076	1.345	1.761	2.145	2.977
15	0.691	0.866	1.074	1.341	1.753	2.131	2.947
16	0.690	0.865	1.071	1.337	1.746	2.120	2.921
17	0.689	0.863	1.069	1.333	1.740	2.110	2.989
18	0.688	0.862	1.067	1.330	1.734	2.101	2.878
19	0.688	0.861	1.066	1.328	1.729	2.093	2.861
20	0.687	0.860	1.064	1.325	1.725	2.086	2.845
21	0.686	0.859	1.063	1.323	1.721	2.080	2.831
22	0.686	0.858	1.061	1.321	1.717	2.074	2.819
23	0.685	0.858	1.061	1.321	1.717	2.074	2.819
24	0.685	0.857	1.059	1.318	1.711	2.064	2.797
25	0.684	0.856	1.058	1.316	1.708	2.060	2.787
26	0.684	0.856	1.058	1.315	1.706	2.056	2.779
27	0.684	0.855	1.057	1.314	1.703	2.052	2.771
28	0.683	0.855	1.056	1.313	1.701	2.048	2.763
29	0.683	0.854	1.055	1.311	1.699	2.045	2.756
30	0.683	0.854	1.055	1.310	1.697	2.042	2.750
40	0.681	0.851	1.050	1.303	1.684	2.021	2.704
50	0.680	0.849	1.048	1.299	1.676	2.008	2.678
60	0.679	0.848	1.046	1.296	1.671	2.000	2.660
120	0.677	0.845	1.041	1.289	1.658	1.980	2.617
∞	0.674	0.842	1.036	1.282	1.645	1.960	2.576

ANALYSIS OF VARIANCE BY F-RATIO

This is a method to assess the relative precision of two sets of measurements.

Calculation

Variance $(s^2) = \dfrac{\Sigma(x - \bar{x})^2}{n - 1}$

for set A and for set B, respectively:

F-ratio $= \dfrac{s^2 \text{ of set A}}{s^2 \text{ of set B}}$

As the ratio must not be less than 1, use the higher variance as the numerator. Then, from the chart (Table 30.2, pp. 586–587) read the value at either 95% or 99% probability (i.e. p=0.05 or p=0.01) for the appropriate degrees of freedom (i.e. n–1) for the two sets of data.

Interpretation

There is a significant difference in variance between the two sets when the calculated ratio is greater than the value read from the chart.

Table 30.2 F Distribution tables
(a) 99% Probability (p=0.01)

d.f. Numerator

d.f. Numerator	1	2	3	4	5	6	7	8	9	10	12	15	20	24	30	40	60	120	∞
1	4052	4999.5	5403	5625	5764	5859	5928	5981	6022	6056	6106	6157	6209	6235	6261	6287	6313	6339	6366
2	98.50	99.00	99.17	99.25	99.30	99.33	99.36	99.37	99.39	99.40	99.42	99.43	99.45	99.46	99.47	99.47	99.48	99.49	99.50
3	34.12	30.82	29.46	28.71	28.24	27.91	27.67	27.49	27.35	27.23	27.05	26.87	26.69	26.60	26.50	26.41	26.32	26.22	26.13
4	21.20	18.00	16.69	15.98	15.52	15.21	14.98	14.80	14.66	14.55	14.37	14.20	14.02	13.93	13.84	13.75	13.65	13.56	13.46
5	16.26	13.27	12.06	11.39	10.97	10.67	10.46	10.29	10.16	10.05	9.89	9.72	9.55	9.47	9.38	9.29	9.20	9.11	9.02
6	13.75	10.92	9.78	9.15	8.75	8.47	8.26	8.10	7.98	7.87	7.72	7.56	7.40	7.31	7.23	7.14	7.06	6.97	6.88
7	12.25	9.55	8.45	7.85	7.46	7.19	6.99	6.84	6.72	6.62	6.47	6.31	6.16	6.07	5.99	5.91	5.82	5.74	5.65
8	11.26	8.65	7.59	7.01	6.63	6.37	6.18	6.03	5.91	5.81	5.67	5.52	5.36	5.28	5.20	5.12	5.03	4.95	4.86
9	10.56	8.02	6.99	6.42	6.06	5.80	5.61	5.47	5.35	5.26	5.11	4.96	4.81	4.73	4.65	4.57	4.48	4.40	4.31
10	10.04	7.56	6.55	5.99	5.64	5.39	5.20	5.06	4.94	4.85	4.71	4.56	4.41	4.33	4.25	4.17	4.08	4.00	3.91
11	9.65	7.21	6.22	5.67	5.32	5.07	4.89	4.74	4.63	4.54	4.40	4.25	4.10	4.02	3.94	3.86	3.78	3.69	3.60
12	9.33	6.93	5.95	5.41	5.06	4.82	4.64	4.50	4.39	4.30	4.16	4.01	3.86	3.78	3.70	3.62	3.54	3.45	3.36
13	9.07	6.70	5.74	5.21	4.86	4.62	4.44	4.30	4.19	4.10	3.96	3.82	3.66	3.59	3.51	3.43	3.34	3.25	3.17
14	8.86	6.51	5.56	5.04	4.69	4.46	4.28	4.14	4.03	3.94	3.80	3.66	3.51	3.43	3.35	3.27	3.18	3.09	3.00
15	8.68	6.36	5.42	4.89	4.56	4.32	4.14	4.00	3.89	3.80	3.67	3.52	3.37	3.29	3.21	3.13	3.05	2.96	2.87
16	8.53	6.23	5.29	4.77	4.44	4.20	4.03	3.89	3.78	3.69	3.55	3.41	3.26	3.18	3.10	3.02	2.93	2.84	2.75
17	8.40	6.11	5.18	4.67	4.34	4.10	3.93	3.79	3.68	3.59	3.46	3.31	3.16	3.08	3.00	2.92	2.83	2.75	2.65
18	8.29	6.01	5.09	4.58	4.25	4.01	3.84	3.71	3.60	3.51	3.37	3.23	3.08	3.00	2.92	2.84	2.75	2.66	2.57
19	8.18	5.93	5.01	4.50	4.17	3.94	3.77	3.63	3.52	3.43	3.30	3.15	3.00	2.92	2.84	2.76	2.67	2.58	2.49
20	8.10	5.85	4.94	4.43	4.10	3.87	3.70	3.56	3.46	3.37	3.23	3.09	2.94	2.86	2.78	2.69	2.61	2.52	2.42
21	8.02	5.78	4.87	4.37	4.04	3.81	3.64	3.51	3.40	3.31	3.17	3.03	2.88	2.80	2.72	2.64	2.55	2.46	2.36
22	7.95	5.72	4.82	4.31	3.99	3.76	3.59	3.45	3.35	3.26	3.12	2.98	2.83	2.75	2.67	2.58	2.50	2.40	2.31
23	7.88	5.66	4.76	4.26	3.94	3.71	3.54	3.41	3.30	3.21	3.07	2.93	2.78	2.70	2.62	2.54	2.45	2.35	2.26
24	7.82	5.61	4.72	4.22	3.90	3.67	3.50	3.36	3.26	3.17	3.03	2.89	2.74	2.66	2.58	2.49	2.40	2.31	2.21
25	7.77	5.57	4.68	4.18	3.85	3.63	3.46	3.32	3.22	3.13	2.99	2.85	2.70	2.62	2.54	2.45	2.36	2.27	2.17
26	7.72	5.53	4.64	4.14	3.82	3.59	3.42	3.29	3.18	3.09	2.96	2.81	2.66	2.58	2.50	2.42	2.33	2.23	2.13
27	7.68	5.49	4.60	4.11	3.78	3.56	3.39	3.26	3.15	3.06	2.93	2.78	2.63	2.55	2.47	2.38	2.29	2.20	2.10
28	7.64	5.45	4.57	4.07	3.75	3.53	3.36	3.23	3.12	3.03	2.90	2.75	2.60	2.52	2.44	2.35	2.26	2.17	2.06
29	7.60	5.42	4.54	4.04	3.73	3.50	3.33	3.20	3.09	3.00	2.87	2.73	2.57	2.49	2.41	2.33	2.23	2.14	2.03
30	7.56	5.39	4.51	4.02	3.70	3.47	3.30	3.17	3.07	2.98	2.84	2.70	2.55	2.47	2.39	2.30	2.21	2.11	2.01
40	7.31	5.18	4.31	3.83	3.51	3.29	3.12	2.99	2.89	2.80	2.66	2.52	2.37	2.29	2.20	2.11	2.02	1.92	1.80
60	7.08	4.98	4.13	3.65	3.34	3.12	2.95	2.82	2.72	2.63	2.50	2.35	2.20	2.12	2.03	1.94	1.84	1.73	1.60
120	6.85	4.79	3.95	3.48	3.17	2.96	2.79	2.66	2.56	2.47	2.34	2.19	2.03	1.95	1.86	1.76	1.66	1.53	1.38
∞	6.63	4.61	3.78	3.32	3.02	2.80	2.64	2.51	2.41	2.32	2.18	2.04	1.88	1.79	1.70	1.59	1.47	1.32	1.00

(b) 95% Probability (p=0.05)

d.f. Numerator

d.f. Numerator	1	2	3	4	5	6	7	8	9	10	12	15	20	24	30	40	60	120	∞
1	161.4	199.5	215.7	224.6	230.2	234.0	236.8	238.9	240.5	241.9	243.9	245.9	248.0	249.1	250.1	251.1	252.2	253.3	254.3
2	18.51	19.00	19.16	19.25	19.30	19.33	19.35	19.37	19.38	19.40	19.41	19.43	19.45	19.45	19.46	19.47	19.48	19.49	19.50
3	10.13	9.55	9.28	9.12	9.01	8.94	8.89	8.85	8.81	8.79	8.74	8.70	8.66	8.64	8.62	8.59	8.57	8.55	8.53
4	7.71	6.94	6.59	6.39	6.26	6.16	6.09	6.04	6.00	5.96	5.91	5.86	5.80	5.77	5.75	5.72	5.69	5.66	5.63
5	6.61	5.79	5.41	5.19	5.05	4.95	4.88	4.82	4.77	4.74	4.68	4.62	4.56	4.53	4.50	4.46	4.43	4.40	4.36
6	5.99	5.14	4.76	4.53	4.39	4.28	4.21	4.15	4.10	4.06	4.00	3.94	3.87	3.84	3.81	3.77	3.74	3.70	3.67
7	5.59	4.74	4.35	4.12	3.97	3.87	3.79	3.73	3.68	3.64	3.57	3.51	3.44	3.41	3.38	3.34	3.30	3.27	3.23
8	5.32	4.46	4.07	3.84	3.69	3.58	3.50	3.44	3.39	3.35	3.28	3.22	3.15	3.12	3.08	3.04	3.01	2.97	2.93
9	5.12	4.26	3.86	3.63	3.48	3.37	3.29	3.23	3.18	3.14	3.07	3.01	2.94	2.90	2.86	2.83	2.79	2.75	2.71
10	4.96	4.10	3.71	3.48	3.33	3.22	3.14	3.07	3.02	2.98	2.91	2.85	2.77	2.74	2.70	2.66	2.62	2.58	2.54
11	4.84	3.98	3.59	3.36	3.20	3.09	3.01	2.95	2.90	2.85	2.79	2.72	2.65	2.61	2.57	2.53	2.49	2.45	2.40
12	4.75	3.89	3.49	3.26	3.11	3.00	2.91	2.85	2.80	2.75	2.69	2.62	2.54	2.51	2.47	2.43	2.38	2.34	2.30
13	4.67	3.81	3.41	3.18	3.03	2.92	2.83	2.77	2.71	2.67	2.60	2.53	2.46	2.42	2.38	2.34	2.30	2.25	2.21
14	4.60	3.74	3.34	3.11	2.96	2.85	2.76	2.70	2.65	2.60	2.53	2.46	2.39	2.35	2.31	2.27	2.22	2.18	2.13
15	4.54	3.68	3.29	3.06	2.90	2.79	2.71	2.64	2.59	2.54	2.48	2.40	2.33	2.29	2.25	2.20	2.16	2.11	2.07
16	4.49	3.63	3.24	3.01	2.85	2.74	2.66	2.59	2.54	2.49	2.42	2.35	2.28	2.24	2.19	2.15	2.11	2.06	2.01
17	4.45	3.59	3.20	2.96	2.81	2.70	2.61	2.55	2.49	2.45	2.38	2.31	2.23	2.19	2.15	2.10	2.06	2.01	1.96
18	4.41	3.55	3.16	2.93	2.77	2.66	2.58	2.51	2.46	2.41	2.34	2.27	2.19	2.15	2.11	2.06	2.02	1.97	1.92
19	4.38	3.52	3.13	2.90	2.74	2.63	2.54	2.48	2.42	2.38	2.31	2.23	2.16	2.11	2.07	2.03	1.98	1.93	1.88
20	4.35	3.49	3.10	2.87	2.71	2.60	2.51	2.45	2.39	2.35	2.28	2.20	2.12	2.08	2.04	1.99	1.95	1.90	1.84
21	4.32	3.47	3.07	2.84	2.68	2.57	2.49	2.42	2.37	2.32	2.25	2.18	2.10	2.05	2.01	1.96	1.92	1.87	1.81
22	4.30	3.44	3.05	2.82	2.66	2.55	2.46	2.40	2.34	2.30	2.23	2.15	2.07	2.03	1.98	1.94	1.89	1.84	1.78
23	4.28	3.42	3.03	2.80	2.64	2.53	2.44	2.37	2.32	2.27	2.20	2.13	2.05	2.01	1.96	1.91	1.86	1.81	1.76
24	4.26	3.40	3.01	2.78	2.62	2.51	2.42	2.36	2.30	2.25	2.18	2.11	2.03	1.98	1.94	1.89	1.84	1.79	1.73
25	4.24	3.39	2.99	2.76	2.60	2.49	2.40	2.34	2.28	2.24	2.16	2.09	2.01	1.96	1.92	1.87	1.82	1.77	1.71
26	4.23	3.37	2.98	2.74	2.59	2.47	2.39	2.32	2.27	2.22	2.15	2.07	1.99	1.95	1.90	1.85	1.80	1.75	1.69
27	4.21	3.35	2.96	2.73	2.57	2.46	2.37	2.31	2.25	2.20	2.13	2.06	1.97	1.93	1.88	1.84	1.79	1.73	1.67
28	4.20	3.34	2.95	2.71	2.56	2.45	2.36	2.29	2.24	2.19	2.12	2.04	1.96	1.91	1.87	1.82	1.77	1.71	1.65
29	4.18	3.33	2.93	2.70	2.55	2.43	2.35	2.28	2.22	2.18	2.10	2.03	1.94	1.90	1.85	1.81	1.75	1.70	1.64
30	4.17	3.32	2.92	2.69	2.53	2.42	2.33	2.27	2.21	2.16	2.09	2.01	1.93	1.89	1.84	1.79	1.74	1.68	1.62
40	4.08	3.23	2.84	2.61	2.45	2.34	2.25	2.18	2.12	2.08	2.00	1.92	1.84	1.79	1.74	1.69	1.64	1.58	1.51
60	4.00	3.15	2.76	2.53	2.37	2.25	2.17	2.10	2.04	1.99	1.92	1.84	1.75	1.70	1.65	1.59	1.53	1.47	1.39
120	3.92	3.07	2.68	2.45	2.29	2.17	2.09	2.02	1.96	1.91	1.83	1.75	1.66	1.61	1.55	1.50	1.43	1.35	1.25
∞	3.84	3.00	2.60	2.37	2.21	2.10	2.01	1.94	1.88	1.83	1.75	1.67	1.57	1.52	1.45	1.39	1.32	1.22	1.00

11. ROUTINE MAINTENANCE OF MICROSCOPES

The microscope is a delicate instrument which must be handled gently. It must be installed in a clean environment, away from chemicals, direct sunlight, heating source or moisture. If the stage is contaminated with saline (in blood transfusion work), it must be cleaned immediately to avoid corrosion. Humidity and high temperatures cause growth of fungus which can damage optical surfaces. As storage in a closed compartment encourages fungal growth, rather than keeping it stored in its wooden box it is generally better to keep it standing in place ready for use, but protected by a light plastic cover. In humid climates it may be necessary to use a drying agent, e.g. calcium chloride in a small container.

CLEANING OF THE MICROSCOPE

Optics

After use the immersion objective should be wiped with lens tissue, absorbent paper, soft cloth or medical cotton wool.

Other lenses (objectives and eyepieces) which are smeared with oil should be wiped with a very little xylol or toluene or the following cleaning solution:

Petroleum ether	40%
Ethanol	40%
Ether	20%

The lenses must *not* be soaked in alcohol as this may dissolve the cement. Contamination of the non-optical parts can be removed with mild detergent; grease and oil are removed with petroleum ether followed by 45% ethanol in distilled water.

The eyepieces must be cleaned from dust with a blower or soft camel hair brush. If dust is inside the eyepiece unscrew the upper lens and clean the inside with the blower or the soft brush.

Condenser and iris

The condenser is cleaned in the same way as the lenses with a soft cloth or tissue moistened with xylol or toluene. The mirror is cleaned with a soft cloth moistened with 96% alcohol. The iris diaphragm is very delicate and if damaged or badly corroded it is usually beyond repair.

Mechanical parts

The microscope controls must never be forced. If any of the controls become stiff, a touch of machine oil may be required. This must be proper machine oil, as vegetable oils become dry and hard. This procedure applies to coarse adjustment, fine adjustment, condenser focusing and mechanical stage. It is recommended periodically to clean and give a touch of oil to all accessible movements. This lubrication not only keeps the parts running smoothly in use but reduces wear and protects the parts against corrosion. The surface of the fixed stage must be kept dry, for if a slide is wet underneath it will be difficult to move, and the increase of pressure put on it can damage the mechanical stage if this is forced.

ADDITIONAL PRECAUTIONS IN HOT CLIMATES

Hot humid climates

In hot humid climates, if no precautions are taken, fungus may develop on the microscope, particularly on the surface of the lenses, in the grooves of the screws and under the paint, and the instrument will soon be useless. This can be prevented as follows.

Every evening place the microscope in a warm cupboard. This is a cupboard with a tight-fitting door, heated by one or two 40-watt light bulbs (for a cupboard just big enough to take 1–4 microscopes one bulb is enough). The bulb is left on continuously, even when the microscope is not in the cupboard. Check that the temperature inside the cupboard is at least 5°C warmer than that of the laboratory.

Hot dry climates

In hot dry climates the main problem is dust. Fine particles work their way into the threads of the screws and under the lenses. This can be avoided as follows:

1. Always keep the microscope under a dustproof plastic cover when not in use.

2. At the end of the day's work, clean the microscope thoroughly by blowing air on it from a rubber bulb.
3. Finish cleaning the lenses with a lens brush or fine paintbrush. If dust particles remain on the surface of the objectives, remove with clean paper.

12. RABBIT BRAIN THROMBOPLASTIN

Freeze-dried rabbit brain thromboplastins are now widely available commercially with a shelf life of at least 2–5 years. Usually, they are calibrated against the WHO International Reference Preparation of thromboplastin and are supplied with an International Sensitivity Index (ISI) and a table converting prothrombin times to International Normalized Ratios (INR).

If a commercial preparation is not available it is possible to prepare a home-made substitute using rabbit brain which does not require freeze drying and which is relatively stable.

ACETONE-DRIED BRAIN POWDER

Strip the membrane off freshly collected rabbit brain, wash free from blood and place in about three times its volume of cold acetone. Macerate for 2–3 min and then filter through absorbent lint (BP or USP grade) on a Büchner funnel. Repeat the extraction 7 times; after two extractions increase the time of exposure to acetone to c 20 min for each subsequent extraction. The material should become 'gritty' by the fourth or fifth extraction. After the last extraction spread the acetone-dried brain on a piece of paper and allow to dry in air for 30 min. Rub through a 1 mm mesh nylon sieve to produce a coarse powder. Dispense into a batch of screw-capped bottles and dry over phosphorus pentoxide in a vacuum desiccator. After drying, screw down the caps tightly and store at 4°C or –20°C. At –20°C the material should be stable for at least 5 yr. 100 g of whole brain yield c 15 g of dried powder.

Preparation of liquid suspension

Dissolve 0.9 g of NaCl and 0.9 g of phenol in 100 ml of water. Suspend 3.6 g of the acetone-dried brain in 100 ml of this phenol-saline solution at 15–20°C and allow to stand at this temperature for 4–5 h, mixing at 30 min intervals. Transfer to a 4°C refrigerator for 24 h with occasional mixing. Thereafter, leave undisturbed at 4°C for 3 h and then decant the supernatant carefully through fine muslin or similar material. The ISI should be not more than 1.4 (see p. 368) and the mean normal prothrombin time 12–13 s. Store the suspension at 4°C. At this temperature it will be stable for at least 6 months, and for at least 7 days at 37°C. It must not be allowed to freeze as freezing results in flocculation of the smooth suspension with deterioration of thromboplastic activity.

13. PTT PHOSPHOLIPID REAGENT

Acetone-dried rabbit brain is suitable for preparing a PTT reagent. Bovine brain may also be used for the PTT reagent, but not for thromboplastin.

Prepare acetone-dried brain powder as described above. Suspend 5 g of the powder in 20 ml of chloroform (analytic grade) in a covered beaker for 1–2 h. Filter through filter paper to obtain a clear filtrate. Wash the brain deposit on the filter paper with 20 ml of chloroform and pool the clear filtrate with the previous filtrate. Evaporate the filtrate to dryness in a beaker of known weight in a water-bath at 60–70°C and weigh the residual deposit: 5 g of dried brain should yield c 1.5 g of phospholipid deposit. Emulsify in saline to give a 5% emulsion; 1.5 g of deposit should provide 30 ml of emulsion. Distribute the emulsion in small volumes in stoppered tubes. At −20°C it should be stable for at least 1 yr.

For use dilute 1 in 100 in saline. For the APTT (PTTK) test (p. 308) mix with an equal volume of 2.5 mg/ml kaolin suspension in imidazole buffer.

---

14. REFERENCE STANDARDS AND REAGENTS

A number of international reference materials for haematology have been established by World Health Organization[5,6] and are held at designated institutions. Except where otherwise indicated, the following are available from: National Institute for Biological Standards and Control (NIBSC), South Mimms, Potters Bar EN6 3QG, UK; Fax (44) 707 646730.

General haematology

Erythropoietin, human, urinary
Erythropoietin, rDNA-derived
Ferritin, human
Haemiglobincyanide★
Hb A_2
Hb F
Transferrin
Vitamin B_{12} in human serum

Immunohaematology

Anti-D immunoglobulin
Anti-A blood typing serum
Anti-B blood-typing serum
Anti-A,B blood-typing serum
Anti-C complete blood-typing serum
Anti-c incomplete blood-typing serum
Anti-D (anti-R_0) incomplete blood-typing serum
Anti-D (anti-Rh_0) complete blood-typing serum★
Anti-E complete blood-typing serum

Immunology

Human serum immunoglobulins IgG, IgA and IgM

Human serum immunoglobulin IgE
Antinuclear factor, homogeneous
FITC-conjugated sheep anti-human IgG, IgM
FITC-conjugated sheep anti-human IgG (anti-γ chain)
Horseradish peroxidase-conjugated sheep anti-human IgG
Human serum complement components C1q, C4, C5, factor B and functional CH_{50}

Coagulation

Anti-thrombin III, plasma
Anti-thrombin III concentrate
Factors II,IX, X concentrate, human
Factor VIII:C concentrate, human
Factors II, VII, IX, X, plasma, human
Factor VIII and von Willebrand factor, plasma
Factor VIIa concentrate
Factor IX concentrate
Heparin, low molecular weight, for molecular calibration
Heparin, porcine
Plasma fibrinogen, human
Plasmin, human
Platelet factor 4
Prekallikrein activator
Protein C, human
Streptokinase
Thrombin, human
α-Thrombin, human
β-Thromboglobulin
Tissue plasminogen activator, human
Urokinase, human

Urokinase, high molecular weight
Thromboplastin, bovine, combined*
Thromboplastin, human, plain*
Thromboplastin, rabbit, plain*

The following Certified Reference Materials have been established by, and can be purchased from: European Union Measurement & Testing

Programme (BCR),[1] rue de la Loi 200, B-1049, Brussels; Fax (32) 2 295 807.

Haemiglobincyanide
Monosized latex particles, 2.2 μm (5.7 fl) and 4.9 μm (60.0 fl)
Thromboplastin, bovine, combined
Thromboplastin, human, plain
Thromboplastin, rabbit, plain

---

*From Central Laboratory of the Netherlands Red Cross Blood Transfusion Service (CLB), Plesmanlaan 125, 1066CX Amsterdam; Fax (31) 20 512 3332

REFERENCES

[1] COMMUNITY BUREAU of REFERENCE (1992). *BCR Reference Materials*. Commission of the European Communities, Brussels.
[2] Hendry, E.B. (1961). Osmolarity of human serum and of chemical solutions of biological importance. *Clinical Chemistry*, **7**, 156.
[3] MOORE, H.C. and MOLLISON, P.L. (1976). Use of a low-ionic-strength medium in manual tests for antibody detection. *Transfusion*, **16**, 291.

[4] WORLD HEALTH ORGANIZATION (1977). *The SI for the Health Professions*. WHO, Geneva.
[5] WORLD HEALTH ORGANIZATION (1991). *Biological Substances: International Standards and Reference Reagents 1990*. WHO, Geneva.
[6] WORLD HEALTH ORGANIZATION (1993). Expert Committee on Biological Standardization, 42nd Report. *WHO Technical Report Series*. WHO, Geneva.

Index

Note — page numbers in italics refer to figures and tables

A antigens, 446
  subgroups, 447
A genes, 446
α globin gene
  cluster, *532*
  probe, 533
A substance secretion tests, 463
Abbott fluorescent microparticle
      enzyme assay using Abbott IMX
      analyser, 424
ABO grouping
  A_1 from A_2 differentiation, 484
  antenatal, 486–7
  auto-immune haemolytic anaemia,
    483, 503, 511–12
  bacterial contamination, 483
  blood transfusion compatibility
    testing, 479, 480–4
  cord blood at delivery, 494
  false negative reactions, 483–4
  false positive results in, 483
  maternal blood at delivery, 494
  microplate method, 482
  mixed-field reactions, 484
  rapid techniques, 489
  reverse, 481
  rouleaux formation, 483
  tube method, 480–1
ABO haemolytic disease of the
      newborn, 104, 495–6
  antenatal prediction, 496
  cord blood testing, 496
  serological investigation, 495–6
ABO incompatibility, 489
  acute intravascular haemolysis, 491
ABO system, 445, 446–8
  antibodies, 447–8
  antigens, 446–7
  secretor status, 447
Acantho–echinocyte, 115
Acanthocytosis, 113–14
  scanning electron microscopy, *119*
Accreditation, 33
Accuracy, 35
Acid citrate dextrose, 36
Acid globin chain electrophoresis, 265

Acid phosphatase reaction, 149–51
  acute lymphoblastic leukaemia, 156
  tartrate resistance, 150–1
Acid-citrate-dextrose (ACD), 6, 575
Acidified serum test, 288
  with additional magnesium, 290
  paroxysmal nocturnal
    haemoglobinuria, 287, 289–90
  significance, 290
Acidosis, 241
Acquired inhibitors of coagulation
    factors *see* Circulating
  anticoagulants, investigation
Activated partial thromboplastin time
    (APTT), 300, 308–9, 311–12
  bleeding disorder, 329, 331
  heparin treatment, 373–4
  inhibitor screen, 339–40
  one-stage assays, 331
  oral anticoagulant treatment, 368
  prolonged, 341–3
Activation peptides, 366
Acute leukaemias, differential
    diagnosis, 154–7
Acute lymphoblastic leukaemia, 124
  acid phosphatase reaction, 151, 156
  characterization, 158
  chromosome abnormalities, 169
  classification, *157*
  cytochemical diagnostic tests, 143
  cytochemistry, 156–7, *157*
  differential diagnosis, 154, 156–7
  FACS scan analysis, *164*
  immunological classification, *160*,
    167–8
  α-naphthol acetate esterase, 152
  naphthol AS acetate reaction, 156
  PAS reaction, *149*, 156
  Sudan black B reaction, 156
  terminal transferase (TdT), 162
Acute myeloblastic (myeloid)
    leukaemia, 145
  cell markers, *164*
  chloracetate esterase reaction, 155
  classification, *155*
  cytochemistry, *155*
  diagnosis, 144
  differential diagnosis, 154–6
  immunological classification, 168

myeloid antigen expression, *165*
  α-naphthol acetate esterase, 152, 156
  naphthol AS acetate esterase, 153
  peroxidase reaction, 155, 156
  pseudo-Pelger cells, 123
  ring sideroblasts, 133
  Sudan black B reaction, 155, 156
Acute phase proteins, 562
Acute phase response tests, 559–64
Adenosine diphosphate (ADP), 235
  platelet aggregation, 322, 323
Adenosine triphosphate (ATP), 224
ADPase, 298
Adrenaline, 322, 324
Afibrinogenaemia
  bleeding time, 319
  investigation, 344
AIDS, mean peroxidase activity index
    (MPXI) increase, 77
Alder-Reilly anomaly, 118, *124*
Aldomet *see* α-Methyldopa
Alkaline globin chain electrophoresis,
    264–5
Alkaline haematin method for
    haemoglobin estimation, 50, 53
Alkaline phosphatase
  anti-alkaline phosphatase method
    (APAAP), 163, 165
  conjugase, 424
Allele-specific oligonucleotide
    hybridization, 539–40
  β-thalassaemia, 542
Allo-antibodies
  co-existing with warm auto-
    antibodies, 513, 515
  screening for 512–13, *514*, 516–17
Allo-antigen systems, 465
Alsever's solution, 6, 575
2-Aminoethyl-*iso*-thiouronium bromide
    (AET) cells, 293
δ-Aminolaevulinic acid, 207
ρ-Aminosalicylic acid, 499
  haemolysis, 525
Ammonium oxalate, 64
cAMP, 300
Amplification refractory mutation
    system (ARMS), 540–1
  β-thalassaemia, 542, *543*
  α-thalassaemia, *543*

593

Anaemia
    diagnosis, 192–3, *194–5*
    haematological investigations,
        192–3
    multifactorial, 192
    secondary, 193
Analysis of variance, 585
Ancrod, 314, 367
Angiotensin II, 298
Anisochromasia, 99, 103
Anisocytosis, 90, 99, *100*
Anti-A$_1$, 448
Anti-A, 445, 447–8
    A substance detection, 463
    reagent, 480
Anti-α, 458
Anti-A,B reagent, 480
Anti-B, 445, 447–8
    B substance detection, 463
    reagent, 480
Anti-C3, 458, 472
Anti-C, 449
Anti-cardiolipin assay, 356
Anti-CD59, 292
Anti-complement, 457–8
    antibodies, 458–9
Anti-D, 449
    haemolytic disease of the newborn,
        493
    measurement, 494
    monoclonal reagents, 485
    reagents, 484
prophylaxis in haemolytic disease of the
        newborn, 495
Anti-DNA antibodies, 568
Anti-E, 449
Anti-EBNA-1, 565
Anti-Γ, 458
Anti-H, 448, 463
Anti-HEMPAS, 290
Anti-I serum, 291
Anti-i specificity, 520
Anti-IgG, 457, 472
IgG subclass antiglobalin reagents,
        507–8
    potency, 458
    reagent, 506
Anti-IgM, 472
    reagent, 506
Anti-Jk^a, 493
Anti-μ, 458
Anti-penicillin antibody detection,
        525–6
Anti-Xa assay, 374, 376–7
Antibody screening for blood
        transfusion, 487–8
Antibody titration, 461–2
Antibody-dependent cell-mediated
        cytotoxicity (ADCC), 450, 451,
        494
Anticoagulants
    collection of blood, 3–4
    mode of action, 6
Anticoagulant treatment, oral control
        of, 367–71

activated partial thromboplastin time
        (APTT), 368
    capillary reagent, 371
    chromogenic substrates, 368
    one-stage prothrombin time of
        Quick, 368, 369
    patient who bleeds, 371
    prothrombin and proconvertin
        (P & P) method, 368
    thromboplastin, 368–71
    thrombotest of Owren, 368
Antiferritin IgG preparation, 440
Antigen demonstration, 163, 165
Antiglobulin test
    direct test (DAT), 457
    false-negatives, 510
    indirect test (IAT), 457
    new technology for antibody
        detection, 460–1
    Rh antibodies, 457–61
    two-stage EDTA-complement
        indirect, 460
    worker assessment, 461
Antinuclear factors
    demonstration, 568–9
    latex-bound
        desoxyribonucleoprotein, 568
    LE-cell test, 568
    radio-immunoassay, 568
α$_2$-Antiplasmin, 303
    chromogenic assay, 357
    congenital deficiency, 360
Antithrombin III, 6, 302
    assay using thrombin, 361–2
    heparin binding, 372
    measurement, 361
    measurement using chromogenic
        assay, 361–2
Aplastic anaemia, 99, 193, 199
    bone marrow biopsy, 177
    neutrophil alkaline phosphatase
        (NAP), 148
    red cell uptake of ^{59}Fe, *401, 402*
    surface counting of ^{59}Fe, 402, *403*
Apparatus cleaning, 32, 580
Arachidonic acid
    metabolism, 299
    platelet aggregation, 322, 324
Arterial thrombosis, 379
Aspirin, 380
Atomic weights, 583
Audit, 33
Auer rods, 145, *146*
Auto-agglutination, 55, 90–1, 116–17
Auto-antibody
    screening tests for auto-immune
        haemolytic anaemia (AIHA),
        512–13, *514*
    types, 500–2
Autohaemolysis, 222–5
Automated counters, 191
    calibration, 79
    impedance, 76
    light scattering, 76
    white cell, 77

Automated differential counters, 75–7
    abnormal sample flagging, 77
    five- to seven-part, 76
    flow cytometry, 77
    three-part, 75, 76
Automated equipment cleaning, 32
    see also Apparatus cleaning
Automated techniques, 68–79
    instrument choice, 69
    semi-automated instruments, 69
Automation, 24
Azure B, 84
Azure B-eosin Y stain, 85, 86, 89, 90

B$_{12}$
    Abbott fluorescent microparticle
        enzyme assay using Abbott IMX
        analyser, 424
    absorption investigation, 427–9
    analogues, 421
    assay method choice, 424–5
    automated non-isotopic assays, *426*
    Baxter Stratus automated
        fluorometric enzyme-linked
        immunoassay,
        423–4
    binding agent, 421
    bound, 422
    CIBA Corning ACS:180 assay, 424
    commercial radioassay kits, *425*
    extraction from serum
        transcobalamins, 421
    intrinsic factor, 421, 423
    neuropathy, 417, 434
    non-specific binding, 421
    plasma binding capacity, 432–3
    protein-bound, 429
    quality control for assays, 425–6
    radioisotope tracer, 422
    reference materials for assays, 425–6
    separation of free from bound, 422
    serum measurement by radioassay,
        420–2
    standards, 421–2
    unsaturated binding capacity, 432–3
    urinary excretion, 428, 429
    whole body counting, 429
B$_{12}$ deficiency, 434
    B$_{12}$ malabsorption, 428–9
    deoxyuridine suppression test, 418
B antigens, 446, 447
B genes, 446
B substance secretion tests, 463
B acute lymphoblastic leukaemia, 157
    antigen expression, 168
B-cell leukaemias, 168
    markers, *161*
B-cell lymphoma
    eosinophilia, 124
    markers, *161*
Bacterial toxin, 104
Barbitone buffer, 577
Barbitone buffered saline, 577
Barbitone-bovine serum albumin
    buffer, 578

Barr body, 170
Basophilia, punctate, 99, 115, *116*
Basophils, 124
    counting chamber method, 63
Baxter Stratus automated fluorometric
        enzyme-linked immunoassay,
        423–4
Bed rest, 397
Bee stings, *112*
Benzidine, 199
Bernard-Soulier syndrome, 127, *321*,
        325
    iso-antibodies, 466
Betke method for Hb F, 281
Biliary obstruction, haptoglobin levels,
        203
Bilirubin, 201
    serum measurement, 205, 206
Biohazard precautions, blood
        collection/handling, 1, 2, 31–2
Blackwater fever
    haemoglobinaemia, 200
    methaemalbuminaemia, 204
Blackfan-Diamond disease, 255
Bleeding disorder
    coagulation factor deficiency/defect,
        325–8
    prolonged APTT and PT, 341–3
Bleeding tendency investigation,
        317–18
Bleeding time, 318–19
    Ivy's method, 318–19
    standardized template method, 318
Blood
    abnormality screening, 191–2
    containers, 2
    defibrination, 3
    defibrination flask, 580
    disorder diagnosis, 191
    donor compatibility test, 409
    quality control materials for counts,
        37–40
    storage, effects on quantitative
        estimation, 46
    temperature, effect on morphology 3
    venous, 7
Blood cells
    examination in plasma, 90–1
    immune destruction mechanisms,
        450–1
    morphology, 4–6, 97–128
    separation, 91–2
    specific cell population separation,
        92
Blood coagulation, 300–2
    cascade, *300*
    contact activation system, 300–1
    factors, 300, *301*
    fibrinogen, 302
    labile factors, 301–2
    limiting mechanism, 302
    tissue factor, 301
Blood counters
    fully automated, 68
    quality control, 39–40

Blood films, 60
    dry, 98–9
    examination, 89–90, 97, 98, *99*
    labelling, 84
    parasites, 89–90
    preparation, 2, 5–6, 83–4
    Romanowsky stain, *87, 88*
    screening for abnormalities, 191–2
    spin method, 83–4
    staining, 84–9, 89–90
    thick, 89–90
Blood group serology
    complement storage, 453
    enzyme-treated red cells, 453–5
    plasma storage, 452–3
    plasma use, 452
    quality control, 452–5
    red cell suspensions, 453
    safety precautions, 452
    sample collection/storage, 452
    serum storage, 452–3
    serum vs plasma, 452
    standard operating procedures, 452
    technique, 452–5
Blood groups
    ABO system, 446–8
    agglutination of red cells by
        antibody, 455–7
    antibody titration, 461–2
    antiglobulin test, 457–61
    Duffy system, 449
    genes, 445
    Kell system, 449
    Kidd system, 449
    lysis of red cells, 456–7
    Rh system, 446–8
Blood loss
    from gastrointestinal tract,
        measurement, 403–4
    survival data correction, 409
Blood transfusion, 479–96
    ABO grouping, 479, 480–4
    allo-antibody specificity, 488
    antibody identification, 488
    antibody screening, 487–8
    blood samples, 480
    clinical history of patient, 479
    close intervals, 490
    CMV negative blood, 490
    compatibility tests in newborn
        infants, 489–90
    cross-matching, 479–80, 488–90
    direct agglutination test, 488
    documentation, 480
    donor-recipient compatibility, 479
    emergency blood issue, 489
    false positive results in ABO
        grouping, 483
    Γ-irradiated blood, 490
    haemolytic reaction, 491–3
    immunological consequences, *491*
    indirect antiglobulin test, 479, 488
    intrauterine, 490
    microplate ABO grouping method,
        482

    papain enzyme tests, 488
    pre-transfusion testing, 479
    reverse grouping, 481
    Rh grouping, 479, 480, 484–7
    rouleaux formation, 483
    safety, 480
    special situation cross-matching,
        489–90
    tube ABO grouping method, 480–1
    two-stage enzyme test, 488
Blood vessel
    endothelial cell function, 297–8
    severe damage, 311
    structure, 297
    subendothelium, 298
Blood volume, 391–7
    calculation, 393
    determination of total, 395–7
    expression of results, 395–7
    measurement, 392–7
    red cell life-span estimation, 409
    repeated measurements, 394
Bohr effect, 245
Bone marrow
    anticoagulant, 179
    aspiration for transplantation, 178
    biopsy, 175–88, 192
    cellularity, 180, 182
    concentration, 179
    diagnostic biopsy, 192
    differential cell counts, 180–1
    DNA extraction, 548
    embedding, 186
    erythroblasts, 181
    examination, 178–80
    imprints, 179
    iron staining, 192
    leuco-erythrogenetic ratio, 181
    lymph follicles, 181
    lymphocytes, 181
    lymphoid cells, 182
    May-Grünwald-Giemsa stain, 187–8
    microtome, 186
    myelofibrosis, 187
    myeloid:erythroid ratio, 181
    myeloid:lymphoid ratio, 181
    myeloid cells, 181
    necrosis, 182–3
    normal values, *181*
    particle preparation, 184
    particle smears, 179
    post-mortem films, 179–80
    quantitative cell counts, 180
    report forms, *183*
    reticulin, 187
    Romanowsky dye, 179
    section preparation, 183–4, 185–8
    silver impregnation, 187
    staining, 187
    trephine biopsy, 185
Bone marrow films, 178–9
    preparation, 84
    reports, 181–3
    staining, 84–9
BRIC–8, 458

Bromelin preparation, 454–5
Buffers, 577–9
Buffy-coat preparation, 91
Burns, severe, 106, *107*
Burr cells, *106*, 114
Business planning, 22–4
n-Butanol stability test, 269–70
Butterfly needle, 1

C3, 450, 458, 459
C4, 458, 459
Capillary blood *see* Peripheral blood
Carboxyhaemoglobin (HbCO), 137,
    210, 252
  demonstration, 212
Carcinogenic reagents, 32
Carcinomatosis
  blue polychromasia, 115
  erythroblasts, 116
Carrier detection, genetic counselling,
    347
CcEe genes, 448
CD55 deficiency, 288
CD59
  deficiency, 288
  flow cytometry analysis, 292
CD-ROM, 27
CDA Type II, 290
Cell destruction, 450
Cell markers
  immunofluorescence tests, 161
  leucocytes, 159–63
  methodology, 159–60
  rosette tests, 160–1
  terminal transferase (TdT), 162
Cellular haemoglobin concentration
    mean (CHCM), 73
Cellulose acetate electrophoresis
  at alkaline pH, 258–60, *261*
  at pH 6.5, 262
Centrifuges
  cleaning, 32
  spillage, 32
Centrifuging speed, 581
Cephalosporin, red cell effects, 525
Chagas disease, 93
α-Chain inclusions in β-thalassaemia
    major, 283
CHCM, automated measurement, 74
Chediak-Higashi syndrome, 118, *121*
Childhood lymphoblastic leukaemia
  acute, 156–7
  PAS, 148
Children, normal haematological
    values, *17*
Chloracetate esterase, 153–4
  acute myeloid leukaemia, 155
Chloroquine stripping technique, 468
Chlorpropamide, 525
Chorionic villus samples, 284
Chromium toxicity, 404
Chromosome 9, 446
Chromosome 11, 252
Chromosome 16, 252
Chromosomes

demonstration, 168–70
haemopoietic malignancy
    abnormalities, *169*
  long, 170
  prometaphase banding, 170
Chronic granulocytic (myeloid)
    leukaemia, *123*, *124*, 157
  basophils, 124
  diagnostic tests, 193
  lymphoblastic transformation, 157
  monocytes, 125
  pseudo-Pelger cells, 123
Chronic lymphocytic leukaemia
  diagnostic tests, 193
  lymphocytes, *125*, 127
  PAS, 148
Chronic lymphoid leukaemia
  chromosome abnormalities, 170
  cytochemical diagnostic tests, 143
Chronic lymphoproliferative disorders,
    158–9
  characterization, 158–9
  membrane phenotype, *158*
Chronic myeloid leukaemia
Chronic myelomonocytic leukaemia,
    157–8
  monocytes, 125
CIBA Corning ACS:180 assay, 424
Circulating anticoagulant
  factor VIII:C level, 331
  investigation, 339–40
Citrate agar electrophoresis at pH 6.0,
    261–2
Citrate-phosphate-dextrose, 6, 36, 575,
    576
Citrate-phosphate-dextrose-adenine
    solution, 576
Citrate-saline buffer, 578
Clauss technique, 345
Clostridium perfringens
  lecithinase, 104
  septicaemia, *105*
Clot lysis time, 357–8
$^{57}CO-B_{12}$, 422
Coagulation
  activation markers, 366
  deficiency/defect, 348
  end-point, 306
  tests, 300
  thrombolytic therapy, 378
Coagulation factors
  deficiency/defect, 325–8
  parallel line bioassays, 326–8
Cobalamin, 417
Cobalt, 428
Cobas Argos 5000 counter, 76
Cobra-venom test, 287
Coefficient of variation (CV), 56–7,
    584
Coincidence correction, 71
Cold agglutinins, 3
  ABO grouping, 483
  auto-immune haemolytic anaemia,
    490
  doubling dilution techniques, *507*

inaccurate RBC counts, 71
MCV errors, 73
thermal range determination, 520
titration, 519, 520
titration end-points, *462*
Cold antibody lysis, 520–2
  in paroxysmal nocturnal
    haemoglobinuria, 287, 291–2
Cold antibody specificity, 519–20
Cold auto-antibodies, 501–2
  agglutination titres, *519*, 520
  lysis, *521*
Cold-haemagglutinin disease (CHAD),
    501, 519, 520
Cold-haemagglutinin syndrome, 200
Collagen, 322, 323
Collection of blood, 1–7
  anticoagulants, 3–4
  biohazard precautions, 1
  mixing, 6
  peripheral, 7
  serum, 2–3
  standard procedure, 3
  standardized conditions, 9
  temperature, 3
  venous, 1–2
Common ALL-antigen, 157
Compatibility, red cell survival, 491
Compatibility tests, 409
  auto-immune haemolytic anaemia,
    490
  intrauterine transfusion, 490
  maternal serum, 489
  newborn infants, 489–90
  transfusions at close intervals, 490
Complement components, 450
Complement-binding antibodies, 452
Computers, 27–8
Congenital ahaptoglobinaemia, 203
Congenital coagulation deficiency/
    defect
  carrier investigation, 347–8
  genotype assignment, 348
  phenotype investigation, 347–8
  replacement therapy monitoring, 348
Congenital dyserythropoietic anaemia,
    100
Congenital NADH methaemoglobin
    reductase deficiency, 252
Contact activation system, 300–1
Containers, 2
  evacuated, 2
Control charts, 40, *41*
Coombs test *see* Direct antiglobulin test
    (DAT)
Coproporphyrin, 207, 209
Cord-blood erythroblasts, 138
Coronary thrombolysis, 379
Corrinoids, 421
Cost-effectiveness, 23–4
Costing, 23
Coulter Counting System, 69
Coumarins, 367
^{51}Cr
  accumulation patterns, 412

^{51}Cr (*Cont'd*)
blood loss, measurement from gastrointestinal tract, 403–4
blood volume, repeated measurements, 394
donor blood compatibility test, 409
labelled red cells, 192
physical separation, 388
platelet life-span measurement, 413–15
red cell destruction site determination, 410–12
red cell labelling, 392, 412
red cell life-span measurement, 404–7, *408*, 409
red cell volume measurement, 392–3
gamma-ray spectrum, *384*
spleen:liver ratio, 411, 412
surface counting studies, 411
Crohn's disease, 125
Cross-matching
blood transfusion, 488–90
direct agglutination test, 489
emergency blood issue, 489
group, antibody screen and save procedure, 488–9
indirect antiglobulin test, 489
routine, 489
special transfusions, 489–90
Cumulative sum method (CUSUM), 40–2
Cyanmethaemoglobin method *see* Haemiglobincyanide method for haemoglobin measurement
Cyanocobalamin, 422
Cytoplasm immunoglobulin markers (CyIg), 159, 161

D antigen, 448, 485, 486, 487
d gene, 448
Dacron grafts, 360
Data
analysis, 9, 40–4
processing, 27–8
statistics, 10–11, 584–5, *586–7*
storage, 27
Decay accelerating factor (DAF)
deficiency, 288
flow cytometry analysis, 292
Delta check, 44
Deoxyuridine suppression test, 418, 426–7
Deviation index, 44–5
Diagnosis, 191
Diagnostic efficiency, 27
3,3'-Diaminobenzidine (DAB) tetrahydrochloride, 144, 145
Diazepoxide, 525
2,3-Diphosphoglycerate, 215, 239–41
measurement, 239–41
normal values, 240
significance of levels, 240–1
Dipyrimadole, 380
Direct antiglobulin test (DAT), 457
agglutination significance, 509

auto-immune haemolytic anaemia, *500*, 503, 505–12
hospital patient positives, 509–10
hypergammaglobulinaemia, 510
normal subject positives, 509
positive, 508–10
qualitative, 506
quantitative, 506–7, *508*
Disinfectants, 32
Disseminated intravascular coagulation, 309, 314, 345–7
factor VIII:C level, 331
fibrin monomer screening test, 346–7
fibrinogen assay, 345–6
fibrinogen/fibrin degradation product detection, 346
latex agglutination method, 346
DL-Dithiothreitol, 264
B_{12} non-specific binding reduction, 421
combined B_{12} folate assay, 422
effect on IgM antibodies
DNA
analysis, 529–30
concentration determination, 548
extraction kits, 548
non-radioactive labelling, 553
nuclear, 530
^{32}P fragment labelling, 552–3
peripheral blood extraction, 530
plasmid, 531
recombinant molecules, 530
Southern blot analysis, 530–8
thermostable polymerase, 538
DNA probes, 531, 551–2
plasmid insert purification, 551
reagents, 551–2
DNA techniques, 529–56
allele-specific oligonucleotide hybridization, 539–40
amplification refractory mutation system (ARMS), 540–1
analysis of DNA, 529–30
analysis of PCR products, 539–40
extraction of genomic DNA, 546–8
G6PD deficiency, 543–4
linkage analysis, 544–6
polymerase chain reaction, 538–9
restriction enzyme digestion, 539
Döhle bodies, 121
Donath-Landsteiner antibody, 502
detection, 522–3
indirect antiglobulin test, 523
specificity, 523
thermal range, 523
titration, 523
Drabkin's reagent, 50
Drepanocytes *see* Sickle cells
D^u phenotype, 485, 486
Duffy system, 449
Dyserythropoiesis, 238
red cell uptake of ^{59}Fe, *401*, *402*
surface counting of ^{59}Fe, 402, *403*
Dysfibrinogenaemia, 309, 310
investigation, 344, 356

E-rosette receptor, 161
Ear-lobe puncture, 6–7
Echinocytes, 114–15
EDTA, 3–4, 6, 49
blood cell degeneration, 5
bone marrow anticoagulant, 179
neutral, 576
neutral buffered, 576
preparation, 576
Ehler's-Danlos syndrome, 319
Elliptocytosis, 101
Embden-Meyerhof pathway, 225
Emergency service, 24
Endothelial cells, 297–8
Eosin, 88–9
Eosin Y, 84
Eosinopenia, 124
Eosinophilia, 124
Eosinophils, *121*, 124
counting chamber method, 62–3
diurnal variation, 16
PAS reaction, 148
Epstein-Barr virus (EBV), 565
Erythroblastaemia, 99, 115–16
Erythroblasts
α-naphthol acetate esterase, 153
PAS reaction, 138
Erythrocyte sedimentation
mechanisms, 561–2
rouleaux formation, 561
Erythrocyte sedimentation rate, 192, 559–63
as acute phase response test, 559–63
estimation (ESR), 4
ICSH standardized method, 561, *562*
modified methods, 560–1
normal range, 560
quality control, 561
sex differences, 563
significance, 562–3
Westergren method, 559–60
Erythrocyte surface area/volume ratio, 216
Erythrocytosis, 252
Erythrokinetics, 397–402, *403*
Erythroleukaemia
PAS reaction, 138, 148, 156
ring sideroblasts, 133
Erythropoiesis
compensatory, 115–16
iron utilization measurement, 401
Erythropoietic porphyria, congenital, 210
Erythropoietic protoporphyria, 210
Erythropoietic stress, 255
Erythropoietin, 571–2
haemoglobin relationship, 571
radio-immunoassay, 571
Escherichia coli, 418
DNA probes, 531
Esterases, 151
Ethylenediamine tetra-acetic acid *see* EDTA
Euglena gracilis, 418

Euglobin lysis time, 357
External quality assessment, 44–6

F distribution tables, *586–7*
F-ratio, 585
Factor 4 assay, 360–1
Factor II, 301, 302
Factor V, 301
  assay, 343
  normal value, 343
Factor V deficiency
  bleeding time, 319
  prolonged APTT and PT, 341
Factor VII, 300, 301, 302
  deficiency, 311
  deficiency/defect investigation, 328
  parallel line bioassay, *326*
Factor VII-tissue factor (TF), 300
Factor VIII, 300, 302
  deficiency, 302, 311
  inhibitors, 340
  X chromosome inactivation, 347
Factor VIII gene
  inheritance, 544
  mutations, 544
  repeat polymorphism, 545–6
Factor VIII:C
  activity, 339
  antibodies, 339
  assay, 326, 327, 333
  concentration, 331
  inheritance, 347
  inhibitor, quantitative measurement,
    340–1
  normal range, 330
  one-stage assay, 329–31
  replacement therapy monitoring, 348
  von Willebrand factor:Ag ratio, 348
Factor IX, 300, 301
  gene mutations, 544
  inhibitors, 341
  X chromosome inactivation, 347
Factor IX deficiency
  APTT prolongation, 329
  inheritance, 347
  nephrotic syndrome, 331
Factor IXa antithrombin III inhibition,
  361
Factor X, 301, 302
  assay, 342–3
  normal value, 343
  prolonged APTT and PT in
    deficiency, 341
  Russell's viper venom, 354, 355
Factor Xa antithrombin III inhibition,
  361
Factor XI, 301, 311
  replacement therapy monitoring, 348
Factor XI deficiency
  APTT prolongation, 329
  bleeding time, 319
Factor XIa antithrombin III inhibition,
  361
Factor XII, 300, 301, 311
Factor XII deficiency, 304

nephrotic syndrome, 331
Factor XIIa antithrombin III
  inhibition, 361
Factor XIII
  clot solubility test, 344–5
  deficiency, 311
Faeces, blood loss, 403, 404
Fanconi's anaemia, 255
Fast Garnet GBC, 149, 150
Favism, 107–8, 225
Fc receptor mediated phagocytosis,
  450
^{59}Fe
  iron absorption, 398–9
  iron distribution, 399
  iron utilization, 400–2
  marrow transit time, 401
  plasma-iron clearance, 399–400
  plasma-iron turnover, 400
  red cell uptake, *401*
  gamma-ray spectrum, *384*
  surface counting, 402, *403*
Ferritin, 131, 201
  assay method selection, 442
  enzyme immunoassay, 440–3
  haemoglobinopathies, 255–6
  infant levels, 443
  serum assay, 439–43
  synthesis, 443
Ferrochelatase, 210
Ferrokinetic patterns, *401, 402*
Fetal loss, second trimester, 352
Fibrin, 300, 302
  D-dimer detection, 349
  degradation products, 309
  deposition, 303
  monomer screening test, 346–7
  plate lysis, 358–9
Fibrinogen, 299, 300, 302
  assay for disseminated intravascular
    coagulation, 345–6
  dry clot weight, 344
  estimation, 344
  plasma viscosity, 563
Fibrinogen/fibrin degradation
  products, 309
Fibrinolytic potential investigation, 357
Fibrinolytic system, 303
  α_2-antiplasmin amidolytic assay,
    359–60
  euglobin lysis time, 357
  fibrin plate lysis, 358
  investigation, 356–60
  plasminogen activator inhibitor
    (PAI-1) assay, 359
  tissue plasminogen activator (t-PA)
    amidolytic assay, 359
  venous occlusion test, 358–9
Fibrinopeptide A, 366
Fibronectin, 298, 299
Field's staining method, 88–9, 90
Filariasis, 93, *95*
Fitzgerald factor, 300
Fletcher factor, 300
Flow cytometry, 77

GPI-linked proteins, 292–5
Flufenamic acid, 525
2,7-Fluorenediamine (FDA), 144–5,
  146
Fluorescein isothiocyanate (FITC),
  138
  labelled antiglobulin reagents, 472
Fluorescence in-situ hybridization
  (FISH), 170
Fluorochromes, 78
Folate
  Abbott fluorescent microparticle
    enzyme assay using Abbott IMX
    analyser, 424
  assay method choice, 424–5
  automated assay methods, 423–6
  automated non-isotopic assays, *426*
  Baxter Stratus automated
    fluorometric enzyme-linked
    immunoassay, 423–4
  binding agent, 422–3
  binding protein, 423
  chloramphenicol-resistant
    Lactobacillus casei assay, 419–20
  CIBA Corning ACS:180 assay, 424
  commercial radioassay kits, *425*
  drug effects on *L.casei* assay, 420
  extraction from serum binder, 422
  microbiological assay, 418–20
  quality control for assays, 425–6
  radioactive tracer, 423
  radioassay measurement, 422–3
  reference materials for assays, 425–6
  separation of free from bound, 423
  standards, 423
Folate deficiency, 417
  B$_{12}$ malabsorption, 428–9
  deoxyuridine suppression test, 418
Formaldehyde, 37
Forssman antibodies, 566
Fructose-1,6-diphosphate, 235
Fuchs-Rosenthal counting chamber, 62

G6DP deficiency, demonstration,
  139–40
G6PD
  assay, 233–5
  enzyme activity calculation, 233
  gene, 234
  normal values, 233–4
  red cell haemolysate, 232
  variants, 235
G6PD deficiency, *135*
  autohaemolysis, 223
  diagnosis, 225
  DNA techniques, 543–4
  fluorescent screening, 227–8
  glutathione levels, 238
  Heinz bodies, 283
  heterozygosity, 234
  heterozygote detection, 229
  methaemoglobin elution, 229–30
  methaemoglobin reduction, 228–9
  screening tests, 225–8
Gaucher's disease, 331

Gaussian distribution, 584
Geiger-Müller counters, 385
General practitioners'laboratory
  services, 30–1
Genetic counselling
  carrier detection, 347
  haemoglobinopathies, 255
Genomic DNA extraction, 546–8
Gibson and Harrison's artificial
  haemoglobin standard, 577
Giemsa stain, 84, 85, 89, 90
Glandular fever see Infectious
  mononucleosis
Glanzmann's disease iso-antibodies,
  466
Glassware, 580
Globin chain
  relative mobility, 266
  synthesis, 193
Globin chain electrophoresis, 264–5,
  266
  acid, 265
  alkaline, 264–5
Globin gene, 249, 250
  cluster organization, 255
  products, 255
Globin gene disorders
  DNA analysis, 284
  fetal diagnosis, 284
  globin chain synthesis, 284
Gloves, 32
β-Glucoronidase, 154
β-Glucosaminidase, 154
Glucose-6-phosphate dehydrogenase
  deficiency see G6PD deficiency
Γ-Glutamylcysteine synthetase, 238
Glutaraldehyde, 37
Glutathione, 226
  concentration calculation, 237–8
  estimation of reduced, 236–8
  infants, 238
  normal range, 238
  oxidized (GSSG), 226, 227
  stability test, 238
  synthetase, 238
Glyceraldehyde-3-phosphate
  dehydroxenase (Ga3DP), 239
Glycerol lysis time tests, 221
Glycine buffer, 578
Glycocalyx, 297
Glycoprotein Ib-IX complex, 299
Glycosylphosphatidylinositol see GPI
Glycosyltransferase, 446
Good safety practice, 31, 32
GPI-linked protein analysis, 288,
  292–3, 294
Graft-versus-host disease, 490
α-Granule deficiency states, 325
Granulocyte
  antigen preparation, 471
  chloracetate esterase, 153
  chloroquine treatment, 473–4
  immunofluorescence test (GIFT),
    470, 471–3
  maturation, 121, 122

myeloperoxidase reaction, 145
non-specific esterases, 151
periodic acid-Schiff (PAS) reaction,
  148
specific esterases, 151
Grey platelet syndrome, 127, 325

H antigens, 447
H body preparation, 193
H substance detection, 463
HAB blood-group genes, 446
Haem
  iron, 252
  pocket, 250
Haemagglutination test, immune
  adherence, 567
Haematocrit, 72–3
  manual techniques, 57–8
Haematological values, 9, 12–14
Haematology analyzers, 29
Haemiglobincyanide (HiCN), 36
Haemiglobincyanide method for
  haemoglobin measurement, 50–2
  reference solution, 51, 52
Haemochromatosis, 443
Haemoglobin, 7
  abnormal pigments, 210–13
  altered oxygen affinity, 252, 271
  n-butanol stability test, 269–70
  catabolic pathway, 198
  catabolism tests, 205–7
  cellulose acetate electrophoresis at
    alkaline pH, 258–60, 261
  cellulose acetate electrophoresis at
    pH 6.5, 262
  chains, 249–50
  citrate agar electrophoresis at pH
    6.0, 261–2
  clinical syndromes with structural
    variants, 251
  electrophoresis methods for variants,
    258–65, 266
  fetal, 137–8
  heat instability test, 268–9
  inadequate formation, 101–3
  instability testing, 268–70
  iso-electric focusing, 262, 263, 264
  isopropanol stability test, 269
  molecule, 249–50
  normal range, 200
  physiological variation, 11, 14–15,
    14–5
  point mutations, 250
  quality assurance, 258
Haemoglobin eslimation
  automated techniques, 69
  Gibson and Harrison's artificial
    standard, 577
  plasma, estimation, 199–201
  raised levels, 200–1
  reference values, 12, 17
  relative mobility, 260, 263, 264, 272
  sample collection, 199–200
  sample preparation, 257–8
  solubility alteration, 250–2

spectrophotometric measurement,
  54
storage effects, 6
structural variant, differential
  diagnosis, 271, 272
structural variants, 249, 250–2,
  256–8
  unstable, 193, 252
  unstable diseases, 135, 263
Haemoglobin C (Hb C), 252
Haemoglobin derivatives, 134–8
  carboxyhaemoglobin, 137
  fetal haemoglobin, 137–8
  methaemoglobin, 137
Haemoglobin estimation
  alkaline haematin method, 50, 53
  manual technique, 50–4
  oxyhaemoglobin method, 50, 52–3
  photoelectric colorimeter method,
    50–3
  spectrometer method, 50–3
Haemoglobin H, 136–7
Haemoglobinaemia, 200
Haemoglobinometer, direct-reading,
  53
Haemoglobinopathies, 250
  patient investigation, 255–6
  red cell inclusions, 283–4
  unstable, 115
Haemolysis
  drug-induced, 120
  extravascular, 450, 492
  intravascular, 450, 491–2
  investigation, 197–8
  site determination, 199
Haemolytic anaemia, 101
  autohaemolysis, 222–5
  chemical-induced, 107
  cold agglutinin titres, 520
  51Cr red cell survival curves, 408
  diagnostic tests, 193, 198
  2,3-diphosphoglycerate, 239–41
  enzyme abnormalities, 215
  enzyme deficiencies in hereditary,
    225–30
  ferrokinetic patterns, 402
  glutathione levels, 326–8
  glycerol lysis time tests, 221
  hereditary, 105, 198–9
  investigation, 197–9
  laboratory methods, 197–213
  membrane abnormalities, 215
  microangiopathic, 106
  osmotic fragility, 220
  oxygen dissociation curve, 241–5
  pyrimidine-5'-nucleotidase screening
    test, 230–1
  pyruvate kinase assay, 235–6
  red cell destruction site
    determination, 410
  red cell elimination, 407
  reticulocytes, 65
  rouleaux formation, 90
  serum bilirubin, 206
  unstable haemoglobin, 107, 108

Haemolytic anaemia, auto-immune, 55, 92, 104, 105, 499
acquired, 199
allo-absorption using papainized cells, 516–17
allo-antibody screening tests in serum, 512–13, *514*, 516–17
antibody elution from red cells, 517–18
auto-antibodies, 500
auto-antibody screening tests in serum, 512–13, *514*
blood group determination, 503, 511–12
blood samples, 502–3
cold agglutinin thermal range determination, 520
cold agglutinin titration, 519, 520
cold antibody, 504
cold antibody lysis, 520–2
cold antibody specificity, 519–20
cold auto-antibodies, *500*, 501–2
cold-type, 490–1
compatibility tests, 490
complement, 507
concentrated ether eluate testing, 510–11
^{51}Cr accumulation patterns, 412
DAT-negative, 510
diagnosis, 500
direct antiglobulin test (DAT), *500*, 503, 505–12
DL-dithiothreitol 524
Donath-Landsteiner antibody detection/titration, 522–3
drug involvement, 505
eluate screening, 518
enzyme-treated group O cells, 518
free antibody demonstration in serum, 512–13, *514*, 515–22
haemoglobinaemia, 200
haemolytic transfusion reactions, 515
IgG, 507
incomplete antibody detection, 505–12
indirect antiglobulin test, 501, 518
manual direct polybrene test, 511
2-mercapto-ethanol treatment, 524
qualitative direct antiglobulin test, 506–7
serological investigation, 503–5
serum samples, 502–3
warm antibody, 504
warm auto-antibody lysis demonstration, 518–19
warm auto-antibody specificity determination, 518
warm type, 490, 500–1
ZZAP reagent in auto-absorption techniques, 515–16
Haemolytic anaemia, drug-induced, 107, *108*, 199, 499, 524–6
anti-penicillin antibody detection, 525–6
antibodies, 467

antibody detection, 526
complement lysis, 524–5
drug-dependent immune, 524–5
extravascular haemolysis, 525
penicillin, 525
red cell damage, 524–5
Haemolytic disease of the newborn, 493–6
ABO, 104, 493
antenatal blood grouping, 486–7
antenatal serology, 493–4
anti-D, 449
anti-D prophylaxis, 494–5
bilirubin level, 206
compatibility tests, 489–90
cord blood tests at delivery, 494
erythroblasts, 116
hyperimmune IgG anti-A/anti-B, 447
Kell antigen, 487
management, 493
maternal blood tests at delivery, 494
prediction, 493
Rh, 486, 487
Haemolytic mechanisms, 198
Haemolytic transfusion reactions, 449, 491–3
auto-immune haemolytic anaemia, 515
delayed, 493
investigation, *491*, 492
red cell allo-antibodies, 515
serological investigations, 492
Haemolytic uraemic syndrome, *106*, 107
Haemopexin, 200
serum levels, 205
Haemophilia A, 311
Bcl I polymorphism, 545
carriers, 347
diagnosis, 544–6
factor VIII:C level, 331
inheritance, 347
linkage analysis, 544–6
Southern blot analysis, 530, 545
Xba I polymorphism, 545
Haemophilia B, 311
carriers, 347
inheritance, 347
Haemosiderin, 131, 133–4, 200, 201
demonstration in urine, 204–5
Haemostasis, 297
acquired thrombotic tendency, *353*
platelet function, 299
vascular disorders, 311, 318
Haemostasis investigation, 303–5
amidolytic assays, 304
chromogenic peptide substrate assays, 304
coagulation assays, 304–5
equipment, 305–6
first-line tests, *310*
immunological methods, 304
laboratory analysis, 303–4
mixing experiments, 311–13

monoclonal antibodies, 304
platelet-poor plasma preparation, 305
polyclonal antibodies, 304
reagents, 306
reptilase time, 314
sample handling, 306
second-line investigations, 310–14
snake venom, 314
technical errors, 305
therapeutic derangement, 367
time bias, 306
venous blood collection, 305
Haemostatic failure
acute, 317
Ham test *see* Acidified serum test
Handbooks, 30
Handling of blood, 1–7
biohazard precautions, 1
Haptoglobin
electrophoresis method, 201–2
radial immunodiffusion method, 202–3
serum estimation, 201–3
Haptoglobin-haemoglobin complex, 203
Hb A$_2$
elution from cellulose acetate, measurement, 274–5
estimation in thalassaemia, 274
high performance liquid chromatography (HPLC), 278–9
interpretation of values, 279
measurement, 193
microcolumn chromatography measurement, 275–8
Hb A, 249
Hb AC
target cells, 256
trait, 109
Hb AE trait, 109, *111*
Hb Bart's, 262
hydrops fetalis, 253–4
Hb C, 252
Hb CC disease, 109
Hb C^{Harlem}, 267
Hb Constant Spring, 250
Hb EE disease, 109, *111*
Hb F, 249
fetal red cells, 494
increase in adult life, 254–5
inherited abnormalities, 255
interpretion of values, 282
intracellular distribution assessment, 281–2
Hb F measurement, 193
acid elution test, 281
alkaline denaturation, 279
estimation, 279–81
immunofluorescent method, 281–2
Jonxis and Visser method, 280
modified Betke method, 279–80
radial immunodiffusion (RID), 280–1

Hb Gower 1, 249
Hb Gower 2, 249
Hb Gun Hill, 250
Hb H
  disease, *136*, 253, 254
  inclusion bodies, 283–4
Hb Köln, 107, *108*, 134, 135, 252
Hb M, 252
  detection, 270–1
Hb Portland, 249
Hb S, 138
  altered solubility, 250–1
  laboratory investigations, *261*
  monoclonal antibody detection, 268
  point mutation, 250
  sickling in whole blood, 266, *267*
  solubility test, 267
  tests, 266–8
Hb S/β-thalassaemia, 109
Hb SC, 251–2
  disease, 109, *110*
Hb SS, 251
  sickle cells, 256
Hb SS disease, 109, 110
  erythroblasts, 116
  scanning electron microscopy, *120*
Hb S^{Travis}, 267
Health and safety, 31–2
Heat instability test, 268–9
Heel blood, 7
Heinz bodies, 68, 107, *108*, *115*, 134–6
  autohaemolysis, 224
  demonstration, 135–6
  red cell inclusions, 283
  staining, 135–6
  unstable haemoglobin, 252
Helmet cells, 107
Help-lines, 30
HEMPAS, 289, 290, 291
  GPI-linked protein expression, 290
Heparin, 4, 6, 311, 367
  antithrombin III binding, 372
  low molecular weight, 372
  preparation, 577
Heparin cofactor II
  anti-Xa assay, 374, 376–7
  assay, 365–6
  deficiency, 365–6
Heparin treatment, 372–3
  activated partial thromboplastin time
      (APTT), 373–4
  dosage, 375
  investigation of patient bleeding
      during, 377
  laboratory control, 372–3
  prophylactic, 375–6
  protamine neutralization test, 374–5
  side effects, 377
  subcutaneous low-dose, 376–7
  therapeutic, 372–3
  thrombin time, 374
Heparinoids, 367
Hepatitis, 31
  antinuclear factors, 568
HEPES buffer, 578

Hereditary elliptocytosis, 101
  ^{51}Cr accumulation patterns, 412
  osmotic fragility, 220
Hereditary ovalocytosis, 101, *102*, *105*
Hereditary persistence of fetal
      haemoglobin (HPFH), 255
  African type, 281, 282
  disorders, 250
Hereditary spherocytosis, *103*, 104, *105*
  acanthocytosis, *113*
  autohaemolysis, 223
  ^{51}Cr accumulation patterns, 412
  ^{51}Cr red cell survival curves, *408*
  2,3-diphosphoglycerate levels, 241
  glycerol lysis time test, 221
  osmotic fragility, 216, 220
  red cell crenation, *112*
  scanning electron microscopy, *119*
Heterophile antibody, 567
High molecular weight kininogen
      (HMWK), 300, 301
  deficiency, 311
High performance liquid
      chromatography (HPLC), 278–9
Hill's constant, 245, 271
Hirudin, 367
Histiocytic lymphoma, 158, 159
HLA antibody
  chloroquine-treated cells, 474
  detection, 468
Hodgkin's disease
  haptoglobin levels, 203
  neutrophil alkaline phosphatase
      (NAP), 148
Homologous restriction factor (HRF)
      deficiency, 288
Howell-Jolly bodies, 78, 116, *117*
  sickle-cell disease, 110
Human immunodeficiency virus
      (HIV), 31
Human resource management, 21–4
Hydrochlorothiazide, 525
Hyperchromasia, 103
Hypergammaglobulinaemia direct
      antiglobulin test (DAT), 510
Hyperglycaemia, 73
Hypergranular promyelocytic
      leukaemia, 155–6
Hypochromasia, 99, 101–3
Hypochromic anaemia, 101
  anisochromasia, 103
  microcytic, 192–3
Hypofibrinogenaemia, 309
  investigation, 344
Hypoplastic anaemia, congenital, 255

^{125}I
  human serum albumin plasma
      volume method, 394
  plasma volume measurement, 392
  spectrum, *384*
^{125}I-labelled folic acid, 423
^{131}I
  human serum albumin plasma
      volume method, 394

plasma volume measurement, 392
Idiopathic thrombocytopenic purpura,
      321
  platelet survival, 414
IgG
  agglutination of sensitized red cells,
      451–2
  red cell auto-antibodies, 507
  warm auto-antibodies, 500
IgG antibodies
  acute extravascular haemolysis, 492
  delayed haemolytic reactions, 493
  in AIHA, 512–13, *514*
Iliac crest puncture, 176
Image analysis, chromosome
      abnormalities, 170
Imidazole-buffered saline, 578
Immune haemolysis, 450
Immunofluorescence tests, cell
      markers, 161
Immunoglobin (Ig) gene, 534
^{111}In
  red cell labelling, 392, 412, 413
  red cell volume measurement, 393–4
  splenic platelet pool, 414
^{113m}In
  red cell labelling, 392, 412, 413
  red cell volume measurement, 393–4
  splenic red cell volume, 397
Indanediones, 367
Indirect antiglobulin test, 479
  blood transfusion, 488
Indomethicine, 525
Infant, normal haematological values,
      17
Infection
  ferrokinetic patterns, *402*
  haptoglobin levels, 203
  lymphocytes, 126
  neutrophils, 121, *122*
Infectious mononucleosis, 126, 499
  diagnosis, 564
  lymphocytes, 126
  monocytes, 125
  Paul-Bunnell test, 546–8
  slide screening test, 564–5
Instrumentation, 24–5, *26*, 27
  carry-over, 25
  comparability, 25, *26*, 27
  disinfection, 32
  equipment evaluation, 24–5, *26*, 27
  laboratory test efficiency, 27
  linearity, 27
  maintenance logs, 27
  precision, 25
Intensive care unit, near-patient
      testing, 29
Interleukin-1, ferritin synthesis, 443
International Normalized Ratio, 368,
      369, 371
  calibration, 370
International reference preparations, 36
International Sensitivity Index, 368,
      369, 371
  calibration, 369–70

602   INDEX

Intrauterine transfusion, compatibility
    tests, 490
Intrinsic factor, 421, 423
    antibody, 429, 430–2
    estimation in gastric juice, 429–30
    normal values, 430
Intrinsic pathway deficiency/defect
    investigation, 329–31
Inulin test, 287
Ionization chambers, 384–5
Iron
    absorption, 398–9
    assessment, 255
    assessment in thalassaemia, 282–3
    children's levels, 443
    distribution, 399
    liberation, 201
    normal serum values, 438
    overload, 443
    radioactive, 398
    serum level measurement, 192,
        437–8
    surface counting of ^{59}Fe, 402, 403
    transport, 131
    utilization, 400–2
Iron deficiency
    ^{59}Fe, 398–9, 401, 402
    hypochromia, 74
    red cell volume distribution (RDW),
        74
Iron deficiency anaemia, 100, 101,
        102, 437–43
    anisochromasia, 103
    ferritin, serum assay, 439–43
    haemosiderin, 133
    iron-binding capacity, 438–9
    osmotic fragility, 219–20
    PAS reaction, 138
    scanning electron microscopy, 120
    schistocytosis, 105
    serum iron estimation, 437–8
    thin red cells, 109
Iron-binding capacity, 192, 438–9
    determination of unsaturated, 439
    estimation of total, 438–9
    haemoglobinopathies, 255
    normal range, 439
    transferrin concentration, 439
Iso-electric focusing, 262, 263, 264
Isopropanol stability test, 269

Jenner-Giemsa stain, 85, 87–8
Jenner's stain, 84
Jk antibodies, 449
Jonxis and Visser method for Hb F,
    280

Kala-azar, 93
Kallikrein, 300, 303
Kaolin
    cephalin clotting time, 308
    clotting time, 352–4
Kell
    antigen in haemolytic disease of the
        newborn, 487

precursor (Kx) absence, 113
    system, 449
Kidd system, 449
Kleihauer acid elution technique,
    494–5

La antigen, 568
Laboratory organization/management,
    21–33
    accreditation, 33
    audit, 33
    business planning, 22–4
    cost-effective working, 23–4
    costing, 23
    customized services, 29–31
    data processing, 27–8
    general practitioners' services, 30–1
    health and safety, 31–2
    human resource management, 21–4
    instrumentation, 24–5, 26, 27
    management structure, 21
    management training, 22
    pre-/post-analytical stages, 28–31
    staff development/appraisal, 21–2
    strategic planning, 22–4
    workload assessment, 23
Lactobacillus casei, 418, 419, 420
Lactobacillus leichmanii, 418
β-Lactoglobulin, 422–3
Lambert-Beer's law, 52
Large granular lymphocyte leukaemia,
    153
    T-cells, 268
Large-cell lymphoma characterization,
    158
Latex spheres, 37
LE body, 569
LE cell
    demonstration, 569–71
    factor, 568
LE cell test, 568, 570–1
    false positives, 571
    interpretation, 570–1
Leishmania, 93
Leishman's stain, 84–5, 88
Leptocytes, 219
Leptocytosis, 109–10
Leuco-erythroblastic anaemia, 116
Leucocyte count, 9
    automated methods, 75, 77
    environmental effects, 16
    manual differential, 60–1
    manual techniques, 59–60
    physiological variations, 15–16
    reference values, 12, 17
Leucocytes, 7
    acid phosphatase reaction, 149–51
    basophils, 63, 124
    buffy coat preparation, 91, 92
    cell markers, 159–63
    chloracetate esterase, 153–4
    cytochemical tests, 143–59
    disorders, 193, 195
    esterase reactions, 151
    lysozyme activity, 154

monocytes, 125, 148
    morphology, 118, 119–20, 121–7
    myeloperoxidase reaction, 144–5,
        146
    α-naphthol acetate esterase, 151–3
    naphthol AS acetate esterase, 153
    neutrophil alkaline phosphatase
        (NAP), 146–8
    nuclear sexing, 170–1
    PAS reaction, 138, 148–9
    reference preparations, 37
    storage effects, 5, 6
    Sudan black B staining, 145–6
    see also Eosinophils; Lymphocytes
Leucocytosis, 143
Leucopenia, 92
Leukaemia
    diagnostic tests, 193
    differential diagnosis, 154–7
    immunological classification, 167–8
    karyotype, 169–70
    mean peroxidase activity index
        (MPXI) increase, 77
Leukaemia/lymphoma syndromes, 268
Leukaemoid reactions, 122, 143
LFA-3 flow cytometry analysis, 292
Limits of agreement, 25, 26, 27
Linkage analysis
    DNA techniques, 544–6
    problems, 545–6
Lipo-oxygenase, 299
Liquid scintillation counters, 385
LISS antiglobulin test, 453
Log normal distribution, 10, 584
Low ionic strength solution (LISS),
    576
Lupus anticoagulant investigation,
    351–6
    anti-cardiolipin assay, 356
    kaolin clotting time, 352–4
    Russell's viper venom time, 354–5
Lymphadenopathy, diagnostic tests, 195
Lymphoblasts, 127
Lymphocytes, 125–7
    physiological variations, 16
    reactive, 126, 127
    transforming, 126
Lymphoid antigen expression, 166
Lymphomas, 127
Lymphoproliferative disorders,
        molecular biological
        abnormalities
    Cβ probe, 535, 537
    Ig gene probes, 535
    Ig gene rearrangement studies, 536,
        537
    JΓ probe, 536
    JH probe, 535, 537
    Southern blot analysis, 530, 534–8
    TCR gene probes, 535–6
    TCR gene rearrangement studies,
        536, 537
Lyonization, 347
Lysozyme activity, 154
McLeod phenotype, 113

Macrocytes, 99–100
Macrocytic anaemias, 193
Macrocytosis, 100, 103
Macrophage activity, 450–1
  cell destruction, 450
  regulation, 451
MAIPA assay, 474–5
  technique, 468
Malaria, 93, *94–5*
  parasites, 78, 85
Malonyldialdehyde, 299
March haemoglobinuria, 200
Marrow puncture needles, 177, *178*
Mast cells, 153
May-Grünwald-Giemsa stain, 85, 86–7
  bone marrow, 187–8
May-Hegglin anomaly, 121
  thrombocytopenia, 127–8
Mean, 584
  calculation, 10
Mean cell haemoglobin concentration
    (MCHC)
  mean patient data for quality control,
    42, *43*, 44
  physiological variation, 14
  reference values, *12*, *17*
  automated methods, 74
  EDTA effects, 4
  manual techniques, 59
Mean cell haemoglobin (MCH)
  mean patient data for quality control,
    42, *43*
  reference values, *17*
  automated methods, 74
  manual techniques, 58–9
Mean cell volume (MCV)
  mean patient data for quality control,
    42, *43*
  megaloblastic anaemia, 417
  physiological variation, 14
  reference values, *12*, *17*
  shape factor, 73
  stored blood, 36
  aperture-impedance systems, 73
  artefacts, 73
  automated techniques, 72–3
EDTA effects, 4
errors, 73
manual techniques, 58–9
Mean peroxidase activity index
    (MPXI), 77
Mean platelet volume (MPV)
  automated methods, 78
Median corpuscular fragility (MCF),
    219
Mediterranean anaemia, 200
Mefenamic acid, 525
Megakaryocytes, 92
Megaloblastic anaemia, 92, 99, 100,
    101, 417–34
  B$_{12}$ absorption investigation, 427–9
  B$_{12}$ neuropathy, 417
  deoxyuridine suppression test, 426–7
  haptoglobin levels, 203
  intrinsic factor antibodies, 430–2

intrinsic factor estimation, 429–30
mean peroxidase activity index
  (MPXI), increase, 77
mean platelet volume (MPV), 78
microbiological assays, 418–20
punctate basophilia, 115
red cell volume distribution (RDW),
  74
response to treatment, 434
schistocytosis, 105
transcobalamin separation, 433–4
Megaloblasts, 92
Membrane glycoproteins, 325
Membrane inhibitor of reactive lysis
    (MIRL) deficiency, 288
2-Mercapto-ethanol, use in
    immunoglobulin investigation,
    524
Metamyelocytes, 61, 92
Methaemalbumin, 200
  measurement, 203–4
Methaemalbuminaemia, 204
Methaemoglobin (Hi), 50, 137, 210
  absorption spectrum, 270
  autohaemolysis, 224
  elution test, 229–30
  measurement, 199, 210–11
  reduction test, 228–9
  variants, 270
Methaemoglobinaemia
  congenital, 270
  congenital NADH methaemoglobin
    reductase deficiency, 252
α-Methyldopa, 499
  auto-immune haemolytic anaemia,
    525
  positive direct antiglobulin test
    (DAT), 510
Methylene blue, polychromed, 88
5-Methyltetrahydrofolate, 417, 418
4-Methylumbelliferyl phosphate, 424
Micro-haematocrit, 57–8
Microcolumn chromatography Hb A$_2$
    measurement
  glycine-potassium cyanide
    developers, 277–8
  Tris-HCl developers, 275–7
Microcytes, 100–1
Microfilariae, 90
Microscope
  magnification, 583
  maintenance, 588–9
Microtrephine biopsy, 175
Miller ocular, 67
Mitogen phytohaemagglutinin (PHA),
    169
Molecular concentrations, 583
Monoclonal antibodies, 163–8
  APAAP method, 163, 165, 167
  diagnostic, 192
  E-rosette receptor, 161
  FACS system, 165
  fixed cell tests, 167
  flow cytometry, 165, 167
  Hb S detection, 268

immunofluorescence method, 165–7
immunoperoxidase techniques, 167
neutrophil antibody assay, 747–5
platelet antibody assay, 747–5
value in diagnosis of leukaemia
Monocytes, 125
  PAS reaction, 148
Mononuclear cells
  atypical, 92
  separation, 159
Mononuclear phagocyte system, 450
Muramidase *see* Lysozyme activity
Myasthenia gravis, 568
Myeloblasts
  myeloperoxidase reaction, 145
  PAS reaction, 148
Myelocytes, 61
  myeloperoxidase reaction, 145
  PAS reaction, 148
Myelodysplasia
  mean peroxidase activity index
    (MPXI), increase, 77
  pseudo-Pelger cells, 123
Myelodysplastic syndromes, 157–8
  cytochemical diagnostic tests, 143
  ring sideroblasts, 133
Myelofibrosis (myelosclerosis), 101, 238
  blue polychromasia, 115
  bone marrow, 187
  diagnostic tests, 195
  erythroblasts, 116
  ferrokinetic patterns, *402*
  PAS reaction, 138
  ring sideroblasts, 133
  surface counting of ^{59}Fe, 402, *403*
Myelogram, 180–1
Myeloid antigen expression, *166*
Myelomatosis
  diagnostic tests, 193
  rouleaux, 117
Myeloperoxidase reaction, 144–5, *146*
Myeloproliferative disorders, chronic,
    157
Myoglobin, demonstration in urine,
    212–13

NADH
  Ga3DP conversion, 239
  pyruvate kinase assay, 235
α-Naphthol acetate esterase, 151–3
  acute myeloid leukaemia, 156
  sodium fluoride inhibition, 152
Naphthol AS acetate
  esterase, 153
  reaction, 156
Naphthol AS-BI phosphate, 149, 150
National External Quality Assessment
    Scheme (NEQAS), 258
Natural killer (NK) cells, 126
Needle biopsy of bone marrow, 175,
    176–84
  aspiration for transplantation, 178
  children, 177
  marrow puncture needles, 177, *178*
  site, 176

Needlestick injury, 31
Nephrotic syndrome, 331
Neubauer counting chamber, 54, *55*
Neutropenia
  auto-immune, 467
  diagnostic tests, 193
  drug-induced antibodies, 467
Neutrophil alkaline phosphatase
    (NAP), 146–8
Neutrophil antibodies
  clinical significance, 465–7
  demonstration, 468–70, 470–6
  drug-induced, 467
  ELISA method, 475
  MAIPA assay, 474–5
Neutrophil platelets
  elution, 470–1
  fluorescent-labelled antiglobulin
    methods, 470–1
Neutrophils, 7
  alkaline phosphatase deficiency, 288
  allo-antigen systems, 465, *466*
  auto-antibodies, 467, 468–9
  cytochemical diagnostic tests, 143
  drumstick nuclear appendage, 118,
    170
  hypersegmented, 123
  nuclear sexing, 170–1
  peroxidase deficiency, 77
  physiological variations, 15–16
  pyknotic, 123–4
  red cell adhesion, 118, *121*
  total neutrophil counts, 61
  see also Polymorphonuclear
    neutrophils
Nicotine adenine dinucleotide
    phosphate (NADP), 225–6
  reduced (NADPH), 226, 227, 233,
    238
Nomifensine haemolysis, 525
Northern blotting technique, RNA
    analysis, 546
NSB-B$_{12}$, 422

O antigens, 446
Occult blood in stools, 192
Ochromonas malhamensis, 418
Oh Bombay phenotype, 446
Oligonucleotide hybridization, allele-
    specific, 539–40
Oral contraceptives, 203
Oriental sore, 93
Osmotic fragility 4, 198
  alternative methods, 219
  curves, *216*, *217*, 219
  factors affecting, 218
  incubated blood, 217–20
  lysis in hypotonic saline, 216–20
  measurement, 216–20
  results, 219–20
Oxygen affinity ($p_{50}O_2$), 244–5
Oxygen dissociation curve, 241–5
  Bohr effect, 245
  calculation, 243–4
  Hill's constant, 245

interpretation, 244–5
measurement, 241–5
pH effects, 244
shift, 241
Oxygen-combining capacity of blood,
    50
Oxyhaemoglobin method for
    haemoglobin estimation, 50,
    52–3

Packed cell volume (PCV), 7
  physiological variation, 11, 14, 15
  reference values, *12*, *17*
  venous, 395
  whole-body, 395
Packed cell volume (PVC) estimation
  automated techniques, 72–3
  blood volume measurement, 391
  EDTA effects, 4
  errors, 73
  manual techniques, 57–8
  micro-haematocrit, 57–8
Pancytopenia, diagnostic tests, 195
Papain, 454
  enzyme tests, 488
  preparation, 454
Papainized cells, allo-absorption,
    516–17
Pappenheimer
  bodies, *115*, 116, 131, *132*
  granular material, 67
Parasites, 93, *94–5*
  blood film examination, 89–90
  wet preparations of blood, 90
Parietal cell antibodies, 432
Paroxysmal cold haemoglobinuria,
    499, 502
  haemoglobinaemia, 200
Paroxysmal nocturnal
    haemoglobinuria, 148, 287–95,
    412
  acidified serum test, 287, 289–90
  autohaemolysis, 223
  cell lysis, 287–8
  cell membrane bound protein
    deficiencies, 288
  clone, 288
  cobra-venom test, 287
  cold-antibody lysis test, 287, 291–2
  flow cytometry, 292–5
  GPI-linked protein analysis, 288,
    292–5
  haemoglobinaemia, 200
  inulin test, 287
  pH lysis curves, *287*, 290
  red cell populations, 288
  red cells, 287–9
  sucrose lysis test, 287, 291
  thrombin test, 287
Paroxysmal nocturnal
    haemoglobinuria-like red cells,
    293
Partial pressure of oxygen (pO_2), 241,
    243
PAS reaction. see Periodic acid-Schiff

(PAS reaction Patient-centred
    care, 30
Paul-Bunnell antibody, 564, 566, 567
Paul-Bunnell test, 546–8
  agglutination, 566–7
  clinical value, 567
  false-positives, 567
  guinea-pig kidney suspension
    preparation, 567–8
  heated ox red cell suspension
    preparation, 567–8
  interpretation, 566–7
  ox red cell suspension preparation,
    568
  quantitative, 565–8
  reagents, 565
  serum absorption, 565–6
  technical factors, 567
Pelger cells, 123
Pelger-Huet anomaly, 123
Penicillin, 499
  haemolytic anaemia, 525
Pentose phosphate pathway, 225
Periodic acid-Schiff (PAS) reaction,
    138
  acute lymphoblastic leukaemia, 156
  chronic lymphocylic leukaemia, 158
  eythroleukaemia, 156
  leucocytes, 148–9
  prolymphocytic leukaemia, 158
Peripheral blood, 6–7
Perls's reaction, 131
  iron stores, *134*
Pernicious anaemia
  antinuclear factors, 568
  bilirubin level, 206
  intrinsic factor antibodies, 430
  neutrophils, 123
  parietal cell antibodies, 432
Peroxidase method
  acute myeloid leukaemia, 155, 156
Phagocytosis, 451
Phenacetin, 499
  haemolysis, 525
Philadelphia (Ph) chromosome, 169
Phosphobilinogen, 207, 209
Phosphate buffer, 578, 579
Phosphoenolpyruvate (PEP), 235
3-Phosphoglycerate, 239
Phosphoglycerate kinase (PGK), 239
Plasma viscosily, 563
Plasma volume, 391
  determination, 394
  Hurley's method, *396*
  ^{131}I-labelled human serum albumin
    method, 394
  measurement, 392, 393
  normal values, 397
  simultaneous measurement with red
    cell volume, 395
Plasma-iron
  clearance, 399–400
  turnover, 400
Plasmid DNA, 531
Plasmin, 303

Plasmin-antiplasmin complex, 303
Plasminogen
    activator, 298, 303
    chromogenic assay, 357
    defect/deficiency investigation,
        356–7
Plasminogen activator inhibitor (PAI-
    1), 303
    assay, 359
    chromogenic assay, 357
Plasminogen activator (t-PA)
    amidolytic assay, 359
    thrombolytic therapy, 378
Plasmodium spp, 93, 94, 95
Platelets, 298–300
    adhesion tests, 319
    adhesion to sub-endothelium, 299
    agglutination, 323, 336
    aggregating agents, 322
    allo-antibodies, 468
    allo-antigen molecular genotyping,
        475–6
    allo-antigen systems, 465
    anisocytosis, 78, 127
    chloroquine treatment, 473–4
    clumping, absence, 6
    coagulant activity, 320
    contractile system, 298–9
    distribution width (PDW), 78
    factor 4, 320
    granular content, 320
    granules, 299
    haemostatic process, 299
    hyperreactivity investigation, 360–1
    immunofluorescence test (PIFT),
        469, 470, 471–3
    investigations, 319–20
    iso-antibodies, 466
    life-span measurement, 413–15
    membrane, 298, 299
    morphology, 127–8
    peroxidase reaction, 143, 156
    reference preparations, 37
    retention tests, 319
    splenic pool, 414–15
    survival, 414
Platelet aggregation, 299–300, 320,
        322–4
    agents, 322
    calculation of results, 324
    inhibition, 298, 300
    interpretation, 322–3
    tests, 319–20
Platelet antibodies
    blood samples, 469
    chloroquine stripping technique, 468
    clinical significance, 465–7
    demonstration, 468–70, 470–6
    drug-induced, 467, 469–70
    ELISA method, 475
    MAIPA assay, 468, 474–5
Platelet antigens, 470–1
Platelet auto-antibodies, 466–7, 468–9
    IgA class, 469
    IgG class, 469

IgM class, 469
    platelet immunofluorescence test,
        469
Platelet count, 7
    automated methods, 77–8
    manual techniques, 63–4
    physiological variation, 16–17
    range, 64
    reference values, 12
    whole blood, 64
Platelet function
    disorders, 311, 319, 324
    investigations, 319–20, 321, 322–5
    substances affecting, 317
Platelet-poor plasma, 320
    preparation, 305
Platelet-rich plasma, 320, 322
Plateletcrit, 78
Pneumonia, atypical, 499
Poikilocytosis, 90, 99, 101
Poisson distribution, 584
Polychromasia, 99, 100, 115
    blue, 115
Polycythaemia, 15
    diagnostic tests, 195
    erythropoietin levels, 571–2
    red cell uptake of ^{59}Fe, 401
    red cell volume, 391
    secondary, 397
    vera, 397
Polymerase chain reaction (PCR),
        538–9
    allele-specific oligonucleotide
        hybridization, 539–40
    amplification refractory mutation
        system (ARMS), 540–1
    haemoglobinopathy investigation,
        541–3
    interpretation, 539
    oligos, 538
    problems, 539
    product analysis, 539–41
    reagents, 553
    restriction enzyme digestion, 540,
        554–5
    sickle-cell disease, 541
    technique, 553–4
    β-thalassaemia, 542
    α-thalassaemia, 542–3
Polymorphonuclear neutrophils, 118,
        121–4
    bacteria, 121, 122
    Döhle bodies, 121
    granules, 118, 121, 123
    hypersegmentation, 123
    nuclei, 121–4
    PAS, 148
    Pelger cells, 123
    vacuoles, 118, 120
Porphyria, 209–10
    cutanea tarda, 209
Porphyrins, 207–10
    biosynthesis, 208
    red cell, 207, 209–10
    urinary, 208, 209–10

Porphyrinuria, 209
Post-transfusion purpura, 467
Precipitin ring, 280, 281
Precision, 35
Pregnancy
    anti-D prophylaxis, 495
    bone marrow, 180, 181
    haptoglobin levels, 203
    Hb F, 255
    leucocytosis, 16
    neutrophils, 122
    plasma volume, 391, 397
    testing schedule for haemolytic
        disease of the newborn, 493
    α-thalassaemia diagnosis, 534
    thalassaemia trait, 282–3
    total blood volume, 397
Prekallikrein deficiency, 311
Prekallikrein/kallikrein, 300, 301
Prenatal diagnosis of globin gene
        disorders, 284
Primaquine sensitivity, 225
Proficiency surveillance, 35–6
Prolymphocytic leukaemia, 148, 158
Promyelocytes, 145
Prostacyclin, 298, 300
Prosthetic valves, 360
Protamine neutralization test, 374–5
Protective clothing, 32
Protein C
    activated resistance, 365
    deficiency investigation, 362–3
    measurement of functional, 363
    system activation, 300
    thrombin cleavage, 302
Protein S, 298, 302
    deficiency investigation, 363–5
    enzyme-linked immunosorbent assay
        of free and total, 364–5
Proteoglycan coat, 297
Prothrombin
    consumption index, 320
    and proconvertin (P & P) method,
        368
    prolonged APTT and PT in
        deficiency, 341
    Taipan venom assay, 342
Prothrombin time, 300, 307–8, 312–13
    interpretation, 307–8
    logarithmic mean, 307
    normal vlaues, 307
    one-stage of Quick, 368, 369
    prolonged, 341–3
    test turnaround time, 29
Protoporphyrin, 207
Prussian blue staining
    iron stores, 134
    test, 131
Pseudo-agglutination, 90
Pseudo-leucocyte preparation, 39–40
Pseudo-Pelger cells, 123
Pseudo-thrombocytopenia, 467
Pseudoxanthoma elasticum, 319
PTT phospholipid reagent, 589–90
Purpura, 6

Pyknocytes, 98
Pyknocytosis, 108–9
Pyrimidine-5'-nucleotidase
    deficiency, 115, *116*, 230–1, 238
    screening test, 230–1
Pyridoxine deficiency, 133
Pyruvate kinase
    activity, 235
    assay, 235–6
    normal values, 236
    variants, 235
Pyruvate kinase deficiency, *136*
    assay results, 236
    autohaemolysis, 223, 224
    diagnosis, 225
    inheritance, 235
    osmotic fragility, 220
    reticulocytosis, 236

Quality assessment, external, 35
Quality assurance, 35–46
    accuracy, 35
    data analysis, 40–4
    duplicate tests, 42
    external quality assessment, 44–6
    precision, 35
    reference preparations, 36–7
    routine programme, 46
Quality control
    aberrant results, 44
    blood count analyzers, 39–40
    correlation check, 44
    internal, 35
    normal data use, 42
    patient data, 42–4
Quality control materials, 37–40
    blood preparation, 37–8
    lysate preparation, 38
    stabilized whole blood control, 38–9
Quinidine, 499
    haemolysis, 525
Quinine, 499
    haemolysis, 525

R binders, 432
R proteins, 429
r-HuEPO, 571
Radial immunodiffusion (RID), 280–1
Radiation
    biological effect, 382–3
    dead-time, 386, 388
    decontamination, 383
    doses, 381–3
    effective dose unit, 383
    forms, 381
    Geiger-Müller counters, 385
    ionization chambers, 384–5
    liquid scintillation counters, 385
    measurement in bulky material, 385
    monitoring, 383
    protection, 383
    ratemeters, 285
    scalers, 385
    scintillation detectors, 384
    thermo-luminescent dose-meter
        badge, 383

timers, 285
Radioactivity
    differential decay, 388
    measurement, 384–7
    mechanical separation of
        radionuclides, 388
    physical decay, 388
    physical separation of radionuclides,
        388
    scanning camera, 386
    scintillation counter, 387–8
    surface counting, 386
    whole-body counting, 386–7
Radioisotope B_{12} dilution assay, 421
Radionuclides, 381
    diagnostic, *382*
    double measurements, 388
    hazards, 381, 383
    imaging, 386
    sources, 383–4
    specific activity, 384
Reagents, reference, 590–1
Recombinant DNA technology for
        thalassaemia, 193
Red blood cell count (RBC), 7
    automated techniques, 69–72
    coincidence correction, 71
    discrimination thresholds, *70*, 71–2
    distribution of cells, 56
    electronic counter reliability, 70–2
    errors, 55–7
    impedance counting, 69–70, 72
    inherent error, 56–7
    light scattering, 70, 72
    manual method, 54–5
    multi-channel instruments, 71–2
    physiological variation, 11, 14–15
    age, 15
    altitude, 15
    diurnal, 15
    ethnic origins, 15
    posture, 15
    smoking, 15
    reference values, *12*
    technical errors, 55–6
Red cell aplasia, 568
Red cell morphology, 98–118
    in disease, 99
    in health, 98
    rouleaux, 98
Red cell life-span
    Ashby survival curve, 407
    ^{51}Cr-labelled, 192
    ^{51}Cr survival curves, *406*, 407, *408*
    differential agglutination method, 404
    disappearance curve, 413
    donor-recipient compatibility for
        survival, 491
    elution rate of ^{51}Cr, 406
    labelled, 392
    labelling for scintillation scanning,
        412
    life-span estimation in vivo, 404–7,
        408, 409
    mean life-span, 407

normal life-span, 409
    radioactivity measurement, 405
    random labelling, 404
    surface counting studies, 411
Red cell volume, 391
    ^{51}Cr method, 392–3
    determination, 392–3
    distribution (RDW), 74
    normal values, 397
    reference range, 74
    simultaneous measurement with
        plasma volume, 395
    splenic, 397
    ^{99m}Tc method, 393
Red cells
    acetyl cholinesterase deficiency, 288
    agglutination by antibody, 455–7
    alcohol excess, 193
    antibody elution, 517–18
    antigen-antibody reactions, 451–2
    antiglobulin test titration scores, 507
    auto-agglutination, 90–1, 116–17
    blood groups, 445–50
    blood volume changes, 409
    bromelin treatment, 455
    cephalosporin effects, 525
    clearance rate of damaged, 413
    complement lysis damage, 524–5
    control samples, 232
    crenation, 110–13, *119*
    cytochemical tests for metabolic
        defects, 139–40
    destruction site determination,
        410–12
    diluting fluid, 55
    enzyme assays, 231–5
    enzyme-treated, 453–5
    ^{59}Fe uptake, *401*
    fetal, 494
    filtration, 232
    folate, 417
    glycolytic pathway, *226*
    haemoglobinization distribution, 75
    haemolysate preparation, 232
    Heinz bodies, 134–5
    hypochromia, 74
    indices in manual techniques, 58–9
    irregularly-contracted, 107–9
    liver disease, 193
    lysis demonstration, 456–7
    macrocytosis, 99
    mass, *396*
    membrane receptor binding, 160–1
    microcytosis, 99
    neutrophil adhesion, 118, *121*
    papain treatment, 454
    paroxysmal nocturnal
        haemoglobinuria, 287–9
    production regulation, 571
    reference preparations, 36–7
    reference values, *17*
    rouleaux, 90–1, 116–17
    sample collection, 231
    scanning electron microscopy, 118,
        119–20

Red cells (*Cont'd*)
  separation from blood samples, 231
  size/shape variation, 99–101
  sizing, 70
  storage effects, 5, 6
  suspensions, 453
  washing, 231–2
Reference limits, 9
Reference preparations, 36–7
Reference ranges, 9–11
Reference reagents, 590–1
Reference standards, 590–1
Reference values, 9, *12–14*
  sample size, 11
Refractory anaemia, 157, 158
Relapsing fever, 90
Relative molecular mass, 583
Reptilase, 314, 367
Resin-embedding techniques, 192
Restriction enzyme digestion, 539
  technique, 554–5
  β-thalassaemia, 542
Reticulin, 65, 187
Reticulocyte count, 66–7, 192
  automated, 68, 78
  errors, 78
  in health, 79
  manual, 66–8
  reference values, *17*
  storage effects, 6
Reticulocytes, 65–6
  erythropoietic activity, 66
  immaturity, 78
  maturation, *65*
  stress, 66
Reticulocytosis
  folate deficiency, 417
  G6PD activity, 234
  polychromasia, 193
  pyruvate kinase deficiency, *136*, 236
Rh antibodies
  anti-IgG, 457
  antiglobulin reactions, 457–61
  comparison of reagents, 459
  cross-match tests of reagents, 459
  monospecific reagents, 458
  new technology for antibody
    detection, 460–1
  polyspecific reagents, 457–8
  reagent specificity, 458
  reference agent, 459
  two-stage EDTA-complement
    indirect antiglobulin test, 460
Rh D antigen, 445
Rh (D) grouping, auto-immune
    haemolytic anaemia, 511–12
Rh (D) haemolytic disease of the
    newborn, 493–4
Rh D-positive genotypes, *487*
Rh grouping
  antenatal, 486–7
  auto-immune haemolytic anaemia,
    503, 511–12
  blood transfusion compatibility
    testing, 479, 480, 484–7

cord blood at delivery, 494
  emergency, 485–6
  false-positive results, 485
  maternal blood at delivery, 494
  microplate method, 485
  rapid techniques, 489
  slide method, 485
  spin tube method, 485
  tube method, 484–5
  weak D phenotype, 485–6
Rh haplotypes, 448
Rh phenotyping, 486, 487
Rh system, 445, 448–50
  antibodies, 449
  antigens, 448–9
  racial differences, 449
Rheumatoid arthritis
  antinuclear factors, 568
  haptoglobin levels, 203
Rifampicin, 525
Ristocetin
  agglutination, 325
  cofactor (RiCoF) activity, 331, 334
  platelet aggregation, 322, 323–4
  response, 127
  sulphate, 322, 323–4
Ristocetin cofactor (RiCoF) assay,
    336–9
  formalin-fixed platelets, 338
  fresh platelet method, 336–7
  normal values, 337
  standard curve, *338*
RNA techniques, 546
R° antigen, 568
Romanowsky effect, 85
Romanowsky stain, 84
  bone marrow, 179, 188
  neutrophils, 118
  peripheral blood cells
  preparation, 85
  siderotic granules, 132
  standardized, 87
Rosette tests, 160–1
Rouleaux formation, 90–1, 98, 116–17
  erythrocyte sedimentation, 561
Russell's viper venom time, 342, 354–5

Safety
  officer, 31
  policy, 31
Salicylazosulphapyridine, 499
  haemolysis, 525
Saline, 576
  barbitone buffered, 577
  imidazole-buffered, 578
  low ionic strength (LISS), 453
  normal ionic strength (NISS), 453
  phosphate buffered, 579
Sample
  collection, 28, 30
  delivery, 28, 30
  recognition, 68
  transit systems, 28, 29
Schilling test, 428, 429
Schistocytes, 98, 105

Schistocytosis, 99, 105–7
Schlesinger's zinc test, 207
Schüffner's dots, 85
Schumm's test, 203–4
Scintillation counter, 387–8
  physical decay correction, 388
  technique, 387–8
  working condition standardization,
    387
Scintillation detector, 384, 410
Scintillation scanning of spleen, 412–13
Screening
  abnormalities, 191–2
  service, 191
Secretor (*Se*) gene, 447
Septicaemia, 121
Serum
  collection, 2–3
  defibrination, 3
Sex chromosome anomalies, 170
Sézary syndrome, 168
Shape factor, 73
Sheehan's syndrome, 331
Sickle cell, 110
  mutation identification, 541
  trait (Hb AS), 251
Sickle cell anaemia
  ^{51}Cr accumulation patterns, 412
  haemoglobinaemia, 200
  homozygous state (Hb SS), 251
Sickle cell disease, 110, 251
  homozygous (Hb SS), 110
  polymerase chain reaction (PCR),
    541
  SC disease, 251–2
  screening of newborn, 268
Sickle haemoglobin (Hb S), 250–1
Sickle stomatocytes, 115
Sickling in whole blood, 266, *267*
Sideroblastic anaemia, 102, 133
  anisochromasia, 103
  PAS reaction, 138
Sideroblasts, 131–4, 133
  ring, 133
Siderocytes, 131–4
  significance, 132–3
Siderotic granules, 131, 132
  staining, 132
Silicone flotation method of Seal, 92
Sjögren's syndrome, 568
Sleeping sickness, 93
Slide cleaning, 580
Smoking, blood value effects, 15, 16
Snake venom, 314
Sodium citrate, 6
Sodium iodide, thallium-activated,
    384, 386
South-East Asia variant of hereditary
    ovalocytosis (SEAHO), 101,
    102
Southern blot analysis, 530–8
  agarose gel electrophoresis, 550
  autoradiography, 551
  background signal, 532
  DNA probes, 531

Southern blot analysis (*Cont'd*)
  haemophilia A, 545
  hybridization, 551
  interpretation, 531–2
  lymphoproliferative disorders, 534–8
  problems, 531–2
  reagents, 548–9
  restriction enzymes, 548–9, 549–50
  Southern transfer, 551
  technique, 548–51
  β-thalassaemia, 534
  zeta globin genes, 532
Spectrophotometry, 54
Spherocytosis, 99, 101, 104, *105*, 111, *112*
Spinous process puncture, 177
Spirochaetes, 90
Spleen scintillation scanning, 412–13
Splenectomy
  acanthocytosis, 113
  effects, 116–17
  Heinz bodies, 283
  siderocytes, 131
  target cells, 109–10, *111*
β-thalassaemia, *120*
Splenic platelet pool, 414–15
Splenomegaly, 397
Spur cell anaemia, 113
Staff
  development/appraisal, 21–2
  multidisciplinary teams, 30
Standard deviation, 10
  control specimens, 40, 41
  duplicate tests, 42
  external quality assessment, 44–5
  variance in red blood cell count, 56
Standard error of mean, 584
Standardization, 36
Statistical procedures, 10–11, 584–5, *586–7*
Stercobilin, 206
Sternum puncture, 176–7
Steroid therapy
  eosinopenia, 124
  haptoglobin levels, 203
Stibophen, 525
Stomato-acanthocytes, 115
Stomatocytosis, 114–15
Strategic planning, 22–4
Streptokinase
  initial dose titration, 378–9
  thrombolytic therapy, 377–8
Sucrose lysis test, 287, 291
Sudan black B reaction, 155, 156
Sudan black staining, 145–6
Sulphaemoglobin (SHb), 50, 210, 252
  measurement, 210, 211–12
Surface membrane immunoglobulin
    molecules (SmIg), 159, 161
  fluorescent antibody staining, 161–2
SWOT analysis, 22
Systemic lupus erythematosus, 92, 499
  antinuclear factors, 568
  haptoglobin levels, 203
  LE cells, 570, 571

T_{50}Cr, 407
T cell receptor (TCR) genes, 534
T acute lymphoblastic leukaemia, 157
  antigen expression, 168
T-cell, 126
  lymphoma, 124
  lymphoproliferation, 151
  α-naphthol acetate esterase, 151
T-cell leukaemias
  immunological classification, 168
  markers, *160*
t-Test, 584, *585*
Taipan venom assay, 342
Target cells, 109–10, *111*
Tart cell, 569
Tartrate resistance, 150–1
^{99m}Tc
  blood volume repeated
      measurements, 394
  derivation, 383
  physical separation, 388
  red cell labelling, 392, 412–13
  red cell volume measurement, 393
  splenic red cell volume, 397
Terminal deoxynucleotidyl transferase
    (TdT), 159, 162
  slide assay, 162–3
Test
  requests, 28
  results, 28, 30
  sensitivity, 27
  specificity, 27
  turnaround time, 28–9
Testing
  near-patient, 29–30
  ward level, 30
Tetrahydrofolate, 417
Tetramethylbenzidine, 199, 200
Thalassaemia syndromes, 100–1, 102, *103*, 252–5
  blood count, 256, 274
  diagnostic tests, 192–3, 256
  haemoglobin synthesis failure, 250
  Hb A_2 estimation, 274
  Hb F value interpretation, 282
  heterozygotes for β chain alleles, 253
  interpretation of Hb A_2 values, 279
  investigation, 272, *273*, 274–9
  iron status assessment, 282–3
  laboratory findings, *254*
  laboratory investigations, *261*
  osmotic fragility, 216, 220
  PAS reaction, 138, 148
  punctate basophilia, 115
  schistocytosis, 105
  sideroblasts, *133*
  structural variants, *254*
  thin red cells, 109
  zinc protoporphyrin assessment, 283
Thalassaemia trait
  pregnancy, 282–3
  red cell volume distribution (RDW), 74
α-Thalassaemia
  α globin gene cluster, *532*

α globin gene probe, 533
amplification refractory mutation
    system (ARMS), *543*
BamH I digests, 533
Bgl II digests, 533
diagnosis, 534
Hb H, 136, 137
Hb H inclusion bodies, 283
polymerase chain reaction (PCR), 534, 542–3
prenatal diagnosis, 534
restriction enzyme fragment sizes, *533*
Southern blot analysis, 530, 532–4
syndromes, 253
β-Thalassaemia, *102*, 103
  allele-specific oligonucleotide
      hybridization, 542
  amplification refractory mutation
      system (ARMS), 542, *543*
  polymerase chain reaction (PCR), 542
  restriction enzyme digestion, 540
  Southern blot analysis, 534
  splenectomy, *120*
  syndromes, 253
β-Thalassaemia major, 253
  α-chain inclusions, 283
  Heinz bodies, 136
  screening of newborn, 268
δβ-Thalassaemia
  heterozygotes, 281
  Southern blot analysis, 534
Thermal injury, 106, *107*
Thrombasthenia, 325
Thrombin, 298, 300
  and antithrombin complex (TAT), 366
  inactivation, 302
  test for paroxysmal nocturnal
      haemoglobinuria, 287
Thrombin time, 309–10
  correction tests, 313–14
  heparin treatment, 374
  venous thrombosis, 378–9
Thrombin-antithrombin complex
    (TAT), 302
Thrombocythaemia, 379
  essential, 78, *127*
Thrombocytopenia
  auto-immune, 466, 469
  bleeding time, 319
  drug-induced immune, 467, 469
  heparin-induced, 377
  severe immune, 127
Thrombocytopenic purpura, *128*
Thrombocytosis, 379
  reactive, 78
β-Thromboglobulin
  assay, 360–1
  plasma assays, 325
  platelet, 320
Thrombolytic therapy, 367, 377–9
  control, 378–9
  heparin treatment, 372–3
  investigation of patient during, 379

Thrombomodulin, 298
Thromboplastin, 307
  calibration, 369–70
  choice, 370–1
  International Normalized Ratio, 371
  International Sensitivity Index, 371
  rabbit brain, 589
  reference, 368–9
  therapeutic range, 370–1
Thrombosis
  coagulation activation markers, 366
  heparin cofactor II deficiency, 365
  thrombin time, 378–9
  venous, 378–9
  young individuals, 352
Thrombotest of Owren, 368
Thrombotic syndromes, inherited
  antithrombin III measurement,
    361–2
  investigation, 361–4
  protein C deficiency, 362–3
  protein C novel cofactor deficiency,
    365
  protein S deficiency, 363–5
Thrombotic tendency 351–6
  investigation, 351, 352
  kaolin clotting time, 352–4
  lupus anticoagulant investigation,
    351–6
  dilute Russell's viper venom time,
    354–5
  haemostasis effects, 353
  hypercoagulability mechanisms, 353
  kaolin clotting time, 352–4
Thromboxane A$_2$, 299
Thromboxane synthetase, 299
Thymidine, tritiated, 426
Thyroiditis, antinuclear factors, 568
Tibia bone marrow biopsy, 177
Tissue factor, 301
  pathway inhibitor (TFPI), 301, 302
Tissue plasminogen activator (t-PA),
    303
  thrombolytic therapy, 378
Tonometer, 242, 243
Total nucleated cell count (TNCC),
    61, 75
Toxic granulation, 118, 121, 121, 123
Toxic reagents, 32

Transcobalamin, 432
  deficiency, 417
  separation, 433–4
Transferrin, 131
  concentration determination, 439
  normal range, 439
  saturation, 439
Trephine biopsy of bone marrow, 175,
    185–8, 192
  section preparation, 185–8
  trephine design, 185
Tris-HCl bovine serum albumin buffer,
    579
Tris-HCl buffer, 579
Tris-HCl/EDTA buffer, 232
Trisodium citrate, 4, 576
Trypanosomiasis, 93, 95
Tube size, 581
Tuberculosis, 125
Tumour cell isolation, 92
Türk cells, 126

Ulcerative colitis, 568
Unsaturated binding capacity of B$_{12}$,
    432–3
Unstable haemoglobin diseases, 135
  Heinz bodies, 283
Urobilin
  measurement, 206–7
  urinary levels, 205
Urobilinogen
  faecal, 205
  measurement, 206–7
Urokinase, 303
  thrombolytic therapy, 377
Uroporphyrin, 207
Uroporphyrinogen cosynthase, 210

Vasoconstriction, 298
Venepuncture, 1–2
Venous blood, 7
  collection, 1–2
Venous thrombosis, 378–9
  see also Thrombosis
Vitamin K, 362, 363
Vitamin K-dependent factors, 301
  synthesis, 367
von Willebrand factor, 298, 302, 320,
    324

deficiency, 329
factor VIII:C level, 331
von Willebrand factor antigen
  electrophoresis, 335–6
  enzyme-linked immunosorbent assay
    (ELISA), 333–4
  ^{125}I labelled antibody, 334
  multimeric analysis, 334–6
  normal range, 333
von Willebrand factor:Ag
  concentration, 331, 332, 333
von Willebrand's disease, 311, 321
  bleeding time, 319
  classification, 331
  investigation, 331–2

Warm auto-antibodies, 500–1
  co-existing with allo-antibodies, 513,
    515
  lysis demonstration, 518–19
  specificity determination, 518
Weibel Palade bodies, 298
Weight units, 581–2
Welcan system, 23
White blood cell count (WBC) see
  Leucocyte count
White blood cell (WBC) control for
  pseudo-leucocyte preparation,
    39
Whole blood viscosity, 563–4
Workload assessment, 23
WORM system, 27
Wright's stain, 85, 132
Wu's peroxidase method, 199

X chromosome, 170
  inactivation, 347

Yaws, 93
Youlden plot, 45

Zeta globin gene, 532
  probe, 533
Zinc protoporphyrin
  haemoglobinopathies, 256
  red cell, 283
ZZAP reagent, 515–16